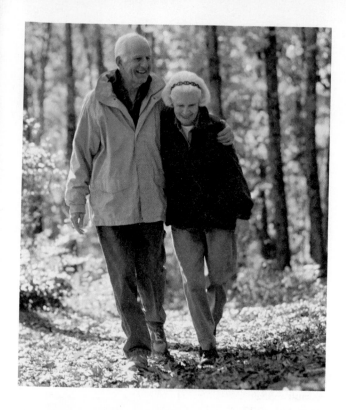

TOPICS OF SPECIAL CONCERN TO MEN

Note: The health issues and conditions listed above include those that disproportionately influence or affect women or men. For more information, see the Index under gender, women, men, and any of the special topics listed here.

DIVERSITY TOPICS RELATED TO ETHNICITY

Note: The health issues and conditions listed above include those that disproportionately influence or affect specific U.S. ethnic groups or for which patterns may appear along ethnic lines. For more information, see the Index under ethnicity, culture, names of specific population groups, and any of the topics listed here.

TEACHING AND LEARNING

Connect Core Concepts in Health is an integrated program designed to personalize the science of personal health and to motivate students to build critical thinking skills and behavior change skills for lifelong health. The new edition of *Connect Core Concepts in Health* combines the expert content and outstanding interactive tools you've come to expect with several exciting new digital resources:

New to Connect for Connect Core Concepts in Health is Connect Insight^{TM}, the first and only analytics tool of its kind. Connect Insight is a series of visual data displays—each framed by an intuitive question to provide at-a-glance information for instructors regarding how a class is doing. Instructors can easily view student performance matched with student activity, and the real-time analytics allow instructors to take action early to keep struggling students from falling behind. Instructors can leverage aggregated information about their courses and students to provide a more personalized teaching and learning experience.

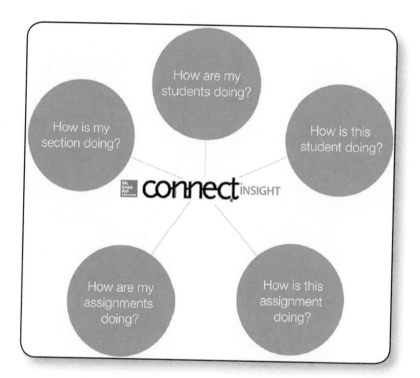

WITH CONNECT CORE CONCEPTS IN HEALTH

SmartBook® is the first and only adaptive reading experience designed to change the way students read and learn. SmartBook creates a personalized reading experience by highlighting the most impactful concepts a student needs to learn at that moment in time. As a student engages with SmartBook, the reading experience continuously adapts by highlighting content based on what the student knows and doesn't know. Use SmartBook's real-time reports to quickly identify the concepts that require more attention from individual students—or the entire class. The end result? Students are more engaged with course content, can better prioritize their time, and come to class ready to participate.

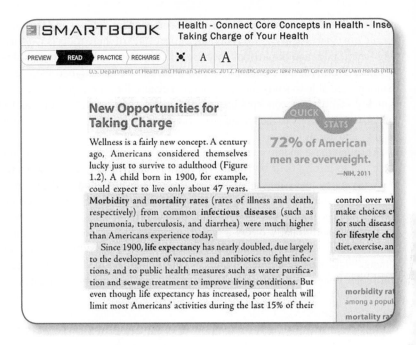

liveWell®, an innovative online multimedia program, is designed to help college students improve their exercise, eating, and stress management habits. liveWell, created by noted behavior change theorist Dr. James Prochaska, is a two-part, self-administered program consisting of (1) an online, personalized assessment of current health-related behaviors and readiness to make meaningful behavior change and (2) a Personal Activity Center (home page) containing activities such as exercise videos and stress management tools matched to each individual's behavior change goals and readiness to change.

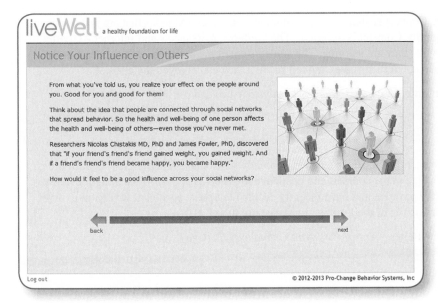

PERSONALIZED AND ADAPTIVE LEARNING

Connect Insight, SmartBook, and *liveWell* complement the existing digital and print instructional tools that make up the *Connect Core Concepts in Health* program. At the center of these tools is **Connect,** McGraw-Hill's digital learning platform, featuring LearnSmart and SmartBook, McGraw-Hill's adaptive learning technology.

LearnSmart is an adaptive study tool designed to strengthen memory recall, increase class retention, and boost grades. Students are able to study more efficiently because they are made aware of what they know and don't know. Real-time reports quickly identify the concepts that require more attention from individual students—or the entire class. **SmartBook** applies adaptive technology to the reading experience, creating a personalized reading plan for each student, based on what that student knows and doesn't know.

Through these adaptive technologies, McGraw-Hill Education authors now have access to student performance data to analyze and to inform their revisions. This data is anonymously collected from the many students who use LearnSmart. Because virtually every text paragraph is tied to several questions that students answer while using LearnSmart, the specific concepts with which students are having the most difficulty are easily pinpointed through empirical data in the form of a "heat map" report. This heat map was used to guide the editorial updates and revisions mentioned on p. xviii.

Connect additionally offers a wealth of interactive online content, including fitness and wellness self-assessment worksheets, video activities on timely health topics such as tattooing and tanning beds, a fitness and nutrition journal, a behavior change workbook, and practice quizzes with immediate feedback. The media-rich e-book contains embedded video clips and full-color images and features note-taking and highlighting functionality.

Instructors have this to say about Connect and McGraw-Hill's adaptive technology:

> " I use this textbook because of Connect. Connect is amazing. I am sure there are other textbooks that are just as good, but I do not switch because the support for Connect is excellent. The Wellness Worksheets and Internet Activities connect my students with the concepts that they are learning. The students email me at the end of the course and tell me how much they learned about themselves and tell me that they had enjoyed the class. "
>
> —Julie Little, *Virginia Highlands Community College*

> " Connect is wonderful! All of my co-workers and I have been very content with Connect and the great opportunities it provides for our students to learn, engage in the courses, and challenge themselves to perform at a high level. We have had very positive feedback with the program and have recently decided to update to the latest version in order to stay on top of the latest and greatest out there! "
>
> —Matthew Belles, *Central Piedmont Community College*

AUTHORITATIVE CONTENT

McGraw-Hill's digital teaching and learning tools are built on the solid foundation of *Connect Core Concepts in Health*'s authoritative, science-based content. *Connect Core Concepts in Health* is written by experts who work and teach in the fields of exercise science, medicine, physical education, and health education. The *Connect content* provides accurate, reliable, current information on key health and wellness topics, while also addressing issues related to mind–body health, research, diversity, gender, and consumer health.

The streamlined pedagogical program for the 14th edition maintains important features on diversity, behavior change, and personal reflection, while integrating some key material into the body of the chapter. All features that appear with a Connect icon offer a linked Connect activity.

Ask Yourself (Questions for Critical Thinking and Reflection) encourage critical reflection on students' own health-related behaviors.

Behavior Change Strategy sections offer specific behavior management/modification plans related to the chapter topic.

Connect to Your Choices sections challenge students to explore their inner motivations for their health choices and to explore ways of translating this awareness into action.

Critical Consumer sections help students to navigate the numerous and diverse set of health-related products currently available.

Diversity Matters features discuss the ways that our personal backgrounds influence our health strengths, risks, and behaviors.

Quick Stats sections focus attention on particularly striking statistics related to the chapter content.

Take Charge boxes challenge students to take meaningful action toward personal improvement.

Tips for Today and the Future end each chapter with a quick, bulleted list of concrete actions readers can take now and in the near future.

Wellness on Campus sections focus on health issues, challenges, and opportunities that students are likely to encounter on a regular basis.

WHAT'S NEW IN CONNECT CORE CONCEPTS IN HEALTH, 14TH EDITION?

All chapters have been updated with the latest data and statistics. In addition, the following topics have been added or significantly revised in every chapter. Revision updates were informed by the heat map data available through LearnSmart. For more on the heat map, see p. xvi.

Chapter	New Coverage	Significant Updates/Revisions
1—Taking Charge of Your Health	• Cultural wellness	
2—Stress: The Constant Challenge		• General adaptation syndrome (GAS) • Personality and stress
3—Psychological Health	• Attention-deficit/hyperactivity disorder (ADHD) • Other psychotherapies: dialectical behavior therapy (DBT), acceptance and commitment therapy (ACT)	• Positive psychology • Post-traumatic stress disorder (PTSD) • Depression treatment • Affordable Care Act and mental health care
4—Intimate Relationships and Communication	• Gender and communication • Sternberg's three dimensions of love • Digital communication and our social networks • Issues and trends in marriage	• Emotional intelligence • Same-sex marriage and civil unions
5—Sexuality, Pregnancy, and Childbirth		• Causes of sexual dysfunction • Treatment of sexual dysfunction • Gender-role flexibility • Origins of sexual orientation • Diagnoses of fetal abnormalities • Complications of pregnancy and pregnancy loss • Choices in childbirth • Postpartum depression
6—Contraception and Abortion	• Long-acting reversible contraception (types, advantages and disadvantages)	• Choices in contraceptive methods • Abortion indicators (lifestyle, fetal, maternal) • Current legal status of abortion • Public debate about abortion
7—Drug Misuse and Addiction	• Prescription drug misuse	• *DSM-5*—updates to abuse and addiction • Synthetic recreational drugs
8—Alcohol and Tobacco	• Alcohol use disorder • Tobacco use disorder • Hookahs/hookah bars	• Who uses tobacco
9—Nutrition Basics	• New research on saturated fats • Global nutrition transitions	• Types of dietary fiber • Dietary Guidelines for Americans
10—Exercise for Health and Fitness	• Pros and cons of interval training • Footwear: Barefoot or minimalist footwear • Cross training to vary workouts	• *Take Charge*: Determining Your Target Heart Rate

Chapter	New Coverage	Significant Updates/Revisions
11—Weight Management	• Energy balance • Evaluation of body weight and body composition • Excess body fat and wellness • Problems associated with very low levels of body fat • Body image • Limits to changes to body weight and shape	• Body composition • Body fat distribution • Heart disease and diabetes
12—Cardiovascular Disease and Cancer	• Gender and CVD • Cardiac rehabilitation for congestive heart failure • Head and neck cancers • Support during cancer therapy	• Blood cholesterol guidelines • Risk factors of CVD that *can* be changed • The role of DNA in causing cancer • Dietary factors in causing cancer • Cancer treatment • Detection and treatment of cancer • Experimental techniques for cancer therapy
13—Immunity and Infection	• Efficacy and safety of vaccines	• Immune system (the inflammatory response) • Types of vaccines • Differentiating between symptoms of cold and flu • Support of your immune system • HIV around the world • Prevention of STIs • HPV—understanding, prevention, treatment • Forms of viral hepatitis
14—Environmental Health	• *Critical Consumer*: Endocrine Disruption (A "New" Toxic Threat)	• Population growth and control • Thinning of the ozone layer • Fracking, water quality and pollution
15—Conventional and Complementary Medicine	• Affordable Care Act of 2010	• 2014 implementation of ACA • Integrative medicine and complementary alternative medicine (CAM) • Pharmaceuticals and the placebo effect • Providers of conventional medicine • Choice of a primary care physician • Health insurance
16—Personal Safety		• School violence • Family and intimate-partner violence
17— The Challenge of Aging		• Alzheimer's disease • *Diversity Matters:* Why Do Women Live Longer? • Long-term care for the elderly • Forms of death • Preparing for retirement • Grief associated with loss of a partner

ACKNOWLEDGMENTS

Connect Core Concepts in Health, 14th edition, has benefited from the thoughtful commentary, expert knowledge, and helpful suggestions of many people. We are deeply grateful for their participation in this project.

Academic Contributors

Philip Takakjian, PhD
Stress: The Constant Challenge and Intimate Relationships and Communication

Michael Ostacher, MD, MPH, MMSc, Stanford University
Psychological Health

Shannon Bertha, PhD, Middlesex County College
Sex and Your Body

Kamilee Christenson, MD, Stanford University
Contraception

Anna Altshuler, MD, MPH, Stanford University
Abortion

Jeroen Vanderhoeven, MD, Swedish Medical Center
Pregnancy and Childbirth

Patrick Zickler, Synergy Enterprises, Inc.
Drug Misuse and Addiction

Marcia Seyler, MPH
Alcohol Misuse and Alcoholism

Omid Fotuhi, PhD, University of Waterloo
Tobacco Use

Frank Franklin, MD, The University of Alabama at Birmingham, and Edmond Kabagambe, PhD, Vanderbilt University
Nutrition Basics

Thomas D. Fahey, EdD, California State University—Chico
Exercise for Health and Wellness

Kim McMahon, MS, RD, LD, Benedictine University and Logan College
Weight Management

Jonathan Schwartz, MD, Stanford University
Cardiovascular Health

Somasundaram Subramaniam, MD, Oncology Fellow, Stanford Cancer Center
Cancer

Martha Zuniga, PhD, University of California, Santa Cruz
Immunity and Infection

Candice McNeil, MD, Stanford University
Sexually Transmitted Infections

Johanna Rochester, PhD, The Endocrine Disruption Exchange
Environmental Health

Robert Jarski, PhD, Professor of Health Sciences and Director of Complementary Medicine and Wellness Program, Oakland University
Conventional and Complementary Medicine

Michael Hoadley, PhD, Eastern Illinois University
Personal Safety

Mary Iten, PhD, University of Nebraska at Kearney
Aging: A Vital Process

Jacob Roth, MD, Chief of Psychiatry, Kaiser Permanente San Jose Medical Center,
Dying and Death

Academic Advisors and Reviewers for the 14th Edition

Matthew Belles, Central Piedmont Community College
Shannon Bertha, Middlesex County College
George Brown, The University of Alabama
Dorinda Cosimano, Kean University
Renee Frimming, University of Southern Indiana
Jeff Goodman, Union College
Chris Harman, California University of Pennsylvania
Emogene Johnson, Norfolk State University
James Ledrick, Grand Valley State University
Julie Little, Virginia Highlands Community College
Donna Lowry, Grand Valley State University
James Metcalf, George Mason University
Clarence Riley, Fort Valley State University
Scott Rogers, College of Southern Idaho
Joshua Searcy, Central State University
Mary Shea, Yosemite Community College District
Jacob Silvestri, Hudson Valley Community College
Shonna Snyder, Gardner Webb University
Susan Stockton, University of Central Missouri

CHAPTER OBJECTIVES

- Describe the dimensions of wellness

- Identify major health problems in the United States today

- Describe the influence of gender, ethnicity, income, disability, family history, and environment on health

- Explain the importance of personal decision making and behavior change in achieving wellness

- List some available sources of health information and explain how to think critically about them

- Describe the steps in creating a behavior management plan to change a health-related behavior

CHAPTER **1**

Taking Charge of Your Health

T he next time you ask someone, "How are you?" and you get the automatic response "Fine," be grateful. If that person had told you how he or she actually felt—physically, emotionally, mentally— you might wish you had never asked. Your friend might be one of the too many people who live most of their lives feeling no better than just all right, or so-so, or downright miserable. Some do not even know what optimal wellness is. How many people do you know who feel great most of the time? Do you?

WELLNESS: NEW HEALTH GOALS

Generations of people have viewed good health simply as the absence of disease, and that view largely prevails today. The word **health** typically refers to the overall condition of a person's body or mind and to the presence or absence of illness or injury. **Wellness** expands this idea of good health to include living a rich, meaningful, and energetic life. Beyond the simple presence or absence of disease, wellness can refer to optimal health and vitality—to living life to its fullest. Although we use the words *health* and *wellness*

interchangeably, there are two important differences. *Health* can be determined or influenced by factors beyond our control, such as our genes, age, and family history. *Wellness* is determined largely by the conscious decisions we make about how we live. These decisions affect the **risk factors** that contribute to disease or injury. We cannot control risk factors such as age and family history, but we can control lifestyle behaviors.

Dimensions of Wellness

Figure 1.1 shows the nine dimensions of wellness.

These dimensions are interrelated and may affect each other, as the following sections explain.

health The overall condition of body or mind and the presence or absence of illness or injury.

TERMS

wellness Optimal health and vitality, encompassing all the dimensions of well-being.

risk factor A condition that increases your chances of disease or injury.

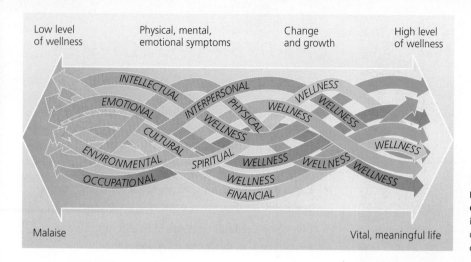

Low level of wellness — Physical, mental, emotional symptoms — Change and growth — High level of wellness

INTELLECTUAL · EMOTIONAL · INTERPERSONAL · PHYSICAL · WELLNESS · WELLNESS · WELLNESS · CULTURAL · WELLNESS · ENVIRONMENTAL · SPIRITUAL · WELLNESS · WELLNESS · WELLNESS · OCCUPATIONAL · WELLNESS · WELLNESS · FINANCIAL

Malaise — Vital, meaningful life

FIGURE 1.1 **The wellness continuum.** The concept of wellness includes vitality in a number of interrelated dimensions, all of which contribute to overall wellness.

Physical Wellness Your physical wellness includes not just your body's overall condition and the absence of disease, but your fitness level and your ability to care for yourself. The higher your fitness level, the higher your level of physical wellness. Similarly, as you develop the ability to take care of your own physical needs, you ensure greater physical wellness. The decisions you make now, and the habits you develop over your lifetime, will help determine the length and quality of your life.

Emotional Wellness Trust, self-confidence, optimism, satisfying relationships, and self-esteem are some of the qualities of emotional wellness. Emotional wellness is dynamic and involves the ups and downs of living. No one can achieve an emotional "high" all the time. Emotional wellness fluctuates with your intellectual, physical, spiritual, cultural, and interpersonal health. Maintaining emotional wellness requires exploring thoughts and feelings. *Self-acceptance* is your personal satisfaction with yourself—it might exclude society's expectations—whereas *self-esteem* relates to the way you think others perceive you; *self-confidence* can be a part of both acceptance and esteem. Achieving emotional wellness means finding solutions to emotional problems, with professional help if necessary.

Intellectual Wellness Those who enjoy intellectual wellness constantly challenge their minds. An active mind is essential to wellness because it detects problems, finds solutions, and directs behavior. Throughout their lifetimes people who enjoy intellectual wellness never stop learning. Often they discover new things about themselves.

Interpersonal Wellness Satisfying and supportive relationships are important to physical and emotional wellness. Learning good communication skills, developing the capacity for intimacy, and cultivating a supportive network are all important to interpersonal (or social) wellness. Social wellness requires participating in and contributing to your community and to society.

Cultural Wellness Cultural wellness refers to the way you interact with others who are different from you in terms of ethnicity, religion, gender, sexual orientation, age, and customs (practices). It involves creating relationships with others and suspending judgment on others' behavior until you have lived with them or "walked in their shoes." It also includes accepting, valuing, and even celebrating the different cultural ways people interact in the world. The extent to which you maintain and value cultural identities is one measure of cultural wellness.

Spiritual Wellness To enjoy spiritual wellness is to possess a set of guiding beliefs, principles, or values that give meaning and purpose to your life, especially in difficult times. The spiritually well person focuses on the positive aspects of life and finds spirituality to be an antidote for negative feelings such as cynicism, anger, and pessimism. Organized religions help many people develop spiritual health. Religion, however, is not the only source or form of spiritual wellness. Many people find meaning and purpose in their lives on their own—through nature, art, meditation, or good works—or their loved ones.

Environmental Wellness Your environmental wellness is defined by the livability of your surroundings. Personal health depends on the health of the planet—from the safety of the food supply to the degree of violence in society. Your physical environment can support your wellness or diminish it. To improve your environmental wellness, you can learn about and protect yourself against hazards in your surroundings and work to make your world a cleaner and safer place.

Financial Wellness Financial wellness refers to your ability to live within your means and manage your money in a way that gives you peace of mind. It includes balancing your income and expenses, staying out of debt, saving for the future, and understanding your emotions about money. See the "Financial Wellness" box.

With stories of home foreclosures, credit card debt, and personal bankruptcies, it has become painfully clear that many Americans do not know how to manage their finances. You can avoid such stress—and gain financial peace of mind—by developing skills that contribute to financial wellness.

Financial wellness means having a healthy relationship with money. It involves knowing how to manage your money, using self-discipline to live within your means, using credit cards wisely, staying out of debt, meeting your financial obligations, having a long-range financial plan, and saving.

Learn to Budget

Although the word *budget* may conjure up thoughts of deprivation, a budget is really just a way of tracking where your money goes and making sure you're spending it on the things that are most important to you. To start one, list your monthly income and your expenditures. If you aren't sure where you spend your money, track your expenses for a few weeks or a month. Then organize them into categories, such as housing, food, transportation, entertainment, services, personal care, clothes, books and school supplies, health care, credit card and loan payments, and miscellaneous. Use categories that reflect the way you actually spend your money. Knowing where your money goes is the first step in gaining control of it.

Now total your income and expenditures. Are you taking in more than you spend, or vice versa? Are you surprised by your spending patterns? Use this information to set guidelines and goals for yourself. If your expenses exceed your income, identify ways to make some cuts. For example, instead of the expense of cable TV, you can stream news and entertainment shows from the Internet through your television or Blu-ray player. Or you can view programs online on Hulu.com and movies on Netflix.com. If you spend money going out at night, consider less expensive options like having a weekly game night with friends or organizing an occasional potluck.

Be Wary of Credit Cards

College students are prime targets for credit card companies: Students tend to be overconfident in their financial decisions and have easy access to credit but little training in finances. Students then may participate in enhanced lifestyles and may compete with peers to consume more. Thus, the government passed the Credit Card Accountability, Responsibility, and Disclosure Act of 2009 to require people age 21 and younger to have a guarantor co-sign their credit card applications to ensure they can make their payments. It was found that students who learn about finance from parents are more likely to pay off their credit card balance in full and regularly.

It is important to understand terms like *APR* (annual percentage rate—the interest you're charged on your balance), *credit limit* (the maximum amount you can borrow), *minimum monthly payment* (the smallest payment your creditor will accept each month), *grace period* (the number of days you have to pay your bill before interest or penalties are charged), and *over-the-limit* and *late fees* (the amounts you'll be charged if you go over your credit limit or make a late payment).

Get Out of Debt

A 2011 study indicated that graduating college students often had debts of $25,250 and that this number would likely increase by several thousand dollars over the next several years. If you have credit card debt, stop using your cards and start paying them off. If you can't pay the whole balance, try to pay more than the minimum payment each month. It can take a very long time to pay off a loan by making only the minimum payments. For example, paying off a credit card balance of $2000 at 10% interest with monthly payments of $20 would take 203 months—17 years. Check out an online credit card calculator like http://money.cnn.com/calculator/pf/debt-free/. Note that by carrying a balance and incurring finance charges, you are also paying back much more than your initial loan.

Start Saving

If you start saving early, the same miracle of compound interest that locks you into years of credit card debt can work to your benefit (for an online compound interest calculator, visit http://www.interestcalc.org). Experts recommend "paying yourself first" every month—that is, putting some money into savings before you start paying your bills, depending on what your budget allows. You may want to save for a large purchase, or you may even be looking ahead to retirement. If you work for a company with a 401(k) retirement plan, contribute as much as you can every pay period.

Become Financially Literate

How well do you manage your money? Most Americans have not received any kind of basic financial training. For this reason, the U.S. government has established the Financial Literacy and Education Commission (MyMoney.gov) to help Americans learn how to save, invest, and manage money better, a skill called financial literacy. Developing lifelong financial skills should begin in early adulthood, during the college years, if not earlier.

SOURCES: Smith, C., and G. A. Barboza. 2013. The role of trans-generational financial knowledge and self-reported financial literacy on borrowing practices and debt accumulation of college students. *Social Science Electronic Publishing, Inc.* (http://ssrn.com/abstract=2342168; Plymouth State University. 2013. *Student Monetary Awareness and Responsibility Today!* (http://www.plymouth.edu/office/financial-aid/smart/); U.S. Financial Literacy and Education Commission. 2013. *MyMoney.gov* (http://www.mymoney.gov).

connect
ACTIVITY
DO IT ONLINE

Occupational Wellness

Occupational wellness refers to the level of happiness and fulfillment you gain through your work. Although high salaries and prestigious titles are gratifying, they alone may not bring about occupational wellness. An occupationally well person enjoys his or her work, feels a connection with others in the workplace, and takes advantage of the opportunities to learn and be challenged. Another important aspect of occupational wellness is recognition from managers and colleagues. An ideal job draws on your interests and passions, as well as your vocational skills, and allows you to feel that you are making a contribution in your everyday work.

TERMS

morbidity rate   The relative incidence of disease among a population.

mortality rate   The number of deaths in a population in a given period of time; usually expressed as a ratio, such as 75 deaths per 1000 members of the population.

infectious disease   A disease that can spread from person to person, caused by microorganisms such as bacteria and viruses.

life expectancy   The period of time a member of a given population is expected to live.

impaired life   The period of a person's life when he or she may not be able to function fully due to disease or disability.

chronic disease   A disease that develops and continues over a long period of time, such as heart disease or cancer.

New Opportunities for Taking Charge

Wellness is a fairly new concept. A century ago, Americans considered themselves lucky just to survive to adulthood (Figure 1.2). A child born in 1900, for example, could expect to live only about 47 years. **Morbidity** and **mortality rates** (rates of illness and death, respectively) from common **infectious diseases** (such as pneumonia, tuberculosis, and diarrhea) were much higher than Americans experience today.

Since 1900, **life expectancy** has nearly doubled, due largely to the development of vaccines and antibiotics to fight infections, and to public health measures such as water purification and sewage treatment to improve living conditions. But even though life expectancy has increased, poor health will limit most Americans' activities during the last 15% of their lives, resulting in some sort of **impaired life** (Figure 1.3). Today a different set of diseases has emerged as our major health threat: Heart disease, cancer, and chronic lower respiratory diseases are now the three leading causes of death for Americans (Table 1.1). Treating such **chronic diseases** is costly and difficult.

The good news is that people have some control over whether they develop chronic diseases. People make choices every day that increase or decrease their risks for such diseases. Each of us can take personal responsibility for **lifestyle choices** that include behaviors such as

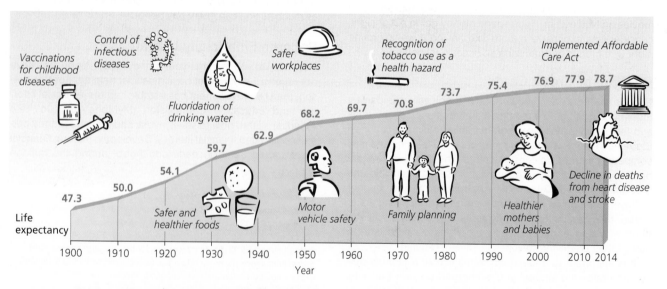

FIGURE 1.2   Public health achievements of the past century. From 1900 to 2000, public health achievements greatly improved Americans' quality of life and dramatically reduced the number of deaths from infectious diseases. In 2013, the government mandated that all Americans be covered by health insurance, a protection already long established in most other industrialized countries.

SOURCES: Hoyert, D. L., and J.Q. Xu. 2012. Deaths: Preliminary Data For 2011. *National Vital Statistics Reports* 61(6). Hyattsville, Md: National Center For Health Statistics; Centers For Disease Control and Prevention. Ten Great Public Health Achievements—United States, 1900–1999. *Morbidity and Mortality Weekly Report* 48(50): 1141; U.S. Department of Health and Human Services. 2012. *Healthcare.Gov: Take Health Care Into Your Own Hands* (http://www.healthcare.gov).

smoking, diet, exercise, and alcohol use. As Table 1.2 makes clear, lifestyle factors contribute to many deaths in the United States, and people can influence their own health risks.

The need to make good choices is especially true for teens and young adults. For Americans ages 15–24, for example, the top three causes of death are unintentional injuries (accidents), suicide, and homicide (Table 1.3).

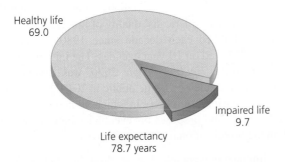

Healthy life
69.0

Impaired life
9.7

Life expectancy
78.7 years

FIGURE 1.3 **Quantity of life versus quality of life.** Years of healthy life as a proportion of life expectancy in the U.S. population.

source: National Center for Health Statistics. 2012. *Healthy People 2010 Final Review.* Hyattsville, MD.

Promoting Health and Preventing Disease

People are a nation's most important resource. A country's creativity, vitality, and prosperity depend on the health of its people. Governments as well as communities find it in their long-term interests to promote health and prevent disease. The World Health Organization (WHO) defines **health promotion** as "the process of enabling people to increase control over their health and its determinants, and thereby improve their health." The primary means of promoting health are public health policies and agencies that identify and discourage unhealthy and high-risk behaviors and that encourage and provide incentives for judicious health behaviors. Many college campuses have health promotion programs or activities.

TERMS

lifestyle choice A conscious behavior that can increase or decrease a person's risk of disease or injury; such behaviors include smoking, exercising, and eating a healthful diet.

health promotion The process of enabling people to increase control over their health and its determinants, and thereby improve their health.

Table 1.1	Leading Causes of Death in the United States, 2011			
RANK	CAUSE OF DEATH	NUMBER OF DEATHS	PERCENTAGE OF TOTAL DEATHS	LIFESTYLE FACTORS
1	Heart disease	596,339	23.7	D I S A
2	Cancer	575,313	22.9	D I S A
3	Chronic lower respiratory diseases	143,382	5.7	■ ■ S ■
4	Stroke	129,180	5.2	D I S A
5	Unintentional injuries (accidents)	118,043	4.9	■ I S A
6	Alzheimer's disease	83,308	3.8	■ ■ ■ ■
7	Diabetes mellitus	68,905	2.8	D I S ■
8	Influenza and pneumonia	53,667	2.1	D I S A
9	Kidney disease	45,731	1.8	■ ■ S ■
10	Intentional self-harm (suicide)	38,285	1.5	■ ■ ■ A
11	Septicemia (systemic blood infection)	35,539	1.4	■ ■ ■ A
12	Chronic liver disease and cirrhosis	33,539	1.3	■ ■ ■ A
13	Hypertension (high blood pressure)	27,477	1.1	D I S A
14	Parkinson's disease	23,107	0.9	■ ■ ■ ■
15	Lung inflammation due to solids and liquids	18,090	0.7	■ ■ ■ A
	All other causes	512,723		■ ■ ■ ■
	All causes	2,512,873	100.0	■ ■ ■ ■

Key				
	D	Diet plays a part.	S	Smoking plays a part.
	I	Inactive lifestyle plays a part.	A	Excessive alcohol use plays a part.

note: Although not among the overall top 15 causes of death, HIV/AIDS (8,352 deaths in 2010) is a major killer. In 2011 HIV/AIDS was the 12th leading cause of death for Americans aged 15–24 years and the 8th leading cause of death for those aged 25–44 years.

source: Hoyert, D. L., and J. Q. Xu. 2012. Deaths: Preliminary data for 2011. *National Vital Statistics Reports* 61(6).

In the United States, the National Institutes of Health (NIH) and the Centers for Disease Control and Prevention (CDC) are federal agencies charged with promoting the public's health. The NIH is the primary federal agency for conducting and supporting medical research. NIH scientists investigate ways to prevent disease as well as the causes, treatments, and cures for common and rare diseases. Composed of 27 institutes and centers, the NIH provides leadership and financial support to researchers in every state as well as around the world. The NIH translates research results into interventions and communicates research findings to patients, health care providers, and the public.

The Healthy People Initiative

The national Healthy People initiative aims to prevent disease and improve Americans' quality of life. *Healthy People* reports, published each decade since 1980, set national health goals based on 10-year agendas. The initiative's most recent iteration, *Healthy People 2020,* was developed in 2008–2009 and released to the public in 2010. *Healthy People 2020* envisions "a society in which all people live long, healthy lives" and proposes the eventual achievement of the following broad national health objectives:

- Eliminate preventable disease, disability, injury, and premature death.
- Achieve health equity, eliminate disparities, and improve the health of all groups.
- Create social and physical environments that promote good health for all.
- Promote healthy development and healthy behaviors across every stage of life.

In a shift from the past, *Healthy People 2020* emphasizes the importance of health determinants—factors that affect the health of individuals, demographic groups, or entire populations. Health determinants are social (including factors such as ethnicity, education level, or economic status) and environmental (including natural and human-made environments). Thus one goal is to improve living conditions in ways that reduce the impact of negative health determinants.

Examples of individual health promotion goals from *Healthy People 2020,* along with estimates of how well Americans are tracking toward achieving those goals, appear in Table 1.4.

VITAL STATISTICS

Table 1.2 Lifestyle and Environmental Contributors to Death among Americans

	NUMBER OF DEATHS PER YEAR	PERCENTAGE OF TOTAL DEATHS PER YEAR
Tobacco	467,000	19.1
Obesity[a]	216,000	8.8
Alcohol consumption[b]	64,000	2.6
Toxic agents[c]	55,000	2.3
Microbial agents[d]	50,003	2.0
Illicit drug use	40,239	1.3
Motor vehicles	34,677	1.1
Firearms	30,867	0.9
Sexually transmitted infections	20,000	0.8

[a]The number of deaths related to obesity is an area of ongoing controversy and research. Recent estimates have ranged from 112,000 to 365,000.

[b]The number of deaths due to alcohol excludes those that indirectly resulted in fatal injury.

[c]Toxic agents include environmental pollutants and chemical agents such as asbestos.

[d]Microbial agents include bacterial and viral infections like influenza and pneumonia.

SOURCES: Danaei, G., et al. 2009. The preventable causes of death in the United States: comparative risk assessment of dietary, lifestyle, and metabolic risk factors. *PLoS Medicine* 6(4): e1000058; Centers for Disease Control and Prevention. 2008. Smoking-attributable mortality, years of potential life lost, and productivity losses—United States, 2000–2004. *Morbidity and Mortality Weekly Report* 57(45): 1226–1228; National Center for Health Statistics. 2012. Deaths: final data for 2009 (data release). *National Vital Statistics Report* 60(3); National Center for Health Statistics. 2012. Deaths: preliminary data for 2011 (data release). *National Vital Statistics Report* 61(6).

VITAL STATISTICS

Table 1.3 Leading Causes of Death among Americans Ages 15–24, 2011

RANK	CAUSE OF DEATH	NUMBER OF DEATHS	PERCENTAGE OF TOTAL DEATHS
1	Accidents:	12,032	40.6
	Motor vehicle	6,984	23.6
	All other accidents	5,048	17.1
2	Suicide	4,688	15.8
3	Homicide	4,506	15.2
4	Cancer	1,609	5.4
5	Heart disease	948	3.2
	All causes	29,605	100.0

SOURCES: National Center for Health Statistics. 2012. Deaths: Preliminary data for 2011. *National Vital Statistics Report* 61(6).

Table 1.4

Select *Healthy People 2020* Objectives

OBJECTIVE	BASELINE (% MEETING GOAL IN 2008)	MOST RECENT PROGRESS (% MEETING GOAL IN 2012)	TARGET (% BY 2020)	PROGRESS
Increase proportion of people with health insurance	83.2	83.1	100.0	O
Increase proportion of people with a primary care provider	76.3 (2007)	77.3 (2011)	83.9	O
Help adults with hypertension get blood pressure under control	43.7	48.9	61.2	+
Reduce proportion of obese adults	33.9	35.3	30.5	−
Reduce proportion of adults who drank excessively in past 30 days	27.1	27.1	24.4	O
Increase proportion of adults who exercise	18.2	20.6	20.1	✓
Reduce proportion of adults who use cigarettes	20.6	18.2	12.0	+
Increase daily intake of vegetables (age adjusted, cup equivalents per 1,000 calories)	0.8 (2001–2004)	0.8 (2007–2010)	1.1	O

✓ Target met   + Improving   O Insignificant or no change   − Getting worse

SOURCE: *Healthy People 2020 Leading Health Indicators: Progress Update,* March 2014 (http://www.healthypeople.gov/2020/LHI/LHI-ProgressReport-ExecSum.pdf)

Health Issues for Diverse Populations

Most health issues concern us all equally. We all need to eat well, exercise, manage stress, and cultivate satisfying personal relationships. We need to know how to protect ourselves from heart disease, cancer, sexually transmitted infections, and injuries. We need to know how to use the health care system.

But some of our differences, as individuals and as members of groups, have important implications for health. Some of us, for example, have a genetic predisposition for developing certain health problems, such as high cholesterol. Some of us have grown up eating foods that raise our risk of heart disease or obesity. Some of us live in an environment that increases the chance that we will smoke cigarettes or abuse alcohol. These health-related differences among individuals and groups can be biological—that is, determined genetically—or cultural—acquired as patterns of behavior through daily interactions with our families, communities, and society. Many health conditions result from a combination of biology and culture.

Health-related differences among groups can be identified and described in the context of several different dimensions. Those highlighted by the Healthy People initiative are sex and gender, ethnicity, income and education, disability, geographic location, and sexual orientation.

When it comes to wellness, **personal responsibility can make the difference.**

QUICK STATS

One in three
Americans reported that in 2013 they delayed seeking medical treatment due to the cost.

—Gallup poll 2013

Sex and Gender   Sex and gender profoundly influence wellness. The WHO defines **sex** as the biological and physiological characteristics that define men and women. These characteristics are related to chromosomes and their effects on reproductive organs and the functioning of the body. Menstruation in women and the presence of testicles in men are examples of sex-related characteristics.

Gender is defined as roles, behaviors, activities, and attributes that a given society considers appropriate for men and women. A person's gender is rooted in biology and physiology, but it is shaped by experience and environment—how society responds to individuals based on their sex. Examples of gender-related characteristics that affect wellness include higher rates of smoking and drinking among men and lower earnings among women (compared with men doing similar work).

Both sex and gender have important effects on wellness, but they can be difficult to separate. For example, in the early 20th

sex   The biological and physiological characteristics that define men and women.

gender   The roles, behaviors, activities, and attributes that a given society considers appropriate for men and women.

TERMS

century, more women began smoking with changes in culturally defined ideas about women's behavior (a gender issue). Because women are more vulnerable to the toxins in tobacco smoke (a sex issue), their cancer rates also increased. Although men are more biologically likely than women to suffer from certain diseases (a sex issue), men are less likely to visit their physicians for regular exams (a gender issue). As a result, 55% of American men have not seen their doctors for checkups in the past year, and 29% of men say they wait as long as possible before seeing a doctor—even when they are sick. About one in three American men don't have a regular health care provider, compared to about one in five American women.

Ethnicity   Compared with the U.S. population as a whole, American ethnic minorities have higher rates of death and disability from many causes (Figure 1.4). These disparities result from a complex mix of genetic variations, environmental factors, and health behaviors.

Some diseases are concentrated in certain gene pools, the result of each ethnic group's relatively distinct history. Sickle-cell disease is most common among people of African ancestry. Tay-Sachs disease afflicts people of Eastern European Jewish heritage and French Canadian heritage. Cystic fibrosis is more common among Northern Europeans. In addition to biological differences, many cultural differences occur along ethnic lines. Ethnic groups may vary in their traditional diets;

their family and interpersonal relationships; their attitudes toward tobacco, alcohol, and other drugs; and their health beliefs and practices. All of these factors have implications for wellness.

The federal government collects population and health information on five broad ethnic minority groups in American society. Each group has some specific health concerns:

• *Latinos* are a diverse group, with roots in Mexico, Puerto Rico, Cuba, and South and Central America. Many Latinos are of mixed Spanish and American Indian descent or of mixed Spanish, Indian, and African American descent. Latinos on average have lower rates of heart disease, cancer, and suicide than the general population, but higher rates of infant mortality and a higher overall birth rate; other areas of concern include gallbladder disease and obesity. At current rates, about one in two Latinas will develop diabetes in her lifetime.

• *African Americans* have the same leading causes of death as the general population, but they have a higher infant mortality rate and lower rates of suicide and osteoporosis. Health issues of special concern for African Americans include high blood pressure, stroke, diabetes, asthma, and obesity. African American men are at significantly higher risk of prostate cancer than men in other groups, and early screening is recommended for them.

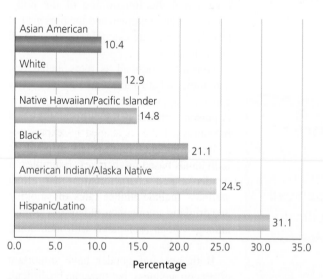

(a) Americans self-reporting health status as fair or poor

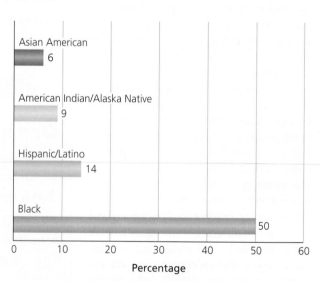

(b) Ethnic groups receiving worse health care than white Americans, based on key core measures

FIGURE 1.4   Self-rated health status and quality of care. White Americans are less likely than most ethnic minorities to report their health status as being fair or poor. Meanwhile, significant percentages of minority groups receive lower-quality health care than white Americans, based on comparisons of key measures of treatment quality.

SOURCES: Centers for Disease Control and Prevention. 2008. Racial/ethnic disparities in self-rated health status among adults with and without disabilities—United States, 2004–2006. *Morbidity and Mortality Weekly Report* 57(39): 1069–1073; U.S. Department of Health and Human Services, Agency for Healthcare Research and Quality. 2010. *2009 National Healthcare Disparities Report.* Rockville, MD: U.S. Department of Health and Human Services, Agency for Healthcare Research and Quality, AHRQ Pub. No. 10-0003.

Among America's ethnic groups, striking disparities exist in health status, access to and quality of health care, and life expectancy.

For example, the estimated life expectancy of black Americans (75.3) is about four years shorter than that of whites (78.8). Blacks also have the highest age-adjusted death rate (898 deaths per 100,000 population) of any ethnic group. Whites have the second-highest death rate (741), followed by Native Americans/Alaska Natives (626), Hispanics (558), and Asian Americans/Pacific Islanders (424).

In studying and attempting to understand the underlying causes of health disparities, it is often helpful to separate the many potential contributing factors.

Income and Education

Poverty and low educational attainment are the most important factors underlying health disparities. However, when groups with similar incomes and levels of education are compared, ethnic disparities persist. Consider the following examples:

- *Overall health.* People living in poverty report worse health than people with higher incomes. Within the latter group, however, African Americans and Latinos rate their health as "bad" more frequently than do whites.

- *Infant mortality.* Rates of infant deaths go down as the education level of mothers goes up. Among mothers who are college graduates, however, African Americans have significantly higher rates of infant mortality than whites, Latinos, and Asian Americans. Overall, the rate of infant mortality among blacks is more than double that of whites, Asian Americans, or Hispanics.

Access to Appropriate Health Care

The Affordable Care Act passed by Congress in 2010 mandated insurance coverage for 40 million Americans

without insurance. Major coverage expansion began in 2014. The legislation will reduce the number of people without access to health care and without information about services and preventive care.

Although people with low incomes have tended to receive poorer-quality health care, disparities among ethnic minorities persist even at higher income levels. For example, among non-poor Americans, many more Latinos than whites or African Americans report no usual source of health care and no health care visits within the past year. Ongoing studies continually find that racial minorities have less access to better health care (such as complex surgery at high-volume hospitals) and receive lower-quality care than whites.

Factors affecting such disparities may include the following:

- *Local differences in the availability of high-tech health care and specialists.* Minorities, regardless of income, may be more likely to live in medically underserved areas.

- *Problems with communication and trust.* People whose primary language is not English are more likely to be uninsured and to have trouble communicating with health care providers. They may also have problems interpreting health information from public health education campaigns. Language and cultural barriers may be compounded by an underrepresentation of minorities in the health professions.

- *Cultural preferences relating to health care.* Groups may vary in their assessment of when it is appropriate to seek medical care and what types of treatments are acceptable.

Culture and Lifestyle

As previously described, ethnic groups may vary in health-related behaviors such as diet, tobacco and alcohol use, coping strategies, and health practices—and these behaviors can have important implications for wellness, both positive and negative. For example, African Americans are more likely to report consuming five or more servings of fruits and vegetables per day than people from other ethnic groups. American Indians report high rates of smoking and smoking-related health problems.

Cultural background can be an important protective factor. For example, poverty is strongly associated with increased rates of depression, but some groups, including Americans born in Mexico or Puerto Rico, have lower rates of mental disorders at a given level of income and appear to have coping strategies that provide special resilience.

Discrimination

Racism and discrimination are stressful events that can cause psychological distress and increase the risk of physical and psychological problems. Discrimination can contribute to lower socioeconomic status and its associated risks. Bias in medical care can directly affect treatment and health outcomes.

Conversely, research shows that better health care results when doctors ask patients detailed questions about their ethnicity. (Most medical questionnaires ask patients to put themselves in a vague racial or ethnic category, such as Asian or Caucasian.) Armed with more information about patients' backgrounds, medical professionals may find it easier to detect some genetic diseases or to overcome language or cultural barriers.

• *Asian Americans* include people who trace their ancestry to countries in the Far East, Southeast Asia, or the Indian subcontinent, including Japan, China, Vietnam, Laos, Cambodia, Korea, the Philippines, India, and Pakistan. Asian Americans have a lower death rate and a longer life expectancy than the general population. They have lower rates of coronary heart disease and obesity. However, health differences exist among these groups. For example, Southeast Asian men have higher rates of smoking and lung cancer, and Vietnamese American women have higher rates of cervical cancer.

• *American Indians and Alaska Natives* typically embrace a tribal identity, such as Sioux, Navaho, or Hopi. American Indians and Alaska Natives have lower death rates from heart disease, stroke, and cancer than the general population, but they have higher rates of early death from causes linked to smoking and alcohol use, including injuries and cirrhosis. Diabetes is a special concern for many groups; for example, the Pimas of Arizona have the highest known prevalence of diabetes of any population in the world.

• *Native Hawaiian and other Pacific Islander Americans* trace their ancestry to the original peoples of Hawaii, Guam, Samoa, and other Pacific Islands. Pacific Islander Americans have a higher overall death rate than the general population and higher rates of diabetes and asthma. Smoking and obesity are special concerns for this group.

Income and Education   Inequalities in income and education underlie many of the health disparities among Americans. In fact, poverty and low educational attainment are far more important predictors of poor health than any ethnic factor. Income and education are closely related, and groups with the highest poverty rates and least education have the worst health status. These Americans have higher rates of infant mortality, traumatic injury, violent death, and many diseases, including heart disease, diabetes, tuberculosis, human immunodeficiency virus (HIV) infection, and some cancers. They are more likely to eat poorly, be overweight, smoke, drink, and use drugs. They are exposed to more day-to-day stressors and have less access to health care services.

Disability   People with disabilities have activity limitations, need assistance, or perceive themselves as having a disability. About one in five people in the United States has some level of disability, and the rate is rising, especially among younger segments of the population. People with disabilities are more likely to be inactive and overweight. They report more days of depression than people without disabilities. Many also lack access to health care services.

Geographic Location   About one in four Americans currently lives in a rural area—a place with fewer than 10,000 residents. People living in rural areas are less likely to be physically active, use safety belts, or obtain screening tests for preventive health care. They have less access to timely emergency services and much higher rates of some diseases and injury-related death than people living in urban areas. They are also more likely to lack health insurance. Children living in dangerous neighborhoods—rural or urban—are four times more likely to be overweight than children living in safer areas.

Sexual Orientation   The 1–5% of Americans who identify themselves as homosexual or bisexual make up a diverse community with varied health concerns. Their emotional wellness and personal safety are affected by factors relating to personal, family, and social acceptance of their sexual orientation. Gay, lesbian, bisexual, and transgender teens are more likely to engage in risky behaviors such as unsafe sex and drug use; they are also more likely to be depressed and to attempt suicide. HIV/AIDS is a major concern for gay men, and gay men and lesbians may have higher rates of substance abuse, depression, and suicide.

CHOOSING WELLNESS

Optimal health comes mostly from a healthy lifestyle—patterns of behavior that promote and support your health now and as you get older. In the pages that follow, you'll find current information and suggestions you can use to build a healthier lifestyle; also, see the "Wellness Matters for College Students" box.

Factors That Influence Wellness

Our behavior, family health history, environment, and access to health care are all important influences on wellness. These factors, which vary for both individuals and groups, can interact in ways that produce either health or disease.

Health Habits   Research continually reveals new connections between our habits and health. For example, heart disease is associated with smoking, stress, a hostile attitude,

Most college students, in their late teens and early twenties, appear to be healthy. But appearances can be deceiving. Each year, thousands of students lose productive academic time to physical and emotional health problems—some of which can continue to plague them for life.

The following table shows the top 10 health issues affecting students' academic performance, according to the Spring 2011 American College Health Association–National College Health Assessment II.

HEALTH ISSUE	STUDENTS AFFECTED (%)
Stress	27.5
Sleep difficulties	19.4
Anxiety	19.1
Cold/flu/sore throat	16.4
Work	13.3
Excessive Internet use/computer games	12.4
Depression	11.9
Concern for a friend/family member	11.0
Relationship difficulties	10.5
Excessive extracurricular activities	9.5

Each of these issues is related to one or more of the dimensions of wellness, and most can be influenced by choices students make daily. Although some troubles—such as the death of a friend—cannot be controlled, students can minimize other physical and emotional concerns by choosing healthy behaviors. For example, there are many ways to manage stress, the top health issue affecting students. By reducing unhealthy choices (such as using alcohol to relax) and by increasing healthy choices (such as using time management techniques), even busy students can reduce the impact of stress on their lives.

The survey also estimated that, based on students' reporting of their height and weight, nearly 33% of college students are either overweight or obese. Although heredity plays a role in determining your weight, lifestyle is also a factor in weight management.

In many studies over the past few decades, a large percentage of students have reported behaviors such as these:

- Overeating
- Snacking on junk food
- Frequently eating high-fat foods
- Using alcohol and binge drinking

Clearly, eating behaviors are often a matter of choice. Although students may not see (or feel) the effects of their dietary habits today, the long-term health risks are significant. Overweight and obese persons run a higher-than-normal risk of developing diabetes, heart disease, and cancer later in life. We now know with certainty that improving your eating habits, even a little, can lead to weight loss and improved overall health.

Other Choices, Other Problems

Students commonly make other unhealthy choices. Here are some examples from the 2011 National College Health Assessment II:

- About 43% of students reported that they did not use a condom the last time they had vaginal intercourse.
- About 16% of students had seven or more drinks the last time they partied.
- About 14% of students had smoked cigarettes at least once during the past month.

What choices do you make in these situations? Remember: It's never too late to change. The sooner you trade an unhealthy behavior for a healthy one, the longer you'll be around to enjoy the benefits.

SOURCE: American College Health Association. 2012. *American College Health Association–National College Health Assessment II: Reference Group Executive Summary Spring 2012*. Hanover, MD: American College Health Association. Reprinted by permission of the American College Health Association.

a poor diet, and being sedentary. Poor health habits take hold before many Americans reach adulthood.

Other habits, however, are beneficial. Regular exercise can help prevent heart disease, high blood pressure, diabetes, osteoporosis, and depression. Exercise can also reduce the risk of colon cancer, stroke, and back injury. A balanced and varied diet helps prevent many chronic diseases. As we learn more about how our actions affect our bodies and minds, we can make informed choices for a healthier life.

Heredity/Family History Your **genome** consists of the complete set of genetic material in your cells—about 25,000 genes, half from each of your parents. **Genes** control the production of proteins that serve both as the structural material for your body and as the regulators of all your body's chemical reactions and metabolic processes. The human genome varies only slightly from person to person,

> **genome** The complete set of genetic material in an individual's cells.
>
> **gene** The basic unit of heredity; a section of genetic material containing chemical instructions for making a particular protein.
>
> TERMS

and many of these differences do not affect health. However, some differences have important implications for health, and knowing your family's health history can help you determine which conditions may be of special concern for you.

Errors in our genes are responsible for about 3500 clearly hereditary conditions, including sickle-cell disease and cystic fibrosis. Altered genes also play a part in heart disease, cancer, stroke, diabetes, and many other common conditions. However, in these more common and complex disorders, genetic alterations serve only to increase an individual's risk, and the disease itself results from the interaction of many genes with other factors. An example of the power of behavior and environment can be seen in the more than 60% increase in the incidence of diabetes that has occurred among Americans since 1990. This huge increase is not due to any sudden change in our genes; it is the result of increasing rates of obesity caused by poor dietary choices and lack of physical activity.

Environment Your environment includes substances and conditions in your home, workplace, and community. Are you frequently exposed to environmental tobacco smoke or the radiation in sunlight? Do you live in an area with high rates of crime and violence? Do you have access to nature? Today environmental influences on wellness also include conditions in other countries and around the globe, particularly weather and climate change, which has attracted much attention worldwide. Most climate scientists agree that human activity—specifically, the burning of fossil fuels for energy and the release of greenhouse gases into the atmosphere—has caused changes that are raising Earth's temperature and threatening the health of the planet and its living systems. The evidence includes melting ice caps, shifting weather patterns, and the threatened extinction of species. Scientists are trying to determine how high Earth's temperature can climb before damage becomes irreversible.

Access to Health Care Adequate health care helps improve both quality and quantity of life through preventive care and the treatment of disease. For example, vaccinations prevent many dangerous infections, and screening tests help identify key risk factors and diseases in their early treatable stages. As described earlier, inadequate access to health care is tied to factors such as low income and lack of health insurance. Cost is one of many issues surrounding the development of advanced health-related technologies.

> Moving in the direction of wellness means **cultivating healthy behaviors and working to overcome unhealthy ones.**

behavior change A lifestyle management process that involves cultivating healthy behaviors and working to overcome unhealthy ones.

TERMS

Taking Personal Responsibility for Your Wellness

In many cases, behavior can tip the balance toward good health, even when heredity or environment is a negative factor. For example, breast cancer can run in families, but it also may be associated with being overweight and inactive. A woman with a family history of breast cancer is less likely to develop the disease if she controls her weight, exercises regularly, and has regular mammograms to help detect the disease in its early, most treatable stage.

Similarly, a young man with a family history of obesity can maintain a normal weight by balancing calorie intake against activities that burn calories. If your life is highly stressful, you can lessen the chances of heart disease and stroke by managing and coping with stress (see the section "Managing Stress" in Chapter 2). If you live in an area with severe air pollution, you can reduce the risk of lung disease by not smoking. You can also take an active role in improving your environment. Behaviors like these can make a difference in how great an impact heredity and environment will have on your health.

REACHING WELLNESS THROUGH LIFESTYLE MANAGEMENT

As you consider the behaviors that contribute to wellness—being physically active, choosing a healthful diet, and so on—you may be doing a mental comparison with your own behaviors. If you are like most young adults, you probably have some healthy habits and some habits that place your health at risk. For example, you may be physically active and have a healthful diet but spend excessive hours playing video games. You may be careful to wear your safety belt in your car but skip meals. Moving in the direction of wellness means cultivating healthy behaviors and working to overcome unhealthy ones. This approach to lifestyle management is called **behavior change**.

As you may already know, changing an unhealthy habit (such as giving up cigarettes) can be harder than it sounds. When you embark on a behavior change plan, it may seem like too much work at first. But as you make progress, you will gain confidence in your ability to take charge of your life. You will also experience the benefits of wellness—more energy, greater vitality, deeper feelings of appreciation and curiosity, and a higher quality of life.

Getting Serious about Your Health

Before you can start changing a wellness-related behavior, you have to know that the behavior is problematic and that you *can* change it. To make good decisions, you need information about relevant topics and issues, including what resources are available to help you change.

Examine Your Current Health Habits

How is your current lifestyle affecting your health today and in the future? Think about which of your current habits enhance your health and which detract from it? Begin your journey toward wellness with self-assessment: Talk with friends and family members about what they have noticed about your lifestyle and your health. Challenge any unrealistically optimistic attitudes or ideas you may hold—for example, "To protect my health, I don't need to worry about quitting smoking until I'm 40 years old" or "Being overweight won't put *me* at risk for diabetes." Health risks are very real and can become significant while you're young; health habits are important throughout life.

Many people consider changing a behavior when friends or family members express concern, when a landmark event occurs (such as turning 30), or when new information raises their awareness of risk. If you find yourself reevaluating some of your behaviors as you read this text, take advantage of the opportunity to make a change in a structured way.

Choose a Target Behavior

Changing any behavior can be demanding. Start small by choosing one behavior you want to change—called a **target behavior**—and working on it until you succeed. Your chances of success will be greater if your first goal is simple, such as resisting the urge to snack between classes. As you change one behavior, make your next goal a little more significant, and build on your success.

Learn about Your Target Behavior

Once you've chosen a target behavior, you need to learn its risks and benefits—both now and in the future. Ask these questions:

• How is your target behavior affecting your level of wellness today?

• Which diseases or conditions does this behavior place you at risk for?

• What effect would changing your behavior have on your health?

As a starting point, use this text and the resources listed in the "For More Information" section at the end of each chapter. See the "Evaluating Sources of Health Information" box for additional guidelines.

Find Help

Have you identified a particularly challenging target behavior or mood—something like alcohol addiction, binge eating, or depression—that interferes with your ability to function or places you at a serious health risk? If so, you may need help to change a behavior or condition that is deeply rooted or too serious for self-management. Don't let the problem's seriousness stop you; many resources are available to help you solve it. On

> To change a behavior, you recognize that **you can take control of your actions.**

campus, the student health center or campus counseling center can provide assistance. To locate community resources, consult the yellow pages, your physician, or the Internet.

Building Motivation to Change

Knowledge is necessary for behavior change, but it isn't usually enough to make people act. Millions of people have sedentary lifestyles, for example, even though they know it's bad for their health. This is particularly true of young adults, who feel healthy despite their unhealthy behaviors. To succeed at behavior change, you need strong motivation. Here are some things to consider.

Examine the Pros and Cons of Change

Health behaviors have short-term and long-term benefits and costs. Consider the benefits and costs of an inactive lifestyle:

• **Short-term.** Such a lifestyle allows you more time to watch TV, use social media, do your homework, and hang out with friends, but it leaves you less physically fit and less able to participate in recreational activities.

• **Long-term.** It increases the risk of heart disease, cancer, stroke, and premature death.

To successfully change your behavior, you must believe that the benefits of change outweigh the costs.

Carefully examine the pros and cons of continuing your current behavior and of changing to a healthier one. Focus on the effects that are most meaningful to you, including those that are tied to your personal identity and values. For example, engaging in regular physical activity and adequate sleep can support an image of yourself as an active person who is a good role model for others. To complete your analysis, ask friends and family members about the effects of your behavior on them. A younger sister may say that your smoking habit influenced her decision to start smoking.

The short-term benefits of behavior change can be an important motivating force. Although some people are motivated by long-term goals, such as avoiding a disease that may hit them in 30 years, most are more likely to be moved to action by shorter-term, more personal goals. Feeling better, doing better in school, improving at a sport, reducing stress, and increasing self-esteem are common short-term benefits of health behavior change.

Boost Self-Efficacy

A big factor in your eventual success is whether you feel confident in your ability to change. **Self-efficacy** refers to your belief in your ability to successfully

---

target behavior   An isolated behavior selected as the object for a behavior change program.

self-efficacy   The belief in your ability to take action and perform a specific task.

TERMS

CRITICAL CONSUMER
Evaluating Sources of Health Information

Believability of Health Information Sources

Surveys indicate that college students are smart about evaluating health information. They trust the health information they receive from health professionals and educators and are skeptical about popular information sources, such as magazine articles and websites.

How good are you at evaluating health information? Here are some tips.

General Strategies

Whenever you encounter health-related information, take the following steps to make sure it is credible:

- **Go to the original source.** Media reports often simplify the results of medical research. Find out for yourself what a study really reported, and determine whether it was based on good science. What type of study was it? Was it published in a recognized medical journal? Was it an animal study or did it involve people? Did the study include a large number of people? What did the authors of the study actually report?

- **Watch for misleading language.** Reports that tout "breakthroughs" or "dramatic proof" are probably hype. A study may state that a behavior "contributes to" or is "associated with" an outcome; this does not prove a cause-and-effect relationship.

- **Distinguish between research reports and public health advice.** Do not change your behavior based on the results of a single report or study. If an agency such as the National Cancer Institute urges a behavior change, however, you should follow its advice. Large, publicly funded organizations issue such advice based on many studies, not a single report.

- **Remember that anecdotes are not facts.** A friend may tell you he lost weight on some new diet, but individual success stories do not mean the plan is truly safe or effective. Check with your doctor before making any serious lifestyle changes.

- **Be skeptical.** If a report seems too good to be true, it probably is. Be wary of information contained in advertisements.

An ad's goal is to sell a product, even if there is no need for it.

- **Make choices that are right for you.** Friends and family members can be a great source of ideas and inspiration, but you need to make health-related choices that work best for you.

Internet Resources

Online sources pose special challenges; when reviewing a health-related website, ask these questions:

- **What is the source of the information?** Websites maintained by government agencies, professional associations, or established academic or medical institutions are likely to present trustworthy information. Many other groups and individuals post accurate information, but it is important to look at the qualifications of the people who are behind the site. (Check the home page or click the "About Us" link.)

- **How often is the site updated?** Look for sites that are updated frequently. Check the "last modified" date of any web page.

- **Is the site promotional?** Be wary of information from sites that sell specific products, use testimonials as evidence, appear to have a social or political agenda, or ask for money.

- **What do other sources say about a topic?** Be cautious of claims or information that appear at only one site or come from a chat room, bulletin board, newsgroup, or blog.

- **Does the site conform to any set of guidelines or criteria for quality and accuracy?** Look for sites that identify themselves as conforming to some code or set of principles, such as those established by the Health on the Net Foundation or the American Medical Association. These codes include criteria such as use of information from respected sources and disclosure of the site's sponsors.

---

take action and perform a specific task. Strategies for boosting self-efficacy include developing an internal locus of control, using visualization and self-talk, and getting encouragement from supportive people.

LOCUS OF CONTROL   Who do you believe is controlling your life? Is it your parents, friends, or school? Is it "fate"? Or is it you? **Locus of control** refers to the figurative "place" a person

> **locus of control**   The figurative "place" a person designates as the source of responsibility for the events in his or her life.
>
> **TERMS**

designates as the source of responsibility for the events in his or her life. People who believe they are in control of their lives are said to have an *internal locus of control.* Those who believe that factors beyond their control determine the course of their lives are said to have an *external locus of control.*

For lifestyle management, an internal locus of control is an advantage because it reinforces motivation and commitment. An external locus of control can sabotage efforts to change behavior. For example, if you believe that you are destined to die of breast cancer because your mother died from the disease, you may view monthly breast self-exams and regular checkups as a waste of time. In contrast, if you believe that you can take action to reduce your risk of breast cancer despite hereditary factors, you will be motivated to follow guidelines for early detection of the disease.

If you find yourself attributing too much influence to outside forces, gather more information about your wellness-related behaviors. List all the ways that making lifestyle changes will improve your health. If you believe you'll succeed, and if you recognize that you are in charge of your life, you're on your way to wellness.

VISUALIZATION AND SELF-TALK One of the best ways to boost your confidence and self-efficacy is to visualize yourself successfully engaging in a new, healthier behavior. Imagine yourself going for an afternoon run three days a week or no longer smoking cigarettes. Also visualize yourself enjoying all the short-term and long-term benefits that your lifestyle change will bring. Create a new self-image: What will you and your life be like when you become a regular exerciser or a nonsmoker?

You can also use *self-talk,* the internal dialogue you carry on with yourself, to increase your confidence in your ability to change. Counter any self-defeating patterns of thought with more positive or realistic thoughts: "I am a strong, capable person, and I can maintain my commitment to change." (See Chapter 3 for more about self-talk.)

ROLE MODELS AND SUPPORTIVE PEOPLE Social support can make a big difference in your level of motivation and your chances of success. Perhaps you know people who have reached the goal you are striving for. They could be role models or mentors for you, providing information and support for your efforts. Gain strength from their experiences, and tell yourself, "If they can do it, so can I." Find a partner who wants to make the same changes you do and who can take an active role in your behavior change program. For example, an exercise partner can provide companionship and encouragement when you might be tempted to skip your workout.

Identify and Overcome Barriers to Change Don't let past failures at behavior change discourage you. They can be a great source of information you can use to boost your chances of future success. Make a list of the problems and challenges you faced in any previous behavior change attempts. To this, add the short-term costs of behavior change that you identified in your analysis of the pros and cons of change. Once you've listed these key barriers to change, develop a practical plan for overcoming each one. For example, if you are not getting enough sleep when you're with certain friends, decide in advance how you will turn down their next late-night invitation.

Enhancing Your Readiness to Change

The transtheoretical, or "stages of change," model has been shown to be an effective approach to lifestyle self-management. According to this model, you move through distinct stages of

action as you achieve your target behavior. First, determine what stage you are in now so that you can choose appropriate strategies to progress through the cycle of change. This will help you enhance your readiness and intention to change. Read the following sections to determine what stage you are in.

Precontemplation At this stage, you think you have no problem and don't intend to change your behavior. For example, your friends have commented that you should exercise more, but you are resistant. You have tried to exercise in the past and now think your situation is hopeless. You are unaware of risks associated with being sedentary; and you also blame external factors like other people for your condition. You believe that there are more important reasons *not* to change than there are reasons to change.

Contemplation You now know you have a problem and within six months intend to do something about. You realize that getting more exercise will help decrease your stress level. You acknowledge the benefits of behavior change but are also aware that the barriers to change may be difficult to overcome. You consider possible courses of action but don't know how to proceed.

Preparation At this stage you plan to take action within a month or you may have already begun to make small changes in your behavior. You may have discovered a place to go jogging but have not yet gone regularly or consistently.

Action You outwardly modify your behavior and your environment. Maybe you start riding your bike to school or work. The action stage requires the greatest commitment of time and energy, and people in this stage are at risk of relapsing into old, unhealthy patterns of behavior. Don't get discouraged. Real change is difficult.

Maintenance You have maintained your new, healthier lifestyle for at least six months by working out and riding your bike. Lapses have occurred, but you have been successful in quickly reestablishing the desired behavior. The maintenance stage can last months or years.

Termination For some behaviors, you may reach the sixth and final stage of termination. At this stage, you have exited the cycle of change and are no longer tempted to lapse back into your old behavior. You have a new self-image and total control with regard to your target behavior.

For ideas on moving forward from stage to stage, see the "Cycle of Stages to Increase Your Level of Exercise" box.

Dealing with Relapse

People seldom progress through the stages of change in a straightforward, linear way. Rather, they tend to move to a certain stage and then slip back to a previous stage before

TAKE CHARGE
Cycle of Stages to Increase Your Level of Exercise

STAGE	PROBLEM	WHAT YOU CAN DO
Precontemplation	Your doctor or friends say you should get more exercise.	Research benefits of exercise. Ask yourself, "Why am I resisting change?" Seek social support. Find an exercise class.
Contemplation	You know you need more exercise because you are stressed out, not sleeping well, and overweight.	Keep a journal of how often you already build exercise into your day (e.g., do you take the stairs instead of the elevator?) and what more you could be doing. Examine what kept you from getting more exercise. Consider what will happen if you do not change your regimen.
Preparation	You plan to get more exercise but have yet to hammer out the details and consistently follow them.	Draw up a plan that includes times, places, and rewards. See yourself jogging/ swimming/playing a team sport, and tell yourself you can succeed at doing these things. Take one day or week at a time. Tell someone about your plan and then how you have followed through with it.
Action	As you adapt to an increase in time and energy spent on exercise, you risk lapsing back into your more sedentary lifestyle.	Change your environment by spending less time in cars or with TVs and computers, and more time walking or biking places. Reward yourself, maybe with a film, massage, or small trip. Keep track of your progress and tell your friends about it.
Maintenance	You have established an exercise routine and sometimes think about quitting it.	Don't let slip-ups set you back. Keep making time to play tennis or take a swim; keep building in exercise to your daily activities such as walking to get groceries and biking to visit a friend.

resuming their forward progress. Research suggests that most people make several attempts before they successfully change a behavior, and four out of five people experience some degree of backsliding. For this reason, the stages of change are best conceptualized as a spiral in which people cycle back through previous stages but are further along in the process each time they renew their commitment (Figure 1.5).

If you experience a lapse (a single slip) or a relapse (a return to old habits), don't give up. Relapse can be demoralizing, but it is not the same as failure; failure means stopping before you reach your goal and never changing your target behavior. During the early stages of the change process, it's a good idea to plan for relapse so you can avoid guilt and self-blame and get back on track quickly.

If relapses keep occurring or you can't seem to control them, you may need to return to a previous stage of the behavior change process. If this is necessary, reevaluate your goals and strategy. A different or less stressful approach may help you avoid setbacks when you try again.

Developing Skills for Change: Creating a Personalized Plan

Once you are committed to making a change, it's time to put together a plan of action. Your key to success is a well-thought-out plan that sets goals, anticipates problems, and includes rewards.

1. Monitor Your Behavior and Gather Data Keep a record of your target behavior and the circumstances surrounding it. Record this information for at least a week or two. Keep your notes in a health journal or notebook or on your computer (see the sample journal entries in Figure 1.6). Record each occurrence of your behavior, noting the following:

- What the activity was.
- When and where it happened.
- What you were doing.
- How you felt at that time.

If your goal is to start an exercise program, track your activities to determine how to make time for workouts.

2. Analyze the Data and Identify Patterns

After you have collected data on the behavior, analyze the data to identify patterns. When are you most likely to overeat? To skip a meal? What events trigger your appetite? Perhaps you are especially hungry at midmorning or when you put off eating dinner until 9:00. Perhaps you overindulge in food and drink when you go to a particular restaurant or when you're with certain friends. Note the connections between your feelings and such external cues as time of day, location, situation, and the actions of others around you.

3. Be "SMART" about Setting Goals

If your goals are too challenging, you will have trouble making steady progress and will be more likely to give up altogether. If, for example, you are in poor physical condition, it will not make sense to set a goal of being ready to run a marathon within two months. If you set goals you can live with, it will be easier to stick with your behavior change plan and be successful.

Experts suggest that your goals meet the "SMART" criteria; that is, your behavior change goals should be

- **Specific.** Avoid vague goals like "eat more fruits and vegetables." Instead state your objectives in specific terms, such as "eat two cups of fruit and three cups of vegetables every day."

- **Measurable.** Recognize that your progress will be easier to track if your goals are quantifiable, so give your goal a number. You might measure your goal in terms of time (such as "walk briskly for 20 minutes a day"), distance ("run two miles, three days per week"), or some other amount ("drink eight glasses of water every day").

- **Attainable.** Set goals that are within your physical limits. For example, if you are a poor swimmer, it might not be possible for you to meet a short-term fitness goal by swimming laps. Walking or biking might be better options.

- **Realistic.** Manage your expectations when you set goals. For example, it may not be possible for a long-time smoker to quit cold turkey. A more realistic approach might

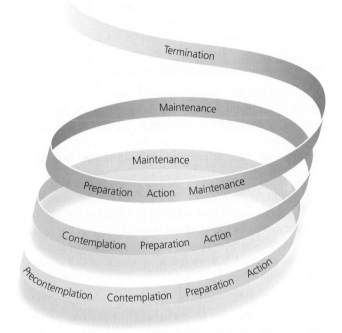

FIGURE 1.5 **The stages of change: A spiral model.**

SOURCE: Adapted from Prochaska, J. O., C. C. DiClemente, & J. C. Norcross. 1992. In search of how people change. *American Psychologist* 47(9): 1102–1114. Copyright © by the American Psychological Association. Reprinted by permission.

Date November 5					Day M TU W TH F SA SU						
Time of day	M/ S	Food eaten	Cals.	H	Where did you eat?	What else were you doing?	How did someone else influence you?	What made you want to eat what you did?	Emotions and feelings?	Thoughts and concerns?	
7:30	M	1 C Crispix cereal 1/2 C skim milk coffee, black 1 C orange juice	110 40 — 120	3	home	reading newspaper	alone	I always eat cereal in the morning	a little keyed up & worried	thinking about quiz in class today	
10:30	S	1 apple	90	1	hall outside classroom	studying	alone	felt tired & wanted to wake up	tired	worried about next class	
12:30	M	1 C chili 1 roll 1 pat butter 1 orange 2 oatmeal cookies 1 soda	290 120 35 60 120 150	2	campus food court	talking	eating w/ friends; we decided to eat at the food court	wanted to be part of group	excited and happy	interested in hearing everyone's plans for the weekend	
M/S = Meal or snack			H = Hunger rating (0–3)								

FIGURE 1.6 **Sample health journal entries.**

be to use nicotine replacement patches or gum for several weeks while getting help from a support group.

- *Time frame–specific.* Give yourself a reasonable amount of time to reach your goal, state the time frame in your behavior change plan, and set your agenda to meet the goal within the given time frame.

Using these criteria, a sedentary person who wants to improve his health and build fitness might set a goal of being able to run three miles in 30 minutes, to be achieved within a time frame of six months. To work toward that goal, he might set a number of smaller, intermediate goals that are easier to achieve. For example, his list of goals might look like this:

WEEK	FREQUENCY (DAYS/WEEK)	ACTIVITY	DURATION (MINUTES)
1	3	Walk < 1 mile	10–15
2	3	Walk 1 mile	15–20
3	4	Walk 1–2 miles	20–25
4	4	Walk 2–3 miles	25–30
5–7	3–4	Walk/run 1 mile	15–20
⋮			
21–24	4–5	Run 2–3 miles	25–30

4. Devise a Plan of Action   Develop a strategy that will support your efforts to change. Your plan of action should include the following steps:

- *Get what you need.* Identify resources that can help you. For example, you can join a community walking club or sign up for a smoking cessation program. You may also need to buy some new running shoes or nicotine replacement patches. Get the items you need right away; waiting can delay your progress.

- *Modify your environment.* If there are cues in your environment that trigger your target behavior, try to control them. For example, if you normally have alcohol at home, getting rid of it can help prevent you from indulging. If you usually study with a group of friends in an environment that allows smoking, try moving to a nonsmoking area. If you always buy a snack at a certain vending machine, change your route so you don't pass by it.

Ask Yourself

QUESTIONS FOR CRITICAL THINKING AND REFLECTION

Think about the last time you made an unhealthy choice instead of a healthy one. How could you have changed the situation, the people in the situation, or your own thoughts, feelings, or intentions to avoid making that choice? What can you do in similar situations in the future to produce a different outcome?

- *Control-related habits.* You may have habits that contribute to your target behavior. Modifying these habits can help change the behavior. For example, if you usually plop down on the sofa while watching TV, try putting an exercise bike in front of the set so you can burn calories while watching your favorite programs.

- *Reward yourself.* Giving yourself instant, real rewards for good behavior will reinforce your efforts. Plan your rewards; decide in advance what each one will be and how you will earn it. Tie rewards to achieving specific goals or subgoals. For example, you might treat yourself to a movie after a week of avoiding snacks. Make a list of items or events to use as rewards. They should be special to you and preferably unrelated to food or alcohol.

- *Involve the people around you.* Tell family and friends about your plan and ask them to help. To help them respond appropriately to your needs, create a specific list of dos and don'ts. For example, ask them to support you when you set aside time to exercise or avoid second helpings at dinner.

- *Plan for challenges.* Think about situations and people that might derail your program and develop ways to cope with them. For example, if you think it will be hard to stick to your usual exercise program during exams, schedule short bouts of physical activity (such as a brisk walk) as stress-reducing study breaks.

5. Make a Personal Contract   A serious personal contract—one that commits you to your word—can result in a better chance of follow-through than a casual, offhand promise. Your contract can help prevent procrastination by specifying important dates and can also serve as a reminder of your personal commitment to change.

Your environment contains powerful cues for both positive and negative lifestyle choices. Identifying and using the healthier options available to you throughout the day is a key part of a successful behavior change program.

Your contract should include a statement of your goal and your commitment to reaching it. The contract should also include details such as the following:

- The date you will start
- The steps you will take to measure your progress
- The strategies you plan to use to promote change
- The date you expect to reach your final goal

Have someone—preferably someone who will be actively helping you with your program—sign your contract as a witness.

Figure 1.7 shows a sample behavior change contract for someone who is committing to eating more fruit every day.

You can apply the general behavior change planning framework presented in this chapter to any target behavior. Additional examples of behavior change plans appear in the Behavior Change Strategy sections at the end of many chapters in this text. In these sections, you will find specific plans for quitting smoking, starting an exercise program, and making other positive lifestyle changes.

Putting Your Plan into Action

When you're ready to put your plan into action, you need commitment—the resolve to stick with the plan no matter what temptations you encounter. Remember all the reasons you have to make the change—and remember that *you* are the boss. Use all your strategies to make your plan work. Make sure your environment is change-friendly, and get as much support and encouragement from others as possible. Keep track of your progress in your health journal and give yourself regular rewards. And don't forget to give yourself a pat on the back—congratulate yourself, notice how much better you look or feel, and feel good about how far you've come and how you've gained control of your behavior.

BEING HEALTHY FOR LIFE

Your first few behavior change projects may never go beyond the planning stage. Those that do may not all succeed. But as you begin to see progress and changes, you'll start to experience new and surprising positive feelings about yourself. You'll probably find that you're less likely to buckle under stress. You may accomplish things you never thought possible—running a marathon, traveling abroad, or finding a rewarding relationship. Being healthy takes extra effort, but the paybacks in energy and vitality are priceless.

Once you've started, don't stop. Remember that maintaining good health is an ongoing process. Tackle one area at a time, but make a careful inventory of your health strengths and weaknesses and lay out a long-range plan. Take on the easier problems first, and then use what you have learned to attack more difficult areas. Keep informed about the latest health news and trends; research is constantly providing new information that directly affects daily choices and habits.

You can't completely control every aspect of your health. At least three other factors—heredity, health care, and environment—play important roles in your well-being. After you quit smoking, for example, you may still be inhaling smoke from other people's cigarettes. Your resolve to eat better foods may suffer a setback when you have trouble finding healthy choices on campus.

But you can make a difference—you can help create an environment around you that supports wellness for everyone. You can support nonsmoking areas in public places. You can speak up in favor of more nutritious foods and better physical fitness facilities. You can provide nonalcoholic drinks at your parties.

You can also work on larger environmental challenges: air and water pollution, traffic congestion, overcrowding and overpopulation, global warming and climate change, toxic

Behavior Change Contract

1. I, __Tammy Lau__, agree to __increase my consumption of fruit from 1 cup per week to 2 cups per day.__

2. I will begin on __10/5__ and plan to reach my goal of __2 cups of fruit per day__ by __12/7__

3. To reach my final goal, I have devised the following schedule of mini-goals. For each step in my program, I will give myself the reward listed.

I will begin to have ½ cup of fruit with breakfast	10/5	see movie
I will begin to have ½ cup of fruit with lunch	10/26	new cd
I will begin to substitute fruit juice for soda 1 time per day	11/16	concert

   My overall reward for reaching my goal will be __trip to beach__

4. I have gathered and analyzed data on my target behavior and have identified the following strategies for changing my behavior: __Keep the fridge stocked with easy-to-carry fruit. Pack fruit in my backpack every day. Buy lunch at place that serves fruit.__

5. I will use the following tools to monitor my progress toward my final goal: __Chart on fridge door__ __Health journal__

   I sign this contract as an indication of my personal commitment to reach my goal: ____Tammy Lau____ __9/28__

   I have recruited a helper who will witness my contract and __also increase his consumption of fruit; eat lunch with me twice a week.__
   ____Eric March____ __9/28__

FIGURE 1.7 **A sample behavior change contract.**

Ask Yourself

?

QUESTIONS FOR CRITICAL THINKING AND REFLECTION

Have you tried to change a behavior in the past, such as exercising more or quitting smoking? How successful were you? Do you feel the need to try again? If so, what would you do differently to improve your chances of success?

and nuclear waste, and many others. These difficult issues need the attention and energy of people who are informed and who care about good health. On every level, from personal to planetary, we can all take an active role in shaping our environment.

connect™

Connect to Your Choices

Have you ever thought about why you make the lifestyle choices you do? Many factors can influence our lifestyle choices, some not as obvious as others. Do you have a lot of the same lifestyle behaviors you had in high school, when you were living at home, such as watching TV or playing video games? Are you strongly influenced by your peers or roommates when it comes to eating and exercise patterns? Do you drink or smoke just because you have the freedom to do so?

What are the external factors that influence your choices about your lifestyle behaviors? What are your inner motivations and core values, and how do they affect your choices? Based on what you learned in this chapter, will you make some different choices in the future? If so, what will they be?

Go online to Connect to complete this activity: www.mcgraw-hillconnect.com

TIPS FOR TODAY AND THE FUTURE

You are in charge of your health. Many of the decisions you make every day have an impact on the quality of your life, both now and in the future. By making positive choices, large and small, you help ensure a lifetime of wellness.

RIGHT NOW YOU CAN:
- Go for a 15-minute walk.
- Have a piece of fruit for a snack.
- Call a friend and arrange a time to catch up with each other.
- Start thinking about whether you have a health behavior you'd like to change. If you do, consider the elements of a behavior change strategy. For example, begin a mental list of the pros and cons of the behavior, or talk to someone who can support you in your attempts to change.

IN THE FUTURE YOU CAN:
- Stay current on health- and wellness-related news and issues.
- Participate in health awareness and promotion campaigns in your community—for example, support smoking restrictions at local venues.
- Be a role model for (or at least be supportive of) someone else who is working on a health behavior you have successfully changed.

SUMMARY

- Wellness is the ability to live life fully, with vitality and meaning. Wellness is dynamic and multidimensional. It incorporates physical, emotional, intellectual, interpersonal, cultural, spiritual, environmental, financial, and occupational dimensions.

- As chronic diseases have become the leading cause of death in the United States, people have recognized that they have greater control over, and greater responsibility for, their health than ever before.

- The Healthy People initiative seeks to achieve a better quality of life for all Americans. The program's broad goals are to eliminate preventable disease, disabilities, injury, and premature death; achieve health equity for all groups; create social and physical environments that promote good health for all; and promote healthy development and healthy behaviors across every stage of life.

- Health-related differences among people that have implications for wellness can be described in the context of gender, ethnicity, income and education, disability, geographic location, and sexual orientation.

- Although heredity, environment, and health care all play roles in wellness and disease, behavior can mitigate their effects.

- To make lifestyle changes, you need information about yourself, your health habits, and resources available to help you change.

- You can increase your motivation for behavior change by examining the benefits and costs of change, boosting self-efficacy, and identifying and overcoming key barriers to change.

- The "stages of change" model describes six stages that people move through as they try to change their behavior: precontemplation, contemplation, preparation, action, maintenance, and termination.

- You can develop a specific plan for change by (1) monitoring your behavior by keeping a journal; (2) analyzing those data; (3) setting specific goals; (4) devising strategies for modifying the environment, rewarding yourself, and involving others; and (5) making a personal contract.

- To start and maintain a behavior change program you need commitment, a well-developed plan, social support, and a system of rewards.

- Although we cannot control every aspect of our health, we can make a difference in helping create an environment that supports wellness for everyone.

FOR MORE INFORMATION

BOOKS

Duhigg, C. 2012. *The Power of Habit: Why We Do What We Do in Life and Business.* New York: Random House. *An entertaining and intelligent exploration of how habits control our lives and how we can take charge of our habits to change our lives; includes both current research and a wealth of real-life stories.*

Komaroff, A. L., ed. 2005. *Harvard Medical School Family Health Guide*. New York: Free Press. *Provides consumer-oriented advice for the prevention and treatment of common health concerns.*

Litin, S. C., ed. 2009. *Mayo Clinic Family Health Book,* 4th ed. New York: HarperCollins. *A complete health reference for every stage of life, covering thousands of conditions, symptoms, and treatments.*

Murat, B., and G. Stewart. 2009. *Do I Need to See the Doctor? The Home-Treatment Encyclopedia—Written by Medical Doctors—That Lets You Decide,* 2nd ed. New York: Wiley. *Fully illustrated, easy-to-read guide to hundreds of common symptoms and ailments, designed to help consumers determine whether they can treat themselves or should seek professional medical attention.*

Prochaska, J. O., J. C. Norcross, and C. C. DiClemente. 1995. *Changing for Good: The Revolutionary Program That Explains the Six Stages of Change and Teaches You How to Free Yourself from Bad Habits*. New York: Morrow. *Outlines the authors' model of behavior change and offers suggestions and advice for each stage of change.*

NEWSLETTERS

Consumer Reports on Health (800-274-7596; http://www.consumerreports.org/health/home.htm)

Harvard Health Publications (877-649-9457; http://www.health.harvard.edu/newsletters/)

Mayo Clinic Health Letter (800-333-9037; http://healthletter.mayoclinic.com)

University of California, Berkeley, Wellness Letter (800-829-9170; http://www.wellnessletter.com)

ORGANIZATIONS, HOTLINES, AND WEBSITES

The Internet addresses listed here were accurate at the time of publication.

Centers for Disease Control and Prevention. Through phone, fax, and the Internet, the CDC provides a wide variety of health information.

http://www.cdc.gov

Federal Deposit Insurance Corporation. Money Smart—A Financial Education Program. "Money Smart for Young Adults" is a free source of information, unaffiliated with commercial interests, that includes eight modules on topics such as "borrowing basics" and "paying for college and cars."

http://www.fdic.gov/consumers/consumer/moneysmart/young. html

Federal Trade Commission: Consumer Protection—Health. Includes online brochures about a variety of consumer health topics, including fitness equipment, generic drugs, and fraudulent health claims.

http://www.ftc.gov/bcp/menus/consumer/health.shtm

Healthfinder. A gateway to online publications, websites, support and self-help groups, and agencies and organizations that produce reliable health information.

http://www.healthfinder.gov

Healthy People 2020. Provides information on Healthy People objectives and priority areas.

http://www.healthypeople.gov

MedlinePlus. Provides links to news and reliable information about health from government agencies and professional associations; also includes a health encyclopedia and information about prescription and over-the-counter drugs.

http://www.nlm.nih.gov/medlineplus/

National Health Information Center (NHIC). Puts consumers in touch with the organizations that are best able to provide answers to health-related questions.

http://www.health.gov/nhic/

National Institutes of Health. Provides information about all NIH activities as well as consumer publications, hotline information, and an A-to-Z listing of health issues with links to the appropriate NIH institute.

http://www.nih.gov

National Wellness Institute. Serves professionals and organizations that promote health and wellness.

http://www.nationalwellness.org

National Women's Health Information Center. Provides information and answers to frequently asked questions.

http://www.womenshealth.gov

Office of Minority Health. Promotes improved health among racial and ethnic minority populations.

http://minorityhealth.hhs.gov

Surgeon General. Includes information on activities of the Surgeon General and the text of many key reports on topics such as tobacco use, physical activity, and mental health.

http://www.surgeongeneral.gov

World Health Organization (WHO). Provides information about health topics and issues affecting people around the world.

http://www.who.int/en

SELECTED BIBLIOGRAPHY

American Cancer Society. 2014. *Cancer Facts and Figures—2014*. Atlanta: American Cancer Society.

American College Health Association. 2013. *American College Health Association—National College Health Assessment II: Reference Group Executive Summary Spring 2011*. Hanover, MD: American College Health Association.

American Heart Association. 2014. *Heart Disease and Stroke Statistics—2014 Update*. Dallas: American Heart Association.

Barr, D. A. 2008. *Health Disparities in the United States: Social Class, Race, Ethnicity, and Health*. Baltimore: The Johns Hopkins University Press.

Bennett, I. M., et al. 2009. The contribution of health literacy to disparities in self-rated health status and preventive health behaviors in older adults. *Annals of Family Medicine* 7(3): 204–211.

Centers for Disease Control and Prevention. 2008. Racial/ethnic disparities in self-rated health status among adults with and without disabilities—United States, 2004–2006. *Morbidity and Mortality Weekly Report* 57(39): 1069–1073.

Centers for Disease Control and Prevention. 2010. *Racial and Ethnic Approaches to Community Health (REACH U.S.): Finding Solutions to Health Disparities, 2010* (http://www.cdc.gov/chronicdisease/resources/publications/AAG/reach.htm).

Everett, B. G, et al. 2013. The nonlinear relationship between education and mortality: An examination of cohort, race/ethnic, and gender differences. *Population Research and Policy Review* 32(6).

Fisher, E. G., et al. 2011. Behavior matters. *American Journal of Preventive Medicine* 40(5): e15–30.

Flegal, K. M., et al. 2010. Prevalence and trends in obesity among U.S. adults, 1999–2008. *Journal of the American Medical Association* 303(3): 235–241.

Herd, P., et al. 2007. Socioeconomic position and health: The differential effects of education versus income on the onset versus progression of health problems. *Journal of Health and Social Behavior* 48(3): 223–238.

Horneffer-Ginter, K. 2008. Stages of change and possible selves: Two tools for promoting college health. *Journal of American College Health* 56(4): 351–358.

KFF. (October 2013) Kaiser Health Tracking Poll, unpublished estimates.

Kohl, H. K., et al. 2011. Healthy people: A 2020 vision for the social determinants approach. *Health Education & Behavior* 38(6): 551–557.

National Center for Health Statistics. 2010. Health behaviors of adults: United States, 2005–07. *Vital and Health Statistics* 10(245).

National Center for Health Statistics. 2011. *Health, United States, 2012. With Special Feature on Socioeconomic Status and Health*. Hyattsville, MD: National Center for Health Statistics.

National Center for Health Statistics. 2012. Deaths: preliminary data for 2011. *National Vital Statistics Report* 61(6).

O'Loughlin, J., et al. 2007. Lifestyle risk factors for chronic disease across family origin among adults in multiethnic, low-income, urban neighborhoods. *Ethnicity and Disease* 17(4): 657–663.

Persky, Susan, et al. 2013. The role of weight, race, and health care experiences in care use among young men and women. *Obesity* 10.1002/oby.20677. [Epub ahead of print]

Pinkhasov, R. M., et al. 2010. Are men shortchanged on health? Perspective on health care utilization and health risk behavior in men and women in the United States. *International Journal of Clinical Practice* 64(4): 475–487.

Printz, C. 2012. Disparities in cancer care: Are we making progress? A look at how researchers and organizations are working to reduce cancer health disparities. *Cancer* 118(4): 867–868.

Rotimi, C. N. 2012. Health disparities in the genomic era: The case for diversifying ethnic representation. *Genomic Medicine* 4(8): 65.

UC Berkeley. 2011 Update. *Evaluating Web Pages: Techniques to Apply and Questions to Ask* (http://www.lib.berkeley.edu/TeachingLib/Guides/Internet/Evaluate.html).

Vaccaro, J. A., and F. G. Huffman. 2012. Reducing health disparities: Medical advice received for minorities with diabetes. *Journal of Health and Human Services Administration* 34(4): 389-417.

Walker, B., and C. P. Mouton. 2008. Environmental influences on cardiovascular health. *Journal of the National Medical Association* 100(1): 98–102.

Williams, D. R. 2012. Miles to go before we sleep: Racial inequities in health. *Journal of Health and Social Behavior* 53(3): 279–295.

Wojno, Marc A. 2013. 12 Things College Students Don't Need. *Kiplinger*, August 29, 2013.

1. I, _____, agree to _____

_____

2. I will begin on _____ and plan to reach my goal of _____

_____ by _____

3. To reach my final goal, I have devised the following schedule of mini-goals. For each step in my program, I will give myself the reward listed.

_____   _____   _____

_____

_____   _____   _____

_____

_____   _____   _____

_____

My overall reward for reaching my goal will be _____

4. I have gathered and analyzed data on my target behavior and have identified the following strategies for changing my behavior:

_____

_____

5. I will use the following tools to monitor my progress toward my final goal: _____

_____

_____

I sign this contract as an indication of my personal commitment to reach my goal: _____

_____

I have recruited a helper who will witness my contract and _____

_____

_____

CHAPTER OBJECTIVES

- Explain what stress is and how people react to it—physically, emotionally, and behaviorally
- Describe the relationship between stress and disease
- List common sources of stress
- Describe techniques for preventing and managing stress
- Put together a plan for successfully managing the stress in your life

Stress: The Constant Challenge

Like the term *wellness, stress* is a word many people use without understanding its precise meaning. Stress is popularly viewed as an uncomfortable response to a negative event, which probably describes *nervous tension* more than the cluster of physical and psychological responses that actually constitutes stress. In fact, stress is not limited to negative situations; it is also a response to pleasurable physical challenges and the achievement of personal goals.

Whether stress is experienced as pleasant or unpleasant depends largely on the situation and the individual. Learning effective responses to stress can enhance psychological health and help prevent a number of serious diseases, and stress management can be an important part of daily life.

---

stressor   Any physical or psychological event or condition that produces physical and emotional reactions.

stress response   The physical and emotional reactions to a stressor.

stress   The general physical and emotional state that the stressor produces.

TERMS

As a college student, you may be in one of the most stressful times of your life. This chapter explains the physiological and psychological reactions that make up the stress response and describes how these reactions can put your health at risk. The chapter also presents methods of managing stress.

WHAT IS STRESS?

In common usage, the term *stress* refers to two different things: situations that trigger physical and emotional reactions (e.g., "That relationship is way too much stress"), *and* the reactions themselves (e.g., "I feel a lot of stress every time I walk into that classroom"). This text uses the more precise term **stressor** for a physical or psychological event that triggers physical and emotional reactions and the term **stress response** for the reactions themselves. A first date and a final exam are examples of stressors; sweaty palms and a pounding heart are symptoms of the stress response. We'll use the term **stress** to describe the general physical and emotional state that accompanies the stress response.

Each individual's experience of stress depends on many factors, including the nature of the stressor and how it is perceived. Stressors take many different forms. Like a fire in your home, some occur suddenly and neither last long nor repeat. Others, like air pollution or quarreling parents, can continue for a long time. The memory of a stressful occurrence can itself be a stressor years after the event, such as the memory of the loss of a loved one. Responses to stressors can include a wide variety of physical, emotional, and behavioral changes. A short-term response might be an upset stomach or insomnia, whereas a long-term response might be a change in your personality or social relations.

Physical Responses to Stressors

Imagine a close call: As you step off the curb, a car careens toward you. With just a fraction of a second to spare, you leap safely out of harm's way. In that split second of danger and in the moments following it, you experience a predictable series of physical reactions. Your body goes from a relaxed state to one prepared for physical action to cope with a threat to your life.

Two systems in your body are responsible for your physical response to stressors: the nervous system and the endocrine system. Through rapid chemical reactions affecting almost every part of your body, you are primed to act quickly and appropriately in time of danger.

The Nervous System   The **nervous system** consists of the brain, spinal cord, and nerves. Part of the nervous system is under voluntary control, as when you tell your arm to reach for a chocolate. The part that is *not* under conscious supervision—for example, the part that controls the digestion of the chocolate—is the **autonomic nervous system.** In addition to digestion, it controls your heart rate, breathing, blood pressure, and hundreds of other involuntary functions.

The autonomic nervous system consists of two divisions:

- The **parasympathetic division** is in control when you are relaxed. It aids in digesting food, storing energy, and promoting growth.
- The **sympathetic division** is activated when your body is stimulated, for example, by exercise, and when there is an emergency, such as severe pain, anger, or fear.

Sympathetic nerves affect nearly every organ, sweat gland, blood vessel, and muscle in order to enable your body to best handle an emergency.

Actions of the Nervous and Endocrine Systems Together   During stress, the sympathetic nervous system triggers the **endocrine system.** This system of glands, tissues, and cells helps control body functions by releasing **hormones** and other chemical messengers into the bloodstream to influence metabolism and other body processes. The nervous system handles very short-term stress, whereas the endocrine system deals with both short-term (*acute*) or long-term (*chronic*) stress. How do both systems work together in an emergency?

Higher cognitive areas in your brain decide that you are facing a threat. The nervous and endocrine systems activate adrenal glands, which are located near the top of the kidneys. These glands release hormones **cortisol** and **epinephrine** (also called adrenaline). These hormones then trigger the physiological changes shown in Figure 2.1, including the following:

- Heart and respiration rates accelerate to speed oxygen through the body.
- Hearing and vision become more acute.
- The liver releases extra sugar into the bloodstream to boost energy.
- Perspiration increases to cool the skin.
- The brain releases **endorphins**—chemicals that can inhibit or block sensations of pain—in case you are injured.

As a group, these nearly instantaneous physiological changes are called the **fight-or-flight reaction.** These changes give you the heightened reflexes and strength you need to dodge a car or deal with other stressors. Although these physiological changes may vary in intensity, the same basic set of physiological reactions occurs in response to any type of stressor—positive or negative, physiological or psychological.

The Return to Homeostasis   Once a stressful situation ends, the parasympathetic division of your autonomic nervous system takes command and halts the stress response.

TERMS

nervous system   The brain, spinal cord, and nerves.

autonomic nervous system   The part of the nervous system that controls certain basic body processes; consists of the sympathetic and parasympathetic divisions.

parasympathetic division   The part of the autonomic nervous system that moderates the excitatory effect of the sympathetic division, slowing metabolism and restoring energy supplies.

sympathetic division   Division of the autonomic nervous system that reacts to danger or other challenges by accelerating body processes.

endocrine system   The system of glands, tissues, and cells that secrete hormones into the bloodstream to influence metabolism and other body processes.

hormone   A chemical messenger produced in the body and transported in the bloodstream to target cells or organs for specific regulation of their activities.

cortisol   A steroid hormone secreted by the cortex (outer layer) of the adrenal gland; also called *hydrocortisone*.

epinephrine   A hormone secreted by the medulla (inner core) of the adrenal gland that affects the functioning of organs involved in responding to a stressor; also called *adrenaline*.

endorphins   Brain secretions that have pain-inhibiting effects.

fight-or-flight reaction   A defense reaction that prepares a person for conflict or escape by triggering hormonal, cardiovascular, metabolic, and other changes.

Pupils dilate to admit extra light for more sensitive vision.

Mucous membranes of nose and throat shrink, while muscles force a wider opening of air passages to allow easier airflow.

Secretion of saliva and mucus decreases; digestive activities have a low priority in an emergency.

Air passages dilate to allow more air into lungs.

Perspiration increases, especially in armpits, groin, hands, and feet, to flush out waste and cool the overheating body by evaporation.

Liver releases sugar into bloodstream to provide energy for muscles and brain.

Muscles of intestines stop contracting because digestion has halted.

Bladder relaxes. Emptying of bladder contents releases excess weight, making it easier to flee.

Blood vessels in skin and internal organs contract; those in skeletal muscles dilate. This increases blood pressure and delivery of blood to where it is most needed.

Endorphins are released to block any distracting pain.

Hearing becomes more acute.

Heart accelerates rate of beating. Strength of contraction increases to allow more blood flow where it is needed.

Digestion halts.

Spleen releases more red blood cells to meet an increased demand for oxygen and to replace any blood lost from injuries.

Adrenal glands stimulate secretion of epinephrine, increasing blood sugar, blood pressure, and heart rate; also spur increase in amount of fat in blood. These changes provide an energy boost.

Pancreas decreases secretions because digestion has halted.

Fat is removed from storage and broken down to supply extra energy.

Voluntary (skeletal) muscles contract throughout the body, readying them for action.

FIGURE 2.1 **The fight-or-flight reaction.** In response to a stressor, the autonomic nervous system and the endocrine system prepare the body to deal with an emergency.

It restores **homeostasis,** a state in which blood pressure, heart rate, hormone levels, and other vital functions are maintained within a narrow range of normal. Your parasympathetic nervous system calms your body down, slowing a rapid heartbeat, drying sweaty palms, and returning breathing to normal. Gradually your body resumes its normal "housekeeping" functions, such as digestion and temperature regulation. Damage that may have been sustained during the fight-or-flight reaction is repaired. The day after you narrowly dodge the car, you wake up feeling fine. In this way, your body can grow, repair itself, and acquire new reserves of energy. When the next crisis comes, you'll be ready to respond again instantly.

The Fight-or-Flight Reaction in Modern Life The fight-or-flight reaction is part of our biological heritage, and it's a survival mechanism that has served humans well. In modern life, however, it is often absurdly inappropriate. Many of the stressors we face in everyday life do not require a physical response—for example, an exam, a mess left by a roommate, or a stoplight. The fight-or-flight reaction prepares the body for physical action regardless of whether a particular stressor necessitates such a response.

Emotional and Behavioral Responses to Stressors

We all experience a similar set of physical responses to stressors, which makes up the fight-or-flight reaction. These responses, however, vary from person to person and from one situation to another. People's perceptions of potential stressors—and of

homeostasis A state of stability and consistency in an individual's physiological functioning. TERMS their reactions to such stressors—also vary greatly. A certain amount of stress, if coped with appropriately, can help promote optimal performance. (Figure 2.2).

Effective and Ineffective Responses

Common emotional responses to stressors include anxiety, depression, and fear. Although emotional responses are determined in part by inborn personality or temperament, we often can moderate or learn to control them. Coping techniques are discussed later in the chapter.

Behavioral responses to stressors—controlled by the **somatic nervous system,** which manages our conscious actions—are entirely under our control. Effective behavioral responses such as talking, laughing, exercising, meditating, learning time management skills, and becoming more assertive can promote wellness and enable us to function at our best. Ineffective behavioral responses to stressors include overeating, expressing hostility, and using tobacco, alcohol, or other drugs.

Personality and Stress
Some people seem to be nervous, irritable, and easily upset by minor annoyances. Others are calm and composed even in difficult situations. Scientists remain unsure just why this is or how the brain's complex emotional mechanisms work. But **personality**—the sum of cognitive, behavioral, and emotional tendencies—clearly affects how people perceive and react to stressors. To investigate the links among personality, stress, and wellness, researchers examine different clusters of characteristics, or "personality types":

- *Type A.* People with Type A personality are overcompetitive, controlling, impatient, and aggressive. Type A people have a higher perceived stress level and more problems coping with stress. They react explosively to stressors and

are upset by events that others would consider only annoyances. Studies indicate that certain characteristics of the Type A pattern—anger, cynicism, and hostility—increase the risk of heart disease.

- *Type B.* The Type B personality is relaxed and contemplative. Type B people are less frustrated by daily events and more tolerant of the behavior of others. They are sometimes described as slow and indecisive.

- *Type C.* The Type C personality is characterized by anger suppression, difficulty expressing emotions, feelings of hopelessness and despair, and an exaggerated response to minor stressors.

- *Type D.* The Type D personality tends toward negative emotional states such as anxiety, depression, and irritability. Type D people also avoid social interactions, worrying that others will react negatively toward them. Having this kind of personality predicts a number of poor health outcomes, including cardiovascular disease.

Depending on the situation, most of us display some of the behaviors characteristic of one or more of the types described.

Researchers have also looked for personality traits that enable people to deal more successfully with stress. One such trait is *hardiness,* a particular form of optimism. People with a hardy personality view potential stressors as challenges and opportunities for growth and learning, rather than as burdens. They see fewer situations as stressful and react less intensely to stress than nonhardy people might. Hardy people are committed to their activities, have a sense of inner purpose and an inner locus of control, and feel at least partly in control of their lives.

The term *resilience* refers to personality traits associated with social and academic success in groups at risk for stress, such as people from low-income families and those with mental or physical disabilities. Resilient people tend to set goals and face adversity through individual effort. There are three basic types of resilience, and each one determines how a person responds to stress:

- *Nonreactive resilience,* in which a person does not react to a stressor
- *Homeostatic resilience,* in which a person may react strongly but returns to baseline functioning quickly
- *Positive growth resilience,* in which a person learns and grows from the stress experience

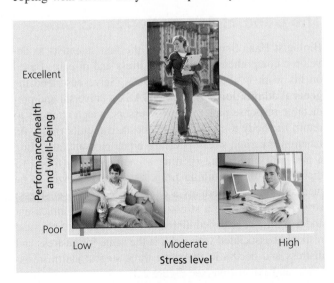

FIGURE 2.2 **Stress level, performance, and well-being.** A moderate level of stress challenges individuals in a way that promotes optimal performance and well-being. Too little stress, and people are not challenged enough to improve; too much stress, and the challenges become stressors that can impair physical and emotional health.

somatic nervous system The branch of the peripheral nervous system that governs motor functions and sensory information, largely under conscious control.

personality The sum of behavioral, cognitive, and emotional tendencies.

TERMS

A person's emotional and behavioral responses to stressors depend on many different factors, including personality, gender, and cultural background. For example, research suggests that women are more likely than men to respond to stressors by seeking social support.

Resilience is associated with emotional intelligence and violence prevention.

You probably can't change your basic personality, but you can change your typical behaviors and patterns of thinking. You can also use positive stress management techniques like those described later in the chapter.

Cultural Background   Young adults from around the world come to the United States for a higher education; most students finish college with a greater appreciation for other cultures and worldviews. The clash of cultures, however, can be a big source of stress for many students—especially when it leads to disrespectful treatment, harassment, or violence. It is important to remember that everyone's reaction to stress is influenced by his or her family and cultural background. Learning to accept and appreciate the cultural backgrounds of other people is both a mind-opening experience and a way to avoid stress over cultural differences.

Gender   Our **gender role**—the activities, abilities, and behaviors our culture expects of us based on our sex—can affect our experience of stress. Some behavioral responses to stressors, such as crying or openly expressing anger, may be deemed more appropriate for one gender than another.

TERMS

gender role   A culturally expected pattern of behavior and attitudes determined by a person's sex.

general adaptation syndrome (GAS)
A pattern of stress responses consisting of three stages: alarm, resistance, and exhaustion.

eustress   Stress resulting from a stressor perceived to be pleasant.

distress   Stress resulting from a stressor perceived to be unpleasant.

Strict adherence to gender roles, however, can limit one's response to stress and can itself become a source of stress. Gender roles can also affect one's perception of a stressor. If a man derives most of his self-worth from his work, for example, retirement may be more stressful for him than for a woman whose self-image is based on several different roles.

Since the American Psychological Association began its yearly "Stress in America" survey in 2007, women have reported a higher level of stress than men. In 2013, women rated their stress level 5.5 on a scale of 1–10, and men averaged 4.8. Women generally reported a significantly higher level of stress than men. The survey also shows that women are more likely than men to try to reduce their stress, although a lower percentage say they were successful than the percent of men who tried to reduce theirs. The women tried to cope with stress more often through behaviors such as reading, spending time with friends, or meditating, in contrast to men, who preferred playing sports.

Experience   Past experiences can profoundly influence the evaluation of a potential stressor. Consider someone who has had a bad experience giving a speech in the past. He or she is much more likely to perceive an upcoming speech as stressful than someone who has had positive public speaking experiences.

STRESS AND HEALTH

According to the American Psychological Association, 76% of the general population report suffering physical symptoms related to stress (such as tense muscles or headaches), and 71% report nonphysical symptoms. The role of stress in health is complex, but evidence suggests that stress can increase vulnerability to many ailments. Several theories have been proposed to explain the relationship between stress and disease.

The General Adaptation Syndrome

Biologist Hans Selye was one of the first scientists to develop a comprehensive theory of stress and disease. Based on his work in the 1930s and 1940s, Selye described the **general adaptation syndrome (GAS),** a universal and predictable response pattern to all stressors, which attempts to return the body to a state of homeostasis (equilibrium). As mentioned earlier, stressors can be either pleasant (attending a party) or unpleasant (getting a bad grade). In the GAS theory, the stress resulting from a stressor perceived to be pleasant although perhaps a challenge is called **eustress;** stress brought on by a stressor perceived to be unpleasant and a hindrance is called **distress.** The sequence of physical responses associated with GAS is the same for eustress and distress and occurs in the same three stages: alarm, resistance, and exhaustion (see Figure 2.3).

•   *Alarm.* The body initially experiences a stressor in a *shock phase.* This is followed by an *antishock phase,* which includes the complex sequence of events brought on by the fight-or-flight response. In these two phases that comprise the

FIGURE 2.3 **The general adaptation syndrome.** During the alarm phase, a lower resistance to injury is evident. With continued stress, resistance to injury is actually enhanced. With prolonged exposure to repeated stressors, exhaustion sets in, with a return of low resistance levels seen during acute stress.

alarm stage, the body is more susceptible to disease or injury because it is using resources and energy to deal with a crisis. Someone in this stage may experience headaches, indigestion, anxiety, and disrupted eating or sleep patterns.

- *Resistance.* Under continued stress, the body develops a new level of homeostasis in which it is more resistant to disease and injury than usual. In this stage, a person can cope with normal life and added stress. However, the body cannot keep this up indefinitely. At some point, the body's resources will become depleted.

- *Exhaustion.* The first two stages of GAS require a great deal of energy. If a stressor persists, or if several stressors occur in succession, general exhaustion sets in. This is not the sort of exhaustion you feel after a long, busy day. Rather, it's a life-threatening type of physiological exhaustion. The body's resources are depleted and the body is unable to maintain normal function. If stage three is extended, long-term damage may result as the body's immune system deteriorates and bodily functions start to break down. The result can manifest itself in illness, ulcers, digestive system trouble, depression, diabetes, cardiovascular problems, and mental illnesses.

Allostatic Load

Although the GAS model is still viewed as a key conceptual contribution to the understanding of stress, some aspects of it are considered outdated. For example, increased susceptibility to disease after repeated or prolonged stress is now thought to be due to the effects of the stress response itself rather than to a depletion of resources (exhaustion state). In particular, long-term overexposure to stress hormones such as cortisol has been linked with health problems. Further, although physical stress reactions promote homeostasis (resistance stage), they also have negative effects on the body. This "wear and tear" on the body that results from long-term exposure to repeated or chronic stress is known as **allostatic load.** The concept of allostatic load helps to explain how frequent activation of the body's stress response, although essential for managing acute threats, can in fact damage the body in the long run. Allostatic

QUICK STATS

45% of American adults have at least one chronic illness.
—Pew Research Center, 2013

Ask Yourself ?

QUESTIONS FOR CRITICAL THINKING
AND REFLECTION

Think of the last time you faced a significant stressor. How did you respond? List the physical, emotional, and behavioral reactions you experienced. Did these responses help you deal with the stress, or did they interfere with your efforts to handle it?

load is generally measured through indicators of cumulative strain on several organs and tissues, but especially on the cardiovascular system.

Psychoneuroimmunology

One of the most fruitful areas of current research into the relationship between stress and disease is **psychoneuroimmunology (PNI).** PNI is the study of the interactions among the nervous system, the endocrine system, and the immune system. The underlying premise of PNI is that stress, through the actions of the nervous and endocrine systems, impairs the immune system and thereby affects health.

A complex network of nerve and chemical connections exists among the nervous and the endocrine systems. In general, increased levels of cortisol are linked to a decreased number of immune system cells, or *lymphocytes.* Epinephrine appears to promote the release of lymphocytes but at the same time reduces their efficiency. Scientists have identified hormone-like substances called *neuropeptides* that appear to translate stressful emotions into biochemical events, some of which impact the immune system, providing a physical link between emotions and immune function.

Different types of stress may affect immunity in different ways. For instance, during **acute stress** (typically lasting between 5 and 100 minutes), white blood cells move into the skin, where they enhance the immune response. During a stressful event sequence, such as a personal trauma and the events that follow, however, there are typically no overall significant immune changes. Chronic (ongoing) stressors such as unemployment have negative effects on almost all

TERMS

allostatic load The "wear and tear" on the body that results from long-term exposure to repeated or chronic stress.

psychoneuroimmunology (PNI) The study of the interactions among the nervous, endocrine, and immune systems.

acute stress Stress immediately following a stressor; may last only minutes or may turn into chronic stress.

functional measures of immunity. **Chronic stress** may cause prolonged secretion of cortisol and may accelerate the course of diseases that involve inflammation, including multiple sclerosis, heart disease, type 2 diabetes, and clinical depression.

Mood, personality, behavior, and immune functioning are intertwined. For example, people who are generally pessimistic may neglect the basics of health care, become passive when ill, and fail to engage in health-promoting behaviors. People who are depressed may reduce physical activity and social interaction, which may in turn affect the immune system and the cognitive appraisal of a stressor. Optimism, successful coping, and positive problem solving, on the other hand, may positively influence immunity.

Although much remains to be learned, it is clear that people who have unresolved chronic stress in their lives or who handle stressors poorly are at risk for a wide range of health problems. In the short term, the problem might be just a cold, a stiff neck, or a stomachache. Over the long term, the problems can be more severe—cardiovascular disease (CVD), high blood pressure, impaired immune function, or a host of other problems.

Cardiovascular Disease

During the stress response, heart rate increases and blood vessels constrict, causing blood pressure to rise. Chronic high blood pressure is a major cause of *atherosclerosis,* a disease in which blood vessels become damaged and caked with fatty deposits. These deposits can block arteries, causing heart attacks and strokes. The stress response can precipitate a heart attack in someone with atherosclerosis. The stress response can also cause stress cardiomyopathy ("broken heart syndrome"), a condition that mimics a heart attack but doesn't block the blood vessels supplying the heart.

Certain emotional responses may increase a person's risk of CVD. As described earlier, people who tend to react to situations with anger and hostility are more likely to have heart attacks than are people with less explosive, more trusting personalities.

Stress has also been linked to other risk factors for CVD, including elevated cholesterol. Inflammation is a key component of the damage to blood vessels that leads to heart attacks. Stress increases inflammation throughout the body. When this happens, messenger molecules are also linked to elevated levels of homocysteine and C-reactive protein (CRP), two compounds that appear to be markers for CVD risk. Stress-related depression and anger are associated with elevated homocysteine levels, and job-related exhaustion is

linked to high CRP levels in some people. Elevated CRP levels have also been implicated in insulin resistance and the development of diabetes, which is in turn a risk factor for CVD. Clearly, stress reduction can improve cardiovascular health. See Chapter 12 for more.

Psychological Problems

Many stressors are inherently anxiety-producing, depressing, or both. Stress has been found to contribute to psychological problems such as depression, panic attacks, anxiety, eating disorders, and posttraumatic stress disorder (PTSD). PTSD, which afflicts war veterans, rape and child abuse survivors, and others who have suffered or witnessed severe trauma, is characterized by nightmares, flashbacks, and a diminished capacity to experience or express emotion. (For information about psychological health, see Chapter 3.)

Altered Immune Function

PNI research helps explain how stress affects the immune system. Some of the health problems linked to stress-related changes in immune function include vulnerability to colds and other infections, asthma and allergy attacks, and flare-ups of chronic diseases such as genital herpes and HIV infection.

Headaches

More than 45 million Americans suffer from chronic, recurrent headaches. Headaches come in various types but are often grouped into the following three categories:

- *Tension headaches.* Approximately 90% of all headaches are tension headaches, characterized by a dull, steady pain, usually on both sides of the head. It may feel as though a band of pressure is tightening around the head, and the pain may extend to the neck and shoulders. Acute tension headaches may last from hours to days, whereas chronic tension headaches may occur almost every day for months or even years. Psychological stress, poor posture, and immobility are the leading causes of tension headaches. There is no cure, but the pain can sometimes be relieved with over-the-counter painkillers and with therapies such as massage, acupuncture, relaxation, hot or cold showers, and rest.

Ask Yourself

QUESTIONS FOR CRITICAL THINKING AND REFLECTION

Have you ever been so stressed that you felt ill in some way? If so, what were your symptoms? How did you handle them? Did the experience affect the way you reacted to other stressful events?

chronic stress Stress that continues for days, weeks, or longer.   TERMS

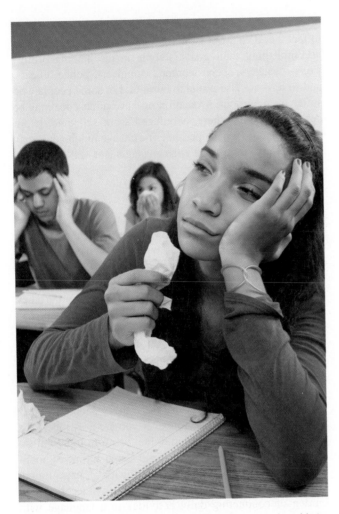

Ongoing stress has been shown to make people more vulnerable to everyday ailments, such as colds and allergies.

- *Migraine headaches.* Migraines typically progress through a series of stages lasting from several minutes to several days. They may produce a variety of symptoms, including throbbing pain that starts on one side of the head and may spread; heightened sensitivity to light; visual disturbances such as flashing lights or temporary blindness; nausea; dizziness; and fatigue. About 70% of migraine sufferers are women. Potential triggers include menstruation, stress, fatigue, atmospheric changes, bright light, specific sounds or odors, and certain foods. The frequency of attacks varies from a few in a lifetime to several per week. Treatment can help reduce the frequency, severity, and duration of migraines. Aerobic exercise is frequently recommended as a treatment for migraine headaches. However, the evidence for the efficacy of exercise to reduce the frequency and severity of migraine headaches is mixed. There is mild evidence that exercise may reduce stress levels, a known trigger for migraine headaches. Researchers have not been able to replicate these findings consistently, however. Several studies have failed to show exercise as an effective treatment for migraine headaches. And for some, exercise itself can trigger migraines.

- *Cluster headaches.* Cluster headaches are extremely severe headaches that cause intense pain in and around one eye. They usually occur in clusters of one to three headaches each day over a period of weeks or months, alternating with periods of remission in which no headaches occur. About 90% of people with cluster headaches are male. There is no known cause or cure for cluster headaches, but a number of treatments are available. During cluster periods, it is important to refrain from smoking cigarettes and drinking alcohol, because these activities can trigger attacks.

Other Health Problems Many other health problems may be caused or worsened by excessive stress, including the following:

- Digestive problems such as stomachaches, diarrhea, constipation, irritable bowel syndrome, and ulcers
- Insomnia and fatigue
- Injuries, including on-the-job injuries caused by repetitive strain
- Menstrual irregularities, impotence, and pregnancy complications

COMMON SOURCES OF STRESS

Recognizing potential sources of stress is an important step in successfully managing the stress in your life.

Major Life Changes

Any major change in your life that requires adjustment and accommodation can be a source of stress. Early adulthood and the college years are associated with many significant changes, such as moving out of the family home. Even changes typically thought of as positive—graduation, job promotion, marriage—can be stressful.

Clusters of life changes, particularly those that are perceived negatively, may be linked to health problems in some people. Personality and coping skills, however, are important moderating influences. People with strong support networks and stress-resistant personalities are less likely to become ill in response to life changes than are people with fewer resources.

Daily Hassles

Although major life changes are stressful, they seldom occur regularly. Researchers have proposed that minor problems—life's daily hassles, such as losing your keys or wallet—can be an even greater source of stress because they occur much more often.

People who perceive hassles negatively are likely to experience a moderate stress response every time they face one. Over time, this can take a significant toll on health. Studies indicate that, for some people, daily hassles contribute to a general decrease in overall wellness.

College Stressors

College is a time of major changes and minor hassles. For many students, college means being away from home and family for the first time. Nearly all students share stresses like the following:

- *Academic stress.* Exams, grades, and an endless workload await every college student but can be especially troublesome for students just out of high school. To learn some proven techniques for overcoming test anxiety, see the Behavior Change Strategy box at the end of this chapter.

- *Interpersonal stress.* Most students are more than just students; they are also friends, children, employees, spouses, parents, and so on. Managing relationships while juggling the rigors of college life can be daunting, especially if some friends or family members are less than supportive.

- *Time pressures.* Class schedules, assignments, and deadlines are an inescapable part of college life. But these time pressures can be drastically compounded for students who also have job or family responsibilities.

- *Financial concerns.* The majority of college students need financial aid not just to cover the cost of tuition but also to survive from day to day while in school. For many, college life isn't possible without a job, and the pressure to stay afloat financially competes with academic and other stressors.

- *Worries about the future.* As college comes to an end, students face the next set of decisions. This decision making means thinking about a career, choosing a place to live, and leaving the friends and routines of school behind. Students may find it helpful to go to the campus career center, where they can talk to counselors and read guides like *What Color Is My Parachute?*, by Richard N. Bolles, now in its 40th edition.

Job-Related Stressors

Americans rate their jobs as a key source of stress in their lives. Various surveys indicate that 40–50% of working Americans say they typically feel tense or stressed out while at work. Tight schedules and overtime leave less time to exercise, socialize, and engage in other stress-proofing activities. Although daily work activities can be stressful enough on their own, stress can be even worse for people who are left out of important decisions relating to their jobs. When workers are given the opportunity to shape how their jobs are performed, job satisfaction goes up and stress levels go down.

If job-related (or college-related) stress is severe or chronic, the result can be **burnout**—a state of physical, mental, and emotional exhaustion. Burnout occurs most often in highly motivated and driven individuals who come to feel that their work is not recognized or that they are not accomplishing their goals. People in the helping professions—teachers, social workers, caregivers, police officers, and so on—are also prone to burnout. For some people who suffer from burnout, a vacation or leave of absence may be appropriate. For others, a reduced work schedule, better communication with superiors, or a change in job goals may be necessary. Improving time management skills can also help.

Social Stressors

Social networks can be real or virtual. Both types can help improve your ability to deal with stress, but any social network can also become a stressor in itself.

Real Social Networks   Although social support is a key buffer against stress, your interactions with others can themselves be a source of stress. The college years, in particular, can be a time of great change in interpersonal relationships. The larger community where you live can also act as a stressor.

Social stressors include prejudice and discrimination. You may feel stress as you try to relate to people of other ethnic or socioeconomic groups. If you are a member of a minority ethnic group, you may feel pressure to assimilate into mainstream society, or to spend as much time as possible with others who share your ethnicity or background. If English is not your first language, you may face the added burden of conducting daily activities in a language with which you are not comfortable. All these pressures can become significant sources of stress. (See the box "Diverse Populations, Discrimination, and Stress.")

Virtual Social Networks   Technology can help you save time, but it can also increase stress. Being electronically connected to work, family, and friends all the time can impinge on your personal space, waste time, and distract you from your current real situation. If you are "always on"—that is, always available by voice or text messaging—some friends or colleagues may think it's all right to contact you anytime, even if you're in class or trying to work, and they may expect an immediate response. The convenience of staying electronically connected comes at a price.

Other Stressors

Have you tried to eat at a restaurant where the food was great, but the atmosphere was so noisy that it put you on edge? This is an example of an environmental stressor—a condition or event in the physical environment that causes stress.

Like the noisy atmosphere of some restaurants, many environmental stressors are mere inconveniences that are easy to avoid. Others, such as pollen or construction noise, may be unavoidable daily sources of stress. For those who live in poor or violent neighborhoods or in a war-torn country, the

---

burnout   A state of physical, mental, and emotional exhaustion.

TERMS

Stress is universal, but an individual's response to stress can vary depending on gender, cultural background, prior experience, and genetic factors. In diverse multiethnic and multicultural nations such as the United States, some groups face special stressors and have higher-than-average rates of stress-related physical and emotional problems. These groups include ethnic minorities, the poor, those with physical or mental disabilities, and those with atypical sexual orientations.

Discrimination occurs when people speak or act according to their prejudices—biased, negative beliefs or attitudes toward some group. A blatant example is painting a swastika on a Jewish studies house. A more subtle example is when an African American student notices that white shopkeepers in a mostly white college town tend to keep a close eye on him.

Recent immigrants to the United States have to learn to live in a new society. Doing so requires a balance between assimilating and changing to be like the majority, and maintaining a connection to their own culture, language, and religion. The process of acculturation is generally stressful, especially when the person's background is radically different from that of the people he or she is now living among.

Both immigrants and minorities that have lived for generations in the United States can face job- and school-related stressors because of stereotypes and discrimination. They may make less money in comparable jobs with comparable levels of education and may find it more difficult to achieve leadership positions.

On a positive note, however, many who experience hardship, disability, or prejudice develop effective goal-directed coping skills and are successful at overcoming obstacles and managing the stress they face.

connect
ACTIVITY
DO IT ONLINE

environment can contain major stressors (see the box "Coping with News of Traumatic Events").

Some stressors are found not in our environment but within ourselves. We pressure ourselves to reach goals and continually evaluate our progress and performance. Striving to reach goals can enhance self-esteem if the goals are reasonable. Unrealistic expectations, however, can be a significant source of stress and can damage self-esteem. Other internal stressors are physical and emotional states such as illness and exhaustion; these can be both a cause and an effect of unmanaged stress.

MANAGING STRESS

You can control the stress in your life by taking the following steps:

- Shore up your support system.
- Improve your communication skills.
- Develop healthy exercise, eating, and sleeping habits.
- Learn to identify and moderate individual stressors.

The effort required is well worth the time. People who manage stress effectively not only are healthier but have more time to enjoy life and accomplish goals.

Social Support

Having the support of friends and family members seems to contribute to the well-being of body and mind. Research supports this conclusion, as the following examples demonstrate:

- Among college students living in overcrowded apartments, a study revealed that those students with a strong social support system were less distressed by their cramped quarters than were the loners who navigated life's challenges on their own.

- Young adults who have strong relationships with their parents tend to cope with stress better than peers with poor parental relationships.

Coping with News of Traumatic Events

We are continually exposed to news of tragic events. Natural disasters, war, terrorism, and poverty are all catastrophic events that we seem to hear about daily. Both experiencing trauma and observing it can result in extreme stress, requiring time and effort to recover. Such events can weaken your sense of security and create uncertainty about how the future may unfold. People react to such news in different ways, depending on their proximity to the event and its recency. People far from the site may suffer emotional reactions simply from watching endless coverage on television.

Responses to trauma include disbelief, shock, fear, anger, resentment, anxiety, mood swings, irritability, sadness, depression, panic, guilt, apathy, feelings of isolation or powerlessness, and many of the symptoms of excess stress. Some people affected by such violence develop posttraumatic stress disorder (PTSD), a more serious condition.

In the case of the 2007 shooting rampage at Virginia Polytechnic Institute and State University (Virginia Tech) that left 32 students and teachers dead, the school and community mobilized quickly to respond to the expected surge in behavioral health needs generated by the attack. Hotline calls and emergency room visits increased dramatically, especially during the second and third weeks following the shootings. Information sources and support groups were established for people grieving the loss of friends, family, neighbors, or colleagues. Volunteers contacted each family that was directly affected by the shootings to offer help in making arrangements and to provide other services.

If you are affected by a disastrous event such as a school shooting or terrorist attack, take these steps:

- Be sure you have the best information about what happened, whether a continuing risk is present, and what you can do to avoid it. That information may be posted on websites or on local radio or TV stations.

- Don't expose yourself to so much media coverage that it overwhelms you.

- Take care of yourself. Use the stress relief techniques discussed in this chapter.

- Share your feelings and concerns with others. Be a supportive listener.

- If you feel able, help others in any way you can, such as by volunteering to work with victims.

- If you feel emotionally distressed days or weeks after the event, consider asking for professional help.

- Many studies show that married people live longer than single people (including those who are divorced, widowed, or never married) and have lower death rates from practically all causes.

Social support can provide a critical counterbalance to the stress in our lives. Give yourself time to develop and maintain a network of people you can count on for emotional support, feedback, and nurturing. If you believe you don't have enough social support, consider becoming a volunteer to help build your network of friends and to enhance your spiritual wellness.

Volunteering

Studies show that not all giving is the same—for example, donating money does not have the same beneficial health effects as volunteering that involves personal contact.

A few simple guidelines can help you get the most out of giving:

- Choose a volunteer activity that puts you in contact with people.
- Make helping voluntary. Obligatory helping can actually increase stress levels.

Ask Yourself

QUESTIONS FOR CRITICAL THINKING AND REFLECTION

What are the top two or three stressors in your life right now? Are they new to your life—as part of your college experience—or are they stressors you've experienced in the past? Do they include both positive and negative experiences (eustress and distress)?

- Volunteer with a group. Sharing your interests with other volunteers increases social support. Volunteering seems to have the most benefits for people who also have other close relationships and social interests.
- Know your limits. Helping that goes beyond what you can handle depletes your own resources and is detrimental to your health.

Communication

Communicating in an assertive way that respects the rights of others—while protecting your own rights—can prevent stressful situations from getting out of control. Better communication skills can help everyone form and maintain healthy relationships. If you typically suppress your feelings, you might want to take an assertiveness training course that can help you identify and change your patterns of communication. If you have trouble controlling your anger, you may benefit from learning anger-management strategies.

Exercise

Exercise helps maintain a healthy body and mind and even stimulates the birth of new brain cells. Regular physical activity can also reduce many of the negative effects of stress. Consider the following examples:

- Taking a long walk can help decrease anxiety and blood pressure.
- A brisk 10-minute walk can leave you feeling more relaxed and energetic for up to two hours.
- People who exercise regularly react with milder physical stress responses before, during, and after exposure to stressors.
- In a study, people who took three brisk 45-minute walks each week for three months reported fewer daily hassles and an increased sense of wellness.

These findings should not be surprising because the stress response mobilizes energy resources and readies the body for physical emergencies. If you experience stress and do not physically exert yourself, you are not completing the energy cycle. You may not be able to exercise while your daily stressors occur—during class, for example, or while sitting in a traffic jam—but you can be active at other times of the day. Physical activity allows you to expend the nervous energy you have built up and trains your body to more readily achieve homeostasis following stressful situations.

It isn't hard to incorporate light to moderate exercise into your day. The important thing is to find an activity that you enjoy so it can become a habit and a regular stress reducer.

Nutrition

A healthful diet gives you an energy bank to draw from whenever you experience stress. Eating wisely also can enhance your feelings of self-control and self-esteem. Learning the principles of sound nutrition is easy, and sensible

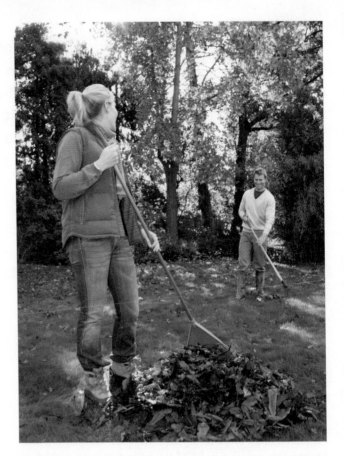

Exercise—even light activity—can be an effective antidote to stress.

eating habits rapidly become second nature when practiced regularly.

Although your diet has an effect on the way your body handles stress, the reverse is also true. Excess stress can negatively affect the way you eat. Many people, for example, respond to stress by overeating; other people skip meals or stop eating altogether during stressful periods. Both responses are not only ineffective (they don't address the causes of stress) but potentially unhealthy.

Sleep

Most adults need seven to nine hours of sleep every night to stay healthy and perform their best. Getting enough sleep isn't just good for you physically. Adequate sleep also improves mood, fosters feelings of competence and self-worth, enhances mental functioning, and supports emotional functioning.

How Sleep Works Sleep occurs in two phases: **rapid eye movement (REM) sleep** and **non–rapid eye movement (NREM) sleep**. A sleeper goes through several cycles of non-REM and REM sleep each night.

> **rapid eye movement (REM) sleep** The portion TERMS of the sleep cycle during which dreaming occurs.
>
> **non–rapid eye movement (NREM) sleep** The portion of the sleep cycle that involves deep sleep; non-REM sleep includes four states of successively deeper sleep.

NREM sleep actually includes four stages of successively deeper sleep. As you move through these stages of sleep, a variety of physiological changes occur:

- Blood pressure drops.
- Respiration and heart rates slow.
- Body temperature declines.
- Growth hormone is released.
- Brain wave patterns become slow and even.

During REM sleep, dreams occur. REM sleep is characterized by the rapid movement of the eyes under closed eyelids. Heart rate, blood pressure, and breathing rate rise, and brain activity increases to levels equal to or greater than those during waking hours. Muscles in the limbs relax completely, resulting in a temporary paralysis.

Sleep and Stress   Stress hormone levels in the bloodstream vary throughout the day and are related to sleep patterns. Peak concentrations occur in the early morning, followed by a slow decline during the day and evening. Concentrations return to peak levels during the final stages of sleep and in the early morning hours. Stress hormone levels are low during non-REM sleep and increase during REM sleep. With each successive sleep cycle during the night, REM sleep lasts a little longer. This increase in REM sleep duration with each sleep cycle may underlie the progressive increase in circulating stress hormones during the final stages of sleep.

Even though stress hormones are released during sleep, it is the *lack* of sleep that has the greatest impact on stress. In someone who is suffering from **sleep deprivation** (not getting enough sleep over time), mental and physical processes steadily deteriorate. A sleep-deprived person experiences headaches, feels irritable, is unable to concentrate, and is more prone to forgetfulness. Poor-quality sleep has long been associated with stress and depression.

> **sleep deprivation**   A lack of sleep over a period of time.   **TERMS**
>
> **insomnia**   A sleep problem involving the inability to fall or stay asleep.
>
> **sleep apnea**   The interruption of normal breathing during sleep.

Most adults need seven to nine hours of sleep every night to stay healthy and perform their best.

Acute sleep deprivation slows the daytime decline in stress hormones, so evening levels are higher than normal. A decrease in total sleep time also causes an increase in the level of stress hormones. Together these changes may cause an increase in stress hormone levels throughout the day and may contribute to physical and mental exhaustion. Extreme sleep deprivation can lead to hallucinations and other psychotic symptoms, as well as to a significant increase in heart attack risk.

Sleep Problems   According to the National Sleep Foundation's 2011 Sleep in America Poll, 14% of American adults sleep an average of less than six hours per night. (Compare this to the recommended seven to nine hours per night.) Although many of us can attribute the lack of sleep to long workdays and family responsibilities, as many as 70 million Americans suffer from chronic sleep disorders—medical conditions that prevent them from sleeping well.

According to National Sleep Foundation polls, more than 50% of adults report having trouble falling asleep or staying asleep—a condition called **insomnia.** The most common causes of insomnia are lifestyle factors, such as high caffeine or alcohol intake before bedtime; medical problems, such as a breathing disorder and stress. About 75% of people who suffer from chronic insomnia report some stressful life event at the onset of their sleeping problems.

Another type of chronic sleep problem, called **sleep apnea,** occurs when a person stops breathing while asleep. Apnea can be caused by a number of factors, but it typically results when the soft tissue at the back of the mouth (such as the tongue or soft palate) "collapses" during sleep, blocking the airway (Figure 2.4). When breathing is interrupted, so is sleep, because the sleeper awakens repeatedly throughout the night to begin breathing again. In most cases, this occurs without the sleeper's even being aware of it. However, the disruption to sleep can be significant, and over time acute sleep deprivation can result from apnea. There are several treatments for apnea, including the use of medications, a special apparatus that helps keep the airway open during sleep, and surgery.

FIGURE 2.4   Sleep apnea. Sleep apnea occurs when soft tissues surrounding the airway relax, "collapsing" the airway and restricting airflow.

During sleep

Tongue   Soft palate   Uvula

Sleep apnea

Blocked airway

Time Management

Learning to manage your time can be crucial to coping with everyday stressors. Overcommitment, procrastination, and even boredom are significant stressors for many people. Along with gaining control of nutrition and exercise to maintain a healthy energy balance, time management is an important element in a wellness program. Try these strategies for improving your time management skills:

• *Set priorities.* Divide your tasks into three groups: essential, important, and trivial. Focus on the first two, and ignore the third.

• *Schedule tasks for peak efficiency.* You've probably noticed you're most productive at certain times of the day (or night). Schedule as many of your tasks for those hours as you can, and stick to your schedule.

• *Set realistic goals and write them down.* Attainable goals spur you on. Impossible goals, by definition, cause frustration and failure. Fully commit yourself to achieving your goals by putting them in writing. (See Chapter 1 for more information about goal setting.)

• *Budget enough time.* For each project you undertake, calculate how long it will take to complete. Then tack on another 10–15%, or even 25%, as a buffer.

• *Break up long-term goals into short-term ones.* Instead of waiting for large blocks of time, use short amounts of time to start a project or keep it moving.

• *Visualize the achievement of your goals.* By mentally rehearsing your performance of a task, you will be able to reach your goal more smoothly.

• *Keep track of the tasks you put off.* Analyze why you procrastinate. If the task is difficult or unpleasant, look for ways to make it easier or more fun.

• *Consider doing your least favorite tasks first.* Once you have the most unpleasant ones out of the way, you can work on the tasks you enjoy more.

• *Consolidate tasks when possible.* For example, try walking to the store so that you run your errands and exercise in the same block of time.

• *Identify quick transitional tasks.* Keep a list of 5- to 10-minute tasks you can do while waiting or between other tasks, such as watering your plants, doing the dishes, or checking a homework assignment.

• *Delegate responsibility.* Asking for help when you have too much to do is no cop-out; it's good time management. Just don't delegate the jobs you know you should do yourself.

• *Say no when necessary.* If the demands made on you don't seem reasonable, say no—tactfully, but without guilt or apology.

• *Give yourself a break.* Allow time for play—free, unstructured time when you can ignore the clock. Don't consider this a waste of time. Play renews you and enables you to work more efficiently.

• *Avoid your personal "time sinks."* You can probably identify your own time sinks—activities like watching television, surfing the Internet, or talking on the phone that consistently use up more time than you anticipate and put you behind schedule. Some days, it may be best to avoid problematic activities altogether; for example, if you have a big paper due, don't sit down for a five-minute TV break if that's likely to turn into a two-hour break. Try a five-minute walk if you need to clear your head.

• *Stop thinking or talking about what you're going to do, and just do it!* Sometimes the best solution for procrastination is to stop waiting for the right moment and just get started. You will probably find that things are not as bad as you feared, and your momentum will keep you going.

Striving for Spiritual Wellness

Spiritual wellness is associated with greater coping skills and higher levels of overall wellness. It is a very personal wellness component, and there are many ways to develop it. Researchers have linked spiritual wellness to longer life expectancy, reduced risk of disease, faster recovery, and improved emotional health. Although spirituality is difficult to study, and researchers aren't sure how or why spirituality seems to improve health, several explanations have been offered:

• *Social support.* Attending religious services or participating in volunteer organizations helps people feel that they are part of a community with similar values and promotes social connectedness and caring.

• *Healthy habits.* Some of the paths to spiritual wellness may encourage healthy behaviors, such as eating a vegetarian diet or consuming less meat and alcohol, and may discourage harmful habits like smoking.

• *Positive attitude.* Spirituality can give a person a sense of meaning and purpose in life, and these qualities create a more positive attitude in the person, which in turn helps her or him cope with life's challenges.

• *Moments of relaxation.* Spiritual practices such as prayer, meditation, and immersion in artistic activities can reduce stress by eliciting the relaxation response.

Spiritual wellness does not require participation in organized religion. Many people find meaning and purpose in other ways. By spending time in nature or working on environmental issues, people can experience continuity with the natural world. Spiritual wellness can come through helping others in your community or by promoting human rights, peace and harmony among people, and opportunities for human development on a global level. Other people develop spiritual wellness through art or their personal relationships.

Spirituality provides an ethical path to personal fulfillment that includes connectedness with self, others, and a higher power or larger reality. Spiritual wellness can make you more aware of your personal values and can help clarify them. Without an awareness of personal values, you might be driven by immediate desires and the passing demands of others. Living according to values means considering your options carefully before making a choice, choosing between options without succumbing to outside pressures that oppose your values, and making a choice and acting on it rather than doing nothing.

Confiding in Yourself through Writing

Keeping a diary is analogous to confiding in others, except that you are confiding in yourself. This form of coping with severe stress may be especially helpful for those who are shy or introverted and find it difficult to open up to others. Although writing about traumatic and stressful events may have a short-term negative effect on mood, over the long term, stress is reduced and positive changes in health occur. A key to promoting health and well-being through journaling is to write about your emotional responses to stressful events. Set aside a special time each day or week to write down your feelings about stressful events in your life.

Cognitive Techniques

Some stressors arise in our own minds. Ideas, beliefs, perceptions, and patterns of thinking can add to our stress level. Each of the following techniques can help you change unhealthy thought patterns to ones that will help you cope with stress. As with any skill, mastering these techniques takes practice and patience.

Think and Act Constructively   Think back to the worries you had last week. How many of them were needless? Think about things you *can* control. Try to stand aside from the problem, consider the positive steps you can take to solve it, and then carry them out. Remember, if you can successfully predict that a stressor will occur, you can better control your response to it. In the evening, try to predict stressful events you might encounter the following day. Then decide how to handle them constructively. This may mean dealing positively with an unpleasant person or figuring out how to stay focused during a boring class. By taking a constructive approach, you can prevent stressors from becoming negative events and perhaps even turn them into positive experiences.

Take Control   A situation often feels more stressful if you feel you're not in control of it. Time may seem to be slipping away before a big exam, for example. Unexpected obstacles may appear in your path, throwing you off course. When you feel your environment is controlling you instead of the other way around, take charge! Concentrate on what is possible to control, and set realistic goals. Be confident of your ability to succeed.

Problem-Solve   Students with greater problem-solving abilities report easier adjustment to university life, higher motivation levels, lower stress levels, and higher grades. When you find yourself stewing over a problem, sit down with a piece of paper and do some problem solving. Try this approach:

1. Define the problem in one or two sentences.
2. Identify the causes of the problem.
3. Consider alternative solutions. Don't just stop with the most obvious one.
4. Weigh positive and negative consequences for each alternative.
5. Make a decision—choose a solution.
6. Make a list of tasks you must perform to act on your decision.
7. Begin to carry out the tasks on your list.
8. Evaluate the outcome and revise your approach if necessary.

Modify Your Expectations   Expectations are exhausting and restricting. The fewer expectations you have, the more you can live spontaneously and joyfully. The more you expect from others, the more often you will feel let down. And trying to meet the expectations others have of you is often futile.

Stay Positive   If you beat up on yourself—"Late for class again! You can't even cope with college! How do you expect to ever hold down a real job?"—try changing your inner dialogue. Talk to yourself as you would to a child you love: "You're a smart, capable person. You've solved other problems; you'll handle this one. Tomorrow you'll simply schedule things so you get to class with a few minutes to spare." (Chapter 3 has more information about self-talk.)

Practice Affirmations   One way of cultivating the positive is to systematically repeat positive thoughts, or *affirmations,* to yourself. For example, if you react to stress with low self-esteem, you might repeat sentences such as "I approve and accept myself completely" and "It matters not what others say, but what I believe." Saying affirmations to yourself every day may make them automatic and help you change the way you react.

Cultivate Your Sense of Humor   When it comes to stress, laughter may be the best medicine. Even a fleeting smile produces changes in your autonomic nervous system

> Problem-solving skills can **improve your motivation, stress level, and grades.**

that can lift your spirits. And a few minutes of belly laughing can be as invigorating as brisk exercise. Hearty laughter elevates your heart rate, aids digestion, eases pain, and triggers the release of endorphins and other pleasurable and stimulating chemicals in the brain. After a good laugh, your muscles go slack; your pulse and blood pressure dip below normal. You are relaxed. Cultivate the ability to laugh at yourself, and you'll have a handy and instantly effective stress reliever.

Focus on What's Important   A major source of stress is trying to store too much data. Forget unimportant details (they will usually be self-evident) and organize important information. One technique you can try is to "chunk" important material into categories. If your next exam covers three chapters from your textbook, consider each chapter a chunk of information. Then break down each chunk into its three or four most important features. Create a mental outline that allows you to trace your way from the most general category down to the most specific details. This technique can be applied to managing daily responsibilities as well.

Relaxation Techniques

The **relaxation response** is a physiological state characterized by a feeling calmness and quiet. This is the opposite of the fight-or-flight reaction. When you call upon a relaxation technique to trigger the relaxation response, your heart rate, breathing, and metabolism slow down, and your blood pressure and oxygen consumption decrease. At the same time, blood flow to the brain and skin increases, and brain waves shift from an alert beta rhythm to a relaxed alpha rhythm. Practiced regularly, relaxation techniques can counteract the debilitating effects of stress.

Progressive Relaxation   Unlike most of the other methods of relaxation, progressive relaxation requires no imagination, willpower, or self-suggestion. You simply tense and relax the muscles in your body, group by group. The technique, also known as deep muscle relaxation, helps you become aware of the muscle tension that occurs when you're under stress. When you consciously relax those muscles, other systems of the body get the message and ease up on the stress response.

Start, for example, with your right fist. Inhale as you tense it. Exhale as you relax it. Repeat. Next, contract and relax your right upper arm. Repeat. Do the same with your left arm. Then, beginning at your forehead and ending at your feet, contract and relax your other muscle groups. Repeat each contraction at least once, breathing in as you tense, breathing out as you relax. To speed up the process, tense and relax more muscles at one time—both arms simultaneously, for instance. With practice, you'll be able to relax very quickly and effectively by clenching and releasing only your fists.

Visualization   Also known as *imagery,* **visualization** lets you daydream without guilt. Next time you feel stressed, close your eyes. Imagine yourself floating on a cloud, sitting on a mountaintop, or lying in a meadow. Involve all your senses; imagine the sounds, the smells, and the other sensations that would be part of the scene. Your body will respond as if the imagery were real. An alternative: Close your eyes and imagine a deep purple light filling your body. Now change the color into a soothing gold. As the color lightens, so should your distress.

You can also use visualization to rehearse for an upcoming event and enhance performance. By experiencing an event ahead of time in your mind, you can practice coping with any difficulties that may arise. Think positively, and you can "psych yourself up" for a successful experience.

Meditation   The need to periodically stop our incessant mental chatter is so great that, from ancient times, hundreds of forms of **meditation** have developed in cultures all over the world. Meditation is a way of telling the mind to be quiet for a while and focus only on what you see and hear. Because meditation has been at the core of many Eastern religions and philosophies, it has acquired an "Eastern" mystique that causes some people to shy away from it. It can be helpful to take a course or acquire some knowledge and background. Whatever philosophical, religious, or emotional reasons may be given for meditation, it is potentially useful for reducing stress. According to a 2008 study, college students who learned how to use meditation for stress management were able to significantly reduce their daily stress levels. Further, those students found it easier to forgive others for perceived wrongdoings and spent less time focusing on negative thoughts.

Meditation helps you tune out the world temporarily, removing you from both internal and external sources of stress. The "thinker" takes time out to become the "observer"—calmly attentive, without analyzing, judging, comparing, or rationalizing. Regular practice of this quiet awareness will subtly carry over into your daily life, encouraging physical and emotional balance no matter what confronts you. For a step-by-step description of a basic meditation technique, see the box "Meditation and the Relaxation Response."

Mindfulness   Another form of meditation, known as *mindfulness meditation,* involves paying attention to physical sensations, perceptions, thoughts, and imagery. Instead

relaxation response   A physiological state characterized by a feeling of calmness and quiet mental alertness.

visualization   A technique for promoting relaxation or improving performance that involves creating or re-creating vivid mental pictures of a place or an experience; also called *imagery*.

meditation   A technique for quieting the mind by focusing on a particular word, object (such as a candle flame), or process (such as breathing).

TERMS

Here is a simple technique for eliciting the relaxation response.

The Basic Technique

1. Pick a word, phrase, or object to focus on. If you like, you can choose a word or phrase that has a deep meaning for you, but any word or phrase will work. Some meditators prefer to focus on their breathing.

2. Take a comfortable position in a quiet environment, and close your eyes if you aren't focusing on an object.

3. Relax your muscles.

4. Breathe slowly and naturally. If you're using a focus word or phrase, silently repeat it each time you exhale. If you're using an object, focus on it as you breathe.

5. Keep a passive attitude. Disregard thoughts that drift in.

6. Continue for 10–20 minutes, once or twice a day.

7. When you're finished, sit quietly for a few minutes with your eyes first closed and then open. Then stand up.

Suggestions

• Allow relaxation to occur at its own pace; don't try to force it. Don't be surprised if you can't quiet your mind for more than a few seconds at a time; it's not a reason for anger or frustration. The more you ignore the intrusions, the easier doing so will become.

• If you want to time your session, peek at a watch or clock occasionally, but don't set a jarring alarm.

• The technique works best on an empty stomach, before a meal or about two hours after eating. Avoid times of day when you're tired—unless you want to fall asleep.

• Although you'll feel refreshed even after the first session, it may take a month or more to get noticeable results. Be patient. Eventually the relaxation response will become so natural that it will occur spontaneously, or on demand, when you sit quietly for a few moments.

connect
ACTIVITY
DO IT ONLINE

of focusing on a word or object to quiet the mind, you observe thoughts that occur without evaluating or judging them. Development of this ability requires regular practice but may eventually result in a more objective view of one's perceptions. It is believed that a greater understanding of one's moment-to-moment thought processes (mindful awareness) provides a richer and more vital sense of life and improves coping. Studies also suggest that people who rate high in mindfulness are less anxious and better able to deal with stress; among people with specific health problems, mindfulness can provide substantial benefits.

Neuroscientist Richard Davidson suggests that mindfulness works by permitting your brain, specifically parts of the prefrontal cortex, to lessen activity in the amygdala, which is responsible for evaluating threats. This helps reduce the likelihood you will overreact and enhances your ability to see potential solutions to problems.

Practicing mindfulness has been shown to be particularly effective in displacing unwanted, bothersome thoughts and allowing relaxation to occur at its own pace.

Yoga   Hatha yoga, the most common yoga style practiced in the United States, emphasizes physical balance and breath control. It integrates components of flexibility, muscular strength and endurance, and muscle relaxation; it also sometimes serves as a preliminary to meditation. A session of

> **QUICK STATS**
>
> **1 in 10** Americans practices yoga in one form or another.
> —Yoga Business Academy, 2011

yoga typically involves a series of postures, each held for a few seconds to several minutes, which involve stretching and balance and coordinated breathing. Yoga can induce the relaxation response and promote body awareness and flexibility. If you are interested in trying yoga, it's best to take a class from an experienced instructor.

Tai Chi   This martial art (in Chinese, *taiji-quan*) is a system of self-defense that incorporates philosophical concepts from Taoism and Confucianism. In addition to self-defense, tai chi aims to bring the body into balance and harmony to promote health and spiritual growth. It teaches practitioners to remain calm and centered, to conserve and concentrate energy, and to manipulate force by becoming part of it—by "going with the flow." Tai chi is considered the gentlest of the martial arts. Instead of quick and powerful movements, tai chi consists of a series of slow, fluid, elegant movements, which reinforce the idea of moving *with* rather than *against* the stressors of everyday life. As with yoga, it's best to start tai chi with a class led by an experienced instructor.

Qigong   (pronounced chee-gung) originates in China and has as its goal the restoration of energy and balance to the body. It is used to relieve stress and chronic pain through various exercises of flowing movements, visualization, and breathing while assuming different postures. Although its popularity is rising, there is no scientific evidence so far that it helps relieve stress or pain.

Biofeedback **Biofeedback** helps people reduce the stress response by enabling them to become more aware of their level of physiological arousal. It involves electrical monitoring of some measure of the physiological stress response, such as perspiration, heart rate, skin temperature, or muscle tension. The subject receives feedback about his or her condition through the use of sound (a tone or music), light, or a meter or dial.

The point of biofeedback training is to learn how relaxation feels, how to induce relaxation, and how to transfer this skill to daily life (without the use of electronic equipment). In addition to monitoring equipment, biofeedback usually also requires the initial help of a therapist, stress counselor, or technician.

Counterproductive Coping Strategies

College is a time when you'll learn to adapt to new and challenging situations and gain skills that will last a lifetime. It is also a time when many people develop counterproductive and unhealthy habits in response to stress. Such habits can last well beyond graduation.

Tobacco Use Cigarettes and other tobacco products contain *nicotine,* a chemical that enhances the actions of neurotransmitters. Nicotine can make you feel relaxed and even increase your ability to concentrate, but it is highly addictive. In fact, nicotine dependence itself is considered a psychological disorder. Cigarette smoke also contains substances that cause heart disease, stroke, lung cancer, and emphysema. These negative consequences far outweigh any beneficial effects, and tobacco use should be avoided. The easiest way to avoid the habit is to not start.

Use of Alcohol and Other Drugs Like nicotine, alcohol is addictive, and many alcoholics find it hard to relax without a drink. Having a few drinks might make you feel temporarily at ease, and drinking until you're intoxicated may help you forget your current stressors. However, using alcohol to deal with stress places you at risk for all the short- and long-term problems associated with alcohol abuse. It also does nothing to address the actual causes of stress in your life. Although limited alcohol consumption may have potential health benefits for some people, many college students have patterns of drinking that detract from wellness.

Using other psychoactive drugs to cope with stress is also usually counterproductive:

• *Caffeine* raises cortisol levels and blood pressure and can make you feel more stressed; caffeine also disrupts sleep. Other stimulants, such as *amphetamines,* can

activate the stress response. They also affect the same areas of the brain that are involved in regulating the stress response.

• Use of *marijuana* causes a brief period of euphoria and decreased short-term memory and attentional abilities. Physiological effects clearly show that marijuana use doesn't cause relaxation; in fact, some neurochemicals in marijuana act to enhance the stress response, and getting high on a regular basis can elicit panic attacks. To compound this, withdrawal from marijuana may also be associated with an increase in circulating stress hormones.

• *Opioids* such as morphine and heroin can mimic the effects of your body's natural painkillers and act to reduce anxiety. However, tolerance to opioids develops quickly, and many users become dependent.

Unhealthy Eating Habits Eating is psychologically rewarding. The feelings of satiation and sedation that follow eating produce a relaxed state. However, regular use of eating as a means of coping with stress may lead to unhealthy eating habits. In fact, a survey by the American Psychological Association revealed that about 25% of Americans use food as a means of coping with stress or anxiety. These "comfort eaters" are twice as likely to be obese as average Americans.

CREATING A PERSONAL PLAN FOR MANAGING STRESS

What are the most important sources of stress in your life? Are you coping successfully with these stressors? No single strategy or program for managing stress will work for everyone, but you can use the principles of behavior management described in Chapter 1 to tailor a plan specifically to your needs.

Identifying Stressors

Before you can learn to manage the stressors in your life, you have to identify them. Many experts recommend keeping a stress journal for a week or two (see Figure 2.5). Each time you feel or express a stress response, record the time and the circumstances in your journal. Note what you were doing at the time, what you were thinking or feeling, and the outcome of your response.

biofeedback A technique in which monitoring devices help a person become conscious of unconscious body processes, such as body temperature or blood pressure, in order to exert some control over them. **TERMS**

STRESS JOURNAL		DATE _1-21-15_
TIME	STRESSOR	REACTION/ COPING STRATEGY
7:45 AM	Tara wouldn't get out of the shower	Yelled at her, started an argument
8:35 AM	Late for class	Slouched in back of room; chewed my nails
11:55 AM	Dad called to discuss credit card debt	Cried, skipped lunch and went out to smoke with Greg
5:30 PM	Power outage at dorm, couldn't study	Took a walk with Tara, made up for arguing this morning, then went to library to study
7:45 PM	Ed called, asked to borrow money	Stayed calm, put down phone and counted to 10, then explained that he already owes me $50.
8:30 PM	Ed called, angry, said he wanted to break up	Argued on phone, then went out with Tara for a drink

FIGURE 2.5 A sample stress journal. Tracking stressful events and reactions can help you understand how you normally cope with stress.

After keeping your journal for a few weeks, you should be able to identify your key stressors and spot patterns in how you respond to them. Take note of the people, places, events, and patterns of thought and behavior that cause you the most stress. You may notice, for example, that mornings are usually the most stressful part of your day. Or you may discover that when you're angry at your roommate, you're apt to respond with behaviors that only make matters worse. Keeping a journal allows you to analyze what produces the most stress in your life and fills in where your conscious memory fails you.

Designing Your Plan

Once you have identified the key stressors in your life, choose the stress reduction techniques that will work best for you and create an action plan for change. Finding a buddy to work with you can make the process more fun and increase your chances of success. Some experts recommend drawing up a formal contract with yourself.

Whether or not you complete a contract, it's important to design rewards into your plan. You might treat yourself to a special breakfast in a favorite restaurant on the weekend (as long as you eat a nutritious breakfast every weekday morning). It's also important to evaluate your plan regularly and redesign it as your needs change. Under times of increased stress, for example, you might want to focus on good eating, exercise, and relaxation habits. Over time, your new stress management skills will become almost automatic. You'll feel better, accomplish more, and reduce your risk of disease.

Getting Help

If the techniques discussed so far don't provide you with enough relief from the stress in your life, you might want to learn more about specific areas to work on. Excellent self-help guides can be found in bookstores or the library. Additional resources are listed in the For More Information section at the end of the chapter.

Your student health center or student affairs office can tell you whether your campus has a peer counseling program. Such programs are usually staffed by volunteer students with special training that emphasizes maintaining confidentiality. Peer counselors can guide you to other campus or community resources or can simply provide understanding.

Support groups are typically organized around a particular issue or problem. In your area, you might find a support group for first-year students; for reentering students; for single parents; for students of your ethnicity, religion, or national origin; for people with eating disorders; or for rape survivors. The number of such groups has increased in recent years as more and more people discover how therapeutic it can be to talk with others who share the same situation.

Short-term psychotherapy can also be tremendously helpful in dealing with stress-related problems. Your student health center may offer psychotherapy on a sliding-fee scale; the county mental health center in your area may do the same. If you belong to any type of religious organization, check to see whether pastoral counseling is available. Your physician can refer you to psychotherapists in your community. Not all therapists are right for all people, so be prepared to have initial sessions with several. Choose the one you feel most comfortable with.

connect™

Connect to Your Choices

Have you ever thought about why you handle stress the way you do? Many factors can influence the choices we make about stress management—some not as obvious as others. Do you try to do too much and then take your frustration out on other people because that's how stress was handled in your family? Do you blow off steam with alcohol on weekends because that's what your friends are doing? Do you dismiss relaxation techniques like yoga, meditation, or deep breathing because you think they're only for a certain type of person?

What are the external factors that influence your choices about stress management? What are your inner motivations and core values, and how do they affect your choices? Based on what you learned in this chapter, will you make some different choices in the future? If so, what will they be?

Go online to Connect to complete this activity:
www.mcgraw-hillconnect.com

TIPS FOR TODAY AND THE FUTURE

For the stress you can't avoid, develop a range of stress management techniques and strategies.

RIGHT NOW YOU CAN:

- Practice a relaxation exercise for 5–10 minutes.
- Visualize a relaxing, peaceful place and imagine yourself experiencing it as vividly as possible. Stay there as long as you can.
- Do some stretching exercises.
- Get out your datebook and schedule what you'll be doing the rest of today and tomorrow. Pencil in a short walk and a conversation with a friend.

IN THE FUTURE YOU CAN:

- Take a class or workshop that can help you overcome a source of stress, such as one in assertiveness training or time management.
- Find a way to build relaxing time into every day. Just 15 minutes of meditation, stretching, or massage can induce the relaxation response.

SUMMARY

- When confronted with a stressor, the body undergoes a set of physical changes known as the fight-or-flight reaction. The sympathetic nervous system and endocrine system act on many targets in the body to prepare it for action.

- Emotional and behavioral responses to stressors vary among individuals. Ineffective responses increase stress but can be moderated or changed.

- Factors that influence emotional and behavioral responses to stressors include personality, cultural background, gender, and past experiences.

- The general adaptation syndrome (GAS) has three stages: alarm, resistance, and exhaustion.

- A high allostatic load characterized by prolonged or repeated exposure to stress hormones can increase a person's risk of health problems.

- Psychoneuroimmunology (PNI) looks at how the physiological changes of the stress response affect the immune system and thereby increase the risk of illness.

- Health problems linked to stress include cardiovascular disease, colds and other infections, asthma and allergies, flare-ups of chronic diseases, psychological problems, digestive problems, headaches, insomnia, and injuries.

- A cluster of major life events that require adjustment and accommodation can lead to increased stress and an increased risk of health problems. Minor daily hassles increase stress if they are perceived negatively.

- Sources of stress associated with college may be academic, interpersonal, time-related, or financial pressures.

- Job-related stress is common, particularly for employees who have little control over decisions relating to their jobs. If stress is severe or prolonged, burnout may occur.

- New and changing relationships, prejudice, and discrimination are examples of interpersonal and social stressors.

- Social support systems help buffer people against the effects of stress and make illness less likely. Good communication skills foster healthy relationships.

- Exercise, nutrition, sleep, and time management are wellness behaviors that reduce stress and increase energy.

- Cognitive techniques for managing stress involve developing new and healthy patterns of thinking, such as practicing problem solving, monitoring self-talk, and cultivating a sense of humor.

- The relaxation response is the opposite of the fight-or-flight reaction. Techniques that trigger it, including progressive relaxation, imagery, meditation, and deep breathing, counteract the effects of chronic stress. Counterproductive coping strategies include smoking, drinking, and unhealthy eating.

- A successful individualized plan for coping with stress begins with the use of a stress journal or log to identify and study stressors and inappropriate behavioral responses. Completing a contract and recruiting a buddy can help your stress management plan succeed.

- Additional help in dealing with stress is available from self-help books, peer counseling, support groups, and psychotherapy.

FOR MORE INFORMATION

BOOKS

Bolles, Richard N. 2012. *What Color Is Your Parachute?* Oregon: Ten Speed Press. *Still probably the most popular guide to exploring the career that is right for you. Now in its 40th edition.*

Davidson, R., and S. Begley. 2012. *The Emotional Life of Your Brain.* New York: Penguin.

Germer, C., R. Siegel, and P. Fulton. 2005. *Mindfulness and Psychotherapy.* New York: The Guilford Press. *A lucid exploration of the applications of mindfulness to clinical psychology.*

Goelitz, J., and R. A. Rees. 2011. *The College De-Stress Handbook: Keeping Cool under Pressure from the Inside Out.* Boulder Creek, CA: Institute of HeartMath. *A brief guide to managing college stress, with tips on recognizing stressors, reducing their intensity, and learning new ways to respond.*

Greenberg, J. 2010. *Comprehensive Stress Management.* 12th ed. New York: McGraw-Hill. *Provides a clear explanation of the physical, psychological, sociological, and spiritual aspects of stress and offers numerous stress management techniques.*

Irwin, M., and K. Vedhara. 2005. *Human Psychoneuroimmunology.* Oxford: University Press. *A survey of the expanding field of psychoneuroimmunology.*

Kabat-Zinn, J. 2011. *Mindfulness for Beginners: Reclaiming the Present Moment—and Your Life.* Louisville, CO: Sounds True. *A distillation of the ideas, attitudes, and practices that constitute the basics of mindfulness and mindful living.*

Keil, R. M. K. 2004. Coping and stress; a conceptual analysis. *Journal of Advanced Nursing* 45(6) 659-665. *A review of the complex interface of stress and coping.*

Ogden, J. 2004. *Health Psychology: A Textbook.* 3rd ed. New York: Open University Press–McGraw-Hill Education, p.259. *A discussion of allostatic load.*

Pennebaker, J. W. 2004. *Writing to Heal: A Guided Journal for Recovering from Trauma and Emotional Upheaval.* Oakland, CA: New Harbinger. *Provides information about using journaling to cope with stress.*

ORGANIZATIONS AND WEBSITES

American Headache Society. Provides information for consumers and clinicians about different types of headaches, their causes, and their treatment.

> http://www.americanheadachesociety.org

The American Institute of Stress. A resource of in-depth information on stress, its causes, and its treatments.

> http://www.stress.org

American Psychiatric Association: Healthy Minds, Healthy Lives. Provides information about mental wellness developed especially for college students.

> http://www.healthyminds.org

American Psychological Association. Provides information about stress management and psychological disorders.

> http://www.apa.org
>
> http://www.apa.org/helpcenter

Association for Applied Psychophysiology and Biofeedback. Provides information about biofeedback and referrals to certified biofeedback practitioners.

> http://www.aapb.org

Benson-Henry Institute for Mind Body Medicine. Provides information about stress management and relaxation techniques.

> http://www.massgeneral.org/bhi

National Institute of Mental Health (NIMH). Publishes brochures about stress and stress management as well as other aspects of mental health.

> http://www.nimh.nih.gov

National Sleep Foundation. Provides information about sleep and how to overcome sleep problems such as insomnia and jet lag.

> http://sleepfoundation.org

SELECTED BIBLIOGRAPHY

American College Health Association. 2011. *American College Health Association–National College Health Assessment II Reference Group Executive Summary, Spring 2011.* Hanover, MD: American College Health Association.

American Psychological Association. 2012. *Mind/Body Health: Stress* (http://www.apa.org/helpcenter/stress.aspx).

American Psychological Association. 2014. *Stress in America: Are Teens Adopting Adults' Stress Habits?* Washington, DC: American Psychological Association.

Bartolomucci, A., and R.Leopardi. 2009. Stress and depression: Preclinical research and clinical implications. *PLoS One* 4(1): e4265.

Busch, V. 2008. Exercise in migraine therapy—Is there any evidence for efficacy? A critical review. *Headache* 48(6): 890–899.

Caldwell, K., et al. 2010. Developing mindfulness in college students through movement-based courses: Effects on self-regulatory self-efficacy, mood, stress, and sleep quality. *Journal of American College Health* 58(5): 433–442.

Centers for Disease Control. 2012. Coping with a disaster or traumatic event: Information for individuals and families (http://emergency.cdc.gov/menta-lhealth/general.asp).

Colton, H. R., and B. M.Altevogt, eds. 2006. *Sleep Disorders and Sleep Deprivation: An Unmet Public Health Problem.* Institute of Medicine Committee on Sleep Medicine and Research. Washington, DC: National Academies Press.

Dallman, M.2010. Stress-induced obesity and the emotional nervous system. *Trends in Endocrinology and Metabolism* 21(3): 159–165.

Darabaneanu, S.2011. Aerobic exercise as a therapy option for migraine: A pilot study. *International Journal of Sports Medicine* 32(6): 455–460.

Flugel Colle, K. F., et al. 2010. Measurement of quality of life and participant experience with the mindfulness-based stress reduction program. *Complementary Therapies in Clinical Practice* 16(1): 36–40.

Fox, S., and M.Duggan. 2013. The diagnosis difference. *Pew Research Internet Project* (http://www.pewinternet.org/2013/11/26/the-diagnosis-difference/).

Freedman, N. 2010. Treatment of obstructive sleep apnea syndrome. *Clinics in Chest Medicine* 31(2): 187–201.

Hefner, J., and D. Eisenberg. 2009. Social support and mental health among college students. *American Journal of Orthopsychiatry* 79(4): 491–499.

Hook, J. N., et al. 2010. Empirically supported religious and spiritual therapies. *Journal of Clinical Psychology* 66(1): 46–72.

Inflammation and anti-inflammatories in depression. 2013. *Bipolar Network News* 17(4) 1–15. *A survey of current therapies.*

Jayson, S. Who's Feeling Stressed? *USA Today,* February 7, 2013.

Kemeny, M.2012. Contemplative/emotion training reduces negative emotional behavior and promotes prosocial responses. *Emoticon* [1528–3542] (12): 338–350.

Kim, B. 2014. *How the Body Works: Overview of the Nervous and Endocrine Systems.* (http://drbenkim.com/nervous-endocrine-system.htm)

National Sleep Foundation. 2011. *2011 Sleep in America Poll.* Washington, DC: National Sleep Foundation.

Nordboe, D. J., et al. 2007. Immediate behavioral health response to the Virginia Tech shootings. *Disaster Medicine and Public Health Preparedness* 1 (Suppl. 1): S31–S32.

Roddenberry, A., and K. Renk. 2010. Locus of control and self-efficacy: Potential mediators of stress, illness, and utilization of health services in college students. *Child Psychiatry and Human Development* 41(4): 353–370.

Sirri, L., et al. 2012. Type A behavior: A reappraisal of its characteristics in cardiovascular disease. *International Journal of Clinical Practice* 66(9): 854–861.

Telles, S., et al. 2009. Effect of a yoga practice session and a yoga theory session on state anxiety. *Perceptual and Motor Skills* 109(3): 924–930.

U.S. Department of Health and Human Services, National Institutes of Health. 2012. *Stress* (http://www.nlm.nih.gov/medlineplus/stress.html).

Do you perform as well as you should on tests? Does anxiety interfere with your ability to study effectively before a test and to think clearly in the test situation? If so, you may be experiencing test anxiety. Two effective methods can help you deal with test anxiety: systematic desensitization and success rehearsal.

Systematic Desensitization

Systematic desensitization is based on the premise that you can't feel anxiety and be relaxed at the same time.

Phase I: Constructing an Anxiety Hierarchy Begin the first phase by thinking of 10 or more situations related to your fear, such as hearing the announcement of the test date in class, studying for the test, reading the test questions, and so on. Write each situation on an index card. On the other side, list several realistic details or prompts that will help you vividly imagine yourself actually experiencing the situation. For example, if the situation is "hearing that 50% of the final grade will be based on the two exams," the prompts might include details such as "sitting in the big lecture auditorium in Baily Hall," "taking notes in my blue notebook," and "listening to Professor Smith's voice."

Next arrange your cards in order, from least tense to most tense situation. Rate each situation on a scale of 0–100, and make sure the distances between items are fairly small and about equal. When you're sure your anxiety hierarchy is a true reflection of your feelings, number the cards.

Phase II: Learning and Practicing Muscle Relaxation The second phase of the program involves learning to relax your muscles and to recognize when they are relaxed (see the description of progressive relaxation in this chapter). As you become proficient at this technique, you'll be able to go into a deeply relaxed state within just a few minutes. When you can do this, go on to the next phase of the program.

Phase III: Implementing the Desensitization Program Use the quiet place where you practiced your relaxation exercises. Sit comfortably and take several minutes to relax completely, and then look at the first card, reading both the brief phrase and the descriptive prompts. Close your eyes and imagine yourself in that situation for about 10 seconds. Then put the card down and relax completely for about 30 seconds. Look at the card again, imagine the situation for 10 seconds, and relax again for 30 seconds.

At this point, evaluate your current level of anxiety about the situation on the card in terms of the rating scale you devised earlier. If your anxiety level is 10 or below, relax for two minutes and go on to the second card. If it's higher than 10, repeat the routine with the same card until the anxiety decreases.

If you have difficulty with a particular item, go back to the previous item and try it again. If you still can't visualize it without anxiety, try to construct three new items with smaller steps between them and insert them before the troublesome item. You should be able to move through one to four items per session.

Sessions can be conducted from twice a day to twice a week and should last no longer than 20 minutes. It's helpful to graph your progress in a way that has meaning for you.

After you have successfully completed your program, you should be desensitized to the real-life situations that previously caused anxiety. If you find that you experience some anxiety in the real situations, take 30 seconds or a minute to relax completely, just as you did when you were practicing.

Success Rehearsal

To practice this variation on systematic desensitization, take your hierarchy of anxiety-producing situations and vividly imagine yourself successfully dealing with each one. Create a detailed scenario for each situation, and use your imagination to experience genuine feelings of confidence. Recognize your negative thoughts ("I'll be so nervous I won't be able to think straight") and replace them with positive ones ("Anxiety will keep me alert so I can do a good job").

Proceed one step at a time, thinking as you go of strategies for success that you can later implement. These might include the following:

- Before the test, find out everything you can about it—its format, the material to be covered, the grading criteria. Ask the instructor for practice materials. Study in advance; don't just cram the night before. Avoid all-nighters.

- Devise a study plan. This might include forming a study group with one or more classmates or outlining what you will study, when, where, and for how long. Generate your own questions and answer them.

- In the actual test situation, sit away from possible distractions, listen carefully to instructions, and ask for clarification if you don't understand a direction.

- During the test, answer the easiest questions first. If you don't know an answer and there is no penalty for incorrect answers, guess. If there are several questions you have difficulty answering, review the ones you have already handled. Figure out approximately how much time you have to cover each question.

- For true-false questions, look for qualifiers such as *always* and *never*. Such questions are likely to be false.

- Avoid worrying about past performance, how others are doing, or the negative consequences of a poor test grade. If you start to become nervous, take some deep breaths and relax your muscles completely for a minute or so.

The best way to counter test anxiety is with successful test-taking experiences. If you find that these methods aren't sufficient to get your anxiety under control, you may want to seek professional help.

CHAPTER OBJECTIVES

- Describe what it means to be psychologically healthy
- Explain how to develop and maintain a positive self-concept and healthy self-esteem
- Discuss the importance of an optimistic outlook, good communication skills, and constructive approaches to dealing with loneliness and anger
- Describe common psychological disorders
- Recognize the warning signs of suicide
- Summarize the different models of human nature on which different therapies are based
- Describe the different types of help available for psychological problems

CHAPTER **3**

Psychological Health

Psychological health contributes to every dimension of wellness. It can be difficult to maintain emotional, social, or even physical wellness if you are not psychologically healthy.

Psychological health, however, is a broad concept—one that is as difficult to define as it is important to understand. That is why the first section of this chapter is devoted to explaining what psychological health is. The rest of the chapter discusses a number of common psychological problems, their symptoms, and their treatments.

DEFINING PSYCHOLOGICAL HEALTH

Psychological health (or *mental health*) can be defined either negatively, as the absence of sickness, or positively, as the presence of wellness. The negative definition concentrates attention on the worst problems and on the people most in need, and it avoids value judgments about the best way to lead our lives. If we think of everyone who is not severely mentally disturbed as being mentally healthy, however, we end up ignoring common problems that can be addressed. Finally, freedom from disorders is only one factor in

psychological wellness. The vast majority of people do not suffer from mental illness, yet they do have to deal with stress, interpersonal conflicts, and difficult emotions. Psychological health refers to the extent to which we are able to function optimally in the face of these challenges.

Positive Psychology

In his book *Toward a Psychology of Being,* psychologist Abraham Maslow adopted a perspective that he called "positive psychology." Maslow developed a *hierarchy of needs* (Figure 3.1): The most important kind is the satisfaction of physiological needs; following this is a feeling of safety, a state of being loved, maintainance of self-esteem, and lastly, self-actualization.

When urgent (life-sustaining) needs—such as the need for food and water—are satisfied, less basic needs take priority. Maslow's conclusions were based on his study of a

psychological health   Mental health, defined   **TERMS**
negatively as the absence of illness or positively as
the presence of wellness.

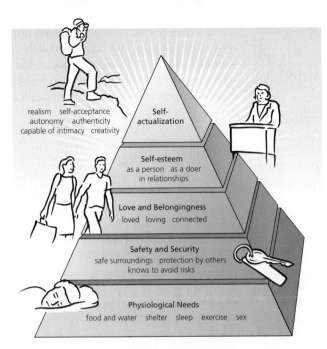

FIGURE 3.1 **Maslow's hierarchy of needs.**

SOURCE: Maslow, A. 1970. *Motivation and Personality,* 2nd ed. New York: Harper & Row.

Ask Yourself

QUESTIONS FOR CRITICAL THINKING AND REFLECTION

Have you ever had a reason to feel concerned about your own psychological health? If so, what was the reason? Did your concern lead you to talk to someone about the issue, or to seek professional help? If you did, what was the outcome, and how do you feel about it now?

rejection. They are open to the pleasure of physical contact and the satisfaction of being close to others—but without being afraid of the risks involved in intimacy, such as the possibility of getting rejected. (Chapters 4 and 5 discuss intimacy in more detail.)

• *Creativity.* Creative people continually look at the world with renewed appreciation and curiosity. Such buoyancy can enhance your creativity.

Self-actualization is an ideal to strive for rather than something most people can reasonably hope to achieve. Maslow himself believed it was achieved quite rarely. Still, fulfilling your own potential is a goal that everyone can work toward.

Influenced by the work of Abraham Maslow, psychologist Martin Seligman suggests that the goal of **positive psychology** is "to find and nurture genius and talent" and "to make normal life more fulfilling" rather than just to identify and treat illness. In other words, it means being able to define positive goals and identify concrete, measurable ways of achieving them.

According to Seligman, we can achieve happiness by traveling different but equally valid roads:

• *The pleasant life.* This life is dedicated to maximizing positive **emotions** about the past, present, and future, and to minimizing pain and negative emotions.

group of visibly successful people who seemed to have lived, or to be living, at their fullest. He suggested that these people had fulfilled a good measure of their human potential and achieved **self-actualization.** Self-actualized people all share certain qualities:

> What a man or woman **can be,** he or she **must be.**
> —A. Maslow, *Motivation and Personality* (1954)

• *Realism.* Self-actualized people know the difference between what is real and what they want. As a result, they can cope with the world as it exists without demanding that it be different; they know what they can and cannot change. Just as important, realistic people accept evidence that contradicts what they want to believe.

• *Acceptance.* Self-accepting people have a positive but realistic **self-concept,** or *self-image.* Such a person typically feels satisfaction and confidence in himself or herself, and thus has healthy **self-esteem.** Self-acceptance also means being tolerant of your own imperfections—an ability that makes it easier to accept the imperfections of others.

• *Autonomy. Autonomous* people can direct themselves, acting independently of their social environment. **Autonomy** is more than physical independence. It is social, emotional, and intellectual independence, as well.

• *Authenticity.* Self-actualized people are not afraid to be themselves. Sometimes, in fact, their capacity for being "real" may give them a certain childlike quality. They respond in a genuine, or *authentic*, spontaneous way to whatever happens, without pretense or self-consciousness.

• *Capacity for intimacy.* People capable of intimacy can share their feelings and thoughts without fear of

self-actualization The highest level of growth in Maslow's hierarchy of needs.

TERMS

self-concept The ideas, feelings, and perceptions a person has about himself or herself; also called *self-image.*

self-esteem Satisfaction and confidence in yourself; the valuing of yourself as a person.

autonomy Independence; the sense of being self-directed.

positive psychology The ability to define positive goals and to identify concrete, measurable ways of achieving them.

emotion A feeling state involving some combination of thoughts, physiological changes, and an outward expression or behavior.

• *The engaged life.* This life involves cultivating positive personality traits (such as courage, leadership, kindness, and integrity) and actively using your talents. "Engagement" also involves cultivating a capacity to "live in the moment" and immerse yourself fully in your activities.

A key to being engaged and successful in life is the positive personality trait of **emotional intelligence.** An emotionally intelligent person can identify and manage his or her own emotions and respond to the emotions of others. People with higher emotional intelligence can perceive their own emotions and can also channel them to reach their intended goals. Psychologists and educators believe that emotional intelligence is not as rooted as abstract intelligence and can be learned.

• *The meaningful life.* Another road to happiness entails working with others toward a meaningful end. Many people find meaning in their connections with and service to families, friends, religious institutions, social causes, and/or work. The happiness to be found by following this path is strongest when meaning comes from more than one source.

Seligman and his colleagues are developing methods of assessing these ways of life and of teaching people how to become happier by adopting one or more of them. They need not be mutually exclusive.

The notion of positive psychology is not without critics. Not everyone accepts the ideas of positive psychology—or even the concept of psychological health—because they involve value judgments that are inconsistent with psychology's scientific status. Defining psychological health requires making assumptions and value judgments about what human goals are desirable, and some think these are matters for religion or philosophy. Positive psychology has also been criticized as promoting a shortsighted denial of reality and unwarranted optimism. In particular, therapists guided by existential philosophy believe that psychological health comes from acknowledging and accepting the painful realities of life.

What Psychological Health Is Not

Psychological health is not the same as psychological normality. Being mentally "normal" simply means being close to average. We can define normal body temperature because a few degrees above or below this temperature means physical sickness, but we cannot measure psychological health this way. Your ideas and attitudes can vary tremendously without your

> Emotional intelligence is not only a positive personality trait but also a **key to being engaged and successful in life.**

losing efficiency or feeling emotional distress. Psychological diversity is actually a valuable asset; with its range of ideas, lifestyles, and attitudes, it allows us to widen our cultural outputs and solve more problems of the social world.

Not seeking help for personal problems does not prove you are psychologically healthy, any more than seeking help proves you are mentally ill or unhealthy. Unhappy people may avoid seeking help for many reasons, and severely disturbed people may not even realize they need help.

Further, we can't say people are "mentally ill" or "mentally healthy" based solely on the presence or absence of symptoms. Consider the symptom of anxiety, for example. Anxiety can help you face a problem and solve it before it becomes too big. Someone who shows no anxiety may be refusing to recognize problems or to do anything about them. A person who is anxious for good reason is likely to be judged more psychologically healthy in the long run than someone who is inappropriately calm.

Finally, we cannot judge psychological health from the way people look. All too often, a person who seems to be OK and even happy suddenly takes his or her own life. At an early age, we learn to conceal our feelings and even to lie about them. We may believe that our complaints put unfair demands on others. Although suffering in silence may sometimes be a virtue, it can also prevent us from getting help.

MEETING LIFE'S CHALLENGES

Life is full of challenges—large and small. Everyone, regardless of heredity and family influences, must learn to cope successfully with new situations and new people.

Growing Up Psychologically

Our responses to life's challenges influence the development of our personality and identity.

Developing an Adult Identity A primary task beginning in adolescence is the development of an adult identity: a unified sense of self, characterized by attitudes, beliefs, and ways of acting that are genuinely our own. People with adult identities know who they are, what they are capable of, what roles they play, and their place among their peers. They have a sense of their own uniqueness but also appreciate what they have in common with others. They view themselves realistically and can assess their strengths and weaknesses without relying on the opinions of others. Achieving an identity also means that we can form intimate relationships with others while maintaining a strong sense of self.

Our identities evolve as we interact with the world and make choices about what we'd like to do and whom we'd like to model ourselves after. Developing an adult identity is particularly

emotional intelligence The capacity to identify and manage your own emotions and the emotions of others.

TERMS

challenging in a heterogeneous, secular, and relatively affluent society like ours, in which many roles are possible, many choices are tolerated, and ample time is allowed for experimenting and making up your mind.

This idea of a core self may seem contradictory with the idea that we are always changing. We show different sides of ourselves, not just as we pass through different ages, but also from one day to the next depending on who we're with or the environment we're in.

Early identities are often modeled after parents and adult caretakers—or the opposite of parents, in rebellion against what they represent. Over time, peers, rock stars, sports heroes, and religious figures are added to the list of possible role models. In high school and college, people often join cliques that assert a certain identity, such as "jocks," "nerds," or "slackers." Although much of our identity is internal—a way of viewing ourselves and the world—certain aspects of it can be external, such as styles of talking and dressing, ornaments like earrings, and hairstyles.

Early identities are rarely permanent. A hardworking student seeking approval one year can turn into a dropout devoted to sleeping all day and partying all night the next year. At some point, however, most of us adopt a more stable, individual identity that ties together the experiences of childhood and the expectations and aspirations of adulthood. However, we don't suddenly assume our final identity and never change after that. Life is more interesting for people who continue evolving into more distinct individuals, rather than being rigidly controlled by their pasts. Identity reflects a lifelong process, and it changes as a person develops new relationships and roles.

"A healthy self-esteem" suggests you regard yourself as **good, competent, and worthy of love.**

Developing an adult identity is an important part of psychological wellness. Without a personal identity, we begin to feel confused about who we are; this situation is called an **identity crisis.** Until we have "found ourselves," we cannot have much self-esteem because a self is not firmly in place.

Developing Intimacy People with established identities can form intimate relationships and sexual unions characterized by sharing, open communication, long-term commitment, and love. Those who lack a firm sense of self may have difficulty establishing relationships because they feel overwhelmed by closeness and the needs of another person. As a result, they experience only short-term, superficial relationships with others and may remain isolated.

Developing Values and Purpose in Your Life
Values are criteria for judging what is good and bad, and they underlie our moral decisions and behavior. The first morality of the young child is to consider "good" to mean what brings immediate and tangible rewards, and "bad" to mean whatever results in punishment. An older child will explain right and wrong in terms of authority figures and rules. But the final stage of moral development, one that not everyone attains, is being able to conceive of right and wrong in more abstract terms such as justice and virtue.

As adults we need to assess how far we have evolved morally and what values we actually have adopted. Without an awareness of our personal values, our lives may be hurriedly driven forward by immediate desires and the passing demands of others. Living according to values means:

- Considering your options carefully before making a choice
- Choosing between options without succumbing to outside pressures that conflict with your values
- Making a choice and acting on it rather than doing nothing

Your actions and how you justify them proclaim to others what you stand for.

Achieving Healthy Self-Esteem

Having a healthy level of self-esteem means regarding your self—which includes all aspects of your identity—as good, competent, and worthy of love. It is a critical component of wellness.

identity crisis   Internal confusion about who you are.   TERMS

values   Criteria for judging what is good and bad, which underlie an individual's moral decisions and behavior.

Developing a Positive Self-Concept Ideally a positive self-concept begins in childhood, based on experiences both within the family and outside it. Children need to develop a sense of being loved and being able to give love and to accomplish their goals. If they feel rejected or neglected by their parents, they may fail to develop feelings of self-worth. They may grow to have a negative concept of themselves.

Another component of self-concept is *integration*. An integrated self-concept is one that you have made for yourself—not someone else's image of you or a mask that doesn't quite fit. Important building blocks of self-concept are the personality characteristics and mannerisms of parents, which children may adopt without realizing it. Later they may be surprised to find themselves acting like one of their parents. Eventually such building blocks may be reshaped and integrated into a new, individual personality.

A further aspect of self-concept is *stability*. Stability depends on the integration of the self and its freedom from contradictions. People who have gotten mixed messages about themselves from parents and friends may have contradictory self-images, which defy integration and make them vulnerable to shifting levels of self-esteem. At times they regard themselves as entirely good, capable, and lovable—an ideal self—and at other times they see themselves as entirely bad, incompetent, and unworthy of love. Neither of these extreme self-concepts allows people to see themselves or others realistically, and their relationships with other people are filled with misunderstandings and ultimately with conflict.

Meeting Challenges to Self-Esteem As an adult, you sometimes run into situations that challenge your self-concept. People you care about may tell you they don't love you or feel loved by you, for example, or your attempts to accomplish a goal may end in failure.

You can react to such challenges in several ways. The best approach is to acknowledge that something has gone wrong and try again, adjusting your goals to your abilities without radically revising your self-concept. Less productive responses are denying that anything went wrong and blaming someone else. These attitudes may preserve your self-concept temporarily, but in the long run they keep you from meeting the challenge.

The worst reaction is to develop a lasting negative self-concept in which you feel bad, unloved, and ineffective—in other words, to become demoralized. Instead of coping, the demoralized person gives up (at least temporarily), reinforcing the negative self-concept and setting in motion a cycle of bad self-concept and failure. In people who are genetically predisposed to depression, demoralization can progress to additional symptoms, which are discussed later in the chapter.

One method for fighting demoralization is to recognize and test the negative thoughts and assumptions you may have about yourself and others. Try to note exactly when an unpleasant emotion—feeling worthless, wanting to give up, feeling depressed—occurs or gets worse, to identify the events or daydreams that trigger that emotion, and to observe whatever thoughts come into your head just before or during the emotional experience. It is helpful to keep a daily journal about such events.

People who are demoralized tend to use all-or-nothing thinking. They overgeneralize from negative events. They overlook the positive and jump to negative conclusions, minimizing their own successes and magnifying the successes of others. They take responsibility for unfortunate situations that are not their fault, then jump to more negative conclusions and more unfounded overgeneralizations. Patterns of thinking that make events seem worse than they are in reality are called **cognitive distortions.**

When you react to a situation, an important piece of that reaction is your **self-talk**—the statements you make to yourself inside your own mind.

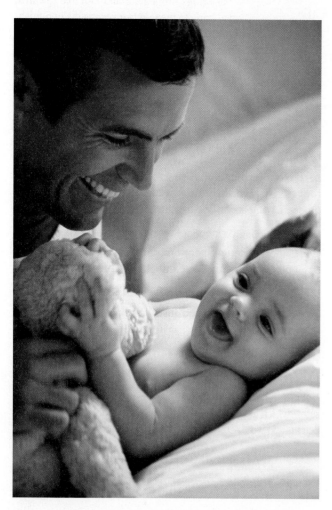

A positive self-concept begins in infancy. The knowledge that he's loved and valued by his parents gives this baby a solid basis for lifelong psychological health.

> **cognitive distortion** A pattern of negative thinking that makes events seem worse than they are.
>
> **self-talk** The statements a person makes to himself or herself.
>
> TERMS

Rational thinking and self-talk will not only help get you through the situation without feeling upset, but also help you avoid damaging your own self-concept.

In your own fight against demoralization, it may be hard to think of a rational response until hours or days after the event that upset you. Responding rationally can be especially hard when you are having an argument with someone else, which is why people often say things they don't mean in the heat of the moment or develop hurt feelings even when the other person had no intention of hurting them.

Once you get used to noticing the way your mind works, however, you may be able to catch yourself thinking negatively and change the process before it goes too far. This approach to controlling your reactions is not the same as positive thinking—which means substituting a positive thought for a negative one. Instead you simply try to make your thoughts as logical and accurate as possible, based on the facts of the situation as you know them, and not on snap judgments or conclusions that may turn out to be false.

Demoralized people can be tenacious about their negative beliefs—so tenacious that they make their beliefs come true in a self-fulfilling prophecy. For example, if you conclude that you are so boring that no one will like you anyway, you may decide not to bother socializing. This behavior could make the negative belief become a reality because you limit your opportunities to meet people and develop new relationships.

For additional tips on changing distorted, negative ways of thinking, see the Take Charge box "Realistic Self-Talk."

Psychological Defense Mechanisms— Healthy and Unhealthy

Sometimes our wishes come into conflict with people in our lives or with our own conscience, and we become frustrated and anxious. If we cannot resolve the conflict by changing the external situation, we try to resolve the conflict internally by rearranging our thoughts and feelings through what are called psychological defenses. Table 3.1 lists some standard **defense mechanisms**. Defense mechanisms can be healthy and adaptive— such as humor and altruism—but sometimes they are what are called maladaptive. The drawback of many of these coping mechanisms is that they succeed temporarily, but make ultimate solutions much harder to find.

Recognizing your own defense mechanisms can be difficult because they've probably become habits, occurring unconsciously. But we all have some inkling about how our minds operate. By remembering the details of conflict situations you have been in, you may be able to figure out which defense mechanisms you used in successful or unsuccessful attempts to cope. Recall a psychologically stressful situation and try to look at yourself as an objective, outside observer would; now analyze your thoughts and behavior in

defense mechanism   A mental mechanism for coping with conflict or anxiety.   TERMS

Table 3.1	Defense and Coping Mechanisms	
MECHANISM	DESCRIPTION	EXAMPLE
Projection	Reacting to unacceptable impulses by denying their existence in yourself and attributing them to others	A student who dislikes his roommate feels that the roommate dislikes him.
Repression	Keeping an unpleasant feeling, idea, or memory out of awareness	The child of an alcoholic, neglectful father remembers only when her father showed consideration and love.
Denial	Refusing to acknowledge to yourself what you really know to be true	A person believes that smoking cigarettes won't harm her because she's young and healthy.
Displacement	Shifting your feelings about a person to another person	A student who is angry with one of his professors returns home and yells at one of his housemates.
Dissociation	Detached from a current experience to avoid emotional distress	Rather than listen to his angry father, Beethoven composes a piece in his mind.
Rationalization	Giving a false, acceptable reason when the real reason is unacceptable	A shy young man decides not to attend a dorm party, telling himself he'd be bored.
Reaction formation	Concealing emotions or impulses by exaggerating the opposite ones	A student struggling with homosexual impulses engages in gay bashing.
Substitution	Replacing an unacceptable or unobtainable goal with an acceptable one	A man in love with an unavailable partner throws himself into training for a marathon.
Passive-aggressive behavior	Expressing hostility toward someone by being covertly uncooperative or passive	A person tells a coworker, with whom she competes for assignments, that she'll help him with a project but then never follows through.
Humor	Finding something funny in unpleasant situations	A student whose bicycle has been stolen thinks how surprised the thief will be when he or she starts downhill and discovers the brakes don't work.
Altruism	Service to others without expecting anything in return	A person who grew up in an upper-class neighborhood volunteers at a foundation that helps people get out of poverty.

Do your patterns of thinking make events seem worse than they truly are? Do negative beliefs you have about yourself become self-fulfilling prophecies? Substituting realistic self-talk for negative self-talk can help you build and maintain self-esteem and cope better with the challenges in your life. Here are some examples of common types of distorted, negative self-talk, along with suggestions for more accurate and rational responses.

COGNITIVE DISTORTION	NEGATIVE SELF-TALK	REALISTIC SELF-TALK
Focusing on negatives	Babysitting is such a pain in the neck; I wish I didn't need the extra money so bad.	This is a tough job, but at least the money's decent and I can study once the kids go to bed.
Expecting the worst	I know I'm going to get an F in this course. I should just drop out of school now.	I'm not doing too well in this course. I should talk to my professor to see what kind of help I can get.
Overgeneralizing	My hair is a mess and I'm gaining weight. I'm so ugly. No one would ever want to date me.	I could use a haircut and should try to exercise more. This way I'll start feeling better about myself and will be more confident when I meet people.
Minimizing	It was nice of everyone to eat the dinner I cooked, even though I ruined it. I'm such a rotten cook.	Well, the roast was a little dry but they ate every bite. The veggies and rolls made up for it. I'm finally getting the hang of cooking!
Blaming others	Everyone I meet is such a jerk. Why aren't people friendlier?	I am going to make more of an effort to meet people who share my interests.
Expecting perfection	I cannot believe I flubbed that solo. They probably won't even let me audition for the orchestra next year.	It's a good thing I didn't stop playing when I hit that sour note. It didn't seem like anyone noticed it as much as I did.
Believing you're the cause of everything	Tom and Sara broke up and it's my fault. I shouldn't have insisted that Tom spend so much time with me and the guys.	It's a shame Tom and Sara broke up. I wish I knew what happened between them. Maybe Tom will tell me at soccer practice. At any rate, it isn't my fault; I've been a good friend to both of them.
Thinking in black and white	I thought that Mike was really cool, but after what he said today, I realize we have nothing in common.	I was really surprised that Mike disagreed with me today. I guess there are still things I don't know about him.
Magnifying events	I stuttered when I was giving my speech today in class. I must have sounded like a complete idiot. I'm sure everyone is talking about it.	My speech went really well, except for that one stutter. I bet most people didn't even notice it, though.

that situation. Having insight into what strategies you typically use can lead to new, less defensive, and more effective ways of coping in the future.

Being Optimistic

Most of us have a predisposition toward optimism or pessimism. **Pessimism** is a tendency to focus on the negative and expect an unfavorable outcome; **optimism** is a tendency to emphasize the hopeful and expect a favorable outcome. Pessimists not only expect repeated failure and rejection but also accept it as deserved. They do not see themselves as capable of success and irrationally dismiss any evidence of their own accomplishments. This negative point of view is learned, typically at a young age from parents and other authority figures. Optimists, on the other hand, consider bad events to be temporary and consider failure to be limited and look forward to new pursuits.

You can learn to be optimistic by recording adverse events in a diary, along with the reactions and beliefs with which you met those events. By doing so, you learn to recognize and dispute the false, negative predictions you generate about yourself, like "The problem is going to last forever and ruin everything, and it's all my fault." Refuting such negative self-talk frees energy for realistic coping.

pessimism The tendency to expect an unfavorable outcome.

optimism The tendency to expect a favorable outcome.

TERMS

Maintaining Honest Communication

Another important area of psychological functioning is communicating honestly with others. It can be very frustrating for us and for people around us if we cannot express what we want and feel. Others can hardly respond to our needs if they don't know what those needs are. We must recognize what we want to communicate and then express it clearly.

Some people know what they want others to do but don't state it clearly because they fear denial of the request, which they interpret as personal rejection. Such people might benefit from assertiveness training: learning to insist on their rights and to bargain for what they want. **Assertiveness** includes being able to say no or yes depending on the situation.

Dealing with Loneliness

It can be hard to strike the right balance between being alone and being with others. Some people are motivated to socialize from fear of being alone. If you discover how to be enjoy being by yourself, you'll be better able to cope with periods when you're forced to be alone—for example, when you are no longer in a romantic relationship or when your usual friends are away on vacation.

Unhappiness with being alone may come from interpreting it as a sign of rejection—that others are not interested in spending time with you. Before you reach such a conclusion, be sure that you give others a real chance to get to know you.

Examine your patterns of thinking: You may harbor unrealistic expectations about other people—for example, that everyone you meet must like you and, if they don't, you must be flawed.

If you decide that you're not spending enough time with people, take action to change the situation. College life provides many opportunities to meet people. If you're shy or introverted, you may have to push yourself to join a group. Look for something you've enjoyed in the past or in which you have a genuine interest.

Dealing with Anger

Anger is a part of the array of normal emotions, yet it is often confusing and difficult to deal

> Defense mechanisms may work right now, **but they can keep you from finding long-term solutions** to conflicts.

with. Some people feel that expressing anger is beneficial for psychological and physical health. However, if angry words or actions damage relationships or produce feelings of guilt or loss of control, they do not contribute to psychological wellness. Some studies have suggested that overtly hostile people seem to be at higher risk for heart attacks. Perhaps the best way to resolve this contradiction is to distinguish between a destructive expression of anger and a reasonable level of self-assertiveness.

At one extreme are people who never express anger or any opinion that might offend others, even when their own rights and needs are being jeopardized. They may be trapped in unhealthy relationships or chronically deprived of satisfaction at work and at home. If you have trouble expressing your anger, consider training in assertiveness and appropriate expressions of anger to help you learn to express yourself constructively.

At the other extreme are people whose anger is explosive or misdirected—such expression of anger can signal a condition called *intermittent explosive disorder (IED)*. It may also be a symptom of a more serious problem—angry outbursts, for instance, are associated with posttraumatic stress disorder. Explosive anger may also happen during periods of intoxication with alcohol or drugs such as amphetamines or cocaine. Explosive anger or rage, like a child's tantrum, renders an individual temporarily unable to think straight or to act in his or her own best interest. During an IED episode, a person may lash out uncontrollably,

assertiveness Expression that is forceful but not hostile. **TERMS**

College offers many antidotes to loneliness in the forms of clubs, organized activities, sports, and just hanging out with friends.

hurting someone else physically or verbally, or destroying property. Anyone who expresses anger this way should seek professional help.

Managing Your Own Anger   If you feel explosive anger coming on, consider the following two strategies to head it off.

First, try to *reframe* what you're thinking at that moment. You'll be less angry at another person if there is a possibility that his or her behavior was not intentionally directed against you. Imagine that another driver suddenly cuts in front of you. You would certainly be angry if you knew the other driver did it on purpose, but you probably would be less angry if you knew he simply did not see you. If you're angry because you've just been criticized, avoid mentally replaying scenes from the past when you received other unjust criticisms. Think about what is happening now, and try to act differently than you would have in the past—less defensively and more analytically.

Second, until you're able to change your thinking, try to *distract* yourself. Use the old trick of counting to 10 before you respond, or start concentrating on your breathing. If necessary, cool off by leaving the situation until your anger has subsided. This does not mean that you should permanently avoid the issues of people who make you angry. Return to the matter after you've had a chance to think clearly about it.

Dealing with Anger in Other People   Anger can be infectious, and it disrupts cooperation and communication. If someone you're with becomes very angry, respond "asymmetrically" by reacting not with anger but with calm. Try to validate the other person by acknowledging that he or she has some reason to be angry: "I totally get that this is making you mad," or "If I were you, I'd be upset, too." This does not mean apologizing if you don't think you're to blame, or accepting verbal abuse. It means that you have considered the other's perspective and that you understand why she might be angry. Finally, if the person cannot be calmed, it may be best to disengage, at least temporarily. After a time-out, you may have better luck trying to solve the problem rationally.

PSYCHOLOGICAL DISORDERS

All of us feel anxious at times. In dealing with anxiety, we may avoid doing something that we want to do or should do. Most of us have periods of feeling down when we

Ask Yourself

QUESTIONS FOR CRITICAL THINKING AND REFLECTION

Think about the last time you were truly angry. What triggered your anger? How did you express it? Do you typically handle your anger in the same manner? How appropriate does your anger management technique seem?

become pessimistic, less energetic, and less able to enjoy life. Many of us are bothered at times by irrational thoughts or odd feelings. Such feelings and thoughts can be normal responses to the ordinary challenges of life, but when emotions or irrational thoughts start to interfere with daily activities and rob us of our peace of mind, they can be considered symptoms of a psychological disorder.

Psychological disorders are generally the result of many factors. Genetic differences, which underlie differences in how the brain processes information and experiences, are known to play an important role, especially in certain disorders such as autism, schizophrenia, and bipolar disorder. However, exactly which genes are involved, and how they alter the structure and chemistry of the brain, is still under study. Learning and life events are important, too: Although one identical twin is often at higher risk of having a disorder if the other has it, the two don't necessarily have the same psychological disorders despite having identical genes. Some people have been exposed to more traumatic events than others, leading either to greater vulnerability to future traumas or, conversely, to the development of better coping skills. Further, what your parents, peers, and others have taught you strongly influences your level of self-esteem and how you deal with frightening or depressing life events (see the box "Ethnicity, Culture, and Psychological Health").

QUICK STATS

26% of adult Americans could be diagnosed with psychological disorders in any given year.

—National Institute of Mental Health, 2012

Anxiety Disorders

Fear is a basic and useful emotion. Its value for our ancestors' survival cannot be overestimated. For modern humans, fear motivates us to protect ourselves and to learn how to cope with new or potentially dangerous situations. We consider fear to be a problem only when it is out of proportion to real danger. **Anxiety** is another word for fear, in particular, fear that is not in response to any definite threat. It becomes a disorder when it occurs almost daily or in life situations that recur and cannot be avoided, interfering with your relationships and the ability to function in social and professional situations.

Specific Phobia   The most common and understandable anxiety disorder, called **specific phobia,** is a fear of something definite like lightning, a particular type of animal, or a

Cultures develop unique ideas about mental health—about what is normal and what is problematic, how symptoms should be interpreted and communicated, whether treatment should be sought, and whether a social stigma is attached to a particular symptom or disorder. Based on their various environmental, cultural, and socioeconomic backgrounds, cultures perceive—categorize and interpret—psychological disorders differently. Climate and geography, as well as other environmental factors such as diet, contribute to a group's health.

These culturally distinct ideas change as the group comes into contact with other groups. For example, Asian immigrants to the United States have often come from *collectivist* cultures that anticipate and care for the needs of each other, so that individuals don't need to request support. In U.S. cultures, usually no group is expected to look after the needs of an individual; rather individuals or their close families bear responsibility to seek help for themselves. For this reason Asian immigrants appear to have more trouble than European Americans asking for explicit social support.

The process by which individuals and groups adapt to each other's cultures, called *acculturation,* is an important influence on health. This adaptation ideally represents an exchange between both cultures, so that they learn how to do things a new way. Acculturation, however, often applies only to immigrants' adopting influences from a dominant culture. When a dominant group takes over the resources of a minority group—for example, a government enforcing an English-only policy on bilingual speakers, thereby increasing the difficulties of the immigrants seeking help—then the socioeconomic status of the adapting group often decreases. As the following examples show, this status change may then further affect the psychological health of the group.

Arctic Native Populations

Studies of native populations around the Arctic (e.g., in northern Canada, Greenland, and Scandinavia) reveal many cases of elevated and chronic stress, accompanied by high blood pressure and cardiovascular risk. This chronic stress is linked to 50 years of rapid socioeconomic change: The population has experienced long-term unemployment, contamination of food, and a multitude of other acculturation problems. As they have acculturated, indigenous people have suffered discrimination, loss of traditional values, and lack of control over their resources. Because they live in climates with less light during winter months, they also experience seasonal affective disorder, a form of depression.

Cultural expressions of their high levels of anxiety and depression include increased incidence of suicide and violence. Adolescents, in particular, among Alaska Natives and Greenland Inuit, have recently had a high number of suicides. Levels of injury and violence reach two to four times as high as national averages.

Latinos in the United States

Latinos in the United States generally are healthier than other U.S. racial and ethnic groups, for example in mortality rates for adults and newborn babies. Still, mortality rates, incidence of chronic illness, and some mental health conditions such as depression vary within the U.S. Latino population, depending on Latino origin or cultural heritage (e.g., Mexican, Puerto Rican, or Cuban).

One of the largest immigrant groups in the United States is from Mexico. Surprisingly, surveys show that these immigrants are psychologically healthier than their own children born in the United States (those who are more acculturated have higher rates of depression). Not all effects of the acculturation process are negative: Latinos get more health care (e.g., cancer screenings) and education, and they increase their perception of how healthy they are. Still, more acculturated Latinos suffer greater substance abuse, worse diet, and poorer birth outcomes (low birth weight and prematurity). Some reasons that more recently arrived immigrants are healthier include maintaining strong family bonds and continuing to use their native languages.

SOURCES: Fisher, E. B. 2014. Peer support in health care and prevention: Cultural, organizational, and dissemination issues. *Annual Review of Public Health* 35:363–83; Leyse-Wallace, R. 2013. *Nutrition and Mental Health.* Boca Raton, FL: CRC Press; Snodgrass, J. J. 2013. Health of indigenous circumpolar populations. *Annual Review of Anthropology* 42: 69–87; Brick, K., et al. 2011. Mexican and Central American immigrants in the United States. Washington, D.C: Migration Policy Institute; Lara, M., et al. 2005. Acculturation and Latino health in the United States: A review of the literature and its sociopolitical context. *Annual Review of Public Health* 26: 367–397.

place. Snakes, spiders, and dogs are commonly feared animals; high or enclosed spaces are often frightening places. Sometimes, but not always, these fears originate in bad experiences, such as being bitten by a snake.

Social Phobia   The 15 million Americans with **social phobia** fear humiliation or embarrassment. Fear of speaking in public is perhaps the most common phobia of this kind. Extremely shy people can have social fears in almost all social situations.

Panic Disorder   People with **panic disorder** experience sudden unexpected surges in anxiety, accompanied by symptoms such as rapid and strong heartbeat, shortness of

social phobia   An excessive fear of being observed by others; speaking in public is the most common example.

panic disorder   A syndrome of severe anxiety attacks accompanied by physical symptoms.

TERMS

breath, loss of physical equilibrium, and a feeling of losing mental control. Such attacks usually begin in a person's early twenties and can lead to a fear of being in crowds or closed places or of driving or flying. Sufferers fear that a panic attack will occur in a situation from which escape is difficult (in an elevator), where the attack could be incapacitating and result in a dangerous or embarrassing loss of control (driving a car or shopping), or where no medical help would be available if needed (alone away from home). Fears such as these lead to avoidance of situations that might cause trouble. The fears and avoidance may spread to a large variety of situations until a person is virtually housebound, a condition called **agoraphobia.** People with panic disorder can often function normally in feared situations if with someone they trust. Panic disorder is different from an occasional **panic attack,** which affects about 40 million American adults age 18 and older every year. This occasional attack of overwhelming anxiety may have no obvious antecedent and usually resolves in an hour or less.

Generalized Anxiety Disorder   A basic reaction to future threats is to worry about them. **Generalized anxiety disorder (GAD)** is a diagnosis given to people whose worries about multiple issues linger more than six months. Worries may involve family, other relationships, work, school, money, and health.

The GAD sufferer's worrying is not completely unjustified—after all, thinking about problems can result in solving them. But this kind of thinking seems to just go

around in circles, and the more you try to stop it, the more you feel at its mercy. The end result is a persistent feeling of nervousness, often accompanied by depression.

Obsessive-Compulsive Disorder   Someone diagnosed with **obsessive-compulsive disorder (OCD)** struggles with obsessions, compulsions, or both.

Obsessions are recurrent, unwanted thoughts or impulses. Unlike the worries of GAD, they are not ordinary concerns but improbable fears such as of suddenly committing an antisocial act or of having been contaminated by germs.

Compulsions are repetitive, difficult-to-resist actions usually associated with obsessions. A common compulsion is hand washing, associated with an obsessive fear of contamination by dirt. Other compulsions are counting and repeatedly checking whether something has been done—for example, whether a door has been locked or a stove turned off.

People with OCD feel anxious, out of control, and embarrassed. Their rituals can occupy much of their time and make them inefficient at work and difficult to live with.

Posttraumatic Stress Disorder (PTSD)   People who suffer from **posttraumatic stress disorder** are reacting to severely traumatic events (events that produce a sense of terror and helplessness) such as physical violence to themselves or their loved ones. Trauma occurs in personal assaults (rape, military combat), natural disasters (floods, hurricanes), and tragedies (fires, airplane or car crashes).

Symptoms include reexperiencing the trauma in dreams and in intrusive memories, trying to avoid anything associated with the trauma, and numbing of feelings. Hyperarousal (being on edge or easily startled), sleep disturbances, and other symptoms of anxiety and depression also commonly occur. Such symptoms can last months or even years. The symptoms of PTSD must last at least a month for the diagnosis to be made. Those whose symptoms have lasted only a month before resolving are considered to have **acute stress disorder.** PTSD symptoms often decrease over time, but up to one-third of PTSD sufferers do not fully recover. Recovery may be slower in those who have previously experienced trauma or who suffer from ongoing psychological problems.

As a result of the Boston Marathon bombing in April 2013, a study by the U.S. Department of Veterans Affairs' National Center for PTSD found that many Boston-area military veterans diagnosed with PTSD experienced flashbacks, unwanted memories, and other psychological effects. The study raises awareness of the effects that tragic events such as terror attacks and mass shootings have on people directly involved but also on those with PTSD and other preexisting psychological conditions. The researchers urge health care systems to be prepared in the future to treat

TERMS

agoraphobia   An anxiety disorder characterized by fear of being alone away from help and by avoidance of many different places and situations; in extreme cases, a fear of leaving home.

panic attack   A brief surge of overwhelming anxiety that usually resolves in an hour or less.

generalized anxiety disorder (GAD)   An anxiety disorder characterized by excessive, uncontrollable worry about all kinds of things and anxiety in many situations.

obsessive-compulsive disorder (OCD)   An anxiety disorder characterized by uncontrollable, recurring thoughts and the performing of senseless rituals.

obsession   A recurrent, irrational, unwanted thought or impulse.

compulsion   An irrational, repetitive, forced action, usually associated with an obsession.

posttraumatic stress disorder (PTSD)   An anxiety disorder characterized by reliving traumatic events through dreams, flashbacks, and hallucinations.

acute stress disorder   An anxiety disorder that resolves in a month or less.

individuals who were either directly or indirectly affected by such tragedies.

Treating Anxiety Disorders Therapies for anxiety disorders range from medication to psychological interventions concentrating on a person's thoughts and behavior. Both drug treatments and cognitive-behavioral therapies are effective in panic disorder, OCD, and GAD. Specific phobias are best treated without drugs.

Attention-Deficit/Hyperactivity Disorder

Attention-Deficit/Hyperactivity Disorder (ADHD) is one of the most common disorders of childhood and adolescence. The main features of ADHD are inattention, hyperactivity, and/or impulsivity. A diagnosis of ADHD is made only if individuals exhibit a persistent pattern of these behaviors; the behaviors must also interfere with the individual's functioning or development, as well as negatively affect school performance, peer relationships, or behavior at home.

To be diagnosed, a person must have symptoms of ADHD before age 12 (even if an adult at first diagnosis). There must also be evidence that the ADHD behaviors are present in two or more settings—for example, at home, school or work; with friends and family; and in other activities. Someone who can pay attention at work but is inattentive only at home usually wouldn't qualify for a diagnosis of ADHD.

ADHD has no cure, and scientists are still working on treatments. They are using tools such as brain imaging to find ways to prevent it. The use of medications is controversial—at best it can relieve some symptoms of the disorder. Other treatments include psychotherapy, education and training, and a combination of treatments.

Mood Disorders

Daily, temporary mood changes typically don't affect our overall emotional state or level of wellness. A person with a **mood disorder,** however, experiences emotional disturbances that are intense and persistent enough to affect normal functioning. The two most common mood disorders are depression and bipolar disorder.

Depression The National Institutes of Health estimate that **depression** strikes nearly 6.7% of Americans annually, making it the most common mood disorder. Depression affects the young as well as adults; about 3% of adolescents aged 13–18 suffer a major depressive episode each year, and nearly 50% of college students report depression severe enough to hinder their daily functioning. Depression tends to be more severe and persistent in blacks than in people of other races. Despite this, fewer than 50% of blacks affected by depression are treated for it.

Almost twice as many women have serious depression as men. Why this is so is a matter of debate. Some experts think much of the difference is due to reporting bias: Women are more willing to admit experiencing negative emotions, being stressed, or having difficulty coping. Women may also be more likely to seek treatment. Other experts point to biologically based sex differences, particularly in the level and action of hormones. It may also be that men are more likely to have symptoms such as anger or irritability when they are depressed, leading them to be misdiagnosed or for the diagnosis to be missed. In addition, women's social roles and expectations are often different from those of men. Women may put more emphasis on relationships in determining self-esteem, so the deterioration of a relationship is a cause of depression that can hit women harder than men. Culturally determined gender roles are more likely to place women in situations where they have less control over key life decisions, and lack of autonomy is associated with depression.

Depression takes different forms but usually involves demoralization and can include the following:

- A feeling of sadness and hopelessness
- Loss of pleasure in doing usual activities
- Poor appetite and weight loss
- Insomnia or disturbed sleep
- Restlessness or fatigue
- Thoughts of worthlessness and guilt
- Trouble concentrating or making decisions
- Thoughts of death or suicide

A person experiencing depression may not have all of these symptoms. Sometimes instead of poor appetite and insomnia, the opposite occurs—eating too much and sleeping too long. (Depression may contribute to weight gain in young women.) People can have multiple symptoms of depression without feeling depressed, although they usually experience a loss of interest or pleasure.

In major depression, symptoms are often severe; a diagnosis of *dysthymic disorder* may apply to people who experience persistent symptoms of mild or moderate depression for two years or longer. In some cases, depression is a clear-cut reaction to specific events, such as the loss of a loved one or

> **attention-deficit/hyperactivity disorder (ADHD)** A disorder characterized by persistent, pervasive problems with inattention and/or hyperactivity to a degree that is not considered appropriate for a child's developmental stage and that causes significant difficulties in school, work, or relationships.
>
> **mood disorder** An emotional disturbance that is intense and persistent enough to affect normal function; two common mood disorders are depression and bipolar disorder.
>
> **depression** A mood disorder characterized by loss of interest, sadness, hopelessness, loss of appetite, disturbed sleep, and other physical symptoms.

TERMS

failing in school or work, whereas in other cases no trigger event is obvious. Regardless of the reason, severe symptoms should be taken seriously. When someone has symptoms of major depression for more than two weeks, even if it is in reaction to a specific event, it is important that they consider treatment. One of the principal dangers of severe depression is suicide, which is discussed later in this chapter.

TREATING DEPRESSION Although treatments are highly effective, only about 35% of people who suffer from depression currently seek treatment. Treatment for depression depends on its severity and on whether the depressed person is suicidal. The best initial treatment for moderate to severe depression is probably a combination of drug therapy and psychotherapy. Newer prescription antidepressants work well, although they may need several weeks to take effect, and patients may need to try multiple medications before finding one that works well. If someone is severely depressed and is at risk of suicide, hospitalization for more intensive treatment to ensure the patient's safety is sometimes necessary. A dysfunctional interaction between neurotransmitters and their receptors is thought to affect some psychiatric disorders (Figure 3.2). The trouble begins when neurotransmitters

electroconvulsive therapy (ECT)   The use of electric shock to induce brief, generalized seizures; used in the treatment of selected psychological disorders.

seasonal affective disorder (SAD)   A mood disorder characterized by seasonal depression, usually occurring in winter, when there is less daylight.

TERMS

(chemicals that transmit messages between nerve cells) misfire and the nerve cells do not properly communicate. Antidepressants work by targeting key neurotransmitters in the brain, including serotonin. When you take an antidepressant such as Prozac, the levels of serotonin increase. This increase has been revealed to help depression and other bodily conditions that serotonin influences, including mood, sexual desire and function, appetite, sleep, memory and learning, temperature regulation, and some social behavior.

To understand how neurotransmitters interact, see Figure 3.2.

When women take antidepressants, they may need a lower dose than men; at the same dosage, blood levels of medication tend to be higher in women. An issue for women who may become pregnant is whether antidepressants can harm a fetus or newborn. The best evidence indicates that the most frequently prescribed types of antidepressants do not cause birth defects, although some studies have reported withdrawal symptoms in some newborns whose mothers used certain antidepressants.

Electroconvulsive therapy (ECT) is effective for severe depression when other approaches have failed, including medications and other electronic therapies such as magnetic stimulation. In ECT, an epileptic-like seizure is induced by an electrical impulse transmitted through electrodes placed on the head. Patients are given an anesthetic and a muscle relaxant to reduce anxiety and prevent injuries associated with seizures. ECT usually includes three treatments per week for two to four weeks.

One type of depression is treated by having sufferers sit with eyes open in front of a bright light source every morning. These patients have **seasonal affective disorder (SAD);**

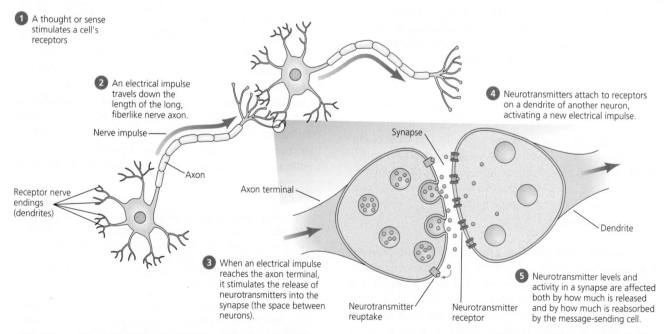

FIGURE 3.2   Nerve cell communication. Nerve cells (neurons) communicate through a combination of electrical impulses and chemical messages. Neurotransmitters such as serotonin and norepinephrine alter the overall responsiveness of the brain and are responsible for mood, levels of attentiveness, and other psychological states. Many psychological issues are related to problems with neurotransmitters and their receptors, and drug treatments frequently target them. For example, the antidepressant drug Prozac increases levels of serotonin by slowing the resorption (reuptake) of serotonin.

their depression worsens during winter months as daylight hours diminish, then improves with the spring and summer. The American Psychiatric Association estimates that 10–20% of Americans suffer symptoms that may be linked to SAD. SAD is more common among people who live at higher latitudes, where there are fewer hours of light in winter. Light therapy may work by extending the perceived length of the day and thus convincing the brain that it is summertime even during the winter months.

Mania and Bipolar Disorder   People who experience **mania,** characteristic of a severe mood disorder called **bipolar disorder,** undergo discrete periods of time when they may be restless, may have excess energy, need little or no sleep, and speak rapidly. Their mood may be elevated (feeling much better than normal) or be abnormally irritable. This is often accompanied by impulsive, pleasure-seeking behavior without regard for the consequences—for example, spending too much money or engaging in risky sexual activity. Many manic people swing between manic and depressive states. This syndrome affects men and women equally.

Antimanic drugs include lithium (a salt that calms manic episodes), mood stabilizers, and antipsychotic medications. Medications to treat depression may also be prescribed.

Schizophrenia

Schizophrenia is a devastating mental disorder that affects a person's thinking and perceptions of reality. People with schizophrenia frequently develop paranoid ideas and false beliefs (delusions), or may have auditory hallucinations (hearing "voices"). People with schizophrenia are often convinced that the voices they hear are "real." The disease can be severe and debilitating or so mild that it's hardly noticeable. Although people are capable of diagnosing their own depression, they usually don't diagnose their own schizophrenia because they often can't see that anything is wrong. This disorder is not rare; in fact, 1 in every 100 people has schizophrenia, most commonly starting in adolescence, which is perhaps what is most tragic and disturbing about the disease—that it starts to affect people in the prime of their lives.

Scientists are uncertain about the exact causes of schizophrenia. Researchers have identified possible chemical and structural differences in the brains of people with the disorder as well as several genes that appear to increase risk.

1 in 100 Americans **is diagnosed with schizophrenia** in their lifetime.

Schizophrenia is likely caused by a combination of genes and environmental factors that occur during pregnancy and development. For example, children born to older fathers have higher rates of schizophrenia, as do children with prenatal exposure to certain infections or medications.

Some general characteristics of schizophrenia include the following:

- *Disorganized thoughts.* Thoughts may be expressed in a vague or confusing way.

- *Inappropriate emotions.* Emotions may be either absent or strong but inappropriate.

- *Delusions.* People with delusions—firmly held false beliefs—may think that their minds are controlled by outside forces, that people can read their minds, that they are great personages like Jesus Christ or the president of the United States, or that they are being persecuted by a group such as the CIA. Paranoid delusions can give people the feeling that they are in grave danger of being harmed.

- *Auditory hallucinations.* Schizophrenic people may hear voices when no one is present. Sometimes these voices tell them to do things (like harm themselves or others), belittle and criticize them, or give individuals a running commentary on someone's thoughts and behaviors. These voices can seem very real to the person hearing them and therefore are quite terrifying.

- *Deteriorating social and work functioning.* Social withdrawal and increasingly poor performance at school or work may be so gradual that they are hardly noticed at first, but over time people suffering from the disease fall far behind their peers—and far behind others' earlier expectations.

None of these characteristics is invariably present. Some schizophrenic people are quite logical except on the subject of their delusions. Others show disorganized thoughts but no delusions or hallucinations.

A schizophrenic person needs help from a mental health professional. Suicide is a risk in schizophrenia, and expert treatment can reduce that risk and minimize the social consequences of the illness by shortening the period when symptoms are active. The key element in treatment is regular medication. At times medication is like insulin for diabetes—it makes the difference between being able to function or not. Sometimes hospitalization is temporarily required to relieve family and friends.

Ask Yourself

QUESTIONS FOR CRITICAL THINKING AND REFLECTION

Have you ever wondered if you were depressed? Try to recall your situation at the time. How did you feel, and what do you think brought about those feelings? What, if anything, did you do to bring about change and to feel better?

mania   A mood disorder characterized by excessive elation, irritability, talkativeness, inflated self-esteem, and expansiveness.

bipolar disorder   A mental illness characterized by alternating periods of depression and mania.

schizophrenia   A psychological disorder that involves a disturbance in thinking and in perceiving reality.

SUICIDE

In the United States, suicide is the third leading cause of death for young people ages 15 to 24 and the 11th leading cause for people of all ages. About 15 attempts are made for every death. In this country, men have much higher suicide rates than women; white men ages 45–54 have the highest suicide rate (Figure 3.3). Whites and Native Americans have higher rates than most other groups, but rates among blacks have been rising. Women attempt three times as many suicides as men, yet men succeed at more than three times the rate of women. Suicide rates among adolescents and young adults and

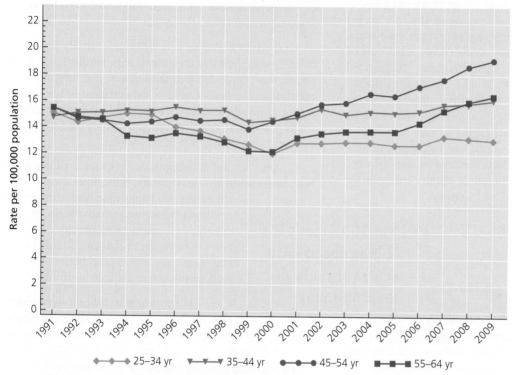

Trends in Suicide Rates* Among Persons Ages 25–64 Years, Both Sexes, by Age Group, United States, 1991–2009

◆—◆ 25–34 yr   ▼—▼ 35–44 yr   ●—● 45–54 yr   ■—■ 55–64 yr

*All rates are age specific. Rates based on less than 20 deaths are not shown as they are statistically unreliable.

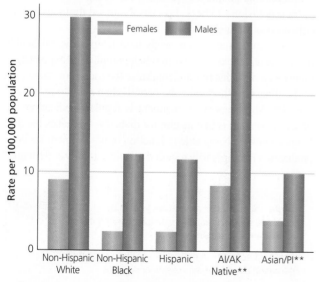

Suicide Rates* Among Persons Ages 25–64 Years, by Race/Ethnicity and Sex, United States, 2005–2009

*All rates are age specific. Rates based on less than 20 deaths are not shown as they are statistically unreliable.

** AI/AK Native: American Indian/Alaskan Native, PI: Pacific Islander

FIGURE 3.3 Rates of suicide per 100,000 people in the United States. The rate of suicide varies by gender, age, and ethnicity. Rates are higher among men than among women at all ages and are higher among whites than other groups. White men ages 45 to 54 have the highest rate of suicide.

SOURCE: Centers for Disease Control and Prevention. 2013–2014. National Suicide Statistics at a Glance. Injury Center. Violence Prevention. Atlanta, GA (http://www.cdc.gov/violenceprevention/suicide/statistics/trends05.html; www.cdc.gov/violenceprevention/suicide/statistics/rates04.html)

In general, people want to be well and healthy and to protect themselves from harm. But many individuals—predominantly in their teens and adolescence—do deliberately harm themselves, although in a nonfatal way. One common method of self-harm is cutting or burning your skin, leaving scars that they hide beneath their clothes.

Self-cutting and other self-injurious behaviors are not aesthetically motivated. Many report seeking the physical sensations (including pain) produced by a self-inflected injury, which may temporarily relieve feelings of tension, perhaps through a release of endorphins.

In 2011 a research group led by Alicia Meuret, an associate professor of psychology at Southern Methodist University, conducted surveys on more than 550 college students and found that over 20% had engaged in self-injury at some point, which is consistent with prevalence estimates in other studies on college populations. In examining differences between self-injurers and non-injurers, individuals that had recently engaged in self-harm were significantly more depressed, anxious, and disgusted with themselves. Compared to non-injurers, self-injurers were roughly 4 times more likely to report a history of physical abuse and 11 times more likely to report a history of sexual abuse.

Self-injury is not the same as a suicide attempt, but individuals who repeatedly hurt themselves are more likely to commit suicide than the general population. In any case, self-injury should be taken seriously. Treatment usually includes group therapy, individual therapy, medication (e.g,, antidepressants), or stress reduction and management skills.

1. **Antidepressants:** One group is called selective serotonin reuptake inhibitors (SSRIs) because of one of their actions; this group includes Prozac (fluoxetine), Paxil (paroxetine), Zoloft (sertraline), Celexa (citalopram), and Lexapro (escitalopram). Another group is called serotonin and norepinephrine reuptake inhibitors (SNRIs) and includes Effexor (venlafaxine) and Cymbalta (duloxetine). Antidepressants that do not fit into these groups include Wellbutrin (buproprion), Serzone (nefazodone), and Remeron (mirtazapine) Another group is called the tricyclics after their chemical structure; it includes Aventyl (nortriptyline) and Elavil (amitriptyline), although these medications are used only infrequently as they may have more side effects than newer antidepressants and can be fatal in overdose due to their effects on heart rhythms.

Surprisingly, these antidepressants are as effective in treating panic disorder and certain kinds of chronic anxiety as they are in treating depression. They may also alleviate the symptoms of OCD. (For more information, see the National Institute of Mental Health's "Mental Health Medications" website at http://www.nimh.nih.gov/health/publications/mental-health-medications/index.shtml).

2. **Mood stabilizers:** Lithium carbonate, Depakote (valproic acid), and Lamictal (lamotrigine) are prescribed as mood stabilizers. They are taken to prevent mood swings that occur in bipolar disorder and certain kinds of schizophrenia.

3. **Antipsychotics:** Older antipsychotics include Haldol (haloperidol) and Prolixin (fluphenazine); newer antipsychotics (sometimes called "atypical") are Clozaril (clozapine), Zyprexa (olanzapine), Risperdal (risperidone), Seroquel (quetiapine), Abilify (aripiprazole), and Geodon (zisprasidone). The drugs reduce hallucinations and disordered thinking in people with schizophrenia, bipolar disorder, and delirium, and they have a calming effect on agitated patients.

4. **Anxiolytics (antianxiety agents) and hypnotics (sleeping pills):** One of the largest and most prescribed classes of anxiolytics is the benzodiazepines, a group of drugs that includes Valium (diazepam), Librium (chlordiazepoxide), Xanax (alprazolam), and Ativan (lorazepam). Dalmane (flurazepam), Restoril (temazepam), and Halcion (triazolam) are benzodiazepines marketed as sleeping aids. Newer hypnotics are Sonata (zaleplon), Ambien (zolpidem), and Lunesta (eszopiclone).

5. **Stimulants:** Ritalin (methylphenidate) and Dexedrine (dextroamphetamine) are most commonly used to treat attention-deficit/hyperactivity disorder (ADHD) in children and less often in adults. Drugs of this type are also marketed under the names Adderall, Strattera, Concerta, Focalin, and Metadate. They are also used against daytime sleepiness in adults, as are purified caffeine (for example, NoDoz) and Provigil (modafinil).

6. **Antidementia drugs:** Dementia is an impairment in memory and thinking that occurs almost exclusively in the elderly. The most common type is Alzheimer's disease (see Chapter 17). Many people with this problem are now prescribed Aricept (donepezil) or Namenda (memantine), although the benefit is often disappointingly small.

among adults over 65 have been falling for the last two decades.

Suicide rarely occurs without warning signs. About 60% of people who commit suicide are depressed. The more symptoms of depression a person has, the greater the risk. Other warning signs include the following:

- Expressing the wish to be dead or revealing contemplated methods

- Increasing social withdrawal and isolation
- A sudden, inexplicable lightening of mood (which can mean the person has decided to commit suicide)

Certain risk factors increase the likelihood of suicide:

- A history of previous attempts
- A suicide by a family member or friend
- Readily available means, such as guns or pills

- A history of substance abuse or eating disorders
- Serious medical problems

If you are severely depressed or know someone who is, expert help from a mental health professional is essential. Don't be afraid to discuss the possibility of suicide with someone you fear is suicidal. You won't give them an idea they haven't already thought of. Asking direct questions is the best way to determine whether someone seriously intends to commit suicide. Encourage your friend to talk and to take positive steps to improve his or her situation.

Most communities have emergency help available, often in the form of a hotline telephone counseling service run by a suicide prevention agency. If you feel there is an immediate danger of suicide, do not leave the person alone. Call for help or take him or her to an emergency room.

Firearms are used in more suicides than homicides. Eighty-three percent of gun-related deaths in the home are the result of suicide, often by someone other than the gun owner. If you learn someone at high risk for suicide has access to a gun, try to convince him or her to put it in safekeeping.

Many psychological disorders have a biological basis in disordered brain chemistry.

tion from a psychiatrist or other medical doctor. All have received U.S. Food and Drug Administration approval as being safe and more effective than a placebo. However, a patient may have to try several drugs before finding one that is effective and has acceptable side effects.

Issues in Drug Therapy The discovery that many psychological disorders have a biological basis in disordered brain chemistry has led to a revolution in the treatment of many disorders, particularly depression. The new view of depression as based in brain chemistry has also lessened the stigma attached to the condition, leading more people to seek treatment. Antidepressants are now among the most widely prescribed drugs in the United States.

Research indicates that, for mild cases of depression, psychotherapy and antidepressants are about equally effective. For major depression, combined therapy is significantly more effective than either type of treatment alone. Therapy can help provide insight into factors that precipitated the depression, such as high levels of stress or a history of abuse. A therapist can also provide guidance in changing patterns of thinking and behavior that contribute to the problem.

MODELS OF HUMAN NATURE AND THERAPEUTIC CHANGE

Human problems such as the psychological disorders discussed in this chapter can be evaluated from at least four different perspectives—biological, behavioral, cognitive, and psychodynamic.

The Biological Model

The *biological model* emphasizes that the mind's activity depends entirely on an organic structure, the brain, whose composition is genetically determined.

Pharmacological Therapy The most important kind of therapy inspired by the biological model is pharmacological therapy, or medication treatment. All require a prescrip-

The Behavioral Model

The *behavioral model* focuses on what people do—their overt behavior—rather than on brain structures and chemistry or on thoughts and consciousness.

Behaviorists analyze behavior in terms of **stimulus, response,** and **reinforcement.** The essence of behavior therapy is to discover what reinforcements keep an undesirable behavior going and then to try to alter those reinforcements.

To change their behavior, fearful people are taught to practice **exposure**—to deliberately and repeatedly enter the feared situation and remain in it until their fear begins to abate.

Although exposure to the real situation works best, exposure in your imagination or through the virtual reality of computer simulation can also be effective. For example, in the case of someone afraid of flying, a simulated scenario would likely be vivid enough to elicit the fear necessary to practice exposure techniques.

The Cognitive Model

The *cognitive model* emphasizes the effect of ideas on behavior and feeling. According to this model, behavior results from complicated attitudes, expectations, and motives rather than from simple, immediate reinforcements.

TERMS

stimulus Anything that causes a response.

response A reaction to a stimulus.

reinforcement Increasing the future probability of a response by following it with a reward.

exposure A therapeutic technique for treating fear; the subject learns to come into direct contact with a feared situation.

Cognitive therapy tries to expose and identify false ideas that produce feelings such as anxiety and depression. For example, a student afraid of speaking in class may harbor thoughts such as "If I begin to speak, I'll say something stupid." In cognitive therapy, such an idea and others like it will be examined critically. If the student prepares, will he or she really sound stupid? Does every sentence said have to be exactly correct and beautifully delivered, or is that an unrealistic expectation? And why does the student care so much about what *they* think? People in cognitive therapy are taught to notice their unrealistic thoughts and to substitute more realistic ones, and they are advised to repeatedly test their assumptions.

The Psychodynamic Model

The *psychodynamic model* also emphasizes thoughts. Proponents of this model, however, do not believe thoughts can be changed directly because they are fed by other unconscious ideas and impulses. Symptoms are not isolated pieces of behavior but the result of a complex set of wishes and emotions hidden by active defenses. In psychodynamic therapy, patients speak as freely as possible in front of the therapist and try to gain an understanding of the basis of their feelings toward the therapist and others. Through this process, patients gain insights that help them overcome their maladaptive patterns. Current therapies of this type tend to focus more on the present (the here and now) than on the past, and the therapist tries to facilitate self-exploration rather than providing explanations.

Evaluating the Models

Ignoring theoretical conflicts among psychological models, therapists have recently developed pragmatic *cognitive-behavioral therapies* that combine effective elements of both models in a single package. For example, the package for treating social anxiety emphasizes exposure as well as changing problematic patterns of thinking. These packages, involving 10 or more individual or group sessions with a therapist and homework between sessions, have been shown to produce significant improvement.

Drug therapy and cognitive-behavioral therapies are also sometimes combined, especially in the case of depression. For anxiety disorders, both kinds of therapy are equally effective, but the effects of drug therapy last only as long as the drug is being taken, while cognitive-behavioral therapies produce longer-term improvement. For schizophrenia, drug therapy is a must, but a continuing relationship with therapists who give support and advice is also indispensable.

Psychodynamic therapies have been attacked as ineffective and endless. Of course effectiveness is hard to demonstrate for therapies that do not focus on specific symptoms. But common sense tells us that being able to open yourself up and discuss your problems with a supportive but objective person who focuses on you and lets you speak freely can enhance your sense of self and reduce feelings of confusion and despair.

Other Psychotherapies

In addition to existing forms of treatment, newer psychotherapies such as *dialectical behavior therapy* (DBT) have become available. Developed by Marsha Linehan, DBT is used to treat people with borderline personality disorder and chronic suicidal behavior, but has since been expanded to treat people with other disorders, such as drug addiction and eating disorders. This therapy uses the principles of standard cognitive-behavioral therapy by encouraging distress tolerance and acceptance of painful feelings and emotions through *mindfulness* (mindful awareness, discussed in Chapter 2), originally derived from Buddhist meditation and other Eastern practices. Mindfulness aims to allow a person to be aware of feelings rather than react to them, and learn techniques to regulate emotions, by decreasing the intensity of emotional reactions. Mindfulness is practiced in group and individual therapy, often involving the use of workbooks and "homework" between sessions.

Another newer therapy called *acceptance and commitment therapy (ACT)* is a scientifically studied psychological intervention that uses acceptance and mindfulness strategies, together with commitment and behavior change strategies, to increase psychological flexibility. **Psychological flexibility** is the process of embracing the present moment fully as a conscious human being, then changing or continuing your behavior in the service of your own chosen values. It was developed in the 1980s by psychologists Steven C. Hayes, Kelly G. Wilson, and Kirk Strosahl.

GETTING HELP

Knowing when you need help dealing with a mental health problem is usually not as difficult as deciding which self-help method or which mental health professional to choose.

Self-Help

A smart way to begin helping yourself is by finding out what you can do on your own. For example, certain behavioral and cognitive approaches can be effective because they all involve becoming more aware of self-defeating actions and ideas and combating them in some way: being more assertive; communicating honestly; raising your self-esteem by counteracting the negative thoughts, people, and actions that undermine it;

> **Psychological flexibility** The process of embracing the present moment fully as a conscious human being, then changing or continuing your behavior in the service of your own chosen values.
>
> TERMS

CRITICAL CONSUMER
Choosing and Evaluating Mental Health Professionals

Mental health workers belong to several different professions and have different roles. Psychiatrists are medical doctors. They are experts in deciding whether a medical disease lies behind psychological symptoms, and they are usually involved in treatment if medication or hospitalization is required. Clinical psychologists typically hold a PhD degree; they are often experts in behavioral and cognitive therapies. Other mental health workers include social workers, licensed counselors, and clergy with special training in pastoral counseling. In hospitals and clinics, various mental health professionals may join together in treatment teams.

Financial considerations are also important. Research the costs of different services and what your health insurance will cover. The Affordable Care Act, also known as Obamacare, has expanded coverage of mental health care; now, with the new law that mandates coverage of individuals up to age 26 by their parents' health insurance, treatments of mental health concerns that start to develop before that age may now be covered (see Chapter 15 for more on the Affordable Care Act). City, county, and state governments often support mental health clinics for those who can afford to pay little or nothing for treatment. Some on-campus services may be free or offered at very little cost.

The cost of treatment is linked to how many therapy sessions will be needed, which in turn depends on the type of therapy and the nature of the problem. Getting this information before you start treatment is important. Many mental health professionals do not accept health insurance payments and only accept direct payments from patients. Psychological therapies focusing on specific problems may require weekly visits for a period of 8–24 sessions, again, depending on the type of therapy. CBT, DBT, and ACT-based therapies are often time-limited, and your therapist can tell you how many sessions to expect. Therapies aiming for psychological awareness and personality change, such as psychodynamic therapies, can last months or years.

Deciding whether a therapist is right for you will require meeting the therapist in person. Before or during your first meeting, find out about the therapist's background and training:

- Does she or he have a degree from an appropriate professional school and a state license to practice?

- Has she or he had experience treating people with problems similar to yours?

- How much will therapy cost?

You have a right to know the answers to these questions and should not hesitate to ask them. After your initial meeting, evaluate your impressions:

- Does the therapist seem like a warm, intelligent person who would be able to help you and seems interested in doing so?

- Are you comfortable with the personality, values, and beliefs of the therapist?

- Is he or she willing to talk about the techniques in use? Do these techniques make sense to you?

If you answer yes to these questions, this therapist may be satisfactory for you. If you feel uncomfortable—and you're not in need of emergency care—it's worthwhile to set up one-time consultations with one or two others before you make up your mind. Take the time to find someone who feels right for you.

Later in your treatment, evaluate your progress:

- Are you being helped by the treatment?

- If you are displeased, is it because you aren't making progress, or because therapy is raising difficult, painful issues you don't want to deal with?

- Can you express dissatisfaction to your therapist? Such feedback can improve your treatment.

The most important predictor of whether or not your therapy will be helpful is how much rapport you feel with your therapist *at the first session*. This has been shown to be true no matter what model of psychotherapy the therapist is practicing. You have to like your therapist and feel that she will be able to help you—if you do, there's a good chance that it will be helpful. If you sense that your therapy isn't working or is actually harmful, thank your therapist for her efforts, and find another. It's extra work for you, but important for your health.

connect™
ACTIVITY
DO IT ONLINE

and confronting, rather than avoiding, the things you fear. Although information from books in the psychology or self-help sections of libraries and bookstores can be helpful, avoid any that make fantastic claims or deviate from mainstream approaches.

Some people find it helpful to express their feelings in a journal. Grappling with a painful experience in this way provides an emotional release and can help you develop more constructive ways of dealing with similar situations in the future. Research indicates that using a journal this way can improve physical as well as emotional wellness.

For some people, religious belief and practice may promote psychological health. Religious organizations provide a social network and a supportive community, and religious practices, such as prayer and meditation, offer a path for personal change and transformation.

Peer Counseling and Support Groups

Sharing your concerns with others is another helpful way of dealing with psychological health challenges. Just being able to share what's troubling you with an accepting, empathetic person can bring relief. Comparing notes with people who have problems similar to yours can give you new ideas about coping.

Many colleges offer peer counseling through a health center or through the psychology or education department. Volunteer students specially trained in maintaining confidentiality are usually those who offer counsel. They may steer you toward an appropriate campus or community resource or simply offer a sympathetic ear.

Many self-help groups work on the principle of bringing together people with similar problems to share their experiences and support one another. Support groups are typically organized around a specific problem, such as eating disorders or substance abuse. Self-help groups may be listed online or in the campus newspaper.

Professional Help

Sometimes self-help or talking to nonprofessionals is not enough. More objective, more expert, or more discreet support is needed, which many people have trouble accepting; often those who most need help are the most unwilling to get it. You may someday find yourself having to overcome your own reluctance, or that of a friend, about seeking help.

In some cases, professional help is optional. Some people are interested in improving their psychological health in a general way by going into individual or group therapy to learn more about themselves and how to interact with others. Seeking professional help for these reasons is a matter of individual choice. In some situations, such as friction among family members or between partners, professional help can mean the difference between a painful divorce and a satisfying relationship.

Professional help is appropriate in any of the following situations:

- Depression, anxiety, or other emotional problems interfere seriously with school or work performance or in getting along with others.

- Suicide is attempted or is seriously considered (see the warning signs listed earlier in the chapter).

Ask Yourself

QUESTIONS FOR CRITICAL THINKING AND REFLECTION

Are you open to discussing the intimate details of your life, your emotions, your fears, your deepest thoughts? Have you ever truly opened up to another person in this manner? Would you be open to this kind of sharing if it meant getting help for a psychological disorder?

TIPS FOR TODAY AND THE FUTURE

Most of life's psychological challenges can be met with self-help and everyday skills. You can take many steps to maintain your mental health.

RIGHT NOW YOU CAN:

- Take a serious look at how you've been feeling recently. If you have any feelings that are especially hard to handle, consider how you can get help with them.
- Think of the way in which you are most creative (an important part of self-actualization), whether it's in music, art, or whatever you enjoy. Try to focus at least an hour each week on this activity.
- Review the list of defense mechanisms in Table 3.1. Have you used any of them recently or consistently over time? Think of a situation in which you used one of those mechanisms and determine how you could have coped with it differently.

IN THE FUTURE YOU CAN:

- Write 100 positive adjectives that describe you. This exercise may take several days to complete. Post your list in a place where you will see it often.
- Record your reactions to upsetting events in your life. Are your reactions and self-talk typically negative or neutral? Decide whether you are satisfied with your reactions and if they are healthy.

Connect to Your Choices

connect™

Have you ever thought about why you approach emotional and psychological problems the way you do? Many factors can influence the choices we make about psychological health, some not as obvious as others. Do you hold in your feelings and hide them from others because that's what was modeled in your family? Do you drink or use drugs when you feel depressed or anxious because you aren't aware of any other options? Do you think getting professional help for a psychological problem is a sign that you're weak or crazy?

What are the external factors that influence your choices about psychological health? What are your inner motivations and core values, and how do they affect your choices? Based on what you learned in this chapter, will you make some different choices in the future? If so, what will they be?

Go online to Connect to complete this activity: www.mcgraw-hillconnect.com

- Symptoms such as hallucinations, delusions, incoherent speech, or loss of memory occur.

- Alcohol or drugs are used to the extent that they impair normal functioning during much of the week, that finding or taking drugs occupies much of the week, or that reducing their dosage leads to psychological or physiological withdrawal symptoms.

SUMMARY

- Psychological health encompasses more than a single particular state of normality. Psychological diversity is valuable among groups of people.

- Defining psychological health as the presence of wellness means that to be healthy you must strive to fulfill your potential.

- Maslow's definition of psychological health centers on self-actualization, the highest level in his hierarchy of needs. Self-actualized people have high self-esteem and are realistic, inner-directed, authentic, capable of emotional intimacy, and creative.

- Crucial parts of psychological wellness include developing an adult identity, establishing intimate relationships, and developing values and purpose in life.

- A sense of self-esteem develops during childhood as a result of giving and receiving love and learning to accomplish goals. Self-concept is challenged every day; healthy people adjust their goals to their abilities.

- Using defense mechanisms to cope with problems can make finding solutions harder. Analyzing thoughts and behavior can help people develop less defensive and more effective ways of coping.

- A pessimistic outlook can be damaging; it can be overcome by developing more realistic self-talk.

- Honest communication requires recognizing what needs to be said and saying it clearly. Assertiveness enables people to insist on their rights and to participate in the give-and-take of good communication.

- People may be lonely if they haven't developed ways to be happy on their own or if they interpret being alone as a sign of rejection. Lonely people can take action to expand their social contacts.

- Dealing successfully with anger involves distinguishing between a reasonable level of assertiveness and gratuitous expressions of anger, heading off rage by reframing thoughts and distracting yourself, and responding to the anger of others with an asymmetrical, problem-solving orientation.

- People with psychological disorders have symptoms severe enough to interfere with daily living.

- Anxiety is a fear that is not directed toward any definite threat. Anxiety disorders include simple phobias, social phobias, panic disorder, generalized anxiety disorder, obsessive-compulsive disorder, and posttraumatic stress disorder.

- Depression is a common mood disorder; loss of interest or pleasure in things seems to be its most universal symptom. Severe depression carries a high risk of suicide, and suicidally depressed people need professional help.

- Symptoms of mania include exalted moods with unrealistically high self-esteem, little need for sleep, and rapid speech. Mood swings between mania and depression characterize bipolar disorder.

- Schizophrenia is characterized by disorganized thoughts, inappropriate emotions, delusions, auditory hallucinations, and deteriorating social and work performance.

- The biological model emphasizes that the mind's activity depends on the brain, whose composition is genetically determined. Therapy based on the biological model is primarily pharmacological.

- The behavioral model focuses on overt behavior and treats psychological problems as bad habits. Behavior change is the focus of therapy.

- The cognitive model considers how ideas affect behavior and feelings; behavior results from complicated attitudes, expectations, and motives, not just from simple reinforcements. Cognitive therapy focuses on changing a person's thinking.

- The psychodynamic model asserts that false ideas are fed by unconscious ideas and cannot be addressed directly. Treatment is based on psychotherapy.

- Help is available in a variety of forms, including self-help, peer counseling, support groups, and therapy with a mental health professional. For serious problems, professional help may be the most appropriate.

FOR MORE INFORMATION

BOOKS

Antony, M. M., and R. P. Swinson. 2008. *The Shyness & Social Anxiety Workbook: Proven, Step-by-Step Techniques for Overcoming Your Fear,* 2nd ed. Oakland, CA: New Harbinger. *Practical suggestions for fears of interacting with people you don't know.*

Grieco, R., and L. Edwards. 2009. *The Other Depression: Bipolar Disorder.* New York: Routledge. *Provides a complete introduction to bipolar disorder, its symptoms, and its current treatments.*

Hayes, Steven. *Acceptance & Commitment Therapy (ACT).* http://contextualscience.org/about_act.

Jenkins, J., D. Keltner, and K. Oatley. 2006. *Understanding Emotions,* 2nd ed. Oxford: Blackwell. *A comprehensive guide to emotions, including current research on the neuroscience of emotions, evolutionary and cultural approaches to emotion, and the expression and communication of emotions.*

Leahy, R. L. 2010. *Beating the Blues Before They Beat You: How to Overcome Depression.* New York: Hay House. *Describes strategies from cognitive-behavioral therapy for changing thinking patterns that contribute to low self-esteem and depression; outlines symptoms, causes, and treatments, including therapy and medication.*

Maslow, A. (1954). *Motivation and Personality.* New York: Harper. pp. 91.

Nathan, P. E., and J. M. Gorman. 2007. *A Guide to Treatments That Work*, 3rd ed. New York: Oxford University Press. *A balanced and comprehensive report on various treatments for psychological disorders.*

Seligman, M. E. 2012. *Flourish: A Visionary New Understanding of Happiness and Well-Being.* New York: Free Press. *The author refines his ideas about learned optimism and happiness, identifying factors that contribute to a satisfying life: positive emotion, engagement, relationships, meaning, and accomplishment.*

ORGANIZATIONS, HOTLINES, AND WEBSITES

American Association of Suicidology. Provides information about suicide and resources for people in crisis.

> http://www.suicidology.org

Anxiety and Depression Association of America (ADAA). Provides information and resources related to anxiety disorders and depression.

> http://www.adaa.org

Cope, Care, Deal. Offers information on mental health issues specifically for teens.

> http://www.copecaredeal.org

Depression and Bipolar Support Alliance (DBSA). Provides educational materials and information about support groups.

> http://www.dbsalliance.org

Mental Health America. Provides consumer information on a variety of issues, including how to find help.

> http://www.nmha.org

NAMI (National Alliance on Mental Illness). Provides information and support for people affected by mental illness.

> 800-950-NAMI (help line)
>
> http://www.nami.org

National Hopeline Network. 24-hour hotline for people who are thinking about suicide or know someone who is; calls are routed to local crisis centers.

> 800-442-HOPE
>
> 800-SUICIDE
>
> http://www.hopeline.com

National Institute of Mental Health (NIMH). Provides helpful information about anxiety, depression, eating disorders, and other challenges to psychological health.

> http://www.nimh.nih.gov

Substance Abuse and Mental Health Services Administration. A one-stop source for information and resources relating to mental health.

> http://samhsa.gov

SELECTED BIBLIOGRAPHY

Agency for Healthcare Research and Quality. 2007. *Antidepressant Medicines: A Guide for Adults with Depression.* Rockville, MD: Agency for Healthcare Research and Quality Publication Number 07-EHC007-2A.

American Psychiatric Association. 2010. *Mental Health* (http://www.healthyminds.org/Main-Topic/Mental-Illness.aspx).

American Psychiatric Association. 2013. *Diagnostic and Statistical Manual of Mental Disorders (DSM-5),* 5th ed. Washington, DC: American Psychiatric Publishing.

Banks, M. V., and K. Salmon. 2012. Reasoning about the self in positive and negative ways: Relationship to psychological functioning in young adulthood. *Memory,* Aug. 17 (epub ahead of print).

Beard, C., et al. 2010. Health-related quality of life across the anxiety disorders: Findings from a sample of primary care patients. *Journal of Anxiety Disorders* 24(6): 559–564.

Carver, C. S., M. F. Scheier, and S. C. Segerstrom. 2010. Optimism. *Clinical Psychology Review* 30(7): 879–889.

Cawood, C. D., and S. K. Huprich. 2011. Late adolescent nonsuicidal self-injury: The roles of coping style, self-esteem, and personality pathology. *Journal of Personality Disorders* 25(6): 765–781.

Centers for Disease Control and Prevention. 2010. Attitudes toward Mental Illness—35 states, District of Columbia, and Puerto Rico, 2007. *Morbidity and Mortality Weekly Report* 59(20): 619–625.

Coryell, W. H. 2006. Clinical assessment of suicide risk in depressive disorder. *CNS Spectrums* 11(6): 455–461.

Dugas, E., et al. 2012. Early predictors of suicidal ideation in young adults. *Canadian Journal of Psychiatry* 57(7): 429–436.

Ferrier-Auerback, A. G., et al. 2010. Predictors of emotional distress reported by soldiers in the combat zone. *Journal of Psychiatric Research* 44(7): 470–476.

Forty, L., et al. 2009. Polarity at illness onset in bipolar I disorder and clinical course of illness. *Bipolar Disorders* 11(1): 82–88.

Greenhoot, A. F., et al. 2012. Making sense of traumatic memories: Memory qualities and psychological symptoms in emerging adults with and without abuse histories. *Memory,* Sept. 4 (epub ahead of print).

Heron, M., et al. 2010. Annual summary of vital statistics: 2007. *Pediatrics* 125(1): 4–15.

Jones, S. H., and G. Burrell-Hodgson. 2008. Cognitive-behavioral treatment of first diagnosis bipolar disorder. *Clinical Psychology & Psychotherapy* 15(6): 367–377.

Kasper, S., et al. 2006. Superior efficacy of St. John's wort extract WS(R) 5570 compared to placebo in patients with major depression: A randomized, double-blind, placebo-controlled, multi-center trial. *BMC Medicine* 4(1): 14.

Klein, D. N., et al. 2012. Predictors of first lifetime onset of major depressive disorder in young adulthood. *Journal of Abnormal Psychology,* Aug. 13 (epub ahead of print).

Lin, Y. R., et al. 2008. Evaluation of assertiveness training for psychiatric patients. *Journal of Clinical Nursing* 17(21): 2875–2883.

Linehan, M. M. 1993. *Cognitive-Behavioral Treatment of Borderline Personality Disorder.* New York: The Guilford Press.

National Institute of Mental Health. 2012. Social phobia (social anxiety disorder) (http://www.nimh.nih.gov/health/topics/social-phobia-social-anxiety-disorder/index.shtml).

National Institute of Mental Health. 2014. Depression (http://www.nimh.nih.gov/health/topics/depression/index.shtml?utm_source=BrainLine.orgutm_medium=Twitter).

Nemeroff, C. B. 2006. The burden of severe depression: A review of diagnostic challenges and treatment alternatives. *Journal of Psychiatric Research,* 25 July [epub ahead of print].

Rickwood, D., and S. Bradford. 2012. The role of self-help in the treatment of mild anxiety disorders in young people: An evidence-based review. *Psychology Research and Behavior Management* 5:25–36.

Rosenthal, B. S., and W. C. Wilson. 2012. Race/ethnicity and mental health in the first decade of the 21st century. *Psychological Reports* 110(2): 645–662.

Rothwell, J. D. 2009. *In the Company of Others: An Introduction to Communication,* 3rd ed. New York: McGraw-Hill.

Saewyc, E. M., and R. Tonkin. 2008. Surveying adolescents: Focusing on positive development. *Pediatrics & Child Health* 13(1): 43–47.

Schatzberg, A. F., J. O. Cole, and C. DeBattista. 2010. *Manual of Clinical Psychopharmacology,* 7th ed. Washington, DC: American Psychiatric Publishing.

Seligman, M. E. P., 2008. Positive health. *Applied Psychology: An International Review* 57, 3–18.

Simon, G. 2009. Collaborative care for mood disorders. *Current Opinion in Psychiatry* 22(1): 37–41.

Simon, G. E., and J. Savarino. 2007. Suicide attempts among patients starting depression treatment with medications or psychotherapy. *American Journal of Psychiatry* 164(7): 1029–1034.

Singh, N. N., et al. 2007. Individuals with mental illness can control their aggressive behavior through mindfulness training. *Behavior Modification* 31(3): 313–328.

Soeteman, D., M. Miller, and J. J. Kim. 2012. Modeling the risks and benefits of depression treatment for children and young adults. *Value in Health* 15(5): 724–729.

Thurber, C. A., and E. A. Walton. 2012. Homesickness and adjustment in university students. *Journal of American College Health* 60(5): 415–419.

Turner, B. J., A. L. Chapman, and B. K. Layden. 2012. Intrapersonal and interpersonal functions of nonsuicidal self-injury: Associations with emotional and social functioning. *Suicide & Life-Threatening Behavior* 42(1): 366–355.

U.S. Food and Drug Administration. 2012. *Medication Guide for Antidepressant Drugs* (http://www.fda.gov/downloads/Drugs/DrugSafety/InformationbyDrugClass/ucm100211.pdf).

Verhaak, P. F., et al. 2009. Receiving treatment for common mental disorders. *General Hospital Psychiatry* 31(1): 46–55.

Williams, D., et al. 2007. Prevalence and distribution of major depressive disorder in African Americans, Caribbean blacks, and non-Hispanic whites. *Archives of General Psychiatry* 64: 305–315.

Williams, J. 2014. "Inside the New York Times Book Review 'My Age of Anxiety.'" *New York Times,* January 24, 2014.

Shyness is often the result of both high anxiety levels and lack of key social skills. To help overcome shyness, you need to learn to manage your fear of social situations and to develop social skills such as appropriate eye contact, initiating topics in conversations, and maintaining the flow of conversations by asking questions and making appropriate responses.

As described in the chapter, repeated *exposure* to the source of your fear—in this case social situations—is the best method for reducing anxiety. When you practice new behaviors, they gradually become easier and you experience less anxiety.

A counterproductive strategy is avoiding situations that make you anxious. Although this approach works in the short term—you eliminate your anxiety because you escape the situation—it keeps you from meeting new people and having new experiences. Another counterproductive strategy is self-medicating with alcohol or drugs. Being under their influence actually prevents you from learning new social skills and new ways to handle your anxiety.

To reduce your anxiety in social situations, try some of the following strategies:

- Remember that physical stress reactions are short-term responses to fear. Don't dwell on them. Remind yourself that they will pass, and they will.

- Refocus your attention away from the stress reaction you're experiencing and toward the social task at hand. Your nervousness is much less visible than you think.

- Allow a warm-up period for new situations. Realize that you will feel more nervous at first, and take steps to relax and become more comfortable. Refer to the suggestions for deep breathing and other relaxation techniques in Chapter 2.

- If possible, take breaks during anxiety-producing situations. For example, if you're at a party, take a moment to visit the restroom or step outside. Alternate between speaking with good friends and striking up conversations with new acquaintances.

- Watch your interpretations. Having a stress reaction doesn't mean that you don't belong in the group, that you're unattractive or unworthy, or that the situation is too much for you. Try thinking of yourself as excited or highly alert instead of anxious.

- Avoid cognitive distortions and practice realistic self-talk. Replace your self-critical thoughts with more supportive ones: "No one else is perfect, and I don't have to be either." "It would have been good if I had a funny story to tell, but the conversation was interesting anyway."

- Give yourself a reality check: Ask if you're really in a life-threatening situation (or just at a party), if the outcome you're imagining is really likely (or the worst thing that could possibly happen), or if you're the only one who feels nervous (or if many other people might feel the same way).

- Don't think of conversations as evaluations. Remind yourself that you don't have to prove yourself with every social interaction. And remember that most people are thinking more about themselves than they are about you.

Starting and maintaining conversations can be difficult for shy people, who may feel overwhelmed by their physical stress reaction. If small talk is a problem for you, try the following strategies:

- Introduce yourself early in the conversation. If you tend to forget names, repeat your new acquaintance's name to help fix it in your mind ("Nice to meet you, Amelia").

- Ask questions and look for shared topics of interest. Simple, open-ended questions like "How's your presentation coming along?" or "How do you know our host?" encourage others to carry the conversation for a while and help bring up a variety of subjects.

- Take turns talking, and elaborate on your answers. Simple yes and no answers don't move the conversation along. Try to relate something in your life—a course you're taking or a hobby you have—to something in the other person's life. Match self-disclosure with self-disclosure.

- Have something to say. Expand your mind and become knowledgeable about current events and local or campus news. If you have specialized knowledge about a topic, practice discussing it in ways that both beginners and experts can understand and appreciate.

- If you get stuck for something to say, try giving a compliment ("Great presentation!" or "I love your earrings.") or performing a social grace (pass the chips or get someone a drink).

- Be an active listener. Reward the other person with your full attention and with regular responses. Make frequent eye contact and maintain a relaxed but alert posture. (See Chapter 4 for more on being an attentive listener.)

- At first, your new behaviors will likely make you anxious. Don't give up—things *will* get easier.

SOURCES: Aron, E. 2010. *The Undervalued Self.* Little, Brown, and Company; Brown, B. 2010. *The Gifts of Imperfection: Let Go of Who You Think You're Supposed to Be and Embrace Who You Are. Your Guide to a Wholehearted Life.* Center City, MN: Hazelden.

CHAPTER 4

CHAPTER OBJECTIVES

- Explain the qualities that help people develop intimate relationships
- Describe different types of love relationships and the stages they often go through
- Identify common challenges of forming and maintaining intimate relationships
- Explain some elements of healthy and productive communication
- Explain the similarities and differences between intimate partners and friends
- List some characteristics of successful families and some potential problems families face

Intimate Relationships and Communication

Human beings need social relationships; we cannot thrive as solitary creatures. Our survival as a species relies on our ability to cherish and support each other, form strong mutual attachments with each other, and create families in which to raise children. Simply put, people need people.

Although we are held together in relationships by a variety of factors, the foundation of many relationships is the ability to both give and receive love. Love in its many forms—romantic, passionate, platonic, parental—is the wellspring from which much of life's meaning and delight flows. In our human culture, love binds us together as partners, parents, children, and friends.

DEVELOPING INTIMATE RELATIONSHIPS

Successful intimate relationships depend on a belief in ourselves and the people around us. We must be willing to share our ideas, feelings, time, and needs and to accept what others want to give us in return. Just as important is the relationship we develop with ourselves—that is, how we generally feel about ourselves, which is the principal element that we bring to all our relationships. What does it mean to have a healthy relationship with ourself?

Self-Concept, Self-Esteem, and Self-Acceptance

To have successful relationships, we must first accept and feel good about ourselves. Having a healthy relationship with yourself means being able to self-soothe, regulate your emotions, and feel comfortable with your own company. The factors that contribute to a healthy sense of self include a positive *self-concept* (how you perceive your self), a healthy level of *self-esteem* (how you feel about your self) and an affirmative *self-acceptance* (how you value your self). Each of these factors allows us to love and respect others.

As discussed in Chapter 3, the roots of our identity and sense of self can be found in childhood, in the relationships we had with our parents and other family members. As adults, we are more likely to have a sense that we are basically lovable, and to view ourselves as worthwhile people who can trust others, if we had the following experiences as babies and children:

- We felt loved, valued, accepted, and respected.
- Adults responded to our needs in appropriate ways.
- Adults gave us the freedom to play, explore, and develop a sense of being separate individuals.

These conditions not only encourage us to develop a positive self-concept and healthy self-acceptance, they also contribute to a basic self-confidence that helps us navigate life's inevitable challenges.

Gender Role and Communication   We also learn in early childhood how to take on a *gender role*—the activities, abilities, and characteristics deemed culturally appropriate for us based on our sex.

In the past, cultural expectations for men have prescribed that they provide for their families; assume aggressive, competitive, and power-oriented behaviors; and solve problems logically. Women have been expected to take care of home and children; be cooperative, supportive, and nurturing; and approach life emotionally and intuitively.

As transgender and feminist movements have progressed, and women have succeeded into more positions of power, expectations are also changing. It is now common for women to work outside the home and for men to participate in more parenting. Studies have shown that girls do not necessarily play cooperatively and that what seemed so ingrained can be changed depending on the messages children receive from caregivers, mass media, and other institutions.

You may have heard that men and women speak different languages, and that this difference is cause for much conflict. Do men speak in a more logical way and women in a more emotional way? Although we can find patterns in some men's and some women's language, this observation does not fit the data of many studies on gendered communication. There is no gene for gendered language—we learn how to speak just as we learn how to become men and women, and we can decide in different situations to communicate differently.

For example, sociolinguist Penny Eckert finds that in early adolescence, girls start using their voices so that in one moment they speak in a very low pitch and in the next a very high one (think ambulance siren). Boys, on the other hand, decrease

their range in pitch, sounding relatively monotone (think robot). These changes represent ways that girls and boys differentiate themselves, preparing to participate in what Eckert calls a heterosexual market. They speak differently so as to fit in socially and to anticipate finding a mate.

Attachment   Another thing we learn in childhood is how to relate to others. Psychologists have suggested that our adult styles of loving may be based on the type of **attachment** we established in infancy with our mother, father, siblings, or other primary caregivers. According to this view, people who are secure in their intimate relationships probably had a secure, trusting, mutually satisfying attachment to their mother, father, or other parenting figure. As adults, they find it relatively easy to get close to others. They don't worry about being abandoned or having someone get too close to them. They feel that other people accept them and are generally well intentioned.

People who run from relationships may have experienced an "anxious/avoidant" attachment as children. In this type of attachment, a parent's responses were either engulfing or abandoning. Anxious/avoidant adults feel uncomfortable being close to others and seek escape from another's control. They're distrustful and fearful of becoming dependent upon and intimate with their partners.

Individuals who endured distant and aloof attachments as children can still establish satisfying relationships later in life. In fact, relationships established during adolescence and adulthood give us the opportunity to work through past

> **attachment**   The emotional tie between an infant and his or her caregiver or between two people in an intimate relationship.
>
> TERMS

The type and strength of our attachment to our parents can affect other relationships throughout our lives.

unresolved issues and conflicts. Human beings can be resilient and flexible. We have the capacity to change our ideas, beliefs, and behaviors. We can learn ways to raise our self-esteem and become more trusting, accepting, and appreciative of others and ourselves. We can acquire the communication and conflict-resolution skills needed to maintain successful relationships. Although it helps to have a good start in life, it may be even more important to begin again, right from where you are.

Friendship

Friendships are the first relationships we form outside the family. The friendships we form in childhood are an important part of our growth. Through them, we learn about tolerance, sharing, and trust. Friendships usually include the following characteristics:

- *Companionship.* The happy and relaxed feeling you have when you're with someone else is *companionship.* Friends typically share common values and interests and plan to spend time together.

- *Respect.* Friends have a basic respect for each other's individuality. Good friends respect each other's feelings and opinions and work to resolve their differences without demeaning or insulting each other. They also show their respect by expressing honest feelings.

- *Acceptance.* Friends accept each other "warts and all." They feel free to be themselves and express their feelings without fear of ridicule or criticism.

- *Help.* Friends know they can rely on each other in times of need. Help may include sharing time, energy, and even material goods.

- *Trust.* Friends are secure in the knowledge that they will not intentionally hurt each other. They feel safe confiding in one another.

- *Loyalty.* Friends can count on one another. In moments of challenge, a friend will stand up for his or her partner rather than join the opposition.

- *Mutuality.* Friends retain their individual identities, but close friendships are characterized by a sense of mutuality—"what affects you affects me." Friends share the ups and downs in each other's lives.

- *Reciprocity.* Friendships are reciprocal. There is give-and-take between friends and the feeling that both share joys and burdens more or less equally.

Intimate partnerships are like friendships in many ways, but they have additional characteristics. These relationships usually include sexual desire and expression, a greater demand for exclusiveness, and deeper levels of

caring. Friendships may be more stable and longer-lasting than intimate partnerships. Friends are often more accepting and less critical than lovers, perhaps because their expectations differ. Like love relationships, friendships bind society together, providing people with emotional support and buffering them from stress.

Love, Sex, and Intimacy

Love is one of the most basic and profound human emotions. It is a powerful force in all our intimate relationships. Love encompasses opposites: affection and anger, excitement and boredom, stability and change, bonds and freedom. Love does not give us perfect happiness, but it can give us more meaning in our lives.

In many kinds of adult relationships, love is closely affected by sexuality. In the past, marriage was considered the only acceptable context for sexual activities, but for many people today, sex is legitimized by love. Many couples, gay and straight, live together in committed relationships. We now use personal standards rather than social norms to make decisions about sex—but those norms are slowly changing.

For most people, love, sex, and commitment are closely linked. Love reflects the positive factors that draw people together and sustain their relationship. It includes trust, caring, respect, loyalty, interest in the other, and concern for the other's well-being. Sex brings excitement and passion to the relationship. It intensifies the relationship and adds fascination and pleasure.

Commitment contributes stability, which helps maintain a relationship. Responsibility, reliability, and faithfulness are characteristics of commitment. Although love, sex, and commitment are related, they are not necessarily connected. One can exist without the others. Despite the various "faces" of love, sex, and commitment, most of us long for a special relationship that contains them all.

Other elements can be identified as features of love, such as euphoria, preoccupation with the loved one, idealization or devaluation of the loved one, and so on, but these tend to be temporary. These characteristics may include **infatuation,** which will fade or deepen into something more substantial. As relationships progress, the central aspects of love and commitment take on more importance.

Psychologist Robert Sternberg proposed that love has three dimensions: intimacy, passion, and a commitment component (Figure 4.1). *Intimacy* refers to feelings of attachment, closeness, connectedness, and bondedness. *Passion* encompasses motivational drives and sexual attraction. *Commitment* relates to the decision to remain together with the ultimate goal of making long-term plans with that person.

infatuation An idealizing, obsessive attraction, characterized by a high degree of physical arousal. **TERMS**

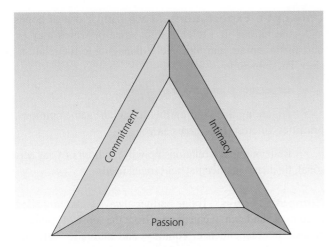

FIGURE 4.1 **The triangular theory of love.**

Different stages and types of love can be understood as different combinations of the three dimensions. Ultimately a relationship based on a single element is less likely to survive than one based on two or three dimensions.

Researchers suggest that men and women have different views of the relationship between love (intimacy) and sex (passion). Although many men report that their most erotic sexual experiences occur in the context of a love relationship, many studies have found that men can separate love from sex more easily than women. Women generally view sex from the point of view of a relationship. Some people believe you can have satisfying sex without love—with friends, acquaintances, or strangers. Although sex with love is an important norm in our culture, it is frequently disregarded in practice, as the high incidence of extrarelational affairs attests.

The Pleasure and Pain of Love The experience of intense love has confused and tormented lovers throughout history. They live in a tumultuous state of excitement, subject to wildly fluctuating feelings of joy and despair. They lose their appetite, can't sleep, and can think of nothing but the loved one. Is this happiness? Misery? Both?

The contradictory nature of passionate love can be understood by recognizing that human emotions have two components: physiological arousal and an emotional explanation for the arousal. Love is just one of many emotions accompanied by physiological arousal. Many unpleasant emotions can also generate arousal, such as fear, rejection, frustration, and challenge. Although experiences like attraction and sexual desire are pleasant, extreme excitement is similar to fear and can be unpleasant. For this reason, passionate love may be too intense for some people to enjoy. Over time, the physical intensity and excitement tend to diminish. When this happens, pleasure may actually increase.

The Transformation of Love Human relationships change over time, and love relationships are no exception. At first, love is likely to be characterized by high levels of passion and rapidly increasing intimacy. After a while

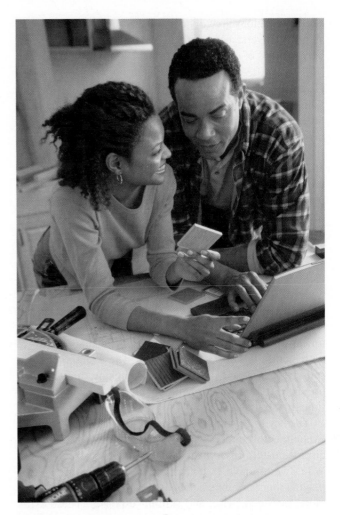

Although passion and physical intimacy often decline with time, other aspects of a relationship—such as commitment—tend to grow as the relationship matures.

passion decreases as we become habituated to it and to the person. The diminishing of romance or passionate love is often experienced as a crisis in a relationship. If a more lasting love fails to emerge, the relationship will likely break up.

Unlike passion, however, commitment does not necessarily diminish over time. When intensity diminishes, partners often discover a more enduring love. They can now move from absorption in each other to a relationship that includes external goals and projects, friends, and family. In this kind of intimate, more secure love, satisfaction comes not just from the relationship itself but also from achieving other creative goals, such as work or child rearing. The key to successful relationships is in transforming passion into an intimate love based on closeness, caring, and the promise of a shared future.

Challenges in Relationships

Many people believe that love naturally makes an intimate relationship easy to begin and maintain, but in fact obstacles arise and challenges occur. Even in the best of circumstances, a loving relationship will be tested. Partners enter a relationship with diverse needs and desires, some of which emerge only at times of change or stress.

Honesty and Openness

At the beginning of a relationship most of us prefer to present ourselves in the most favorable light. Although sharing thoughts and feelings can be emotionally risky, honesty is necessary to achieve the freedom for the next step of the relationship. Over time, you and your partner will learn more about each other and feel more comfortable sharing. In fact, intimate familiarity with your partner's life is a key characteristic of successful long-term relationships.

Emotional Intelligence

In his book *Emotional Intelligence—Why It Can Matter More Than IQ,* Daniel Goleman argues that classical IQ is *not* destiny and that our traditional view of intelligence is too narrow. He asserts that the traditional view ignores a range of abilities vital to how well we function in life. Goleman illuminates the factors at work when people with high IQs flounder and those with modest IQs do remarkably well. These factors include self-awareness, self-discipline, and empathy, and they add up to a different way of being intelligent known as "emotionally intelligent."

The key to developing emotional intelligence lies in cultivating the overarching skill of mindfulness—the ability to dispassionately observe thoughts and feelings as they occur. When we are able to note and observe emotions without judging them or immediately acting on them, we can make more measured, wise, and skillful responses. These skills can be particularly helpful when we are involved in an argument or a conflict with someone with whom we have a close personal relationship.

Mindfulness can be cultivated by paying more attention to the operation of our minds, slowing down our lives enough to make more detailed observations, and staying in the moment as we go about our day-to-day activities. Although we often have limited control over external events, we have a great deal of ability to discipline, focus, and train our minds. Practicing mindfulness and developing emotional intelligence will improve your sense of self and the quality of your relationships, and may even result in the peace of mind that many people find so elusive.

Unequal or Premature Commitment

When one person in an intimate partnership becomes more serious about the relationship than the other, it can be difficult to maintain it without someone feeling hurt. Sometimes a couple makes a premature commitment, and then one of the partners has second thoughts and wants to break off the relationship. Eventually both partners recognize that something is wrong, but each is afraid to tell the other. It may be painful but necessary to resolve this conflict by stepping up and saying, "We have a problem, can we have an honest talk about it?" Such problems usually can be resolved only by honest and sensitive communication.

Unrealistic Expectations

Each partner brings hopes and expectations to a relationship, some of which may be unrealistic, unfair, and ultimately damaging to the relationship. These include:

- Expecting your partner to change.

- Assuming that your partner has all the same opinions, priorities, interests, and goals as you.

- Believing that a relationship will fulfill all of your personal, financial, intellectual, and social needs.

Competitiveness

If one partner always feels compelled to compete and win, it can detract from the sense of connectedness, interdependence, equality, and mutuality between partners. The same can be said for a perfectionistic need to be right in every instance—to "win" every argument.

If competitiveness is a problem for you, ask yourself if your need to win is more important than your partner's feelings or the future of your relationship. Try noncompetitive activities or an activity where you are a beginner and your partner excels. Accept that your partner's views may be just as valid and important to your partner as your own views are to you.

Balancing Time Together and Apart

You may enjoy time together with your partner, but you may also want to spend time alone or with other friends. If you or your partner interpret time apart as rejection or lack of commitment, it can damage the relationship. Talk with your partner about what time apart means and share your feelings about what you expect from the relationship in terms of time together. Consider your partner's feelings carefully, and try to reach a compromise that satisfies both of you.

Differences in expectations about time spent together can mirror differences in ideas about emotional closeness. Any romantic relationship involves giving up some degree of autonomy in order to develop an identity as a couple. But remember that every person is unique and has different needs for distance and closeness in a relationship.

Jealousy

Jealousy is the angry, painful response to a partner's real, imagined, or possible involvement with a third person. Some people think that the existence of jealousy proves the existence of love, but jealousy is actually a sign of insecurity or possessiveness.

In its irrational and extreme forms, jealousy can destroy a relationship by its insistent demands and attempts at control. Jealousy is a factor in precipitating violence in dating relationships among both high school and college students, and abusive spouses often use jealousy to justify their violence.

People with a healthy level of self-esteem are less likely to feel jealous. When jealousy occurs in a relationship, it's important for the partners to communicate clearly with each other about their feelings. In this sense, jealousy can offer partners the chance to look closely at issues like possessiveness, insecurity, and low self-esteem and thereby strengthen the relationship by working through jealousy.

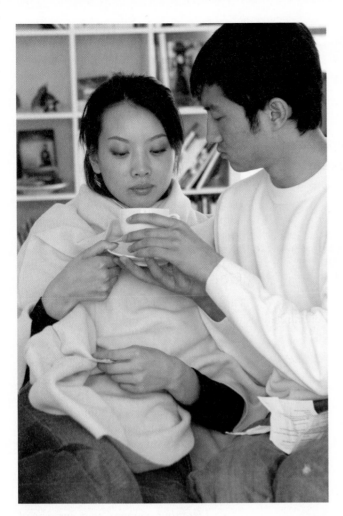

Supportiveness is a sign of commitment and compassion and is an important part of any healthy relationship.

Supportiveness   Another key to successful relationships is the ability to ask for and give support. Partners need to know that they can count on each other during difficult times.

Unhealthy Relationships

Everyone should be able to recognize when a relationship is unhealthy. Relatively extreme examples of unhealthy relationships are those that are physically or emotionally abusive or that involve codependency.

Even relationships that are not abusive or codependent can still be unhealthy. If your relationship lacks love and respect and places little value on the time you and your partner have spent together, it may be time to get professional help or to end the partnership. Further, if your relationship is characterized by communication styles that include criticism, contempt, defensiveness, and withdrawal—despite real efforts to repair these destructive patterns—the relationship may not be salvageable.

Spiritual leaders suggest that relationships are unhealthy when you feel that your sense of spontaneity, your potential for inner growth and joy, and your connection to your spiritual life is deadened. There are negative physical and mental consequences of being in an unhappy relationship. Although breaking up is painful and difficult, it is ultimately better than living in a toxic relationship.

Ending a Relationship

Even when a couple starts out with the best of intentions, an intimate relationship may not last. Some breakups occur quickly following direct action by one or both partners, but many occur over an extended period as the couple goes through a cycle of separating and reconciling.

Ending an intimate relationship is usually difficult and painful. Both partners may feel attacked and abandoned, but feelings of distress are likely to be more acute for the rejected partner. If you are involved in a breakup, the following suggestions may help make the ending easier:

- Give the relationship a fair chance before breaking up.

- Be fair and honest.

- Be tactful and compassionate, and admit your own contributions to the problem.

- If you are the rejected person, give yourself time to resolve your anger and pain.

- Recognize the value in the experience.

Use the recovery period following a breakup for self-renewal. Redirect more of your attention to yourself, and reconnect with people and areas of your life that may have been neglected as a result of the relationship. Time will help heal the pain of the loss of the relationship.

Finally, be aware of the tendency or impulse to "rebound" quickly into another relationship. Although a new relationship may mute the pain of a breakup, forming a relationship in order to avoid feeling pain is not a good strategy. Too often, rebound relationships fail because they were designed to be "lifeboats" or because one or both of the partners is not truly ready to be close to someone else again.

COMMUNICATION

The key to developing and maintaining any type of intimate relationship is good communication. Miscommunication creates frustration and distances us from our friends and partners.

Nonverbal Communication

Even when we're silent, we're communicating. We send messages when we look at someone or look away, lean forward or sit back, smile or frown. Especially important forms of nonverbal communication are touch, eye contact, and proximity. If someone we're talking to touches our hand or arm, looks into our eyes, and leans toward us when we talk, we get the message that the person is interested in us and cares about what we're saying. If a person keeps looking around the room while we're talking or takes a step backward, we get the impression the person is uninterested or wants to end the conversation.

The ability to interpret nonverbal messages correctly is important to the success of relationships. It's also important, when sending messages, to make sure our body language agrees with our words. When our verbal and nonverbal messages don't correspond, we send a mixed message.

Attunement, or tuning into each other's tone of voice, is important. More than any other cue, tone of voice conveys most accurately a person's emotional state. Our effectiveness at connecting or reconnecting emotionally with another depends on the accuracy of our attunement.

How we feel when communicating with another can give the listener important data about the speaker. If "out of nowhere" we begin to feel sad, anxious, or angry, it's possible that these are emotional states the other person is communicating. A simple example would be feeling sad when communicating with a grieving friend.

Digital Communication and Our Social Networks

The Internet enables us to communicate more rapidly, but some experts question whether this capability is affecting interpersonal relations generally and, specifically, our ability to relate to others in person. In 2011 psychologist Sherry Turkle argued that Internet, texting, and other electronic means are alienating and damaging to "real-world" relationships.

But surveys by the Pew Internet and American Life Project found that technology users had larger and more diverse core discussion networks and were just as involved in their communities as people who communicate face-to-face.

QUICK STATS

32.2% of college students say their intimate relationships have been traumatic or hard to handle at least once in the past year.

—American College Health Association, 2011

The Internet is a tool that affords certain—though wide-ranging—types of communication (the brief immediacy of a tweet is very different from an extended conversation over Skype). People worry about the effect of the technologies because they change our environment and the size and makeup of our social networks. But for many who are long distance or who have little time to see each other face-to-face, digital communication is crucial and maintains some relationships that would otherwise be altogether lost.

Communication Skills

Three skills essential to good communication in relationships are self-disclosure, listening, and feedback:

- *Self-disclosure* involves revealing personal information that we ordinarily wouldn't reveal because of the risk involved. It usually increases feelings of closeness and moves the relationship to a deeper level of intimacy. Friends often disclose the most to each other, sharing feelings, experiences, hopes, and disappointments. Married couples sometimes share less and may make unwarranted assumptions because they think they already know everything about each other.

The sources of conflict for couples change over time but primarily revolve around these issues: **finances, sex, children, in-laws, and housework.**

- *Listening* requires that we spend more time and energy trying to fully understand another person's "story" and less time judging, evaluating, blaming, advising, analyzing, or trying to control. Empathy, warmth, respect, and genuineness are qualities of skillful listeners. Attentive listening encourages friends or partners to share more and, in turn, to be attentive listeners. To connect with other people and develop real emotional intimacy, listening is essential.

- *Feedback*, a constructive response to another's self-disclosure, is the third key to good communication. Giving positive feedback means acknowledging that the friend's or partner's feelings are valid—no matter how upsetting or troubling—and offering self-disclosure in response. If, for example, your partner discloses unhappiness about your relationship, it is more constructive to say that you're concerned or saddened by that and want to hear more about it than to get angry, blame, try to inflict pain, or withdraw. Self-disclosure and feedback can open the door to change, whereas other responses block communication and change. (For tips on improving your skills, see the box "Guidelines for Effective Communication.")

Ask Yourself

QUESTIONS FOR CRITICAL THINKING AND REFLECTION

Have you ever ended an intimate relationship? If so, how did you handle it? How did you feel after the breakup? How did the breakup affect your former partner? Did the experience help you in other relationships?

Getting Started

- When you want to have a serious discussion with your partner, choose a private place and a time when you won't be interrupted or rushed.

- Face your partner and maintain eye contact. Use nonverbal feedback to show that you are interested and involved.

Being an Effective Speaker

- State your concern or issue as clearly as you can.

- Use "I" statements rather than statements beginning with "you." When you use "I" statements, you take responsibility for your feelings. "You" statements are often blaming or accusatory and will probably get a defensive or resentful response. The statement "I feel unloved," for example, sends a clearer, less blaming message than the statement "You don't love me."

- Focus on a behavior, not the whole person. Be specific about the behavior you like or don't like. Avoid generalizations beginning with "you always" or "you never." Such statements make people feel defensive.

- Make constructive requests. Opening your request with "I would like" keeps the focus on your needs rather than your partner's supposed deficiencies.

- Avoid blaming, accusing, and belittling. Even if you are right, you have little to gain by putting your partner down. When people feel criticized or attacked, they are less able to think rationally or solve problems constructively.

- Ask for action ahead of time, not after the fact. Tell your partner what you would like to have happen in the future; don't wait for him or her to blow it and then express anger or disappointment.

Being an Effective Listener

- Provide appropriate nonverbal feedback (nodding, smiling, making eye contact, and so on).

- Don't interrupt.

- Listen reflectively. Don't judge, evaluate, analyze, or offer solutions (unless asked to do so). Your partner may just need to sort out his or her feelings. By jumping in to "fix" the problem, you may cut off communication.

- Don't give unsolicited advice. Giving advice implies that you know more about what a person needs to do than she or he does; therefore, it often evokes anger or resentment.

- Clarify your understanding of what your partner is saying by restating it in your own words and asking if your understanding is correct. "I think you're saying that you would feel uncomfortable having dinner with my parents and that you'd prefer to meet them in a more casual setting. Is that right?" This type of specific feedback prevents misunderstandings and helps validate the speaker's feelings and message.

- Be sure you are really listening, not off somewhere in your mind rehearsing your reply. Try to tune in to your partner's feelings as well as the words. Accurately reflecting the other person's feelings is often a more powerful way of connecting than just reframing his or her thoughts.

- Let your partner know that you value what he or she is saying and want to understand. Respect for the other person is the cornerstone of effective communication.

Conflict and Conflict Resolution

Conflict is natural in intimate relationships. No matter how close two people become, they still remain separate individuals with their own needs, desires, past experiences, and ways of seeing the world. In fact, the closer the relationship, the more differences and the more opportunities for conflict.

Conflict itself isn't dangerous to a relationship. In fact, it may indicate that the relationship is growing. But if it isn't handled constructively, conflict can damage—and ultimately destroy—the relationship.

Conflict is often accompanied by anger—a natural emotion—but one that can be difficult to handle. If we express anger aggressively, we risk creating distrust, fear, and distance. If we act it out without thinking things through, we can cause the conflict to escalate. If we suppress anger, it turns into resentment and hostility. The best way to handle anger in a relationship is to recognize it as a symptom of

something that requires attention and needs to be changed. When angry, partners should exercise restraint so as not to become abusive. It is important to express anger skillfully and not in a way that is out of proportion to the issue at hand. The best time to express yourself is almost certainly when you are not boiling over with strong emotions.

The sources of conflict for couples change over time but primarily revolve around these issues: finances, sex, children, in-laws, and housework.

Although there are numerous theories on and approaches to conflict resolution, the following strategies can be helpful; just remember that different couples communicate in different ways around conflict.

1. *Clarify the issue.* Take responsibility for thinking through your feelings and discovering what's really bothering you. Agree that one partner will speak first and have the chance to speak fully while the other listens.

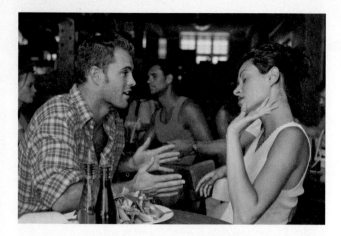

Conflict is an inevitable part of any intimate relationship. How can we resolve our conflicts in constructive ways?

Then reverse the roles. Try to understand your partner's position fully by repeating what you've heard and asking questions to clarify or elicit more information. Agree to talk only about the topic at hand and not get distracted by other issues. Sum up what your partner has said.

2. *Find out what each person wants.* Ask your partner to express his or her desires. Don't assume you know what your partner wants, and don't speak for him or her.

3. *Determine how you both can get what you want.* Brainstorm to come up with a variety of options.

4. *Decide how to negotiate.* Work out a plan for change. For example, one partner will do one task and the other will do another task. Be willing to compromise, and avoid trying to "win."

5. *Solidify the agreements.* If necessary, go over the plan and write it down, to ensure that you both understand and agree to it.

6. *Review and renegotiate.* Decide on a time frame for trying out your plan, and set a time to discuss how it's working. Make adjustments as needed.

To resolve conflicts, partners have to feel safe in voicing disagreements. They have to trust that the discussion won't get out of control, that they won't be abandoned, and that the partner won't take advantage of their vulnerability. Partners should follow some basic ground rules when they argue, such as avoiding ultimatums, resisting the urge to give the silent treatment, refusing to "hit below the belt," and not using sex to smooth over disagreements.

When you argue, maintain a spirit of goodwill and avoid being harshly critical or contemptuous. Remember—you care about your partner and want things to work out. See the disagreement as a difficulty that the two of you have together rather than as something your partner does to you. Finish serious discussions on a positive note by expressing your respect and affection for your partner and your appreciation for having been listened to. If you and your partner find that you argue again and again over the same issue, it may be better to stop trying to resolve that problem and instead come to accept the differences between you.

PAIRING AND SINGLEHOOD

Although most people eventually marry or commit to a partner, everyone spends some time as a single person, and nearly all people make some attempt, consciously or unconsciously, to find a partner. Intimate relationships are as important for singles as for couples.

Choosing a Partner

Most men and women select partners for long-term relationships through a fairly predictable process, although they may not be consciously aware of it. First attraction is based on easily observable characteristics: looks, dress, social status, and reciprocated interest. Studies have shown that most people pair with someone who

- Lives in the same geographic area
- Comes from a similar ethnic and socio-economic background
- Has a similar educational status
- Leads a lifestyle like theirs
- Has (what they think is) the same level of physical attractiveness as themselves

Once the euphoria of romantic love winds down, personality traits and behaviors become more significant factors in how partners view each other. The emphasis shifts to basic values and future aspirations regarding career, family, and children. At some point, they decide whether the relationship feels viable and is worthy of their continued commitment.

Perhaps the most important question for potential mates to ask is, "How much do we have in common?" Although differences add interest to a relationship, similarities increase the chances of a relationship's success. Differences can affect a relationship in the areas of values, religion, ethnicity, attitudes toward sexuality and gender roles, socioeconomic status, familiarity with each other's culture, and interactions with the extended family. But acceptance and communication skills go a long way toward making a relationship work, no matter how different the partners.

Dating

Every culture has certain rituals for pairing and finding mates. Parent-arranged marriages, still the norm in many cultures, are often stable and permanent. Although the American cultural norm is personal choice in courtship and

> An important question for potential mates to ask is, **"How much do we have in common?"**

Physical attraction plays a strong role in the initial choosing of a partner. People tend to gravitate toward others who share similar characteristics, such as appearance, ethnicity, education, and socioeconomic background.

For many college students today, group activities have replaced dating as a way to meet and get to know potential partners.

mate selection, the popularity of dating services and online matchmaking suggests that many people want help finding a suitable partner.

Many people find romantic partners through some form of dating. They narrow the field through a process of getting to know each other. Dating often revolves around a mutually enjoyable activity, such as seeing a movie or having dinner. Casual dating may then evolve into steady or exclusive dating, then engagement, and finally marriage.

In recent years, traditional dating has given way to a more casual form of getting together in groups. Two people may begin to spend more time together, but often with other couples or groups. If sexual involvement develops, it is more likely to be based on friendship, respect, and common interests than on expectations related to gender roles. In this model, mate selection may progress from getting together to living together to marriage.

Among some teenagers and young adults, dating has been supplanted by *hooking up*—casual sexual activity without any relationship commitment. For more about this trend, see the box "Hooking Up."

Online Relationships

Connecting with people online has advantages and drawbacks. It allows people to communicate in a relaxed way, try out different personas, and share things they might not share when face-to-face with family or friends. It's easier to put yourself out there without too much investment; you can get to know someone from the comfort of your own home, set your own pace, and start and end relationships at any time. With millions of singles using dating sites that let them describe exactly what they are seeking, the Internet can increase a person's chance of finding a good match.

QUICK STATS

40 million adult Americans have tried using an online dating service.

—Statistic Brain, 2012

However, participants often misrepresent themselves, pretending to be very different—older or younger or even of a different sex—than they really are. Investing time and emotional resources in such relationships can be painful. In rare cases, online romances become dangerous or even deadly.

Because people have greater freedom to reveal only what they want to, users should also be aware of a greater tendency to idealize online partners. If your online friend seems perfect, take that as a warning sign. You may search for perfection, find fault quickly, and not give people a chance; conversely, you may act on impulse with insufficient information.

Relationship sites also remove an important and powerful source of information from the process: chemistry and in-person intuition. Much of our communication is transmitted through body language and tone, which aren't obvious in text messages and can't fully be captured even by web cams and microphones. Consider these questions. Are you comfortable in disclosing personal information about yourself? Is there a balance in the amount of time spent talking by each of you? Is the other person

Hooking Up

A current trend among teenagers, young adults, and college students is *hooking up*—having casual sexual encounters with acquaintances or strangers with no commitment or investment in a relationship. The sexual activity can be anything from kissing to intercourse, but the key element is the lack of emotional intimacy. Although casual sex is not new, the difference today is that hooking up seems to be the main form of sexual activity for many people, as opposed to sexual activity within a relationship. Some data indicate that more than 80% of college students have had at least one hookup experience. If dating occurs at all, it happens after people have had sex and become a couple.

Hooking up most likely has its roots in the changing social and sexual patterns of the 1960s. Since then, changes in college policies have contributed to the shift, such as the move away from colleges acting *in loco parentis* (in the place of parents), the trend toward coed dorms, and the increase in the percentage of women in student populations and the decreased availability of men. This behavior addresses the desire for "instant intimacy," but also protects the participants from the risk or responsibility of emotional involvement.

Because hooking up is often fueled by alcohol, it is associated with sexual risk taking and negative health effects, including the risk of acquiring a sexually transmitted disease. According to the Centers for Disease Control and Prevention (CDC) in 2007, young adults aged 15 to 24 had rates of chlamydia that were 4 to 5.5 times the overall incidence rate for the general population. Hooking up can also have adverse emotional and mental health consequences, including sexual regret, negative emotional reactions, psychological distress, depression, and anxiety. Women are more likely to suffer these reactions after hooking up, but men experience them too. Biological anthropologists suggest that having sex—even casual sex—sets off hormones that cause feelings of bonding and attachment, which are inevitably thwarted in a hookup.

On some campuses, a backlash against hooking up has taken place. In some cases, individuals are deciding they don't want to be part of the hookup culture. In other cases, groups and organizations have formed to call for a return to traditional dating or at least some middle ground between dating and hooking up that doesn't have the potential to cause physical and emotional distress.

SOURCES: Downing-Matibag, T. M., and B. Geisenger. 2009. Hooking up and sexual risk taking among college students: a health belief model perspective. *Qualitative Health Research* 19(9): 1196–1209; Bachtel, M. Is dating really dead? Emerging evidence on the college hookup culture and health issues. *Action Newsletter, American College Health Association* 49(2): 16–18; Chen, S. 2010. No hooking up, no sex for some coeds (http://www.cnn.com/2010/LIVING/04/19/college.anti.hookup.culture/index.html?hpt Sbin).

respecting your boundaries? Just as in face-to-face dating, online relationships require you to use common sense and to trust your instincts.

If you pursue an online relationship, the following may help you have a positive experience and stay safe:

• To improve your chances of meeting people interested in you as a person, avoid sexually oriented websites. Some sites that seem like dating sites are actually used for "hooking up"—that is, arranging meetings for casual sex—rather than for building relationships. Inspect each site thoroughly before registering or providing any information about yourself. If you aren't comfortable with a site's content or purpose, close your web browser and clear out its cache and its store of cookies. (If you don't know how to do this, check your browser's help section for instructions.)

• Know what you are looking for as well as what you can offer someone else. If you are looking for a relationship, make that fact clear. Find out the other person's intentions.

• Don't post photos unless you are completely comfortable with potential consequences (e.g., they might be downloaded by others).

• Don't give out personal information, including your real full name, school, or place of employment, until you feel sure that you are giving the information to someone who is trustworthy.

• Set up a second e-mail account for sending and receiving dating-related e-mails.

• If someone does not respond to a message, don't take it personally. There are many reasons why a person may not pursue the connection. Don't send messages to an unresponsive person; doing so could lead to an accusation of stalking. If someone stops responding, drop the interaction completely.

• Before deciding whether to meet an online friend in person, arrange to talk over the phone a few times.

• Don't agree to meet someone face-to-face unless you feel comfortable about it. Always meet initially in a very public place—a museum, a coffee shop, or a restaurant. Consider bringing along a friend to increase your safety, and let others know where you will be.

If you pursue online relationships, don't let them interfere with your other personal relationships and social activities. Online dating can become addictive. To protect your emotional and personal wellness, use the Internet to widen your circle of friends, not shrink it.

Living Together

According to the U.S. Census Bureau, about 5.4 million opposite-sex couples and 700,000 same-sex couples live together in the United States. The Human Rights Campaign, however, estimates that the number of same-sex couples in the United States is closer to 1.6 million. Living together, or **cohabitation,** is one of the most rapid and dramatic social changes that has occurred in our society. By age 30, about half of all men and women will have cohabited. Several factors are involved in this change, including greater acceptance of premarital sex, increased availability of contraceptives, the tendency for people to wait longer before getting married, and a larger pool of single and divorced individuals.

Are there advantages to living together over marriage? For one thing, it may give the partners a greater sense of autonomy. Not bound by the social rules and expectations that are part of marriage, partners may find it easier to keep their identities and more of their independence. Cohabitation doesn't incur the same obligations as marriage. If things don't work out, the partners may find it easier to leave a relationship that hasn't been legally sanctioned.

But living together has drawbacks, too. In many cases, the legal protections of marriage are absent, such as health insurance benefits and property and inheritance rights. These considerations can be particularly serious if the couple has children. Couples may feel social or family pressure to marry or otherwise change their living arrangements, especially if they have young children. The general trend, however, is toward legitimizing nonmarital partnerships; for example, some employers, communities, and states now extend benefits to unmarried domestic partners.

Although many people choose cohabitation as a kind of trial marriage, unmarried partnerships tend to be less stable than marriages. A 2010 survey conducted by the National Center for Health Statistics revealed that cohabitation is much less likely than marriage to survive the one-, three-, and five-year milestones.

Same-Sex Partnerships

Regardless of **sexual orientation,** most people look for love in a committed relationship. Gay couples have many similarities with **straight** couples. According to one study, most gay men and lesbians have experienced at least one long-term relationship with a single partner. Like any intimate relationship, same-sex partnerships provide intimacy, passion, and security.

Same-sex partnerships tend to be more egalitarian (equal) and less organized around traditional gender roles. Same-sex couples put greater emphasis on partnership than on role assignment. Domestic tasks are shared or split, and both partners usually support themselves financially.

Another difference between straight (heterosexual) and gay (homosexual) relationships is that same-sex partners often have to deal with societal hostility or ambivalence toward their relationship, in contrast to the societal approval and rights given to heterosexual couples (see the box "Same-Sex

Marriage and Civil Unions"). *Homophobia,* which is fear or hatred of homosexuals, can be obvious, as in the case of violence or discrimination, or subtle, such as how same-sex couples are portrayed in the media. Additional stress can arise if an LGB (lesbian, gay, or bisexual) individual belongs to a family or ethnic group that doesn't accept her or his sexual orientation.

People with diverse sexual orientations and gender identities are often grouped together in the category "LGBT," "LGBTQ," or "LGBTQI," where T is for transgender, Q is for questioning or queer, and I is for intersex. Transgender individuals—people whose biological sex doesn't match their gender identity—and intersex individuals—people born with ambiguous genitals—may be heterosexual, homosexual, or bisexual, or they may feel that current definitions of sexual orientation and gender are too narrow to apply to them.

Singlehood

Despite the popularity of marriage, a significant and growing number of adults in our society never marry. Currently more than 116 million single individuals—the largest group of unmarried adults—have never been married (Figure 4.2).

Several factors contribute to the growing number of single people. One is the changing view of singlehood, which is increasingly being viewed as a legitimate alternative to marriage. Education and careers are delaying the age at which young people are marrying. The median age for marriage is now 28.2 years for men and 26.1 years for women. More young people are living with their parents as they complete their education, seek jobs, or strive for financial independence. Many other single people live together without being married. Gay people who would marry their partners if they were legally permitted to do so are counted among the single population. High divorce rates mean more singles, and people who have experienced divorce may have more negative attitudes about marriage and more positive attitudes about singlehood.

Being single, however, does not mean living without the benefit of close relationships. Single people date, enjoy active and fulfilling social lives, and have a variety of sexual

cohabitation   Living together in a sexual relationship without being married.   TERMS

sexual orientation   A consistent pattern of emotional and sexual attraction based on biological sex; it exists along a continuum that ranges from exclusive heterosexuality (attraction to people of the other sex) through bisexuality (attraction to people of both sexes) to exclusive homosexuality (attraction to people of one's own sex).

Straight   Attraction to people of the other sex; heterosexual.

In its legal definitions, marriage is an institution in which couples derive legal and economic rights and responsibilities from state and federal statutes. The U.S. General Accountability Office says more than 1000 federal laws make distinctions based on marriage. Marital status affects many aspects of life, such as social security benefits, federal tax status, inheritance, and medical decision making.

The push for legal recognition of same-sex partnerships has gone on for decades. Supporters of same-sex marriage rights have met opposition at the local, state, and federal levels, in both the public and private sectors. However, on June 26, 2013, the U.S. Supreme Court ruled that the federal government must recognize same-sex marriages performed by states that allow them. At the time of this writing, 20 states have legalized same-sex marriage—nine by court decision, eight through state legislature, and three by popular vote. The recent rulings by federal judges affect several federal rights, one of which is that a U.S. citizen may now petition for a same-sex spouse to immigrate to the United States. Although the majority of states (31 at the time of this writing) have passed laws and amendments that effectively ban same-sex marriage, challenges to these bans are working their way through the judicial system.

Opponents of civil unions and same-sex marriage offer several arguments

against such unions. For example, opponents claim that the purpose of marriage is to procreate, that the Bible forbids same-sex unions, that homosexuals are seeking special rights, that same-sex unions are bad for children and families, and that most Americans oppose such unions. The primary argument is that same-sex marriage undermines the sanctity and validity of marriage as it is traditionally understood and thus undermines society. The underlying assumption of this position is that homosexual behavior is a choice and that people can change their orientation, though the process may be difficult.

Proponents of civil unions and same-sex marriage believe that sexual orientation is outside the control of the individual and results from genetic and environmental factors that create an unchangeable orientation. The issue of same-sex union is then seen as one of basic civil rights, in which a group is being denied rights—to publicly express their commitment to one another, to provide security for their children, and to receive the legal and economic benefits afforded to married heterosexual couples—on the basis of something as unalterable as skin color. According to a 2013 Gallup poll, public opinion in favor of allowing same-sex couples to marry has more than doubled since 1997 and now constitutes a clear majority.

Opponents and proponents of same-sex marriage agree that marriage is healthy for both men and women and is the main social institution promoting family values.

SOURCES: ProCon.org. 2014. *Gay Marriage.* (http://gaymarriage.procon.org/view.resource. php?resourceID=004857); U.S. Government Accountability Office. 2004. *Defense of Marriage Act: Update to Prior Report.* (http://www.gao.gov/products/GAO-04-353R).

connect™
ACTIVITY
DO IT ONLINE

---

experiences and relationships. Other advantages of being single include more opportunities for personal and career development without concern for family obligations and more freedom and control in making life choices. Disadvantages include a lack of companionship and loneliness, as well as economic hardships (particularly for single women). Single men and women alike experience some discrimination and often are pressured to get married.

Nearly every adult has at least one episode of being single, whether prior to marriage, between marriages, following divorce or the death of a spouse, or for his or her entire life. How enjoyable and valuable this single time is

depends on several factors, including how deliberately the person has chosen it; how satisfied the person is with his or her social relationships, standard of living, and job; how comfortable the person feels when alone; and how resourceful and energetic the person is about creating an interesting and fulfilling life.

MARRIAGE

The majority of Americans marry at some time in their lives. Marriage continues to remain popular because it satisfies several basic needs. There are many important social, moral, economic, and political aspects of

> **QUICK STATS**
>
> Just over **2 million** marriages took place in the United States in 2009.
>
> —National Center for Health Statistics, 2010

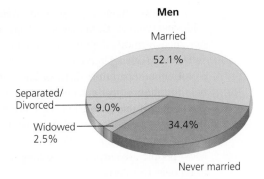

Men

Married

52.1%

Separated/Divorced —— 9.0%

Widowed 2.5%

34.4%

Never married

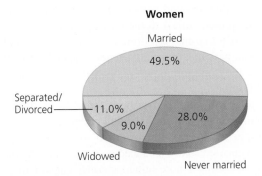

Women

Married

49.5%

Separated/Divorced —— 11.0%

9.0%

28.0%

Widowed

Never married

FIGURE 4.2 Marital status of the U.S. population aged 15 years and older, 2011.

U.S. Census Bureau. 2012. *America's Families and Living Arrangements: 2011* (http://www.census.gov/population/www/socdemo/hh-fam/cps2011.html).

marriage, all of which have changed over the years. In the past people married mainly for practical reasons, such as raising children or forming an economic unit. Today people marry more for personal, emotional reasons.

The Benefits of Marriage

The primary functions and benefits of marriage are those of any intimate relationship: affection, personal affirmation, companionship, sexual fulfillment, and emotional growth. Marriage also provides a setting in which to raise children, although an increasing number of couples choose to remain childless, and people can also choose to raise children without being married. Marriage is also important for providing for the future. By committing themselves to the relationship, people establish themselves with lifelong companions as well as some insurance for their later years.

Research shows that good marriages have myriad positive effects on individuals' health.

Issues and Trends in Marriage

Marital roles and responsibilities have undergone profound changes over time. Many husbands share domestic tasks, and many wives work outside the home. While women still take most of the responsibility for home and children even when they work, and while men still suffer more job-related stress

Ask Yourself

QUESTIONS FOR CRITICAL THINKING AND REFLECTION

How do you define "commitment" in a relationship? Is it simply a matter of staying faithful to a partner, or is there more? In your own relationships, what signs of commitment do you look for from your partner? What signs of commitment does your partner see in you?

and health problems than women do, the trend is toward an equalization of responsibilities in the home.

What about love? Although we might like to believe otherwise, love is not enough to make a successful marriage. The recognition of this has led to some recent trends in marriage, including couples choosing not to marry, couples marrying later–after a lengthy cohabitation, and couples marrying without a formal marriage certificate.

The following relationship characteristics appear to be the best predictors of a happy marriage:

- The partners have realistic expectations about their relationship.
- Each feels good about the personality of the other.
- Partners develop friendships with other couples.
- They communicate well.
- They have effective ways of resolving conflicts.
- They agree on religious/ethical values.
- They have an egalitarian role relationship.
- They have a good balance of individual versus joint interests and leisure activities.

Once married, couples must provide each other with emotional support, negotiate and establish marital roles, establish domestic and career priorities, handle their finances, make sexual adjustments, manage boundaries and relationships with their extended family, and participate in the larger community.

The Role of Commitment

Studies show that commitment not only brings stability to a relationship but is essential to overcoming the inevitable ups and downs experienced in relationships. Commitment is based on conscious choice rather than on feelings, which, by their very nature, are transitory. Commitment is a promise of a shared future—a promise to be together, come what may. No matter how they feel, committed partners put effort and energy into the relationship. They take time to attend to their partners, give compliments, and deal with conflict when necessary. Commitment has become an important concept in recent years. To many people, commitment is the most important part of a relationship.

Separation and Divorce

Divorce is fairly common in the United States (Figure 4.3). Those who have never experienced divorce personally—either their own or that of their parents—almost certainly have friends or relatives who have. The high rate of divorce in the United States may reflect our extremely high expectations for emotional fulfillment and satisfaction in marriage. It may also indicate that our culture no longer embraces the permanence of marriage.

The process of divorce usually begins with an emotional separation. Often one partner is unhappy and looks for a more satisfying relationship. Dissatisfaction increases until the unhappy partner decides he or she can no longer stay. Physical separation follows, although it may take some time for the relationship to be over emotionally.

Except for the death of a spouse or family member, divorce may be the greatest stress-producing event in life. Studies show that divorced women are more likely to develop

> To many people, **commitment is a more important goal** than living together or marriage.

heart disease than married, remarried, or widowed women. Both men and women experience turmoil, depression, and lowered self-esteem during and after divorce. People experience separation distress and loneliness for about a year and then begin a recovery period of one to three years. During this time they gradually construct a postdivorce identity, along with a new pattern of life. Most people are surprised how long it takes to recover from divorce.

Children are especially vulnerable to the trauma of divorce, and sometimes counseling is appropriate to help them adjust to the change. However, recent research has found that children who spend substantial time with both parents are usually better adjusted than those in sole custody and are as well-adjusted as their peers from intact families.

Coping with divorce has been found to be difficult for children at any age, including adult children.

Despite the distress of separation and divorce, the negative effects are usually balanced sooner or later by the possibility of finding a more suitable partner, constructing a new life, and developing new aspects of the self. About 75% of all people who divorce remarry, often within five years. One result of the high divorce and remarriage rate is a growing number of stepfamilies.

FAMILY LIFE

American families are very different today than they were even a few decades ago. Currently 69% of children under the age of 18 live with both parents (either married or unmarried), whereas 27% of children live with a single parent. The remaining 4% of children live in a household where neither parent is present.

Becoming a Parent

Few new parents are prepared for the job of parenting, yet they literally must assume the role overnight. They must quickly learn how to hold and feed a baby, change diapers, and differentiate a cry of hunger from a cry of pain or fear. No wonder the birth of the first child is one of the most stressful transitions for any couple.

Even couples with an egalitarian relationship before their first child is born find that their marital roles become more traditional with the arrival of the new baby. The father typically becomes the primary provider and protector, and the mother typically becomes the primary nurturer. Most research indicates that mothers have to make greater changes in their lives than fathers do. Although men today spend more time caring for their infants than ever before, women still take the ultimate responsibility for the baby. Women are usually the ones who make job changes, either quitting work

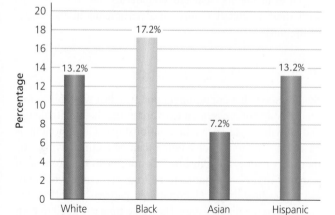

FIGURE 4.3 Percentage of separated and divorced Americans, 2011.

U.S. Census Bureau. 2012. *America's Families and Living Arrangements: 2011* (http://www.census.gov/population/www/socdemo/hh-fam/cps2011.html).

or reducing work hours in order to stay home with the baby for several months or more. Many mothers juggle the multiple roles of mother, homemaker, and employer/employee and feel guilty that they never have enough time to do justice to any of these roles.

Parenting

Parents may wonder about the long-term impact of each decision they make on their child's well-being and personality. According to parenting experts, no one action or decision (within limits) will determine a child's personality or development. Instead the *parenting style,* or overall approach to parenting, is most important. Parenting styles vary according to the levels of two characteristics of the parents:

- *Demandingness* encompasses the use of discipline and supervision, the expectation that children act responsibly and maturely, and the direct reaction to disobedience.

- *Responsiveness* refers to a parent's warmth and intent to facilitate independence and self-confidence in a child by being supportive, connected, and understanding of the child's needs.

Several parenting styles have been identified. Each style emerges according to the parents' balance of demandingness and responsiveness. Here are some examples:

- *Authoritarian* parents are high in demandingness and low in responsiveness. They give orders and expect obedience, giving very little warmth or consideration to their children's special needs.

- *Authoritative* parents are high in both demandingness and responsiveness. They set clear boundaries and expectations, but they are also loving, supportive, and attuned to their children's needs.

- *Permissive* parents are high in responsiveness and low in demandingness. They do not expect their children to act maturely but instead allow them to follow their own impulses. They are very warm, patient, and accepting, and they are focused on not stifling their child's innate creativity.

- *Uninvolved* parents are low in both demandingness and responsiveness. They require little from their children and respond with little attention, frequency, or effort. In extreme cases, this style of parenting might reach the level of child neglect.

At each stage of the family life cycle, the relationship between parents and children changes. And with those changes come new challenges. The parents' primary responsibility to a baby is to ensure its physical well-being around the clock. As babies grow into toddlers and begin to walk and talk, they begin to be able to take care of some of their own physical needs. For parents, the challenge at this stage is to strike a balance between giving children the freedom to explore and setting limits that will keep the children safe and secure. As children grow toward adolescence, parents need to give them increasing independence and gradually be willing to let them risk success or failure on their own.

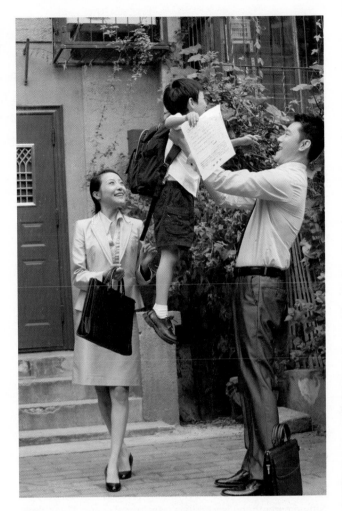

Setting clear boundaries, holding children to high expectations, and responding with warmth to children's needs are all positive parenting strategies.

Marital satisfaction for most couples tends to decline while the children are in school. Reasons include the financial and emotional pressures of a growing family and the increased job and community responsibilities of parents in their thirties, forties, and fifties. Once the last child has left home, marital satisfaction can increase because the parents have more time to focus on each other.

Single Parents

According to the U.S. Census Bureau, about 27% of all children under 18 live with only one parent. In some single-parent families, the traditional family life cycle is reversed and the baby comes before the marriage. In these families, the single parent is usually a teenage mother. Data reported in 2011 indicate that 25% were white, 55% were black, and 29% were Hispanic.

Economic difficulties are the primary problem for single mothers, especially for unmarried mothers who have not finished high school and have difficulty finding work. Divorced mothers usually experience a sharp drop in income the first few years on their own, but if they have job skills or education they usually can eventually support themselves and their children. Other problems for single mothers are the often-conflicting demands of being both father and mother and the difficulty of satisfying their own needs for adult companionship and affection.

Financial pressures are also a complaint of single fathers, but they do not experience them to the extent that single mothers do. Because they are likely to have less practice than mothers in juggling parental and professional roles, they may worry that they do not spend enough time with their children. Because single fatherhood is not as common as single motherhood, however, the men who choose it are likely to be stable, established, and strongly motivated to be with their children.

Research about the effect on children of growing up in a single-parent family is inconclusive. Evidence seems to indicate that these children tend to have less success in school and in their careers than children from two-parent families, but these effects may be associated more strongly with lower educational attainment of the single parent than with the absence of the second parent. Two-parent families are not necessarily better if one of the parents spends little time relating to the children or is physically or emotionally abusive.

Stepfamilies

Single parenthood is usually a transitional stage: About three out of four divorced women and about four out of five divorced men will ultimately remarry. Rates are lower for widowed men and women, but overall almost half the marriages in the United States are remarriages for the husband, the wife, or both. If either partner brings children from a previous marriage into the new family unit, a stepfamily (or "blended family") is formed.

Stepfamilies are significantly different from primary families and should not be expected to duplicate the emotions and relationships of a primary family. Research has shown that healthy stepfamilies are less cohesive and more adaptable than healthy primary families; they have a greater capacity to allow for individual differences and accept that biologically related family members will have emotionally closer relationships. Stepfamilies gradually gain more of a sense of being a family as they build a history of shared daily experiences and major life events.

Successful Families

Family life can be extremely challenging. A strong family is not a family without problems; it's a family that copes successfully with stress and crisis. Successful families are intentionally connected—members share experiences and meanings.

QUICK STATS

4% of American children live in a home where neither parent is present.

—U.S. Census Bureau, 2012

An excellent way to build strong family ties is to develop family rituals and routines—organized, repeated activities that have meaning for family members. Families with regular routines and rituals have healthier children, more satisfying marriages, and stronger family relationships. Some of the most common routines identified in research studies are dinnertime, a regular bedtime, and household chores; common rituals include birthdays, holidays, and weekend activities. Family routines may even serve as protective factors, balancing out potential risk factors associated with single-parent families and families with divorce and remarriage. Incorporating a regular family mealtime into a family's routine allows parents and children to develop closer relationships and leads to better parenting, healthier children, and better school performance.

Although there is tremendous variation in American families, experts have proposed that six major qualities or themes appear in strong families:

1. *Commitment.* The family is very important to its members. Sexual fidelity between partners is included in commitment.

2. *Appreciation.* Family members care about one another and express their appreciation. The home is a positive place for family members.

3. *Communication.* Family members spend time listening to one another and enjoying one another's company. They talk about disagreements and attempt to solve problems.

4. *Time together.* Family members do things together—often simple activities that don't cost money.

5. *Spiritual wellness.* The family promotes sharing, love, and compassion for other human beings.

6. *Stress and crisis management.* When faced with illness, death, marital conflict, or other crises, family members pull together, seek help, and use other coping strategies to meet the challenge.

It may surprise some people that members of strong families are often seen at counseling centers. They know that the smartest thing to do in some situations is to get help.

Ask Yourself

QUESTIONS FOR CRITICAL THINKING AND REFLECTION

Do you think of your own family as successful? Why or why not? Either way, what could you do to make your relationships in your family more successful? Are you comfortable talking to your family about these issues?

Connect to Your Choices

Have you ever thought about why you handle your relationships the way you do? Many factors can influence the relationship choices we make—some not as obvious as others. Do you avoid intimate relationships because you don't want to replicate the patterns you saw in your parents' relationship? Are you frequently disappointed with your relationships because they aren't as blissful or as exciting as the relationships you see in movies or on TV? Do you go along with your partner's ideas because you're not sure what you want?

What external factors influence your choices about relationships? What are your inner motivations and core values, and how do they affect your choices? Based on what you learned in this chapter, will you make some different choices in the future? If so, what will they be?

Go online to Connect to complete this activity:
www.mcgraw-hillconnect.com

TIPS FOR TODAY AND THE FUTURE

A balanced life includes ample time for nourishing relationships with friends, family, and intimate partners.

RIGHT NOW YOU CAN:

- Seek out an acquaintance or a new friend and arrange a coffee date to get to know the person better.
- Call someone you love and tell him or her how important the relationship is to you. Don't wait for a crisis.

IN THE FUTURE YOU CAN:

- Think about the conflicts you have had in the past with your close friends or loved ones and consider how you handled them. Decide whether your conflict management methods were helpful. Using the suggestions in this chapter and Chapter 3, determine how you could better handle similar conflicts in the future.
- Think about your prospects as a parent. What kind of example have your parents set? How do you feel about having children in the future (if you don't have children already)? What can you do to prepare yourself to be a good parent?

SUMMARY

- Healthy intimate relationships are an important component of the well-being of both individuals and society. Many intimate relationships are held together by love.

- Successful relationships begin with a positive sense of self and reasonably high self-esteem. Personal identity, gender roles, and attachment styles are all rooted in childhood experiences.

- Characteristics of friendship include companionship, respect, acceptance, help, trust, loyalty, and reciprocity.

- Love, sex, and commitment are closely linked ideals in intimate relationships. Love includes trust, caring, respect, and loyalty. Sex brings excitement, fascination, and passion to the relationship.

- Common challenges in relationships relate to issues of self-disclosure, commitment, expectations, competitiveness, balance of time together and apart, and jealousy.

- Partners in successful relationships have strong communication skills and support each other in difficult times.

- The keys to good communication in relationships are self-disclosure, listening, and feedback.

- Conflict is inevitable in intimate relationships; partners need to find ways to negotiate their differences.

- People usually choose partners like themselves. If partners are very different, acceptance and good communication skills are especially necessary to maintain the relationship.

- Most Americans find partners through dating or getting together in groups. Cohabitation is a growing social pattern that allows partners to get to know each other intimately without being married.

- Gay and lesbian partnerships are similar to heterosexual partnerships, with some differences. Partners often don't conform to traditional gender roles, and they may experience societal hostility or ambivalence rather than approval of their partnerships.

- Singlehood is a growing option in our society. Advantages include greater variety in sex partners and more freedom in making life decisions; disadvantages include loneliness and possible economic hardship, especially for single women.

- Marriage fulfills many functions for individuals and society. It can provide people with affection, affirmation, and sexual fulfillment; a context for child rearing; and the promise of lifelong companionship.

- Love isn't enough to ensure a successful marriage. Partners must be realistic, feel good about each other, have communication and conflict resolution skills, share values, and balance their individual and joint interests.

- When problems can't be worked out, people often separate and divorce. Divorce is traumatic for all involved, especially children, but the negative effects are usually balanced in time by positive ones.

- At each stage of the family life cycle, relationships change. Marital satisfaction may be lower during the child-rearing years and higher later.

- Many families today are single-parent families. Problems for single parents include economic difficulties, conflicting demands, and time pressures.

- Stepfamilies are formed when single, divorced, or widowed people remarry and create new family units. Stepfamilies gradually gain more of a sense of being a family as they build a history of shared experiences.

- Important qualities of successful families include commitment to the family; appreciation of family members; communication; time spent together; spiritual wellness; and effective methods of dealing with stress.

FOR MORE INFORMATION

For resources in your area, check your campus directory for a counseling center or peer counseling program, or search online.

BOOKS

Brooks, J. B. 2010. *The Process of Parenting*, 8th ed. New York: McGraw-Hill. *Demonstrates how parents and caregivers can translate their love and concern for children into effective parenting behavior.*

DeGenova, M. K., et al. 2010. *Intimate Relationships, Marriages, and Families*, 8th ed. New York: McGraw-Hill. *A comprehensive introduction to relationships.*

Goleman, D. 1995. *Emotional Intelligence: Why it can matter more than IQ*. New York: Bantam Books. *Redefines what it means to be intelligent.*

Jones, D. 2014. *Love Illuminated: Exploring Life's Most Mystifying Subject (with the Help of 50,000 Strangers)*. New York: William Morrow/HarperCollins.

Lewis, T., F. Amni, and R. Lannon. 2000. *A General Theory of Love*. New York: Random House. *A lucid exploration of the biopsychosocial nature of love and interconnectedness of people.*

McKay, M., P. Fanning, and K. Paleg. 2007. *Couple Skills: Making Your Relationship Work*, 2nd rev. ed. New York: New Harbinger. *A comprehensive guide to improving communication, resolving conflict, and developing greater intimacy and commitment in relationships.*

Miller, R., 2011. *Intimate Relationships*, 6th ed. New York: McGraw-Hill. *A balanced presentation of both the positive and the problematic aspects of intimate relationships.*

Olson, D., J. DeFrain, and L. Skogrand. 2010. *Marriages and Families: Intimacy, Diversity, and Strengths*, 7th ed. New York: McGraw-Hill. *A comprehensive introduction to relationships and families.*

Sears, W., and M. Sears. 2001. *The Attachment Parenting Book: A Commonsense Guide to Understanding and Nurturing Your Child*. Boston: Hachette Book Group. *A style of parenting that encourages a strong early attachment and advocates parental responsiveness to babies' dependency needs.*

ORGANIZATIONS AND WEBSITES

American Association for Marriage and Family Therapy. Provides information about a variety of relationship issues and referrals to therapists.

http://www.aamft.org

Association for Couples in Marriage Enrichment (ACME). An organization that promotes activities to strengthen marriage; a resource for books, tapes, and other materials.

http://www.bettermarriages.org

Conflict Resolution Information Source. Provides links to a broad range of Internet resources for conflict resolution. Information covers interpersonal, marriage, family, and other types of conflicts.

http://www.crinfo.org

Family Education Network. Provides information about education, safety, health, and other family-related issues.

http://www.familyeducation.com

The Gottman Relationship Institute. Includes tips and suggestions for relationships and parenting, including an online relationships quiz.

http://www.gottman.com

Parents without Partners (PWP). Provides educational programs, literature, and support groups for single parents and their children. Search the online directory for a referral to a local chapter.

http://www.parentswithoutpartners.org

Pew Research Center. Surveys Americans about issues and attitudes and analyzes publications in mass media and social science research.

http://www.pewresearch.org

United States Census Bureau. Provides current statistics on births, marriages, and living arrangements.

http://www.census.gov

U.S. General Accountability Office. Acts like a "congressional watchdog," investigating how the federal government spends taxpayer money.

http://www.gao.gov

See also the listings for Chapters 3 and 8.

SELECTED BIBLIOGRAPHY

American College Health Association. 2011. *American College Health Association–National College Health Assessment II Reference Group Executive Summary, Spring 2011*. Hanover, MD: American College Health Association.

Centers for Disease Control and Prevention, National Center for Health Statistics. 2010. Births, marriages, divorces, and deaths: Provisional data for 2009. *National Vital Statistics Reports* 58(25).

Centers for Disease Control and Prevention, National Center for Health Statistics. 2010. Marriage and cohabitation in the United States: A statistical portrait based on cycle 6 (2002) of the National Survey of Family Growth. *Vital and Health Statistics* 23(28): 1–46.

Centers for Disease Control and Prevention, National Center for Health Statistics. 2011. *Health, United States, 2010*. Hyattsville, MD: National Center for Health Statistics.

Christakis, N. A., et al. 2006. Mortality after hospitalization of a spouse. *New England Journal of Medicine* 354(7): 719–730.

Eckert, P., and S. McConnell-Ginet. 2013. *Language and Gender*, 2nd ed. New York: Cambridge University Press.

Federal Interagency Forum on Child and Family Statistics. 2011. *America's Children: Key National Indicators of Well-Being, 2011*. Washington, DC: U.S. Government Printing Office.

Goodwin, M. H. 2006. *The Hidden Life of Girls: Games of Stance, Status, and Exclusion*. Oxford: Blackwell.

Kirschenbaum, H., and V. Henderson. 1989. *The Carl Rogers Reader*. Boston: Houghton Mifflin.

McPherson, M., L. Smith-Lovin, and M. Brashears. 2006. Social isolation in America: Changes in core discussion networks over two decades. *American Sociological Review* 71: 353–375.

National Conference of State Legislatures. 2012. *Defining Marriage: Defense of Marriage Acts and Same-Sex Marriage Laws* (http://www.ncsl .org/issues-research/human-services/same-sex-marriage-overview.aspx).

Pleis, J. R., and M. Lethbridge-Cejku. 2007. Summary health statistics for U.S. adults: National Health Interview Survey, 2006. *Vital and Health Statistics* 10(235): 1–153.

Roisman, G. I., et al. 2008. Adult romantic relationships as contexts of human development: A multimethod comparison of same-sex couples with opposite-sex dating, engaged, and married dyads. *Developmental Psychology* 44(1): 91–101.

Salovey, P., et al., ed. 2004. *Emotional Intelligence: Key Readings on the Mayer and Salovey Model.*

Schoen, R., et al. 2007. Family transitions in young adulthood. *Demography* 44(4): 807–820.

Tufekci, Z. 2014. The social Internet: Frustrating, enriching, but not lonely. *Public Culture* 26(1):13–23.

Turkle, S. 2011. *Alone Together: Why We Expect More from Technology and Less from Each Other*. New York: Basic Books.

Yarber, W., B. Sayad, and B. Strong. 2010. *Human Sexuality: Diversity in Contemporary America,* 7th ed. New York: McGraw-Hill.

CHAPTER 5

CHAPTER OBJECTIVES

- Describe the structure and function of the female and male sex organs
- Explain the changes in sexual functioning that occur over the course of a person's life
- Describe how the sex organs function during sexual activity
- Identify common causes of sexual problems
- Outline the factors that influence sexual behavior and the various ways human sexuality can be expressed
- Describe guidelines for safe, responsible sexual behavior
- Describe the physical changes a pregnant woman typically experiences
- Identify the stages of fetal development
- List the important components of good prenatal care
- Describe the process of labor and delivery

Sexuality, Pregnancy, and Childbirth

Humans are sexual beings. Sexual activity is the source of our most intense physical pleasures, a central ingredient in many of our intimate emotional relationships, and the key to reproduction.

Sexuality is more than just sexual behavior. It is a complex, interacting group of biological characteristics and acquired behaviors people learn while growing up in a particular family, community, and society. Sexuality includes biological sex (being biologically male or female), gender (masculine and feminine behaviors), sexual anatomy and physiology, sexual functioning and practices, and social and sexual interactions with others. Our individual sense of identity is powerfully influenced by our sexuality. We think of ourselves in fundamental ways as male and female; heterosexual and homosexual; single, attached, married, and divorced. Sexuality should be thought of as a spectrum, rather than as a binary system of either/or.

Basic information about the body, sexual functioning, and sexual behavior is vital to sexual wellness. Once we understand the facts, we have a better basis for evaluating the messages we get and for making informed, responsible choices about our sexual activities.

SEXUAL ANATOMY

Despite their different appearances, the sex organs of men and women arise from the same structures and fulfill sex-specific but parallel functions. Each person has a pair of

---

sexuality A dimension of personality shaped by biological, psychosocial, and cultural forces and concerning all aspects of sexual behavior.

TERMS

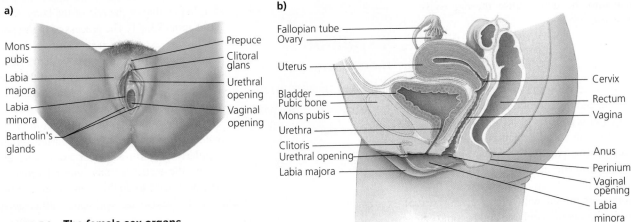

a)

Mons pubis
Labia majora
Labia minora
Bartholin's glands

Prepuce
Clitoral glans
Urethral opening
Vaginal opening

b)

Fallopian tube
Ovary
Uterus
Bladder
Pubic bone
Mons pubis
Urethra
Clitoris
Urethral opening
Labia majora

Cervix
Rectum
Vagina
Anus
Perinium
Vaginal opening
Labia minora

FIGURE 5.1   The female sex organs.
(a) An external view of the vulva. (b) An internal view of the vulva.

gonads: ovaries in females and testes in males. The gonads produce **germ cells** and sex hormones. The germ cells are **ova** (eggs) in females and **sperm** in males. Ova and sperm are the basic units of reproduction; their union results in the creation of a new life.

Female Sex Organs

The external sex organs, or genitals, of the female are called the **vulva** (Figure 5.1). The vulva, commonly confused with the vagina, includes the *mons pubis*, *labia majora* and *minora*, clitoris, and urethral and vaginal openings. The *mons pubis,* a rounded mass of fatty tissue over the pubic bone, becomes covered with hair during puberty (biological maturation). Below it are two paired folds of skin called the *labia majora* (outer lips) and the *labia minora* (inner lips). Enclosed within these folds are the *clitoris*, the opening of the urethra, and the opening of the vagina.

The **clitoris** is highly sensitive to stimulation and plays an important role in female sexual arousal, orgasm, and pleasure. The clitoris consists of 8,000 nerve endings concentrated in the glans, or head. The clitoris may be externally visible between the labia. It then extends internally into the anterior wall of the vagina (Figure 5.1b). Inside the clitoris, spongy, erectile tissue fills with blood during sexual excitement, creating engorgement of the genitals. The clitoral hood, or **prepuce,** covers the glans and is formed from the upper portion of the inner lips.

The female **urethra** is a duct that leads directly from the urinary bladder to its opening between the clitoris and the opening of the vagina. The urethra conducts urine from the bladder to the outside of the body. Women have a much shorter urethra than men and as a result are more likely to suffer from urinary tract infections or UTIs. Both males and females should urinate after sexual activity to cleanse this tube.

Some women are able to expel fluid or ejaculate during sexual activity. If so, the fluid exits the urethra, not the vagina. This fluid has been tested and is typically not urine, although some remnants of urine have been found simply because urine travels out of the same tube. This fluid is consistent and similar to prostatic fluid in men.

The **vagina** is the passage that leads to the internal reproductive organs. It is the female structure used for sexual intercourse and penetration. It is a potential birth canal and serves as a passageway for the menstrual fluid to be expelled. Located about 1–2 inches internally in the vagina, is the Grafenberg- or *G-spot*. This spot—or more accurately, region—is the root of the clitoris and can be highly sensitive in some women. Projecting into the upper part of the vagina is the **cervix,** which is the opening of the **uterus**—or *womb*—where a fertilized egg is implanted and develops into a *fetus*.

A pair of **fallopian tubes** (or *oviducts*) extends from the top of the uterus. The end of each oviduct surrounds

TERMS

gonads   The primary reproductive organs that produce germ cells and sex hormones; the ovaries and testes.

germ cells   Sperm and ova (eggs).

ovum   A germ cell produced by a female, which combines with a male germ cell (sperm) to create a fetus; plural, *ova*. Also called an *egg*.

sperm   A germ cell produced by a male, which combines with a female germ cell (ovum) to create a fetus.

vulva   The external female genitals, or sex organs.

clitoris   The highly sensitive female genital structure, whose only function is for sexual pleasure.

prepuce   The foreskin of the clitoris or penis.

urethra   The duct that carries urine from the bladder to the outside of the body.

vagina   The canal leading from the female genitals to the internal reproductive organs; the birth canal.

cervix   The opening of the uterus in the upper part of the vagina.

uterus   The hollow, thick-walled, muscular organ in which the fertilized egg develops; the *womb*.

fallopian tube   A duct that guides a mature ovum from the ovary to the uterus; also called an *oviduct*.

an **ovary** and guides the mature ovum down into the uterus after the egg exits the ovary.

Male Sex Organs

A man's external sex organs, or genitals, are the penis and the scrotum (Figure 5.2).

The **penis** consists of the glans, often referred to as the head, which is typically the most sensitive part of the penis. The shaft extends from the head to the body of the penis and is made up of spongy tissue that becomes engorged with blood during sexual excitement, causing the organ to enlarge and become erect.

The **scrotum** is a pouch that contains a pair of sperm-producing male gonads, called **testes.** The scrotum maintains

QUICK STATS

15 million or more sperm per milliliter of semen is considered a normal sperm count.

—Mayo Clinic
(www.mayoclinic.org), 2012

the testes at a temperature approximately 5°F below that of the rest of the body—that is, at about 93.6°F. The process of sperm production is extremely heat-sensitive. In hot temperatures, the muscles in the scrotum relax and the testes move away from the heat of the body. This ability to regulate the temperature of the testes is important because elevated testicular temperature can interfere with normal sperm production. Men should regularly perform testicular exams and examine the testes for any unusual growths. The best place to do this is in the shower because it is warm and the scrotal sac will hang further away from the body.

The male urethra is a tube that runs through the entire length of the penis. The urethra carries both urine and **semen** (sperm-carrying fluid) to the opening at the tip of the penis. The **Cowper's glands** are two small structures flanking the urethra. During sexual arousal, these glands excrete a clear, mucus-like fluid that appears at the tip of the penis. This preejaculatory fluid is thought to help lubricate the urethra to facilitate the passage of sperm and flush out any remaining urine in the tube. The release of preejaculatory fluid is an involuntary reflex and may contain sperm, so withdrawal of the penis before ejaculation is not a reliable form of contraception. It is also possible to contract a sexually transmitted infection from preejaculatory fluid.

Starting at about age 14, males begin producing sperm, around 400 million per day. The sperm take the following journey:

1. Sperm are produced inside a maze of tiny, tightly packed tubules within the testes. As they begin to mature, sperm flow into a single storage tube called the **epididymis,** which lies on the surface of each testis.

2. Sperm move from each epididymis into another tube— called the **vas deferens.**

> **TERMS**
>
> **ovaries**   The paired female reproductive glands that produce ova (eggs) and sex hormones; ovaries are the female gonads.
>
> **penis**   The male genital structure consisting of the glans and shaft, spongy tissue that becomes engorged with blood during sexual excitement.
>
> **scrotum**   The loose sac of skin and muscle fibers that contains the testes.
>
> **testis**   One of two male gonads, the site of sperm production; plural, *testes*. Also called *testicle.*
>
> **semen**   The fluid that carries sperm out of the male penis during ejaculation.
>
> **Cowper's gland**   In the male reproductive system, a small organ that produces preejaculatory fluid.
>
> **epididymis**   A storage duct for maturing sperm, located on the surface of each testis.
>
> **vas deferens**   A tube that carries sperm from the epididymis through the prostate gland to the seminal vesicles; plural, *vasa deferentia.*

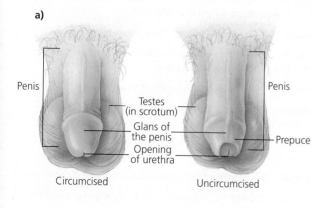

a)

Penis

Testes
(in scrotum)

Glans of
the penis

Opening
of urethra

Circumcised

Penis

Prepuce

Uncircumcised

b)

Bladder

Pubic bone

Vas deferens

Corpus spongiosum

Penis

Urethra

Glans

Opening of urethra

Seminal vesicle

Rectum

Prostate

Cowper's gland

Anus

Epididymis

Testis

Scrotum

FIGURE 5.2   The male sex organs.
(a) An external view. (b) An internal view.

3. The two *vasa deferentia* eventually merge into a pair of **seminal vesicles,** whose secretions provide nutrients for the sperm. The sperm then pass through an organ called the **prostrate gland,** where they pick up a milky fluid and become semen.

4. On the final stage of their journey, sperm flow into the **ejaculatory ducts.** Although urine and semen share a common passage, they are prevented from mixing together by muscles that control their entry into the urethra.

The smooth, rounded tip of the penis is the highly sensitive **glans,** an important component in sexual arousal (Figure 5.2a shows a frontal view; Figure 5.2b shows a side view). The glans is partially covered by the foreskin, or prepuce, a retractable fold of skin that is removed by **circumcision** in about 55% of newborn males in the United States. Circumcision is performed for cultural, religious, and hygienic reasons. Rates of circumcision vary widely among different groups (see the box "Genital Alteration").

HORMONES AND THE REPRODUCTIVE LIFE CYCLE

The sex hormones produced by the ovaries or testes have a major influence on the development and function of the reproductive system throughout life. In addition to their effects on reproductive organs, sex hormones influence many other organs in the body, including the brain.

Both males and females produce testosterone, estrogens, and progestogens; however, the quantity differs in the male and female bodies. The male sex hormones, made by the testes, are called **androgens,** the most important of which is *testosterone*. Males will produce lower levels of estrogen and progesterone. The female sex hormones, produced by the ovaries, belong to two groups: **estrogens** and **progestogens.** The ovaries also produce a small amount of testosterone. The **adrenal glands** also produce sex hormones in both males and females.

Sex hormones are regulated by the hormones of the **pituitary gland,** located at the base of the brain. This gland in turn is controlled by hormones produced by the **hypothalamus** in the brain.

Ask Yourself

QUESTIONS FOR CRITICAL THINKING AND REFLECTION

What are your personal views on circumcision? Who or what has influenced those opinions? Are the bases of your views primarily cultural, moral, or medical? If you had a son, would you circumcise him?

Endocrine-disrupting chemicals (EDCs), are examples of substances from the environment that act like hormones and disrupt normal endocrine activity, particularly activity related to reproduction and development. The most studied EDCs are environmental estrogens, which mimic the female sex hormone estrogen and can duplicate or exaggerate its effects. Other EDCs can block estrogen, mimic or block androgens (male sex hormones), or otherwise alter hormonal responses in the body.

Differentiation of the Embryo

How do we become a "girl" or a "boy" embryo? All human cells typically contain 23 pairs of chromosomes. In 22 of the pairs, the two partner chromosomes match. But in the 23rd pair, called the **sex chromosomes,** one comes from the mother and one from the father. Mothers contribute an X and fathers an X or a Y. Therefore, it is the father's sex chromosome that determines the sex of the child: Females are XX and males are XY, and this genetic fact occurs at the moment of conception.

Abnormalities sometimes occur in the sex chromosomes; the two most common disorders of sex chromosomes are Klinefelter's syndrome and Turner's syndrome. Klinefelter's syndrome, a condition where a male carries two or more

---

TERMS

seminal vesicle   A tube leading from the vas deferens to the ejaculatory duct; secretes nutrients for the semen.

prostate gland   A male reproductive organ; produces some of the fluid in semen, which helps transport and nourish sperm.

ejaculatory duct   A tube that carries mature sperm to the urethra so they can exit the body upon ejaculation.

glans   The head of the penis or the clitoris.

circumcision   Surgical removal of the foreskin of the penis.

androgens   Male sex hormones, produced by the testes.

estrogens   A class of female sex hormones, produced by the ovaries, that bring about sexual maturation at puberty and maintain reproductive functions.

progestogens   A class of female sex hormones, produced by the ovaries, that sustain reproductive functions.

adrenal glands   Endocrine glands, located over the kidneys, that produce sex hormones.

pituitary gland   An endocrine gland at the base of the brain that produces hormones and regulates the release of hormones—including sex hormones—by other glands.

hypothalamus   A region of the brain above the pituitary gland whose hormones control the secretions of the pituitary; also involved in the control of many bodily functions, including hunger, thirst, temperature regulation, and sexual functions.

sex chromosomes   The X and Y chromosomes, which determine an individual's biological sex.

DIVERSITY MATTERS
Genital Alteration

The alteration of the appearance and function of children's genitalia, either shortly after birth or as part of a puberty rite, provokes much controversy worldwide. The most common form of genital alteration is male circumcision—the removal of the foreskin of the penis. Circumcision is a relatively minor surgical procedure that is performed for a variety of cultural, religious, aesthetic, and medical reasons. Worldwide an estimated one-third of males are circumcised. In the United States a little more than one-half of male newborns are circumcised (from a high of nearly 90% in the 1960s); over time, fewer American parents are having their sons circumcised.

Currently no major medical group in the United States recommends the routine circumcision of male infants. The procedure, though minor, carries some medical risks, including bleeding, infection, damage to the penis, and even death. Circumcision causes pain to the infant, although most pain can be alleviated with appropriate use of local anesthetic. Circumcision may change the sensitivity of the penis, and some critics claim that it can diminish a man's sexual pleasure. Opponents of circumcision point to the fact that most of the world's men are uncircumcised; why perform surgery, they ask, when there is no clear need for it?

On the other side of the debate, there are a number of health benefits of circumcision. Proponents argue that it promotes cleanliness and reduces the risk of urinary tract infections in newborns and sexually transmitted infections in later life. In 2012 the American Academy of Pediatrics announced that it now supported circumcision among newborns because the "preventive health benefits of elective circumcision of male newborns outweigh the risks of the procedure." Studies conducted in developing countries have shown that circumcision can reduce a man's risk of acquiring human immunodeficiency virus (HIV), herpes simplex virus type 2, human papillomavirus (HPV), and genital ulcer disease through heterosexual contact. Male circumcision has also been shown to lower HPV, genital ulcer disease, bacterial vaginosis, and trichomoniasis among female partners. However, STI education, the practice of abstinence or low-risk sexual behaviors, or using barrier methods such as condoms have a far greater impact on the transmission of STIs than does circumcision.

Far more controversial is the practice of female genital cutting (FGC), also called female genital mutilation or modification. FGCs range from removal of the external genitalia (including the clitoris and labia) to sowing up the labia but leaving a small opening through which urine and menstrual fluid can pass. A common explanation is that FGC controls a woman's sexuality and ensures she remain a virgin before marriage. Other explanations refer to an empowerment for girls: Through the bonding and educational experiences surrounding the ceremonies, girls attain a status similar to cohorts of boys the same age who are undergoing circumcision. These explanations are cultural rather than medical.

Each year about 3 million female children undergo FGC, usually between infancy and age 15, and about 140 million women worldwide are estimated to have had some form of genital cutting. FGC is often performed under unsterile conditions and without adequate anesthesia. Serious complications are common and include severe pain, infection, bleeding, and death. Common long-term health issues include infertility, difficulties with childbirth, and problems with urinary and sexual function.

The World Health Organization has come out strongly against FGC, declaring it a violation of the human rights of girls and women. FGC is now illegal in many countries, including the United States, but it is still performed on large numbers of girls where the cultural tradition persists.

SOURCES: Boyle, E. H., and A. C. Corl. 2010. Law and culture in a global context: Interventions to eradicate female genital cutting. *Annual Review of Law and Social Science* 6:195–215. Centers for Disease Control and Prevention. 2011. Trends in in-hospital newborn male circumcision—United States, 1999–2010. *Morbidity and Mortality Weekly Report* 60(34): 1167–1168; World Health Organization. 2012. *Female Genital Mutilation* (http://www.who.int/topics/female_genital_mutilation/en/); Tobian, Aaron A. R., et al. 2014. Male circumcision: A globally relevant but under-utilized method for the prevention of HIV and other sexually transmitted infections. *Annual Review of Medicine* 65:293–306.

X chromosomes in addition to the Y chromosome, occurs in about 1 in 1000 males and causes infertility and underdeveloped genitalia. Turner's syndrome occurs in about 1 in 2500 females. Women with Turner's have only a single complete X chromosome. These women are usually not able to have children and can sometimes have other medical problems.

TERMS

puberty The period of biological maturation during adolescence; in this stage of development, the individual becomes capable of sexual reproduction.

progesterone The most important female sex hormone for pregnancy; regulates the menstrual cycle and sustains pregnancy.

Female Sexual Maturation

Although humans are typically sexually differentiated at birth, the differences between males and females are accentuated at **puberty,** the period during which the reproductive system matures, secondary sex characteristics develop, and the bodies of males and females begin to appear more distinctive. The changes of puberty are induced by testosterone in the male and estrogen and **progesterone** in the female.

Puberty in Females The first sign of puberty in girls is breast development, followed by a rounding of the hips and buttocks. As the breasts develop, hair appears in the pubic region and later in the underarms. Shortly after the onset of breast development, girls show an increase in growth rate. Breast development usually begins between ages 8 and 13, and the time of rapid body growth occurs between ages 9 and 15.

The Menstrual Cycle A major landmark of puberty for young women is the onset of the **menstrual cycle,** the monthly ovarian cycle that leads to menstruation (loss of blood and tissue lining the uterus) in the absence of pregnancy. The timing of **menarche** (the first *menstrual period*) varies with several factors, including ethnicity, genetics, and nutritional status. The current average age of menarche in the United States is around 12½ years of age, but menstruation may also normally start several years earlier or later.

The day of the onset of bleeding is considered to be day 1 of the menstrual cycle. For the purposes of our discussion, a cycle of 28 days will be used; however, normal cycles vary in length from 21 to 35 days. The menstrual cycle consists of the following four phases:

1. MENSES During **menses**, characterized by the menstrual flow, blood levels of hormones from the ovaries and the pituitary gland are relatively low. This phase of the cycle usually lasts from day 1 to about day 5.

2. ESTROGENIC PHASE The estrogenic phase begins when the menstrual flow ceases and the pituitary gland begins to produce increasing amounts of follicle-stimulating hormone (FSH) and luteinizing hormone (LH). Under the influence of FSH, an egg-containing ovarian **follicle** begins to mature, producing increasingly higher amounts of estrogen. Stimulated by estrogen, the **endometrium** (the uterine lining) thickens with large numbers of blood vessels and uterine glands.

3. OVULATION A surge of a potent estrogen called *estradiol* from the follicle causes the pituitary gland to release a large burst of LH and a smaller amount of FSH. The high concentration of LH stimulates the developing follicle to release its ovum. This event is known as **ovulation**. After ovulation, the follicle is transformed into the **corpus luteum**, which produces progesterone and estrogen. Ovulation theoretically occurs about 14 days prior to the onset of menstrual flow, with the window of greatest fertility occurring from a few days before ovulation to about one day after. This information has been used to attempt to predict the most fertile time during the menstrual cycle for fertility treatments and natural family planning methods. However, a recent study showed that even women with regular menstrual cycles often have unpredictable ovulation, and can actually be fertile on any day of the month, including during menstruation. The "window of fertility" is especially unpredictable in teenagers and women who are approaching menopause.

4. PROGESTATIONAL PHASE During the progestational phase of the cycle, the amount of progesterone secreted from the corpus luteum increases and remains high until the onset of the next menses. Under the influence of estrogen and progesterone, the endometrium continues to develop, readying itself to receive and nourish a fertilized ovum. When pregnancy occurs, the fertilized egg produces the hormone human chorionic gonadotropin (HCG), which maintains the corpus luteum. Thus levels of ovarian hormones remain high and the uterine lining is preserved, preventing menses.

If pregnancy does not occur, the corpus luteum degenerates, and estrogen and progesterone levels gradually fall. Below certain hormonal levels, the endometrium can no longer be maintained, and it begins to slough off, initiating menses. As the levels of ovarian hormones fall, a slight rise in LH and FSH occurs, and a new menstrual cycle begins.

Menstrual Problems Menstruation is a normal biological process, and physical or emotional symptoms associated with the menstrual cycle are very common. Many women experience menstrual cramps, the severity of which tends to vary from cycle to cycle. **Dysmenorrhea,** discomfort associated with menstruation, can include any combination of the following symptoms: lower abdominal cramps, backache, vomiting, nausea, bloating, diarrhea, headache, and fatigue. Many of these symptoms can be attributed to uterine muscular contractions caused by chemicals called *prostaglandins*. Nonsteroidal anti-inflammatory drugs (NSAIDs) such as ibuprofen (Motrin, Advil) often relieve dysmenorrhea by blocking the effects of prostaglandins. Oral contraceptives are also effective in reducing dysmenorrheal symptoms in most women.

Many women experience transient emotional symptoms prior to the onset of their menstrual flow. Depending on their severity, these symptoms may be categorized along a continuum: **premenstrual tension, premenstrual syndrome (PMS),**

TERMS

menstrual cycle The monthly ovarian cycle, regulated by hormones; in the absence of pregnancy, menstruation occurs.

menarche The first menstrual period, experienced by most young women at some point during adolescence.

menses The portion of the menstrual cycle characterized by menstrual flow.

follicle A saclike structure within the ovary, in which an egg (ovum) matures.

endometrium The lining of the uterus.

ovulation The release of a mature egg (ovum) from an ovary.

corpus luteum The part of the ovarian follicle left after ovulation, which secretes estrogen and progesterone during the second half of the menstrual cycle.

dysmenorrhea Painful or problematic menstruation.

premenstrual tension Mild physical and emotional changes associated with the time before the onset of menses.

premenstrual syndrome (PMS) A disorder characterized by physical discomfort, psychological distress, and behavioral changes that begin after ovulation and cease when menstruation begins.

and **premenstrual dysphoric disorder (PMDD).** Premenstrual tension symptoms are mild and may include negative mood changes and physical symptoms such as abdominal cramping and backache. More severe symptoms are classified as PMS; very severe symptoms that impair normal daily and social functioning are classified as PMDD. All three conditions share a definite pattern. Symptoms appear prior to the onset of menses and disappear within a few days after the start of menstruation. Premenstrual tension is quite common, PMS affects about 1 in 5 women, and PMDD affects fewer than 1 in 10 women.

Symptoms associated with PMS and PMDD can include breast tenderness, water retention (bloating), headache, fatigue, insomnia or excessive sleep, appetite changes, food cravings, irritability, anger, increased interpersonal conflict, depression, anxiety, tearfulness, inability to concentrate, social withdrawal, and the sense of being out of control or overwhelmed.

Despite many research studies, the causes of PMS and PMDD are still unknown, and it is unclear why some women are more vulnerable than others. Research has focused on a variety of substances in the body that may fluctuate with the menstrual cycle. Most researchers agree that PMS is probably caused by a combination of hormonal, neurological, genetic, dietary, and psychological factors.

The following strategies provide relief for many women with premenstrual symptoms, and all of them can contribute to a healthy lifestyle at any time:

- *Limit salt intake.* Salt promotes water retention and bloating.
- *Exercise.* Women who exercise may experience fewer symptoms before and after menstrual periods.
- *Don't use alcohol or tobacco.* Alcohol and tobacco may aggravate certain symptoms of PMS and PMDD.
- *Eat a nutritious diet.* Choose a low-fat diet rich in complex carbohydrates from vegetables, fruits, and whole-grain breads, cereals, and pasta. Get enough calcium from calcium-rich foods and, if needed, supplements. Minimize your intake of sugar and caffeine, and avoid chocolate, which is rich in both.
- *Relax.* Stress reduction is always beneficial, and stressful events can trigger PMS symptoms. Try relaxation techniques during the premenstrual time. Orgasms also help reduce stress and relieve cramping.

If you suffer persistent premenstrual symptoms, keep a daily diary to track the types of symptoms, their severity, and their correlation with your menstrual cycle. See your physician for an evaluation and learn about treatments that are available only by prescription.

Selective serotonin reuptake inhibitors (SSRIs), such as Prozac and Zoloft, are often used to treat PMS and PMDD. Until recently, women using SSRIs took the medication throughout the entire menstrual cycle, but taking the medication during just the progestational phase of the cycle is effective in some women. However, these medications are not without side effects and may negatively affect sexual functioning—specifically causing low desire as well as difficulty with arousal and attaining orgasm.

Other drug treatments for PMS and PMDD include certain oral contraceptives, diuretics to minimize water retention, and NSAIDs such as ibuprofen. A number of vitamins, minerals, and other dietary supplements have also been studied for PMS relief. Only one supplement, calcium, has been shown to provide relief in rigorous clinical studies; several others show promise, but more research is needed.

Male Sexual Maturation

Reproductive maturation of boys occurs about two years later than that of girls; it usually begins at about age 10 or 11. Testicular growth is usually the first obvious sign of sexual maturity in boys. The penis also grows at this time, reaching adult size by about age 18. Pubic hair starts to develop after the genitals begin increasing in size, with underarm and facial hair gradually appearing. Hair on the chest, back, and abdomen increases later in development. Facial hair often continues to get thicker and darker for several years after puberty. The voice deepens as a result of the lengthening and thickening of the vocal cords.

Boys grow taller for about six years after the first signs of puberty, with a very rapid period of growth about two years after puberty starts. Largely because of the influence of testosterone, muscle development and bone density are much greater in males than in females. By adulthood, men on average have one and a half times the lean body mass of women, and nearly half the body fat.

Ask Yourself

QUESTIONS FOR CRITICAL THINKING AND REFLECTION

Think about your own experience as you matured during puberty and adolescence. In what ways did these changes affect your life? How did they contribute to the person you are today?

---

premenstrual dysphoric disorder (PMDD) **TERMS**
A severe form of PMS, characterized by symptoms serious enough to interfere with daily activities and relationships.

Aging and Human Sexuality

Hormone production and sexual functioning change as we age. Although sexual functioning may diminish as one ages, sexuality and sensuality can continue to be a source of great pleasure and satisfaction. A recent study of sexuality in older Americans found that three-fourths of 57- to 64-year-olds were sexually active (defined as having had at least one sexual partner in the last year). Half of those people ages 65–74, and about one-fourth of people ages 75–85, remained sexually active. People who remain healthy and active are much more likely to continue to be sexually active in their older years.

Menopause As a woman approaches age 50, her ovaries gradually cease to function and she enters **menopause,** the cessation of menstruation (Table 5.1). For some women, the associated drop in hormone production causes troublesome symptoms. The most common physical symptom of menopause is the hot flash, a sensation of warmth rising to the face from the upper chest, with or without perspiration and chills. During a hot flash, skin temperature can rise by more than 10 degrees. Other menopausal symptoms can include vaginal dryness, low libido, painful intercourse, night sweats, insomnia, thinning of head hair, and mood changes. Osteoporosis—decreasing bone density—can develop, making older women more vulnerable to fractures.

As a result of decreased estrogen production during menopause, the vaginal walls become thin, and lubrication in response to sexual arousal diminishes. Sexual intercourse may become painful. Hormonal treatment or the use of lubricants during intercourse can minimize these problems.

Cross-cultural studies comparing Japanese with North American women dispel the idea that hot flashes and other menopausal reactions are universal. A diet of fish and vegetables, an exercise regimen of cycling, walking, or farming, and cultural ideas about the meaning of bodily changes positively affected the Japanese experience of menopause among the women studied.

In Western medicine, it became common to prescribe postmenopausal women estrogen for relief from hot flashes, vaginal dryness, bone loss, and a host of other symptoms.

Although sexual physiology changes as people get older, many men and women readily adjust to these alterations.

menopause The cessation of menstruation, occurring gradually around age 50.

TERMS

Table 5.1	Reproductive Aging in Women	
AGE*	SIGNS & SYMPTOMS—WHAT'S HAPPENING	STAGE OF REPRODUCTION
9–15	First period; variable menstrual cycles	Menarche; beginning reproductive years
16–30	Regular menstrual cycle; fertility peaking	Reproductive years
31–42	Regular menstrual cycle; fertility progressively declining	Reproductive years
Early 40s	Lengths of menstrual cycle vary increasingly	Menopausal transition
Late 40s–early 50s	2 or more skipped periods; hot flashes, irritability, and sleep disturbance; bone loss begins	Menopausal transition
51	Final period, i.e., no period for 12 months	Menopause
50s and beyond	Vaginal dryness, bone loss. Hot flashes can persist (for a few women, into their 60s and 70s).	Postmenopause

*Women vary a great deal in the ages at which they go through these stages. The average length of menopause and the transition leading up to it is four years, but for some women symptoms may last only a few months, and for others, 10 years.

SOURCE: American Society for Reproductive Medicine. 2012. *Reproductive Aging in Women.* (http://www.reproductivefacts.org).

However, doctors discovered that giving estrogen alone to postmenopausal women resulted in higher rates of endometrial cancer. To alleviate this problem, it became customary to prescribe estrogen with a progestogen (called *hormone replacement therapy*, or *HRT*), since this combination reduced the risk for uterine cancer as well as reduced menopausal symptoms. The medical community was taken by surprise in 2002 when a large study showed that women taking a common form of estrogen/progestogen therapy had higher rates of cardiovascular disease, blood clots, and breast cancer than postmenopausal women not taking hormones. Prescriptions for HRT plummeted after this news. Breast cancer rates dropped over the next few years, but experts are not sure whether the decline in breast cancer was due to the decrease in HRT or to other factors.

In the past several years, reanalysis of the data and information from newer studies have resulted in a more individualized approach to HRT. It appears that younger women who have become menopausal within the past 5 years are more likely to benefit from HRT and less likely to have serious side effects than older women. Current forms of HRT include low-dose estrogen, sometimes in the form of a patch, cream, or vaginal ring, designed to treat specific symptoms of menopause and with a reduced risk of side effects.

Aging Male Syndrome   Between the ages of 35 and 65, men experience a gradual decline in testosterone production, resulting in the aging male syndrome, sometimes referred to as *male menopause* or *andropause*. Some experts prefer the term *aging male syndrome* because the process is much more gradual than female menopause. Symptoms vary widely, but most men experience at least some of the following symptoms as they age: loss of muscle mass, increased fat mass, decreased sex drive, erectile problems, depressed mood, irritability, difficulties with concentration, increased urination, loss of bone mineral density, and sleep difficulties. In some cases, men who have low testosterone may benefit from carefully prescribed testosterone replacement therapy.

As men get older, they depend more on direct physical stimulation for sexual arousal. They take longer to achieve an erection and find it more difficult to maintain; orgasmic contractions are less intense. Older men with erectile dysfunction often use prescribed medications such as Viagra that increase blood flow to the penis, resulting in a firmer erection.

Unlike women, who are born with all the eggs they will ever have and stop being fertile at menopause, men continue to produce sperm throughout their lives and can sometimes father children well into their eighties and even nineties. Starting at about age 30, however, men become gradually less fertile. The pregnancy rate drops to 50% for couples with a man over age 35, regardless of the woman's age. Men over age 40 are more likely to produce children with health problems such as autism, schizophrenia, and Down syndrome.

Men over 40 are more likely to **produce children with health problems** such as autism, schizophrenia, and Down syndrome.

SEXUAL FUNCTIONING

Sexual activity is based on stimulus and response. Erotic stimulation leads to sexual arousal (excitement), which may culminate in the intensely pleasurable experience of orgasm. Pleasure comes from engaging the genitals, and it also comes from engaging the entire body and mind.

Sexual Stimulation

Physical stimuli excite us directly; some people believe psychological stimuli—thoughts, fantasies, desires, perceptions—excite us even more. Regardless of the source of eroticism, all stimulation has a physical basis, to which the brain gives meaning.

Physical Stimulation   Physical stimulation comes through the senses: We are aroused by things we see, hear, taste, smell, and feel. The most obvious and effective physical stimulation is touching. Even though culturally defined practices vary and different people have different preferences, most sexual encounters eventually involve some form of touching with hands, lips, and body surfaces. Kissing, caressing, fondling, and hugging are as much a part of sexual encounters as they are a part of expressing affection.

The most intense form of stimulation typically involves the genitals. The clitoris and the glans of the penis are particularly sensitive to such stimulation. Other highly responsive areas include the vaginal opening, nipples, breasts, insides of the thighs, buttocks, anal region, scrotum, lips, armpits, and earlobes. Such sexually sensitive areas, or erogenous zones, are especially susceptible to sexual arousal for most people, most of the time. Often, though, what determines the response is not *what* is touched but how, for how long, and by whom. Under the right circumstances, touching any part of the body can cause sexual arousal and even orgasm.

Psychological Stimulation   Sexual arousal also has an important psychological component, regardless of the nature of the physical stimulation. Fantasies, ideas, memories of past experiences, and mood can all generate sexual excitement.

Arousal is also powerfully influenced by emotions and attitudes about sex. How you feel about sex, the person you are with, and how the person feels about you matter tremendously in how sexually responsive you are likely to be. Even the most direct forms of physical stimulation carry emotional overtones. Kissing, caressing, and fondling express affection and caring. The emotional charge they give to a sexual interaction plays a significant role in sexual arousal—for some, as significant as the purely physical stimulation achieved by touching.

The Sexual Response Cycle

Men and women respond physiologically with a predictable set of reactions, regardless of the nature of the stimulation. Two physiological mechanisms explain most genital and bodily reactions during sexual arousal and orgasm. These mechanisms are **vasocongestion** and muscular tension. Vasocongestion is the engorgement of tissues that results when more blood flows into an organ than is flowing out. Thus the penis and the clitoris become erect on the same principle that makes a garden hose become stiff when the water is turned on. Increased muscular tension culminates in rhythmic muscular contractions during orgasm.

Four phases characterize the sexual response cycle:

1. In the *excitement phase,* in men, the penis becomes erect as its tissues become engorged with blood. The testes expand and are pulled upward within the scrotum. In women, the clitoris, labia, and vaginal walls are similarly engorged with blood. Tension increases in the vaginal muscles, and the vaginal walls become moist with lubricating fluid.

2. The *plateau phase* is an extension of the excitement phase. Reactions become more marked. In men, the penis becomes harder, and the testes become larger. In women, the uterus rises, causing the inner one-third of the vaginal canal to lengthen and "tent" open near the cervix while the outer one-third of the vagina swells, and vaginal lubrication increases.

3. In the *orgasmic phase,* or **orgasm,** rhythmic contractions occur along the man's penis, urethra, prostate gland, seminal vesicles, and muscles in the pelvic and anal regions. These involuntary muscular contractions lead to the ejaculation of semen**,** which consists of sperm cells from the testes and secretions from the prostate gland and seminal vesicles. In women, contractions occur in the lower part of the vagina and in the uterus, as well as in the pelvic region and the anus. Some women may also expel fluid out of the urethra, known as female ejaculation.

4. In the *resolution phase,* all the changes initiated during the excitement phase are reversed. Excess blood drains from tissues, the muscles in the region relax, and the genital structures return to their unstimulated states. Males experience a *refractory period,* or period of time following orgasm in which more stimulation will not cause arousal.

More general physical reactions accompany the genital changes in both men and women. Beginning with the excitement phase, nipples become erect, the woman's breasts begin to swell, and in both sexes the skin of the chest becomes flushed; these changes are more marked in women. The heart rate doubles by the plateau phase, and respiration becomes faster. During orgasm, breathing becomes irregular and the person may moan or cry out. A feeling of warmth leads to increased sweating during the resolution phase. Deep relaxation and a sense of well-being pervade the body and the mind as dopamine and oxytocin are released during the response cycle.

Male orgasm is marked by the ejaculation of semen. After ejaculation, men enter a refractory period. Women do not have this period and may immediately experience one or more orgasms.

Sexual Problems

Both physiological and psychological factors can interfere with sexual functioning. Many diseases specifically affect the sex organs. Any illness that affects your general health is likely to also affect your ability to function sexually. These problems may be due to physical problems, psychological issues, or a combination of both.

Common Sexual Health Problems   Medical conditions that affect women's sexual organs include the following:

• *Vaginitis* (inflammation of the vagina) is a common problem that can be caused by a variety of organisms: *Candida* (yeast infection), *Trichomonas* (trichomoniasis), and the overgrowth of a variety of bacteria (bacterial vaginosis). Symptoms include vaginal discharge, vaginal irritation, and pain during intercourse. Vaginitis is treated with a variety of topical and oral medications.

• *Vulvodynia,* or chronic and unexplained vulvar pain, affects between 15 and 18 percent of women in the United States. Patients describe their pain as "burning," "knifelike," and "raw." Because the condition presents diagnostic challenges, it's not uncommon for women and their sexual partners to wait five to seven years for a diagnosis and appropriate treatment.

• *Endometriosis* is the growth of endometrial-like tissue outside the uterus. It can cause serious problems if left untreated because endometrial tissue can scar and partially or completely block the oviducts, causing infertility (difficulty conceiving) or sterility (the inability to conceive). Endometriosis is treated with medication and/or surgery.

• *Pelvic inflammatory disease (PID)* is an infection of the uterus, oviducts, or ovaries caused when microorganisms spread to these areas from the vagina. Approximately 50–75% of PID cases are caused by sexually transmitted organisms associated with diseases such as gonorrhea and chlamydia. PID can cause scarring of the oviducts, resulting in infertility or sterility. Symptoms include abdominal and pelvic pain, fever, and possibly pain during intercourse.

---

vasocongestion   The accumulation of blood in tissues and organs by more blood flowing into an area than flowing out.

orgasm   The discharge of accumulated sexual tension with characteristic genital and bodily manifestations and a subjective sensation of intense pleasure; may include ejaculation for men and women.

TERMS

Sexual health problems affecting men include the following:

- *Prostatitis* is an inflammation or infection of the prostate gland that can be acute (sudden) or chronic (gradual and long lasting). The symptoms of *acute bacterial prostatitis* usually appear suddenly and may include fever, chills, flu-like symptoms, pain in the lower back or groin, problems with urination, and painful ejaculation. Acute prostatitis is treated with antibiotics. *Chronic prostatitis* can be caused by infection or inflammation of the prostate and is sometimes difficult to diagnose and treat.

- *Prostate cancer* is the second most common cancer in men, especially older men. Men over 40 should have routine prostate exams done by a physician.

- *Testicular cancer* occurs most commonly in men in their twenties and thirties. A rare cancer, it has a very high cure rate if detected early. Every man should perform testicular self-exams regularly.

- *Epididymitis* is an inflammation of the epididymis (the coiled tube located on the top and back of each testicle). The most common cause of epididymitis is infection, often sexually transmitted. Symptoms include tenderness over the testicle, swelling, fever, and pain with ejaculation. The treatment is antibiotics.

- *Testicular torsion* occurs when the spermatic cord, which supplies blood to the testicle, becomes twisted. Decreased blood flow to the testicle causes severe, sudden pain, and if not treated quickly, it can cause permanent damage to the testicle. Testicular pain should be evaluated by a medical professional promptly; sudden, severe pain is a medical emergency.

Sexual health problems affecting both women and men include *systemic diseases*—illnesses that affect organs throughout the body. A common example is diabetes, which often results in sexual dysfunction because of poor blood flow to the sexual organs, along with impaired sensation and nerve function. Sexual difficulties are frequently the first sign of serious health problems because any disease that affects the cardiovascular, nervous, or endocrine system is likely to have an impact on sexual functioning.

Sexual Dysfunctions The term **sexual dysfunction** encompasses disturbances in sexual desire, performance, or satisfaction. Many physical conditions and drugs can interfere with sexual functioning. Psychological causes and relationship problems can be important factors as well. Sexual satisfaction is highly individual, so no one should feel that it is necessary to live up to a particular standard of sexual performance or "normalcy." Only you can determine if some aspect of your sexuality is creating a problem for you or your partner.

COMMON SEXUAL DYSFUNCTIONS Common sexual difficulties that men may experience are low desire, erectile dysfunction, premature ejaculation, and delayed ejaculation. **Erectile dysfunction** (previously called *impotence*) is the inability to achieve or maintain an erection sufficient for sexual activity. Erectile dysfunction occurs in men of all ages but becomes much more common as men age. **Premature ejaculation** (ejaculation before or just after penetration) is also common, especially among younger men. If the problem is persistent and bothersome to the man and his partner, there are numerous treatments. **Delayed ejaculation** is the inability to ejaculate after an erection is achieved. Many men experience occasional difficulty achieving an erection or ejaculating because of excessive alcohol consumption, legal or illicit drugs, fatigue, or stress.

Female sexual problems generally involve a lack of desire to have sex, the failure to become physically aroused and lubricated even when sex is desired, the inability to have an orgasm (**orgasmic dysfunction**), or pain during sexual penetration. All of these problems can have physical and psychological components. Many medical problems can influence a woman's desire and ability to respond sexually. Factors such as hormonal birth control, menopause, and antidepressants can negatively affect sexual functioning. Psychological and social issues such as relationship difficulties, family stresses, depression, shame, guilt, and past sexual trauma are all frequent causes of sexual dysfunction for both women and men.

> . . . family stresses, depression, shame, guilt, and past sexual trauma are all **frequent causes of sexual dysfunction for both women and men.**

Women are more likely to achieve orgasm from stimulation to the clitoris, through self-stimulation, manual stimulation with a partner, oral sex, or use of a vibrator than through sexual intercourse. In general, the inability to experience orgasm under certain circumstances is a problem only if the woman considers it so.

Dyspareunia (painful intercourse) is a common symptom in women with many possible causes. Infection, lack of lubrication, endometriosis, past sexual trauma, fear of penetration, menopause, and scarring due to childbirth are a few common reasons for pain during intercourse. In some women, *vaginismus* (the involuntary contractions of pelvic

---

sexual dysfunction A disturbance in sexual desire, performance, or satisfaction that causes distress.

TERMS

erectile dysfunction The inability to achieve or maintain an erection sufficient for sexual activity.

premature ejaculation Involuntary orgasm before or shortly after the penis enters the vagina, mouth, or anus; ejaculation that takes place sooner than desired.

delayed ejaculation The inability to ejaculate when you wish to during sexual activity.

orgasmic dysfunction The inability to experience orgasm.

muscles) makes sexual penetration difficult to impossible. This condition may also include discomfort with inserting a tampon or finger or discomfort during a pelvic exam.

CAUSES OF SEXUAL DYSFUNCTION   For even an inkling of what might be causing a specific sexual dysfunction, the first step is to have a physical examination. This exam should evaluate an individual's overall health and explore a possible medical cause for the dysfunction. Heart disease and diabetes, for example, reduce blood flow and therefore have a negative effect on arousal for both men and women. In men, up to 80% of all erectile problems are thought to be due to physical factors, particularly vascular problems involving restriction of blood flow. Smoking affects blood flow in the genitals (and throughout the body of both men and women) and is an independent risk factor.

Alcohol and many prescription and nonprescription drugs can inhibit sexual response. In particular, antidepressant drugs (especially SSRIs, such as Prozac) are believed to cause sexual dysfunction in up to 50% of people. Sometimes drugs such as Viagra and Cialis are used to counteract the side effects of antidepressants.

Other common medications that can inhibit sexual response include certain drugs that treat high blood pressure.

TREATING SEXUAL DYSFUNCTION   Most forms of sexual dysfunction are treatable. For erectile dysfunction in particular, many treatments are available. Viagra (sildenafil citrate), Cialis (tadalafil), and Levitra (vardenafil) work by enhancing the effects of nitric oxide, a chemical that relaxes smooth muscles in the penis. The relaxed muscles increase blood flow and allow a natural erection to occur in response to sexual stimulation. The medications are generally safe for healthy men, but they should not be used by men who have a high risk of heart attack or stroke. They are effective in about 70% of users, but there are potential side effects, including headaches, indigestion, facial flushing, back pain, visual and hearing disturbances, and changes in blood pressure.

Viagra use by men between the ages of 18 and 45 has risen dramatically—possibly due to use of the drug for recreational purposes. The drug may cut the refractory period in men who do not have erectile dysfunction; younger men may also be using it to cope with performance anxiety or the effects of other drugs, such as antidepressants.

Although Viagra is not approved by the FDA for use by women, a growing number of women are trying the drug to help increase blood flow to the genitals, which is necessary for arousal and orgasm. Recent studies have shown that the drug can sometimes help women with sexual dysfunction caused by use of antidepressant drugs.

Other treatments for erectile dysfunction in men are available. Prostaglandin E1 (Alprostadil) dilates blood vessels. It can be injected into the penis or placed into the tip of the penis as a tiny suppository about the size of a grain of rice. It works by relaxing the smooth muscles lining the blood vessels in the penis. Alprostadil in a cream form that can be applied to the penis is currently awaiting FDA approval. There are also vacuum devices that pull blood into the penis, and in cases where other treatments are unsuccessful, penile implants can be used. Exercise may also help improve erectile function, especially exercises that target the muscles of the pelvic floor.

With greater awareness of symptoms of testosterone deficiency, more men are seeking treatment for testosterone deficiency with hormone replacement therapy. Symptoms of low testosterone include low libido, fatigue, anemia, increased body fat, reduced muscle mass, and mild depression.

Even when there is a physical reason for sexual dysfunction, emotional and social factors frequently compound the problem. Many people with no obvious physical disorder have sexual problems because of psychological and social issues.

Too often sexual difficulties are treated with drugs when nondrug strategies may be more appropriate. Psychosocial causes of dysfunction include troubled relationships, a lack of sexual skills, ineffective stimulation, irrational attitudes and beliefs, anxiety, prior learning and experiences, and psychosexual trauma such as sexual abuse or rape. Many of these problems can be addressed through sex therapy or counseling.

Premature ejaculation is an example of a common sexual problem that often responds well to nondrug therapy. On average, men typically ejaculate between 2 and 10 minutes after intercourse begins, but most men periodically ejaculate more quickly. Several nondrug techniques are frequently helpful for men who habitually ejaculate sooner than they would like. Kegel exercises, which strengthen and improve control of the pelvic muscles, as well as practicing **masturbation** (genital self-stimulation) to extend arousal, are often helpful. Certain antidepressants delay ejaculation and are sometimes prescribed for this purpose.

Women who seek treatment for orgasmic dysfunction often have not learned what types of stimulation will excite them and bring them to orgasm. Most sex therapists treat this problem with masturbation. Women are taught about their own anatomy and sexual responses and then are encouraged to experiment with masturbation, focusing on the clitoris, until they experience orgasm. Vibrators, once taboo, are becoming more and more common and are helpful devices during masturbation or intercourse. Once women can masturbate to orgasm, they can transfer this learning to other sexual behaviors including those with a partner.

> Any disease affecting the cardiovascular, nervous, or endocrine systems **may also affect sexual functioning.**

masturbation   Self-stimulation for the purpose of sexual arousal and orgasm.   TERMS

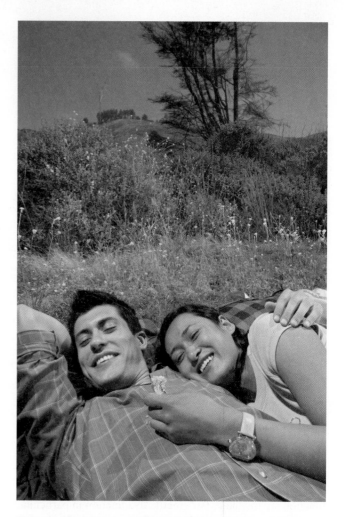
Substances being tested for the treatment of female sexual dysfunction include prostaglandin creams and testosterone patches. Testosterone replacement is currently being used "off-label" to treat low desire in women, because there has not been an FDA testosterone approved for women. A prostaglandin cream that improves blood flow to the clitoris is currently being developed and may be available to treat female sexual arousal disorder in the future. Other options are a vibrator and a device that creates suction over the clitoris to increase blood flow and sensitivity.

Dyspareunia and vaginismus are treated first by diagnosing and treating any underlying physical cause of the problem. The use of generous amounts of lubricant during sexual activity is important. Sexual therapy for vaginismus often involves gradual desensitization techniques including the use of dilators. Dilators range in size and are inserted into the vagina in order to relax the vaginal muscles, to stop the involuntary spasms, and for the vagina to gradually stretch. Recently, the FDA approved a procedure using Botox injections, a chemical that paralyzes muscles, which has been successful in relaxing the pelvic muscles in some women with vaginismus.

SEXUAL BEHAVIOR

Many behaviors stem from sexual impulses, and sexual expression takes a variety of forms. Probably the most basic aspect of sexuality is reproduction. But sexual excitement and satisfaction are aspects of sexual behavior separate from reproduction. The intensely pleasurable sensations of arousal and orgasm are probably the strongest motivators for human sexual behavior. People are infinitely varied in the ways they seek to experience erotic pleasure. Our behavior is shaped by the interplay of our biological predispositions and our life experiences.

Sexual Orientation

Sexual orientation often refers to whom a person is emotionally connected to (love), romantically attached to (relationship), sexually attracted to (desire), and behaviorally intimate with (sex). For many, the pattern is consistent, exclusively heterosexual or

This couple's physical experiences together will be powerfully affected by their emotions, ideas, values, and the quality of their relationship.

exclusively homosexual for all categories: love, relationship, desire, and sex. For others, there may be more variation. As indicated in Chapter 4, sexual orientation exists along a continuum that ranges from exclusive heterosexuality (attraction to people of the other sex) through bisexuality (attraction to people of both sexes) to exclusive homosexuality (attraction to people of your own sex). The terms *straight* and *gay* are often used to refer to heterosexuals and homosexuals, respectively, and female homosexuals are also referred to as *lesbians*. In recent years, the term *queer* has been reclaimed as a self-identifier by some elements of the gay community.

Sexual orientation involves feelings and self-concept, and individuals may or may not express their sexual orientation in their behavior. In national surveys, about 2–6% of men identify themselves as homosexuals and about 2% of women identify themselves as lesbians. Gauging the accuracy of these estimates is difficult because people may not tell the truth in surveys that probe very sensitive and private aspects of their lives. In addition, people's expressed sexual orientations may be quite different from their actual sexual practices. For example, some people identify as heterosexual, but most of their sexual partners may be of their own sex.

Whom am I sexually attracted to?

- What are the characteristics that usually attract me to someone in a physical way?

- How comfortable am I with the people I find sexually attractive? What would I change if I could? Do I feel safe when I am with them?

- Are the people I am usually sexually attracted to the same types of people that I could envision having a long-term, stable relationship with? Why or why not?

What sexual behaviors are comfortable for me right now?

- What has influenced my comfort level with these behaviors?

- What am I not entirely comfortable with, but would be willing to experiment with in order to please a partner? What level of trust would I need to establish with that partner in order to proceed? What would we need to talk about ahead of time?

- What exactly do I say in order to make my comfort level clear to my partner? What do I do if my partner tries to push me beyond my comfort level?

How can I express my sexual needs, desires, and concerns to a potential sexual partner?

- When would be the best time to talk about these needs, desires, and concerns?

- How do I start the conversation?

- What will I do if my needs are not being met or my concerns are not taken seriously?

What preparations do I need to make in order to engage in the safest sex possible?

- If I am engaging in heterosexual sexual activity, I need to obtain birth control. Have I consulted a health professional to figure out the best method of birth control for myself and my partner? Do I know how to employ this method correctly? Have we discussed what we plan to do if a pregnancy occurs?

- If I am engaging in any type of sexual activity with a partner, I need protection from STIs. Have I consulted a health professional to figure out the best method of STI protection for myself and my partner? Do I know how to employ this method correctly? Have I discussed with my partner his or her sexual history, including information about risky behavior and STIs?

- What do I need from my partner in order to ensure that I feel emotionally safe before, during, and after our sexual behavior together?

- Do I engage in any behaviors that cause me to participate in sexual activity that I wouldn't otherwise be comfortable with, such as excessive drinking or drug use? What do I need to do in order to reduce or eliminate these behaviors?

connect
ACTIVITY
DO IT ONLINE

So far, most studies on the origin of sexual orientation have focused on males. The factors that determine sexual orientation in women may be even more complex. Although genes appear to be the most important determinant of sexual orientation, further research is required to fully undertand the complex interactions that exist.

Varieties of Human Sexual Behavior

Some sexual behaviors are aimed at self-stimulation only, whereas other practices involve interaction with a partner. Some people choose not to express their sexuality at all.

Celibacy   Continuous abstention from sexual activities, called **celibacy,** can be a conscious and deliberate choice, or it can be necessitated by circumstances. Health considerations and religious and moral beliefs may lead some people to celibacy, particularly until marriage or until an acceptable partner appears. Many people use the related term *abstinence* to refer to avoidance of just one sexual activity—intercourse.

Autoeroticism   The most common sexual behavior for humans is masturbation. Masturbation is one form of **autoeroticism;** another is **erotic fantasy,** or creating imaginary experiences that range from fleeting thoughts to elaborate scenarios. Orgasms originate in our brain as it gives meaning to stimulation and pleasure. Using functional MRI (fMRI) scans to map orgasms in the brain, researchers at Rutgers University found that at the time of orgasm every part of our brain lights up and is engaged. No other activity produces the same brain response.

	TERMS
celibacy Continuous abstention from sexual activity.	
autoeroticism Behavior aimed at sexual self-stimulation.	
erotic fantasy Sexually arousing thoughts and daydreams.	

Touching and Foreplay Touching is integral to sexual experiences, whether in the form of massage, kissing, fondling, or holding. Our entire body surface is a sensory organ, and touching almost anywhere can enhance intimacy and sexual arousal. Touching can convey a variety of messages, including affection, comfort, and a desire for further sexual contact.

During arousal, many partners manually and orally stimulate each other by touching, stroking, and caressing their partner's genitals. People vary greatly in their preferences for the type, pace, and vigor of such **foreplay.** Working out the details to accommodate each other's pleasure is a key to enjoying these activities. Direct communication about preferences can enhance sexual pleasure and protect both partners from physical and psychological discomfort.

Oral-Genital Stimulation **Cunnilingus** (the stimulation of the female genitals with the lips and tongue) and **fellatio** (the stimulation of the penis with the mouth) are common practices. Oral sex may be practiced either as part of foreplay or as a sex act culminating in orgasm. Although prevalence varies in different populations, 90% of men, 88% of women, and more than 50% of teens report that they have engaged in oral sex. Like all acts of sexual expression between two people, oral sex requires the cooperation and consent of both partners.

Anal Intercourse According to the CDC, about 36% of males and 31% of women have engaged in anal sex. Some men and women find they are able to achieve orgasm through anal sex.

Because the anus is composed of delicate tissues that tear easily with friction, anal intercourse can be one of the riskiest of sexual behaviors for the transmission of HIV and all other sexually transmitted infections. If people are monogamous, up to date with their STI status, or use barrier devices such as condoms, the risk becomes lower. The use of condoms is highly recommended for anyone engaging in anal sex.

Sexual Intercourse Men and women engage in vaginal intercourse to fulfill sexual and psychological needs, as well as to reproduce. Data from a 2006–2008 study by the National Center for Health Statistics find that 97% of men aged 15–44 and 98% of women in the same age group reported having had vaginal intercourse. The most common heterosexual practice is the man inserting his erect penis into the woman's lubricated vagina after sufficient arousal. Among both men and women, one of the most popular reasons to have sex was to express emotional attachment to their partner.

The use of force and coercion in sexual relationships is one of the most serious problems in human interactions. The most extreme manifestation of **sexual coercion**—forcing a person to submit to another's sexual desires—is rape, but sexual coercion occurs in many subtler forms, such as sexual harassment.

Commercial Sex

Conflicting feelings about sexuality are apparent in the attitudes of Americans toward commercial sex: prostitution and sexually oriented materials in a variety of formats. Our society supposedly disapproves of prostitution, but it also provides prostitutes with their customers. Pornography is readily available and widely viewed in our society, although many people are concerned about its ubiquitous nature and the blurring of pornography with popular culture.

Pornography Derived from the Greek word meaning "the writing of prostitutes," **pornography** (*porn*) is now often defined as obscene literature, art, or movies. A major problem in identifying pornographic material is that different people and communities have different opinions about what

One of the commonly stated reasons for having sex is **to express emotional attachment to your partner.**

TERMS

foreplay Kissing, touching, and any form of oral or genital contact.

cunnilingus Oral stimulation of the female genitals.

fellatio Oral stimulation of the penis.

sexual intercourse Sexual relations involving genital union; also called coitus; also known as making love.

sexual coercion The use of physical or psychological force or intimidation to make a person submit to sexual demands.

pornography The depiction of sexual activities in pictures, writing, or other material with the intent to arouse.

Ask Yourself

QUESTIONS FOR CRITICAL THINKING AND REFLECTION

What do you consider to be appropriate, moral sexual behavior? What behaviors do you think are inappropriate or immoral? What experiences have shaped your views of such behaviors? Have they changed in the past five years? What do you think they will be like five years from now?

is obscene, as obscenity is typically a judgment by someone who finds it offensive. Differing definitions of obscenity have led to many legal battles over potentially pornographic materials. Currently the sale and rental of pornographic materials is restricted so that only adults can legally obtain them; however, the Internet is difficult to regulate, and many minors may have access to pornographic materials online. Child pornography or showing children who are not 18 years old naked and/or in sexual acts is illegal.

Much of the debate about pornography focuses on whether it is harmful. Some people argue that adults who want to view pornographic materials in the privacy of their own homes should be allowed to do so. Others feel that the exposure to explicit sexual material can lead to delinquent or criminal behavior, such as rape or the sexual abuse of children. Currently there is no reliable evidence that pornography by itself leads to violence or rape, and debate is likely to continue.

Online Porn and Cybersex   The appearance of thousands of sexually oriented websites has expanded the number of people with access to pornography, and has made it more difficult for authorities to enforce laws regarding porn. Of special concern is the increased availability of child pornography, which previously could be acquired only with great difficulty and at great legal risk. Online porn is now a multibillion-dollar industry.

Hundreds of thousands of people also use the Internet to engage in **cybersex,** or *virtual sex.* Cybersex is erotic interaction between people who are communicating over the Internet. Although many people view cybersex as a safe form of sexual expression, it is not without problems. It can be addictive, and some cybersex addicts report spending more than 50 hours a week online for sexual purposes. People who become addicted to cybersex or viewing online porn may become isolated and perform poorly at work or school. Their addiction may also have a negative impact on their interpersonal relationships.

"Sexting," sending provocative photos from cell phone to cell phone, has become popular, sometimes with serious consequences. Images can end up traveling from person to person by cell phone and from there onto social networking websites like Facebook. These images can haunt individuals years later when they are viewed by potential employers or partners. Some teens have found themselves charged with child pornography and have even faced jail time as a result of forwarding a sexually explicit photo of an underaged person to a friend. Teens who have found pictures of themselves engaging in sexual activity posted or sent around have faced adverse effects. Some have even committed suicide.

Prostitution   The exchange of sexual services for money is **prostitution**. Prostitutes may be men, women, or children, and the buyer of a prostitute's services is nearly always a man. Except in parts of Nevada, prostitution is illegal in the United States. Most customers are white, middle-class, middle-aged, and married. Although they come from a wide variety of backgrounds, prostitutes are usually motivated to join the profession because of money.

Acquired immunodeficiency syndrome (AIDS) and other STIs are major concerns for prostitutes and their customers. Many prostitutes are injection drug users or are involved with men who are. The rate of HIV infection among prostitutes varies widely, but in some parts of the country it is as high as 25–50%. Unfortunately many prostitutes are children. The majority, both female and male, began working as prostitutes before they were 16 years of age. A majority also report that they were sexually abused as children. Many prostitutes start out as child runaways, escaping abusive homes and turning to prostitution as a way to survive.

Responsible Sexual Behavior

Healthy sexuality is an important part of adult life. It can be a source of pleasurable experiences and emotions and an important part of intimate partnerships. But sexual behavior also carries many responsibilities, as well as potential consequences such as pregnancy, STIs, and emotional changes in the relationship.

Open, Honest Communication   Each partner needs to clearly indicate what sexual involvement means to him or her. Does it mean love, fun, a permanent commitment, or something else? The intentions of both partners should be clear. For strategies on talking about sexual issues with your partner, see the box "Communicating about Sexuality."

Agreed-On Sexual Activities   No one should pressure or coerce a partner. Sexual behaviors should be consistent with the sexual values, preferences, and comfort level of both partners. Everyone has the right to refuse sexual activity at any time, including married couples.

Sexual Privacy   Intimate relationships involving sexual activity are based on trust, and that trust can be violated if partners reveal private information about the relationship to others. Sexual privacy also involves respecting other people—not engaging in activities in the presence of others that would make them uncomfortable.

Safe Sex   Both partners should be aware of and practice safe sex to guard against STIs. Many sexual behaviors carry the risk of STIs, including HIV infection. Partners should be honest about their health and any medical conditions and work out a plan for protection.

Contraception Use   If pregnancy is not desired, contraception should be used during sexual intercourse. Both partners need to take responsibility for protecting against unwanted pregnancy. Partners should discuss contraception before sexual involvement begins.

---

cybersex   Erotic interaction between people who are not in physical contact, conducted over a network such as the Internet; also called *virtual sex.*

prostitution   The exchange of sexual services for money or goods.

TERMS

TAKE CHARGE
Communicating about Sexuality

To talk with your partner about sexuality, follow the general suggestions for effective communication in Chapter 4. Getting started may be the most difficult part. Some people feel more comfortable if they begin by talking about talking—that is, initiating a discussion about why people are so uncomfortable talking about sexuality. Talking about sexual histories—how partners first learned about sex or how family and cultural background influenced sexual values and attitudes—is another way to get started. Reading about sex can also be a good beginning: Partners can read an article or book and then discuss their reactions.

Be honest about what you feel and what you want from your partner. Cultural and personal obstacles to discussing sexual subjects can be difficult to overcome, but self-disclosure is important for successful relationships. Research indicates that when one partner openly discusses attitudes and feelings, the other partner is more likely to do the same. If your partner seems hesitant to open up, try asking open-ended or either/or questions: "Where do you like to be touched?" or "Would you like to talk about this now or wait until later?"

If something is bothering you about your sexual relationship, choose a good time to initiate a discussion with your partner. Be specific and direct but also tactful. Focus on what you actually observe rather than on what you think the behavior means. "You didn't touch or hug me when your friends were around" is an observation. "You're ashamed of me around your friends" is an inference about your partner's feelings. Try focusing on a specific behavior that concerns you rather than on the person as a whole—your partner can change behaviors but not his or her entire personality. For example, you could say "I'd like you to take a few minutes away from studying to kiss me" instead of "You're so caught up in your work, you never have time for me."

If you are going to make a statement that your partner may interpret as criticism, try mixing it with something positive: "I love being with you, but I feel annoyed when you... ." Similarly, if your partner says something that upsets you, don't lash back. An aggressive response may make you feel better in the short run, but it will not help the communication process or the quality of the relationship.

If you want to say no to some sexual activity, say no unequivocally. Don't send mixed messages. If you are afraid of hurting your partner's feelings, offer an alternative if it's appropriate: "I am uncomfortable with that. How about . . . ?"

If you're in love, you may think that the sexual aspects of a relationship will work out magically without discussion. However, partners who never talk about sex deny themselves the opportunity to increase their closeness and improve their relationship.

Sober Sex   The use of alcohol or drugs in sexual situations increases the risk of unplanned, unprotected sexual activity. Such consequences are particularly true for young adults, many of whom binge-drink during social events. The link between intoxication and unsafe sex is illustrated by a recent study that found states with higher drinking ages and higher beer taxes have lower rates of STIs. Alcohol and drugs impair judgment and should not be used in association with sexual activity. Be honest with yourself; if you need to drink in order to engage in sexual activities, maybe it's time to rethink your social life and relationships.

According to the Coalition to Prevent Substance Abuse:

- As many as 70% of college students admit to having engaged in sexual activity primarily as a result of being under the influence of alcohol, or to having sex they wouldn't have had if they had been sober.

- 90% of all campus rapes occur when alcohol has been used by either the assailant or the victim.

- At least one out of five college students abandons safe sex practices when they're drunk, even if they do protect themselves when they're sober.

- One in twelve college males admit to having committed acts that meet the legal definition of rape or acquaintance rape.

- 55% of female students and 75% of male students involved in acquaintance rape admit to having been drinking or using drugs when the incident occurred.

- 60% of college women infected with STIs, including genital herpes and AIDS, report they were under the influence of alcohol at the time they had intercourse with the infected person.

- Female college freshman are at the highest risk for sexual assault between the first day of school and Thanksgiving break.

Ask Yourself

QUESTIONS FOR CRITICAL THINKING AND REFLECTION

If you are sexually active or plan to become active soon, how open have you been in communicating with your partner? Are you aware of your partner's feelings about sex and his or her comfort level with certain activities? Do you and your partner share the same views on contraception, STI prevention, and ethical issues about sex?

UNDERSTANDING FERTILITY

Conception is a complex process. Although many couples conceive easily, others face a variety of difficulties.

Conception

The process of conception begins with the union of the nucleus of a woman's egg cell (ovum) and the nucleus of a man's sperm cell—a process called **fertilization**. Every month during a woman's fertile years, her body prepares itself for conception and pregnancy. In one of her ovaries, an egg matures and is released from its follicle. The egg, about the size of a pinpoint, travels through an oviduct, or fallopian tube, to the uterus in three to four days. The endometrium, which is the lining of the uterus, has already thickened for the implantation of a **fertilized egg,** that is, a *zygote*. If the egg is not fertilized, it lasts about 24 hours and then disintegrates. The woman's body then expels the egg's remains and the uterine lining during menstruation.

Fertilization Sperm cells are produced in the man's testes and ejaculated from his penis into the woman's vagina during sexual intercourse. Sperm cells are much smaller than eggs. The typical ejaculate contains millions of sperm, but only a few complete the journey through the uterus and up the fallopian tube to the egg.

Of those that reach the egg, only one will penetrate its hard outer layer. As sperm approach the egg, they release enzymes that soften this outer layer. Enzymes from hundreds of sperm must be released in order for the egg's outer layer to soften enough to allow one sperm cell to penetrate. The first sperm cell that bumps into a spot that is soft enough can swim into the egg cell. It then fuses with the nucleus of the egg, and fertilization occurs. The sperm's tail, its means of locomotion, gets stuck in the egg's outer membrane and drops off, leaving the sperm's head inside the egg. The egg then undergoes chemical change that makes it impenetrable by other sperm.

The ovum carries the hereditary characteristics of the mother and her ancestors; sperm cells carry the hereditary characteristics of the father and his ancestors. Each parent cell—egg or sperm—contains 23 chromosomes, each of which contains **genes,** which are packages of biochemical instructions for the developing baby. Genes provide the blueprint for a unique individual based on the functional and health characteristics of his or her ancestors.

Twins In the usual course of events, one egg and one sperm unite to produce one fertilized egg and one baby. But if the ovaries release two or more eggs during ovulation and if both eggs are fertilized, twins develop. The development of two or more fetuses in the same pregnancy is called *multiple gestation* and leads to a *multiple birth*. These twins will be no more alike than siblings from different pregnancies because each will have come from a different fertilized egg.

Twins who develop this way are referred to as **fraternal (dizygotic) twins;** they may be the same sex or different sexes. About 70% of twins are fraternal.

Twins can also develop from the division of a single fertilized egg into two cells that develop separately. Because these babies share all genetic material, they will be **identical (monozygotic) twins.**

The most serious complication of multiple births is preterm delivery (delivery before the fetuses are adequately mature). The higher the number of fetuses that a woman carries, the earlier in gestation she will deliver.

Infertility

About 2 million American couples have difficulty conceiving. **Infertility** is defined as the inability to conceive after trying for a year or more. Infertility affected about 6% of reproductive-aged American women (15–44 years) in the United States in 2010 (the most recent year for which reliable statistics are available). Over 1 million women seek treatment for infertility each year. Although the focus is often on women (where the cause of infertility is found in 50% of cases), one-fourth (26%) of the factors contributing to infertility are male, and in one-third (35%) of infertile couples, both partners have problems. Therefore, it is important that both partners be evaluated.

Female Infertility One-third of cases of female infertility usually results from one of two key causes—tubal blockage (14%) or failure to ovulate (21%). An additional one-third (37%) of cases of female infertility is due to anatomical abnormalities, benign growths in the uterus, thyroid disease, and other uncommon conditions; the remaining 28% of cases are unexplained.

Blocked oviducts are most commonly the result of *pelvic inflammatory disease (PID),* a serious complication of several sexually transmitted infections. One study found that of 100,000 women aged 20–24 who were diagnosed with PID, 16,800 (1 of every 6) went on to have problems with

---

TERMS

fertilization The initiation of biological reproduction; the union of the nucleus of an egg cell with the nucleus of a sperm cell.

fertilized egg The egg after penetration by a sperm; a *zygote*.

gene The basic unit of heredity; a section of a chromosome containing biochemical instructions for making a particular protein.

fraternal (dizygotic) twins Twins who develop from separate fertilized eggs; such twins are not genetically identical.

identical (monozygotic) twins Twins who develop from the division of a single zygote; such twins are genetically identical.

Infertility The inability to conceive after trying for a year or more.

infertility. Most cases of PID are associated with untreated cases of chlamydia or gonorrhea. More than 2.5 million cases of PID are treated each year, but physicians estimate that just as many may go untreated because of an absence of symptoms. Tubal blockages can also be caused by prior surgery or by *endometriosis,* which is typically treated with hormonal therapy and surgery.

Age also impacts fertility. Beginning around age 30, a woman's fertility naturally begins to decline. Age is probably the main factor in ovulation failure. Exposure to toxic chemicals, cigarette smoke, or radiation also appears to reduce fertility, as do genetic factors identifiable in your family history.

Male Infertility The leading causes of male infertility can be divided into four main categories: hypothalamic pituitary disease (1–2%), testicular disease (30–40%), disorders of sperm transport or posttesticular disorders (10–20%), and unexplained (40–50%). Some acquired disorders of the testes can lead to infertility, such as damage from drug use (including marijuana), smoking, infection, or environmental toxins.

Treating Infertility The cause of infertility can be determined for about 85% of infertile couples. Most cases of infertility are treated with conventional medical therapies. Surgery can repair oviducts, remove endometriosis, and correct anatomical problems in men and women. Fertility drugs can help women ovulate, but may cause multiple births. If these conventional treatments don't work, couples can turn to **assisted reproductive technology (ART)** techniques, as described in the following sections. According to 2011 estimates from the CDC, about 1–3% of births in the United States and Europe are the result of ART treatments.

Most infertility treatments are expensive and emotionally draining, and their success is hard to predict. Some infertile couples choose not to try to have children, whereas others turn to adoption. One measure you can take to avoid infertility is to protect yourself against STIs and get prompt treatment for any disease you contract. Couples

who are ready should consider trying to conceive prior to the woman's late 30s to decrease the probability of age-related infertility.

INTRAUTERINE INSEMINATION Male infertility can sometimes be overcome by collecting and concentrating the man's sperm and introducing the semen by syringe into a woman's vagina or uterus, a procedure known as **artificial (intrauterine) insemination.** To increase the probability of success, the woman is often given fertility drugs to induce ovulation prior to the insemination procedure. The sperm can be provided by the woman's partner or a donor. Donor sperm are also used by single women and lesbian couples who want to conceive using artificial insemination. The success rate is about 5–20%. The wide range is due to age-related influences.

IVF A surgical technique used to overcome infertility, **in vitro fertilization (IVF),** involves surgically removing mature eggs from a woman's ovary and pairing the harvested eggs with sperm outside the woman's body (*in vitro*), in a laboratory dish. If eggs are successfully fertilized, one or more of the resulting embryos are inserted into the woman's uterus. The remaining embryos can then be frozen for future use.

There are disadvantages to IVF. Success rates determined by live birth rates vary from about 4% to 40% depending on age. It costs more than $10,000 per procedure and may require five or more attempts to produce one live birth. IVF also increases the chance of twins or triplets, which in turn increases the risk of premature birth and maternal complications, including pregnancy-related hypertension and diabetes.

GESTATIONAL CARRIER (FORMERLY KNOWN AS SURROGACY) A *gestational carrier (GC)* is a fertile woman who agrees to carry a fetus for an infertile couple. The GC agrees to be artificially inseminated by the father's sperm or to undergo IVF with the couple's embryo, to carry the baby to term, and to give it to the couple at birth. In return, the couple pays her for her services and medical costs (typically around $50,000). As of 2011, less than 1% of all ART in the United States is performed through gestational carriers.

TERMS

assisted reproductive technology (ART) Advanced medical techniques used to treat infertility.

artificial (intrauterine) insemination The introduction of semen into the vagina by artificial means.

in vitro fertilization (IVF) Combining eggs and sperm outside the body and inserting one or more fertilized eggs into the uterus.

trimester One of the three 3-month periods of pregnancy.

PREGNANCY

Pregnancy is usually discussed in terms of **trimesters**—three periods of about three months (or 13 weeks) each. During the first trimester, the mother experiences a few physical changes and some fairly common symptoms. During the second trimester, often the most peaceful time of pregnancy, the mother gains weight, looks noticeably pregnant, and may experience a general sense of well-being if

Women have access to a variety of over-the-counter home pregnancy tests today, but generally speaking, these tests all work in the same way to determine whether a woman is pregnant. Pregnancy tests are designed to detect the presence of the hormone **human chorionic gonadotropin (HCG)**, a hormone produced by the implanted fertilized egg, which is discussed in this chapter. Because the placenta releases HCG, the hormone can be detected in her urine or blood when a woman is pregnant.

Home pregnancy tests have become extremely accurate since their introduction in 1975. In a 2001 study, researchers found that the highest possible screening sensitivity for an HCG-based pregnancy test is 90% when taken on the first day of a missed period. In 10% of women, the fertilized egg may not have implanted in the uterine wall by the first day of a missed period. The researchers estimated that when taken seven days after the first day of a missed period, the highest

possible screening sensitivity of a home pregnancy test is 97%. The typical test provides accurate results 99% of the time.

A clinical blood test is more accurate but not necessarily more sensitive than a home pregnancy test. That is, it cannot detect pregnancy sooner than a urine test.

If you use a home pregnancy test, be aware of the limitations. If you're comfortable waiting, a sensitive test taken a week after your period is due will almost certainly give you accurate results. If you elect to take the test as early as the day after you've missed your period, remember that a negative result isn't 100% certain. A positive result may mean either a viable pregnancy or a pregnancy destined to end shortly after it began. With either of those results, you should plan to test again a week later, just to be sure. For that reason, it's a good idea to buy tests in pairs; Most commercially available home testing products come as multiple-test kits.

she is happy about having a child. The third trimester is the hardest for the mother because she must breathe, digest, excrete, and circulate blood for herself and the growing fetus.

Changes in the Woman's Body

Hormonal changes begin as soon as an egg is fertilized, and for the next 9 months the woman's body nourishes the fetus and adjusts to its growth (Figure 5.3).

Early Signs and Symptoms Early recognition of pregnancy is important, especially for women with medical conditions or nutritional deficiencies. The following symptoms are not absolute indications of pregnancy, but they are reasons to visit a gynecologist, and maybe take a home pregnancy test (see the box "Home Pregnancy Tests"):

• *A missed menstrual period.* When a fertilized egg implants in the uterine wall, the endometrium is retained to nourish the embryo.

• *Slight bleeding.* Following implantation of the fertilized egg into the endometrial lining, slight bleeding occurs in about 14% of pregnant women. Because this happens about when a period is expected, about 2 weeks after ovulation, the bleeding is sometimes mistaken for menstrual flow. It usually lasts only a few days.

human chorionic gonadotropin (HCG) A hormone produced by a fertilized egg that can be detected in the urine or blood of the mother shortly after conception.

TERMS

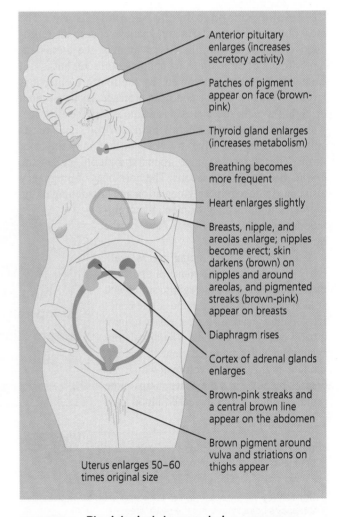

- Anterior pituitary enlarges (increases secretory activity)
- Patches of pigment appear on face (brown-pink)
- Thyroid gland enlarges (increases metabolism)
- Breathing becomes more frequent
- Heart enlarges slightly
- Breasts, nipple, and areolas enlarge; nipples become erect; skin darkens (brown) on nipples and around areolas, and pigmented streaks (brown-pink) appear on breasts
- Diaphragm rises
- Cortex of adrenal glands enlarges
- Brown-pink streaks and a central brown line appear on the abdomen
- Brown pigment around vulva and striations on thighs appear

Uterus enlarges 50–60 times original size

FIGURE 5.3 Physiological changes during pregnancy.

- *Nausea.* About 50–90% of pregnant women feel increased nausea, probably in reaction to surging levels of progesterone and other pregnancy hormones. Although this nausea is often called *morning sickness,* some women have it all day long. It frequently begins during the 6th week and disappears by the 12th week. In some cases it continues throughout the pregnancy.

- *Breast tenderness.* Some women experience breast tenderness, swelling, and tingling, usually described as different from the tenderness experienced before menstruation.

- *Increased urination.* Increased frequency of urination can occur soon after the missed period.

- *Sleepiness, fatigue, and emotional upset.* These symptoms result from hormonal changes. Fatigue can be surprisingly overwhelming in the first trimester but usually improves significantly around the third month of pregnancy.

The first reliable physical signs of pregnancy can be distinguished about 4 weeks after a woman misses her menstrual period. Increased uterine growth and blood flow contribute to softening of the uterus just above the cervix, called *Hegar's sign,* and a bluish discoloration to the cervix and labia minora, termed *Chadwick's sign.*

Continuing Changes in the Woman's Body The most obvious changes during pregnancy occur in the reproductive organs. During the first 3 months, the uterus enlarges to about three times its nonpregnant size, but it still cannot be felt in the abdomen. By the fourth month, it is large enough to make the abdomen protrude. By the seventh or eighth month, the uterus pushes up under the rib cage, which makes breathing slightly more difficult. The breasts enlarge and are sensitive; by week 8, they may tingle or throb. The pigmented area around the nipple, called the *areola*, darkens and broadens. The hormones of pregnancy also contribute to hyperpigmentation and broadening of the nipple, and for some women, hyperpigmentation may show in the face, or the midline of the abdomen.

Other changes are going on as well. Early in pregnancy, the muscles and ligaments attached to bones begin to soften and stretch. The joints between the pelvic bones loosen and spread, making it easier to have a baby but harder to walk. The circulatory system becomes more efficient to accommodate higher blood volume, which increases by 50%, and the heart pumps more rapidly. Much of the increased blood flow goes to the uterus and placenta (the organ that exchanges nutrients and waste between mother and fetus). The mother's lungs also become more efficient, and her rib cage widens to permit her to inhale up to 40% more air.

The average weight gain during a healthy pregnancy is 27.5 pounds, although actual weight change varies with the individual. About half of the weight gain is directly related to the baby (such as the fetus and placenta); the rest accumulates over the woman's body as fluid and fat.

Changes during the Later Stages of Pregnancy
By the end of the 6th month, the increased needs of the fetus place a burden on the mother's lungs, heart, and kidneys. Her back may ache from the pressure of the baby's weight and from having to throw her shoulders back to keep her balance while standing. Her body retains more water, perhaps up to three extra quarts of fluid. Her legs, hands, ankles, or feet may swell, and she may be bothered by leg cramps, heartburn, or constipation. Despite discomfort, both her digestion and her metabolism are working at top efficiency.

Near term, the uterus prepares for childbirth with a series of preliminary contractions, called **Braxton Hicks contractions**. Unlike true labor contractions, *Braxton Hicks contractions* are irregular with short duration; they are also often painless. To the mother, a contraction may initially feel only as though her abdomen is hard to the touch. As the delivery date approaches, true labor contractions become more frequent, regular, and intense and ultimately result in labor.

In the 9th month, increased joint laxity coupled by a softening cervix allows the baby to settle deeper into the pelvis. This process, called **lightening,** produces a visible change in the mother's abdominal profile. Pelvic pressure increases, and pressure on the diaphragm lightens. Breathing becomes easier; urination becomes more frequent. Sometimes, after a first pregnancy, lightening does not occur until labor begins.

Emotional Responses to Pregnancy

Rapid changes in hormone levels can cause a pregnant woman to experience unpredictable emotions. During the first trimester, the pregnant woman may fear that she may miscarry or that the child will not be normal. During the second trimester, the pregnant woman can feel early fetal movements, and worries about miscarriages usually begin to diminish. The third trimester is the time of greatest physical stress during the pregnancy. Because some women feel physically awkward and sexually unattractive, they may experience periods of depression. But many also feel a great deal of happy excitement and anticipation.

Braxton Hicks contractions A pattern of late pregnancy uterine contractions that are irregular in timing, short in duration, and painless and ultimately result in labor.

lightening A process in which the uterus sinks down because the baby's head settles into the pelvic area.

TERMS

FIGURE 5.4 **A chronology of milestones in prenatal development.**

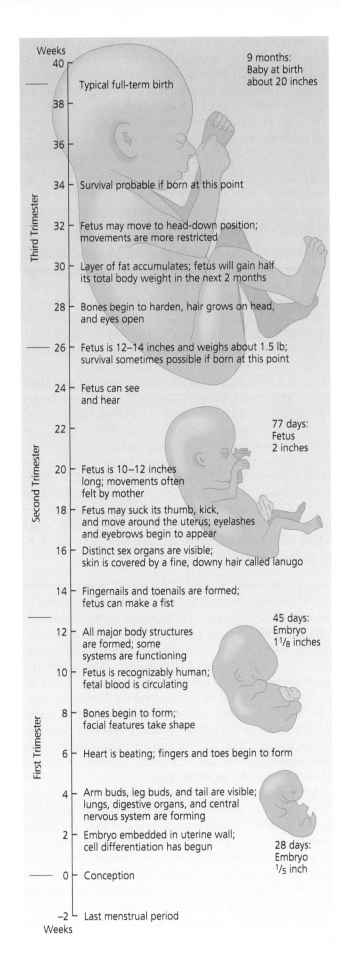

Weeks
40
9 months:
Baby at birth
about 20 inches

Typical full-term birth

38

Third Trimester

36

34 — Survival probable if born at this point

32 — Fetus may move to head-down position; movements are more restricted

30 — Layer of fat accumulates; fetus will gain half its total body weight in the next 2 months

28 — Bones begin to harden, hair grows on head, and eyes open

26 — Fetus is 12–14 inches and weighs about 1.5 lb; survival sometimes possible if born at this point

24 — Fetus can see and hear

Second Trimester

22
77 days:
Fetus
2 inches

20 — Fetus is 10–12 inches long; movements often felt by mother

18 — Fetus may suck its thumb, kick, and move around the uterus; eyelashes and eyebrows begin to appear

16 — Distinct sex organs are visible; skin is covered by a fine, downy hair called lanugo

14 — Fingernails and toenails are formed; fetus can make a fist

12 — All major body structures are formed; some systems are functioning
45 days:
Embryo
1 1/8 inches

10 — Fetus is recognizably human; fetal blood is circulating

8 — Bones begin to form; facial features take shape

6 — Heart is beating; fingers and toes begin to form

First Trimester

4 — Arm buds, leg buds, and tail are visible; lungs, digestive organs, and central nervous system are forming

2 — Embryo embedded in uterine wall; cell differentiation has begun
28 days:
Embryo
1/5 inch

0 — Conception

−2 — Last menstrual period
Weeks

Fetal Development

Now that we've seen what happens to the mother's body during pregnancy, let's consider the development of the fetus (Figure 5.4).

The First Trimester   About 30 hours after an egg is first fertilized, the cell divides, and this process of cell division repeats many times. As the cluster of cells drifts along the oviduct, several different kinds of cells emerge. The entire set of genetic instructions is passed to every cell, but each cell follows only a specific subset of the instructions; if this were not the case, there would be no different organs or body parts. For example, all cells carry genes for hair color and eye color, but only the cells of the hair follicles and irises (of the eye) respond to that information.

On about the fourth day after fertilization, the cluster of rapidly developing cells arrives in the uterus as a **blastocyst,** or a mostly hollow sphere of about 32–128 cells. The blastocyst attaches to the uterine wall on the 6th or 7th day, allowing for implantation into the nourishing uterine lining.

The blastocyst becomes an **embryo** by about the end of the second week after fertilization. The inner cells of the blastocyst separate into three layers. One layer becomes inner body parts—the digestive and respiratory systems; the middle layer becomes muscle, bone, blood, kidneys, and sex glands; and the third layer becomes the skin, hair, and nervous tissue.

The outermost shell of cells becomes the supporting structures of the pregnancy: the **placenta, umbilical cord,** and **amniotic sac.** A network of blood vessels called *chorionic villi* eventually forms the placenta. The human placenta allows a two-way exchange of nutrients and waste materials between the mother and the fetus. The placenta brings oxygen and nutrients to the fetus and transports waste products out. The placenta does not provide a perfect barrier between the fetal circulation and the maternal circulation, however. Some blood cells are exchanged, and certain substances,

TERMS

blastocyst   A stage of embryonic development, days 4–7, before the cell cluster becomes the embryo and placenta.

embryo   The stage of development between blastocyst and fetus; about weeks 2–8.

placenta   The organ through which the fetus receives nourishment and empties waste via the mother's circulatory system; after birth, the placenta is expelled from the uterus.

umbilical cord   The cord connecting the placenta and fetus, through which nutrients pass.

amniotic sac   A membranous pouch enclosing and protecting the fetus; also holds amniotic fluid.

such as alcohol, pass freely from the maternal circulation through the placenta to the fetus.

The period between weeks 2 and 9 is a time of rapid differentiation and change. All major body structures are formed during this time, including the heart, brain, liver, lungs, and sex organs. Eyes, nose, ears, arms, and legs also appear. Some organs begin to function, as well; the heart begins to beat, and the liver starts producing blood cells. Because body structures are forming, the developing organism is vulnerable to damage from environmental influences such as drugs and infections.

By the end of the second month, the fetal brain sends out impulses that coordinate the functioning of its other organs. The embryo is now a fetus, and most further changes will be in the size and refinement of working body parts. In the third month, the fetus becomes active. By the end of the first trimester, at 13 weeks, the fetus is about an inch long and weighs less than one ounce.

The Second Trimester

To grow during the second trimester, to about 14 inches and 1.5 pounds, the fetus requires large amounts of food, oxygen, and water, which come from the mother through the placenta. All body systems are operating, and the fetal heartbeat can be heard with a stethoscope. By the 4th or 5th month, the mother can detect early fetal movements that may feel like "flutters." Against great odds, a fetus born at 24–26 weeks (the end of the second trimester) has a greater than 50% chance of survival.

The Third Trimester

The fetus gains most of its birth weight during the last three months of the pregnancy. Some of the weight is brown fat under the skin that insulates the fetus and supplies food. *Brown fat* is a special fat rich with blood supply found in hibernating mammals and newborns and is associated with protection against hypothermia. The fetus also takes in other nutrients; about 85% of the calcium and iron the mother consumes goes into the fetal bloodstream.

The fetus may live if it is born during the 7th month, but it needs the fat layer acquired in the 8th month and time for organs—especially the respiratory and digestive organs—to develop. It also needs the immunity supplied by the antibodies in the mother's blood during the final three months. The antibodies protect the fetus against many of the diseases to which the mother has acquired immunity.

Diagnosing Fetal Abnormalities About 3% of babies are born with a major birth defect. Information about the health and sex of a fetus can be obtained prior to birth through prenatal testing.

NONINVASIVE SCREENING TESTS Traditionally, blood is taken from the mother at 16–19 weeks of pregnancy and analyzed for four hormone levels—human chorionic gonadotropin (HCG), unconjugated estriol, alpha-fetoprotein (AFP), and inhibin-A. These four hormones levels, the **quadruple marker screen (QMS),** can be compared to appropriate standards, and the results are used to estimate the probability that the fetus has particular anomalies. This type of test is a screening test rather than a diagnostic test; in the case of abnormal QMS results, parents may choose further testing such as an amniocentesis or ultrasonography.

A newer noninvasive screening test, **cell free DNA,** uses small fragments of fetal DNA identified in the maternal serum typically after 10 weeks of pregnancy. Currently, this DNA is primarily used to identify chromosomal disorders, such as Down syndrome, in women with elevated risk for *aneuploidy* (an abnormal number of chromosomes in the fetus) such as pregnant women over age 35, or in cases where the fetus is known to be at risk for a particular chromosomal or genetic defect.

INVASIVE DIAGNOSTIC TESTS **Chorionic villus sampling (CVS)** is a diagnostic test that can be performed in weeks 10 through 12 of pregnancy for high-risk women or women with abnormal screening results. This procedure involves removing a tiny section of the chorionic villi, which contain fetal cells that can be analyzed. For later diagnosis, **amniocentesis** is typically performed between 16 and 22 weeks and removes fluid from around the developing fetus. The fluid contains skin cells that can be cultured for analysis. This analysis can include genetic analyses for chromosomal disorders but also for some genetic diseases, like Tay-Sachs disease. Because the genetics are known, the sex of the fetus can also be determined.

Ultrasonography (also called *ultrasound*) uses high-frequency sound waves to create a **sonogram,** or visual image, of the fetus in the uterus. Sonograms show the fetus's position, size, and gestational age, and identify the presence of certain anatomical problems. Sonograms can sometimes be used to determine the sex of the fetus. Sonograms are considered safe for a pregnant woman and the fetus, but the U.S. Food and Drug Administration (FDA) advises against "keepsake" sonograms performed for no medical purpose.

> TERMS
>
> **quadruple marker screen (QMS)** A measurement of four hormones, used to assess the risk of fetal abnormalities.
>
> **cell free DNA** A newer measurement of fetal genetic material in the maternal blood supply, used to assess the risk of fetal genetic conditions with potentially greater accuracy.
>
> **chorionic villus sampling (CVS)** Surgical removal of a tiny section of chorionic villi to be analyzed for genetic defects.
>
> **amniocentesis** A process in which amniotic fluid is removed and analyzed to detect possible birth defects.
>
> **ultrasonography** The use of high-frequency sound waves to view the fetus in the uterus; also known as *ultrasound*.
>
> **sonogram** The visual image of the fetus produced by ultrasonography.

Ultrasonography provides information about the position, size, and physical condition of a fetus in the uterus.

First-trimester screening for Down syndrome combines ultrasound evaluation of nuchal translucency (the thickness of the back of the fetus's neck) with maternal blood testing. This test can be done between the 10th and 14th weeks of pregnancy. This can be combined with serum testing at 16 weeks for a sequential screen to improve the sensitivity of noninvasive screening tests. If results indicate an increased risk of abnormality, further diagnostic studies such as amniocentesis can be done for confirmation.

Researchers are developing new fetal screening techniques that are less invasive and that can be done earlier in pregnancy. One such test, MaterniT21, is a laboratory-developed test that analyzes maternal blood for cell free fetal DNA as early as 10 weeks. It can detect increased levels of chromosome 21, which indicate a fetus with Down syndrome.

Fetal Programming   Prenatal testing techniques look for chromosomal, genetic, and other anomalies that typically cause immediate problems. A new area of study known as *fetal programming theory* focuses on how conditions in the womb may influence the risk of adult diseases. For example, researchers have linked low birth weight to an increased risk of heart disease, high blood pressure, obesity, diabetes, and schizophrenia. High birth weight in female infants, however, has been linked to an increased risk of breast cancer in later life.

Although fetal programming theory is not yet embraced by all scientists, these studies emphasize that everything that occurs during pregnancy can have an impact on the developing fetus. In the future, people may be able to use information about their birth weight and other indicators of gestational conditions just as they now can use family history and genetic information—to alert them to special health risks and to help them improve their health.

The Importance of Prenatal Care

Adequate prenatal care—as described in the following sections—is essential to the health of both mother and baby. All physicians recommend that women start getting regular prenatal checkups as soon as they become pregnant. Typically this means one checkup per month during the first 8 months, then one checkup per week during the final month. About 84% of pregnant women begin receiving adequate prenatal care during the first trimester; about 3.5% wait until the last trimester or receive no prenatal care at all.

Regular Checkups   In the woman's first visit to her obstetrician, she will be asked for a detailed medical history of herself and her family. Her obstetrician will note any hereditary conditions that may assume increased significance during pregnancy. The tendency to develop gestational diabetes (diabetes during pregnancy only), for example, can be inherited; appropriate treatment during pregnancy reduces the risk of serious harm.

The woman is given a complete physical exam and is informed about appropriate diet. She returns for regular checkups throughout the pregnancy, during which her blood pressure and weight gain are measured, her urine is analyzed, and the fetus's size and position are monitored.

Blood Tests A blood sample is taken during the initial prenatal visit to determine blood type and detect possible anemia or Rh incompatibilities. The **Rh factor** is a blood protein. If an Rh-positive father and an Rh-negative mother conceive an Rh-positive baby, the baby's blood will be incompatible with the mother's blood. This condition is completely treatable with a serum called *Rh-immune globulin*, which coats Rh-positive cells as they enter the mother's body and prevents her immune system from recognizing them and forming antibodies. Blood may also be tested for evidence of hepatitis B, syphilis, rubella immunity, thyroid problems, and, with the mother's permission, HIV infection.

Prenatal Nutrition A nutritious diet throughout pregnancy is essential for both the mother and her unborn baby. Not only does the baby get all its nutrients from the mother, but it also competes with her for nutrients not sufficiently available to meet both their needs. When a woman's diet is low in iron or calcium, the fetus receives most of it, and the mother may become deficient in the mineral. To meet the increased nutritional demands of her body, a pregnant woman shouldn't just eat more; she should make sure that her diet is nutritionally adequate.

To maintain her own health and help the fetus grow, a pregnant woman typically needs to consume about 250–500 extra calories per day. Breastfeeding an infant requires even more energy—about 500 or more calories per day. To ensure that she's getting enough calories and nutrients, a pregnant woman should talk to her physician or a registered dietician about her dietary habits and determine what changes she should make.

Some physicians prescribe high-potency vitamin and mineral supplements to pregnant and lactating women. Supplements can help boost the levels of nutrients available to mother and child, helping with fetal development while ensuring that the mother doesn't become nutrient-deficient. Pregnant and lactating women, however, should not take supplements without the advice of their physicians because some vitamins, such as vitamin A, can be harmful if taken in excess. Pregnant women also should not take herbal dietary supplements without consulting a physician.

Two vitamins—vitamin D and the B vitamin folate—are particularly important to pregnant women. Pregnant women who don't get enough vitamin D are more likely to deliver low-birth-weight babies. Chronic vitamin D deficiency has been linked to other health problems, including heart disease.

If a woman doesn't get the recommended daily amount of folate, both before and during pregnancy, her child has an increased risk of neural tube defects, including spina bifida.

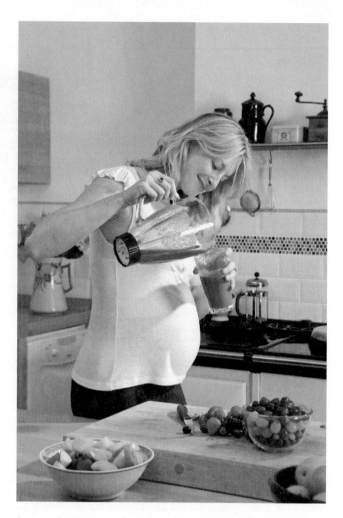

A woman's dietary needs change during pregnancy, so it's important to eat a nutritionally sound diet.

Any woman capable of becoming pregnant should get at least 400 μg (0.4 mg) of folic acid (the synthetic form of folate) daily from fortified foods and/or supplements, in addition to folate from a varied diet. Pregnant women should get 1000 μg every day.

Food safety is another special dietary concern for pregnant women because foodborne pathogens can be especially dangerous to them and their unborn children. Germs and parasites such as *Listeria monocytogenes* and *Toxoplasma gondii* are both particularly worrisome. To avoid them, pregnant women should avoid eating undercooked and ready-to-eat meats and should be sure to thoroughly wash produce before eating it. Pregnant women should also follow the FDA's recommendations for consumption of fish and seafood. For complete information about nutrition and food safety, see Chapter 9.

Avoiding Drugs and Other Environmental Hazards
Everything the mother ingests may eventually reach the fetus in some proportion. In addition to the food the mother eats, the drugs she takes and the chemicals she is exposed to affect the fetus. Some drugs harm the fetus but not the mother because the fetus is in the process of developing and

---

Rh factor A protein found in blood; Rh incompatibility between a mother and fetus can jeopardize the fetus's health.

TERMS

because the proper dose for the mother is a proportionately massive dose for the fetus.

During the first trimester, when the major body structures are rapidly forming, the fetus is extremely vulnerable to environmental factors such as viral infections, radiation, drugs, and other **teratogens**, any of which can cause **congenital malformations,** or birth defects. The most susceptible body parts are those growing most rapidly at the time of exposure. The rubella (German measles) virus, for example, can cause congenital malformation of nerves supplying the eyes and ears in the first trimester, leading to blindness or deafness, but exposure to it later in the pregnancy does no damage. Similarly, excess retinoic acid (Vitamin A) exposure in the first trimester can lead to spontaneous abortion and fetal malformations such as microcephaly and cardiac anomalies. Another example is the class of medications known as anti-epileptics (such as valproic acid), which is associated with cleft palate and neural tube defect. The most common congenital malformations identified are open neural tube, congenital cardiac defects, urinary tract defects, skeletal abnormalities, and cleft palates. Women on medications known to cause birth defects must take care to avoid pregnancy (see Chapter 6 on contraception and abortion).

ALCOHOL Alcohol is a potent teratogen. Getting drunk just one time during pregnancy may be enough to cause brain damage in a fetus. A high level of alcohol consumption during pregnancy is associated with spontaneous miscarriage and stillbirth. Fetuses born to mothers who have consumed alcohol are at risk for **fetal alcohol syndrome (FAS).** A baby born with FAS is likely to be characterized by a small head and body size, unusual facial features, congenital heart defects, defective joints, impaired vision, mental impairment, and abnormal behavior patterns. Researchers doubt that any level of alcohol consumption is safe, and they recommend total abstinence during pregnancy.

TOBACCO Smoking is a preventable risk factor associated with miscarriage, low birth weight, preterm birth, infant death, and other pregnancy complications. The mechanism for this damage is theorized to be direct damage to genetic material. Nicotine, the active ingredient of cigarette smoke, impairs oxygen delivery to the fetus and leads to faster fetal heart rates and reduced fetal breathing.

CAFFEINE Caffeine, a powerful stimulant, puts both mother and fetus under stress by raising the level of the hormone epinephrine. Caffeine also reduces the blood supply to the uterus. A pregnant woman should limit her caffeine intake to no more than the equivalent of two cups of coffee per day.

DRUGS Some prescription drugs, such as some blood pressure medications, can harm the fetus, so they should be used only under medical supervision. Antidepressant use in pregnancy can lead to withdrawal symptoms in newborns after delivery. Newborns may become fussy with high-pitched, irritable cries, and develop difficulty feeding.

Recreational drugs, such as cocaine, are thought to increase the risk of major birth defects. Marijuana is associated with preterm birth and stillbirth. Methamphetamine use is associated with underweight babies.

STIs AND OTHER INFECTIONS Infections, including those that are sexually transmitted, are another serious problem for the fetus. Such infections can pose a threat before, during, and after birth. Rubella, syphilis, gonorrhea, hepatitis B, Group B streptococcus (GBS), herpes, and HIV are among the most dangerous infections for the fetus. Treatment of the mother or immunization of the baby just after birth can help prevent problems from many infections. Women at risk for HIV infection should be tested before or during pregnancy because early treatment can dramatically reduce the chance that the virus will be passed to the fetus. Some experts advocate universal HIV screening for pregnant women.

Prenatal Activity and Exercise Physical activity during pregnancy contributes to mental and physical wellness (see the box "Physical Activity during Pregnancy"). Women can continue working at their jobs until late in their pregnancy, provided the work isn't so physically demanding that it jeopardizes their health. At the same time, pregnant women need more rest and sleep to maintain their own well-being and that of the fetus.

Kegel exercises, to strengthen the pelvic floor muscles, are recommended for pregnant women. These exercises are performed by alternately contracting and releasing the muscles used to stop the flow of urine. Each contraction should be held for about five seconds. Kegel exercises should be done several times a day for a total of about 50 repetitions daily.

TERMS

teratogen An agent or influence that causes physical defects in a developing fetus.

congenital malformation A physical defect existing at the time of birth, either inherited or caused during gestation.

fetal alcohol syndrome (FAS) A combination of birth defects caused by excessive alcohol consumption by the mother during pregnancy.

Physical Activity during Pregnancy

Maintaining a regular routine of physical activity throughout pregnancy can help a mother-to-be stay healthy and feel her best. Regular exercise can improve posture and decrease common pregnancy-related discomforts, such as backaches and fatigue. There is also evidence that physical activity may prevent gestational diabetes, relieve stress, and build stamina that can be helpful during labor and delivery.

A woman who was physically active before pregnancy should be able to continue her favorite activities in moderation, except for those that carry a risk of trauma, or unless there is a medical reason to reduce or stop exercise.

The American Congress of Obstetricians and Gynecologists (ACOG) offers advice regarding exercise during pregnancy. For example, downhill skiing or contact sports such as hockey, basketball, or soccer place pregnant women at risk for falls or abdominal trauma and need to be avoided. In general, experts encourage low-impact aerobic activities such as walking or swimming over high-impact exercise. Physicians and pregnant women alike have concerns about exercise intensity. A good rule of thumb is to never exercise more than allows you to comfortably talk with a friend. If a pregnant exercising woman is out of breath, she should slow down! Experts also recommend proper hydration and dress to avoid overheating.

A woman who has never exercised regularly can safely start an exercise program during pregnancy after consulting with her health care provider. A routine of regular walking is considered a safe way to start exercising during pregnancy. The ACOG recommends that any pregnant woman who exercises should stop exercising if she experiences any of the following warning signs:

- Vaginal bleeding
- Increased shortness of breath
- Dizziness or feeling faint
- Headache
- Pain in the chest or calves
- Contractions
- Decreased fetal movement
- Leakage of amniotic fluid

SOURCES: ACOG Committee on Obstetric Practice. 2002 (reaffirmed 2009). Committee opinion: Exercise during pregnancy and the postpartum period. *Obstetrics and Gynecology* 99(1): 171–173; Physical Activity Guidelines Advisory Committee. 2008. *Physical Activity Guidelines Advisory Committee Report, 2008.* Washington, DC: U.S. Department of Health and Human Services.

Preparing for Birth   Childbirth classes are almost a routine part of the prenatal experience for both mothers and fathers today. These classes typically teach the details of the birth process as well as relaxation techniques to help deal with the discomfort of labor and delivery. The mother learns and practices a variety of techniques so she will be able to choose what works best for her during labor when the time comes. The father or her partner typically acts as a coach, supporting her emotionally and helping her with her breathing and relaxing. He or she remains with the mother throughout labor and delivery, even when a cesarean section is performed.

Complications of Pregnancy and Pregnancy Loss

Complications can arise in pregnancy for a myriad of reasons: *maternal diseases and exposures* such as diabetes, hypertension, or tobacco use; *placental factors,* including abruption or placenta previa; or *fetal conditions* such as genetic conditions like Down syndrome or cystic fibrosis. Each

complication benefits from early diagnosis, counseling, and, if possible, corrective action.

Ectopic Pregnancy   In an **ectopic pregnancy,** the fertilized egg implants and begins to develop outside the uterus, usually in an oviduct (Figure 5.5). As the limited space of the oviduct cannot accommodate the rapid growth of a fertilized egg, ectopic pregnancies pose high risk of emergent bleeding through tubal rupture. Although ectopic pregnancies account for only 1–2% of all pregnancies, they contribute 3–4% of all maternal deaths.

Ectopic pregnancies usually occur because of occlusion (blockage) of the fallopian tube, most often as a result of pelvic inflammatory disease, although smoking also increases a woman's risk for ectopic pregnancy. The embryo may spontaneously abort, or the embryo and placenta may continue to expand until they rupture the oviduct. Sharp pain on one side of the abdomen or in the lower back, usually in about the 7th or 8th week of pregnancy, may signal an ectopic pregnancy, and there may be irregular bleeding.

Surgical removal of the embryo and the oviduct may be necessary to save the mother's life, although microsurgery can sometimes be used to repair the damaged oviduct. If diagnosed early, before the oviduct ruptures, ectopic pregnancy can often be successfully treated without surgery with the chemotherapeutic agent methotrexate.

> **ectopic pregnancy**   A pregnancy in which the embryo develops outside the uterus, usually in an oviduct.
>
> TERMS

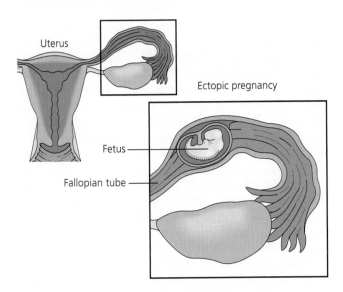

FIGURE 5.5 **Ectopic pregnancy in a fallopian tube.**

Women with preeclampsia without severe features may be monitored closely as outpatients and placed on home bed rest. More severe cases may require hospitalization for close medical management and early delivery.

Placenta Previa   In **placenta previa,** the placenta either completely or partially covers the cervical opening, preventing the mother from delivering the baby vaginally. As a result, the baby must be delivered by cesarean section. Risk factors include prior cesarean delivery, multiple pregnancies, intrauterine surgery, smoking, multiple gestations, and advanced maternal age.

Placental Abruption   In **placental abruption,** a normally implanted placenta prematurely separates from the uterine wall. Patients experience abdominal pain, vaginal bleeding, and uterine tenderness. The condition also increases the risk of fetal death. The risk factors for developing a placental abruption are maternal age, smoking, cocaine use, multiple gestation, trauma, preeclampsia, hypertension, and premature rupture of membranes.

Spontaneous Abortion   A spontaneous abortion, or miscarriage, is the termination of pregnancy before the 20th week. Most miscarriages—about 60%—are due to chromosomal abnormalities in the fetus. Certain occupations that involve exposure to chemicals or radiation may increase the likelihood of a spontaneous abortion. One miscarriage doesn't mean that later pregnancies will be unsuccessful, and about 70–90% of women who miscarry eventually become pregnant again.

> A miscarriage doesn't mean future pregnancies will fail. **Up to 90% of women who miscarry become pregnant again.**

Gestational Diabetes   During gestation, about 7–18% of all pregnant women develop **gestational diabetes (GDM),** in which the body loses its ability to use insulin properly. In these women, diabetes occurs only during pregnancy. Women diagnosed with GDM have an increased risk of developing type 2 diabetes later in life. It is important to accurately diagnose and treat GDM because it can lead to preeclampsia, polyhydramnios (increased levels of amniotic fluid), large fetuses, birth trauma, operative deliveries, perinatal mortality, and neonatal metabolic complications. All women in pregnancy are therefore advised to test for GDM. When a diagnosis of GDM is made, treatment can be in the form of diet and exercise modification, or medication.

Stillbirth   The terms *fetal death, fetal demise, stillbirth,* and *stillborn* all refer to the delivery of a fetus that shows no signs of life. Risk factors for stillbirth include smoking, advanced maternal age, obesity, multiple gestations, and chronic disease. Race is also a factor; black women have twice as many stillbirths as white women. Although some attribute the increased risk for stillbirth among black women to the corresponding increased risk of preterm delivery, other reasons for race-based health care disparities may include poor access to care, infection, and the combined effects of racism and poverty.

Preterm Labor and Birth   When a pregnant woman goes into labor before the 37th week of gestation, she is said to undergo *preterm labor.* About 30–50% of preterm labors

Preeclampsia   A disease unique to pregnancy, **preeclampsia** is characterized by elevated blood pressure and the appearance of protein in the urine. Left untreated, preeclampsia will worsen over time, resulting in symptoms including headache, right upper-quadrant abdominal pain, vision changes (referred to as *scotomata*), and notable increased swelling and weight gain. One of the most severe outcomes of untreated preeclampsia is the onset of seizures, a condition called **eclampsia.** Other potential complications of preeclampsia are liver and kidney damage, bleeding, fetal growth restriction, and even fetal death.

TERMS

preeclampsia   A condition of pregnancy characterized by high blood pressure and protein in the urine.

eclampsia   A severe, potentially life-threatening form of preeclampsia, characterized by seizures.

placenta previa   A complication of pregnancy in which the placenta covers the cervical opening, preventing the mother from delivering the baby vaginally.

placental abruption   A complication of pregnancy in which a normally implanted placenta prematurely separates from the uterine wall.

gestational diabetes (GDM)   A form of diabetes that occurs during pregnancy.

resolve themselves, with the pregnancy continuing to full term. In other cases, interventions may be required to delay labor and allow gestation to continue.

Around the world, an estimated 13 million babies are born prematurely—before 37 completed weeks of gestation—each year. In 2012, 11.6% of babies were born prematurely in the United States. The rate has increased by 9% since 2000 and by 20% since 1990. Preterm birth rates vary widely among racial and ethnic groups.

Preterm birth is the leading direct cause of newborn death, accounting for about one-third of all infant deaths. More than 1 million preterm newborns die annually in the United States. Preterm birth is also the main risk factor for newborn illness and death from other causes, particularly infection. Babies born prematurely appear to be at a higher risk of long-term health and developmental problems, including delayed development and learning problems.

Risk factors for preterm birth include lack of prenatal care, smoking, drug use, stress, personal health history, infections or illness during pregnancy, obesity, exposure to environmental toxins, a previous preterm birth, and the carrying of multiple fetuses. However, only about half the women who give birth prematurely have any known risk factors.

Labor Induction If pregnancy continues well beyond the baby's due date, it may be necessary to induce labor artificially. This is one of the most common obstetrical procedures and is typically offered to pregnant women who have not delivered and are 7–14 days past their due dates.

Low Birth Weight and Premature Birth A **low-birth-weight (LBW)** baby is one that weighs less than 5.5 pounds at birth. LBW babies may be **premature** (born before the 37th week of pregnancy) or full-term. Babies who are born small even though they're full-term are referred to as *small-for-dates* or *small-for-gestational-age* babies. Low birth weight affected 8.0% of babies born in 2012 in the United States. About half of all cases are related to teenage pregnancy, cigarette smoking, poor nutrition, and poor maternal health. Other maternal factors include drug use, stress, depression, and anxiety. Adequate prenatal care is the best way to prevent LBW. Full-term LBW babies tend to have fewer problems than premature infants.

Infant Mortality The U.S. rate of **infant mortality,** the death of a child at less than 1 year of age, is near its lowest point ever; however, it remains far higher than rates in most of the developed world. Poverty and inadequate health care are key causes.

Forty-six percent of infant death is due to one of three leading factors: congenital abnormalities, prematurity/low birth weight, and **sudden infant death syndrome (SIDS)**. SIDS is defined by a sudden and unexpected death of a child less than 1 year of age not explained by thorough investigation including autopsy. More than 2000 babies died of SIDS in 2010, the latest year for which statistics are available.

Research suggests that abnormalities in the brain stem, the part of the brain that regulates breathing, heart rate, and other basic functions, underlie the risk for SIDS. Risk is greatly increased for infants with these innate differences if they are exposed to environmental risks such as tobacco smoke, alcohol, substance use, and, most importantly, sleeping stomach-side down. Because infants developmentally change how they sleep between 2 and 4 months, this is a time period of particular risk. Additionally, suffocation risk increases with the presence of many items common to cribs: fluffy pillows, mattresses, or plush toys. Therefore, existing recommendations recommend allowing babies to sleep back down, on a firm sleep surface, without soft bedding, plush toys, or additional clothing that might cause overheating. Parental avoidance of tobacco smoke, alcohol, and illicit drugs is important. Several studies have found that the use of a pacifier significantly reduces the risk of SIDS.

CHILDBIRTH

By the end of the ninth month of pregnancy, most women are tired of being pregnant; both parents are eager to start a new phase of their lives. Most couples find the actual process of birth to be an exciting and positive experience.

Choices in Childbirth

Many parents-to-be today can choose the type of practitioner and the environment they want for the birth of their child. A high-risk pregnancy is best handled by a specialist physician, but for low-risk pregnancies, many options are available.

In 2012, 98.6% of babies in the United States were delivered in hospitals. Physicians performed 91.6% of all deliveries and certified nurse-midwives performed 7.6% of them. Although physicians typically deliver in hospital settings,

TERMS

low birth weight (LBW) Weighing less than 5.5 pounds at birth, often the result of prematurity.

premature Born before the 37th week of pregnancy.

infant mortality The death of a child at less than 1 year of age.

sudden infant death syndrome (SIDS) The sudden death of an apparently healthy infant during sleep.

nurse-midwives may attend deliveries in free standing birth centers where the environment may feel more comfortable while still remaining close to the medical resources of a hospital.

In 2012, 1.4% of American women elected to give birth at home or in birth facilities that offer low-technology care. In 2011, the American Congress of Obstetricians and Gynecologists recommended against homebirth. The American Academy of Pediatrics notes that, although hospital or freestanding accredited birth centers are the safest place to give birth, every infant should have access to the birth setting that is best for him or her. However, the American College of Nurse-Midwives supports out-of-hospital births for low-risk, healthy women.

Health care providers will need to assess maternal and fetal health and make decisions together with prospective parents about appropriate care providers and location. It is important for prospective parents to discuss all aspects of labor and delivery with their provider beforehand so they can learn what to expect and can state their preferences.

Labor and Delivery

The birth process occurs in three stages (Figure 5.6). **Labor** begins when hormonal changes in both the mother and the baby cause strong, rhythmic uterine **contractions** to begin. These contractions exert pressure on the cervix and cause the lengthwise muscles of the uterus to pull on the circular muscles around the cervix, causing effacement (thinning) and dilation (opening) of the cervix. The contractions also pressure the baby to descend into the mother's pelvis, if it hasn't already. The entire process of labor and delivery usually takes between 2 and 36 hours, depending on the size of the baby, the baby's position in the uterus, the size of the mother's pelvis, the strength of the uterine contractions, the number of prior deliveries, and other factors. The length of labor is generally shorter for second and subsequent births.

The First Stage of Labor   The first stage of labor averages 13 hours for a first birth, although there is a wide variation among women. It begins with cervical effacement and dilation and continues until the cervix is completely dilated. Contractions usually last about 30 seconds and occur every 15–20 minutes at first, more often later. The prepared mother relaxes as much as possible during these contractions to allow labor to proceed without being blocked by tension. Early in the first stage, a small amount of bleeding may occur as a plug of slightly bloody mucus that blocked the opening of

labor   The act or process of giving birth to a child, expelling it with the placenta from the mother's body by means of uterine contractions.

contraction   Shortening of the muscles in the uterine wall, which causes effacement and dilation of the cervix and assists in expelling the fetus.

TERMS

(a)

(b)

(c)

FIGURE 5.6   Birth: labor and delivery. (a) The first stage of labor; (b) the second stage of labor; delivery of the baby; (c) the third stage of labor: expulsion of the placenta.

the cervix during pregnancy is expelled. In some women, the amniotic sac ruptures and the fluid rushes out; this is sometimes referred to as "breaking the bag of water."

The last part of the first stage of labor, called **active labor,** is characterized by strong and frequent contractions, much more intense than in the early stages of labor. Contractions may last 60–90 seconds and occur every 1–3 minutes. During active labor the cervix opens completely, to a diameter of about 10 centimeters. When the head of the fetus is curled, to present its smallest diameter, it measures 9–10 centimeters. Therefore, a completely dilated cervix should permit the passage of the fetal head.

The Second Stage of Labor

The second stage of labor begins with complete cervical dilation and ends with the delivery of the baby. The baby is slowly pushed down, through the bones of the pelvis, past the cervix, and into the vagina, which it stretches open. The mother bears down with the contractions to help push the baby down and out. Some women find this the most difficult part of labor; others find that the contractions and bearing down bring a sense of relief. The baby's head and body turns to fit through the narrowest parts of the passageway, and the soft bones of the baby's skull move together and overlap as it is squeezed through the pelvis. When the top of the head appears at the vaginal opening, the baby is said to be *crowning.*

As the head of the baby emerges, the physician or midwife will check to ensure that the umbilical cord is not around the neck. With a few more contractions, the baby's shoulders and body emerge. As the baby is squeezed through the pelvis, cervix, and vagina, amniotic fluid in the lungs is forced out by the pressure on the baby's chest. Once this pressure is released as the baby emerges from the vagina, the chest expands and the lungs fill with air for the first time. The baby will appear wet and often is covered with a cheesy substance. The baby's head may be oddly shaped at first, due to the molding of the soft plates of bone during birth, but it usually takes on a more rounded appearance within 24 hours.

The Third Stage of Labor

In the third stage of labor, the uterus continues to contract until the placenta is expelled. This stage usually takes 5–30 minutes. It is important that the entire placenta be expelled; if part remains in the uterus, it may cause bleeding and infection. Breastfeeding soon after delivery helps control uterine bleeding because it stimulates the secretion of a hormone that makes the uterus contract.

The baby's physical condition is assessed with the **Apgar score,** a formalized system for assessing the baby's physical condition and whether there is need for medical assistance. Heart rate, respiration, color, reflexes, and muscle tone are individually rated with a score of 0–2, and a total score between 0 and 10 is given at 1 and 5 minutes after birth. A score of 7–10 at 5 minutes is considered normal. Most newborns are also tested for 29 specific disorders, some of which are life-threatening. The American Academy of Pediatrics endorses these tests, but they are not routinely performed in every state.

Pain Relief during Labor and Delivery

Women vary in how much pain they experience in childbirth. First babies are typically the most challenging to deliver because the birth canal has never stretched to this extent before. It is recommended that women and their partners learn about labor and what kinds of choices are available for pain relief. Childbirth preparation courses are a good place to start, and communicating with one's obstetrician or midwife is essential to assessing pain relief options. Pain can be modified through staying active in labor, laboring in water, and the use of different breathing and relaxation techniques including hypnosis.

Medical pain relief can come in the form of intravenous narcotics, which are short-acting and can be used only in early labor. If a baby is born under the influence of narcotic, it can appear floppy and without vigor. The most commonly employed medical intervention for pain relief is the *epidural injection.* This procedure involves placing a thin plastic catheter between the vertebrae in the lower back. Medication that reduces the transmission of pain signals to the brain is given through this catheter. Regional anesthetic drugs are given in low concentration to minimize weakening of the leg muscles so that the mother can effectively push during the birth. The advantage of the epidural is that the medication is used in low amounts in the confined space of the spinal column, protecting the fetus from the effect of the medication. The mother is awake and is an active participant in the birth.

Local anesthesia is available for repair of any tear or **episiotomy** (a surgical incision of the perineum to allow easier delivery of the baby) if the mother has not used an epidural for the labor.

Cesarean Delivery

In a **cesarean section,** the baby is removed through a surgical incision in the abdominal wall and uterus. Cesarean sections are necessary when a baby cannot be delivered vaginally—for example, if the baby's head is bigger than the mother's pelvis or if the baby is not head down at the time of labor. If the mother has a serious health condition such as high blood pressure, a cesarean may be safer for her than labor and a vaginal delivery. Cesareans are more common among women who are overweight or have diabetes. Other reasons for cesarean delivery include

---

active labor The last part of the first stage of labor, during which the cervix becomes fully dilated; characterized by intense and frequent contractions.

TERMS

Apgar score A formalized system for assessing a newborn's need for medical assistance.

episiotomy An incision made in the perineum to widen the vaginal opening to facilitate birth and prevent uncontrolled tearing during delivery.

cesarean section A surgical incision through the abdominal wall and uterus, performed to deliver a fetus.

abnormal or difficult labor, fetal distress, and the presence of a dangerous infection like herpes that can be passed to the baby during delivery.

Repeat cesarean deliveries are also very common. About 90% of American women who have had one child by cesarean have subsequent children delivered the same way. Although the risk of complications from a vaginal delivery after a previous cesarean delivery is low, there is a small (1%) risk of serious complication to the mother and baby if the previous uterine scar opens during labor (uterine rupture). For this reason, women and their physicians may choose to deliver by elective repeat cesarean.

Like any major surgery, cesarean section carries a longer recovery period and additional risks. Most cesarean deliveries are performed with regional anesthetic, which permits the mother to remain awake for the surgery with her partner present.

The Postpartum Period

The **postpartum period,** a stage of about three months following childbirth, is a time of critical family adjustments. Parenthood begins literally overnight, and the transition can cause considerable stress.

Breastfeeding **Lactation,** the production of milk, begins about three days after childbirth. Prior to that time (sometimes as early as the second trimester), **colostrum** is secreted by the nipples. Colostrum contains antibodies that help protect the newborn from infectious diseases, and is also high in protein.

The American Academy of Pediatrics recommends breastfeeding exclusively for six months, then in combination with solid food until the baby is one year of age, and

then for as long after that as a mother and baby desire. Currently only 11% of U.S. mothers breastfeed exclusively for six months. Human milk is perfectly suited to the baby's nutritional needs and digestive capabilities, and it supplies the baby with antibodies. Breastfeeding decreases the incidence of infant infection and diarrhea and appears to decrease diabetes and childhood obesity.

Breastfeeding is beneficial to the mother as well. It stimulates contractions that help the uterus return to normal more rapidly, contributes to post-pregnancy weight loss, and may reduce the risk of breast and ovarian cancers. For women who want to breastfeed but who have problems, help is available from support groups, books, or lactation consultants and health care providers.

However, bottlefeeding can also provide adequate nutrition, and when bottlefed, it is easier to tell how much milk an infant is taking in. Additionally, bottlefed infants tend to sleep longer. Whether breastfeeding or bottlefeeding, both can be part of loving, secure parent-child relationships.

When a mother doesn't nurse, menstruation usually begins within about 10 weeks. Breastfeeding can prevent the return of menstruation for six months or longer because the hormone prolactin, which aids milk production. However, ovulation—and pregnancy—can occur before menstruation returns, so breastfeeding is not a reliable contraceptive method; if a woman wishes to avoid pregnancy, she should use a reliable method of birth control.

Postpartum Depression The physical stress of labor, blood loss, fatigue, decreased sleep, fluctuating postpartum hormone levels, and anxieties of becoming a new parent all contribute to emotional instability postpartum. About 50–80% of new mothers experience "baby blues," characterized by episodes of sadness, weeping, anxiety, headache, sleep disturbances, and irritability.

About 9–16% of new mothers experience **postpartum depression** which is characterized by a prolonged period of anxiety, guilt, fear, or self-blame; these feelings prevent the new mother from normal participation in everyday life or the normal care of her newborn. Fortunately, postpartum depression can be effectively prevented and treated. Women with a history of depression or depression during pregnancy can benefit from early referral to an appropriate mental health care provider. Rest is a key component of recovery. The

Breastfeeding can enhance the bond between mother and child. The American Academy of Pediatrics recommends breastfeeding exclusively for six months and then in combination with solid food until the baby is at least one year of age.

postpartum period The period of about three months after delivering a baby.　　　TERMS

lactation The production of milk.

colostrum A yellowish fluid secreted by the mammary glands around the time of childbirth until milk comes in, about the third day.

postpartum depression An emotional low that may be experienced by the mother following childbirth.

What are some early signs or symptoms of depression? Consider ways you might start a conversation about depression or help a new mother find access to help. What kind of things might you say or do?

connect™

Connect to Your Choices

Have you ever thought about why you handle your sexuality and sexual relationships the way you do? Have you ever thought about where you get your ideas and plans about having children? Many factors can influence our ideas, some not as obvious as others. Do you feel you have to be sexually active because your peers and potential partners are? Do you assume you will have children one day because it's an expected life path? Are you influenced by media portrayals of sex and parenthood?

What are the external factors that influence your choices about your sexuality and children? What are your inner motivations and core values, and how do they affect your choices? Based on what you learned in this chapter, will you make some different choices in the future? If so, what will they be?

Go online to Connect to complete this activity: www.mcgraw-hillconnect.com

TIPS FOR TODAY AND THE FUTURE

*

A healthy sexual life built on acceptance of yourself and good communication with your partner is integral to wellness, as is recognizing that parenthood means making responsible choices and preparing for it long before pregnancy.

RIGHT NOW YOU CAN:
- Deal with any sexual question or problem you've been avoiding. A good place to start is by talking with your doctor. Don't be afraid or embarrassed to ask questions.
- If you're in a sexual relationship, consider the information you and your partner have shared about sex. Are you comfortable that you and your partner know enough about each other to have a safe, healthy sexual relationship?
- Take some time to think about whether you really *want* to have children. Cut through the cultural, societal, family, and personal expectations that may stand in the way of making the decision you really want to make.
- Think of one thing your mother or father did as a parent that you particularly liked; if you become a parent, consider how you can be sure to do the same thing for your children.

IN THE FUTURE YOU CAN:
- If you're in a sexual relationship, or if you plan to begin one, open (or reopen) a dialogue with your partner about sex. Make time to talk at length about the responsibilities and consequences of a sexual relationship.
- Make behavioral changes that can improve your prospects as a parent. For example, you may need to adopt healthier eating habits or start exercising more consistently.
- If you want to be a parent someday, start looking at the many sources of information about pregnancy, childbirth, and parenting. This is a good idea for anyone—man or woman—who plans to have a family.

mother's support system should offer to take on important responsibilities to allow the mother to rest and recover, as well as to encourage her to continue outside interests.

Some men also seem to get a form of postpartum depression, characterized by anxiety about their changing roles and feelings of inadequacy. Both mothers and fathers need time to adjust to their new roles as parents.

Attachment Another feature of the postpartum period is the development of attachment—the strong emotional tie that grows between the baby and the adult who cares for the baby. Parents can foster secure attachment relationships in the early weeks and months by responding sensitively to the baby's true needs. Parents who respond appropriately to the baby's signals of gazing, looking away, smiling, and crying establish feelings of trust in their child. They feed the baby when she's hungry, for example; respond when she cries; interact with her when she gazes, smiles, or babbles; and stop stimulating her when she frowns or looks away. A secure attachment relationship helps the child develop and function well socially, emotionally, and mentally.

For most people, the arrival of a child creates a deep sense of joy and accomplishment. However, adjusting to parenthood requires effort and energy. Talking with friends and relatives about their experiences during the first few weeks or months with a baby can help prepare new parents for the period when the baby's needs may require all the energy that both parents have to expend. But the pleasures of nurturing a new baby are substantial, and many parents look back on this time as one of the most significant and joyful of their lives.

SUMMARY

- The female external sex organs are referred to as the vulva; the clitoris plays an important role in sexual arousal and orgasm because of the high concentration of nerve endings. The vagina leads to the internal female sex organs, including the uterus, oviducts or fallopian tubes, and ovaries.

- The male external sex organs are the penis and the scrotum; the glans of the penis is an important site of sexual arousal because of the high concentration of nerve endings. Male internal sexual structures include the testes, epididymis, vasa deferentia, seminal vesicles, Cowper's gland, ejaculatory duct, and prostate gland.

- The menstrual cycle has four phases: menses, the estrogenic phase, ovulation, and the progestational phase.

- The ovaries gradually cease to function as women approach age 50 and enter menopause. The pattern of male sexual responses changes with age, and testosterone production gradually decreases.

- Sexual activity is based on stimulus and response. Stimulation may be physical or psychological.

- The sexual response cycle has four stages: excitement, plateau, orgasm, and resolution.

- Physical and psychological problems can both interfere with sexual functioning. Treatment for sexual dysfunction first addresses any underlying medical conditions and then looks at psychosocial problems.

- Responsible sexuality includes open, honest communication; agreed-on sexual activities; sexual privacy; contraception use; safe sex practices; sober sex; and the taking of responsibility for consequences.

- Fertilization is a complex process culminating when a sperm penetrates the membrane of the egg released from the woman's ovary. Infertility affects about 6% of the reproductive-age population of the United States.

- During pregnancy, the uterus enlarges until it pushes up into the rib cage; the breasts enlarge and may secrete colostrum; the muscles and ligaments soften and stretch; and the circulatory system, lungs, and kidneys become more efficient.

- The fetal anatomy is almost completely formed in the first trimester and is refined in the second; during the third trimester, the fetus grows and gains most of its weight, storing nutrients in fatty tissues.

- Prenatal tests available include ultrasound and both noninvasive screening and invasive diagnostic testing such as amniocentesis or chorionic villus sampling.

- Pregnancy usually proceeds without major complications. Problems that can occur include ectopic pregnancy, spontaneous abortion, preeclampsia, low birth weight, and preterm birth.

- The first stage of labor begins with contractions that exert pressure on the cervix, causing effacement and dilation. The second stage begins with complete cervical dilation and ends when the baby emerges. The third stage of labor is expulsion of the placenta.

- During the postpartum period, the mother's body begins to return to its prepregnancy state, and she may begin to breastfeed. Both mother and father must adjust to their new roles as parents as they develop a strong emotional bond with their baby.

FOR MORE INFORMATION

BOOKS

Amato, P. and M. Blott. 2013. *Pregnancy Day by Day.* New York: DK Publishing.

American College of Obstetricians and Gynecologists. 2005. *Your Pregnancy and Birth,* 4th ed. Washington, DC: ACOG. *Advice on conception, pregnancy, prenatal care, and delivery options.*

American Dietetic Association. 2009. *Expect the Best: Your Guide to Healthy Eating Before, During, and After Pregnancy.* New York: Wiley. *Provides up-to-date dietary information and meal-planning guides for women who want to get pregnant, are pregnant, or have had a baby.*

Bogle, K. 2008. *Hooking Up: Sex, Dating and Relationships on Campus.* New York: New York University Press. *A sociologist looks at the "hookup" culture on college campuses today.*

Erickson-Schroth, L. ed. 2014. *Trans Bodies, Trans Selves.* Oxford: Oxford University Press.

Kelly, G. F. 2011. *Sexuality Today,* 10th ed. New York: McGraw-Hill. *An accessible approach that highlights cross-cultural examples, popular topics and issues, and case studies featuring college-age individuals.*

Lees, C., et al. 2007. *Pregnancy and Birth: Your Questions Answered.* London: Dorling Kindersley. *Answers hundreds of common questions about conception, pregnancy, and delivery.*

Marcus, E. 2005. *Is It a Choice? Answers to 300 of the Most Frequently Asked Questions about Gays and Lesbian People,* 3rd ed. San Francisco: HarperOne. *Candid and informative information on coming out, family roles, and politics.*

Mayo Clinic. 2011. *Mayo Clinic Guide to a Healthy Pregnancy,* 1st ed. Intercourse, PA: Good Books. *An authoritative reference manual written by a team of pregnancy experts.*

Meston, C., and D. Buss. 2009. *Why Women Have Sex.* New York: Times Books. *Fascinating, readable, yet scholarly book about all aspects of female sexuality, especially sexual desire.*

Taverner, W. J. 2009. *Taking Sides: Clashing Views on Controversial Issues in Human Sexuality,* 11th ed. New York: McGraw-Hill. *Includes pro and con position statements on sexuality issues relating to biology, behavior, and legal and social issues.*

Wynbrandt, J. 2008. *Encyclopedia of Genetic Disorders and Birth Defects,* 3rd ed. New York: Facts on File, Inc. *A detailed overview of many types of birth defects, both inherited and noninherited.*

ORGANIZATIONS AND WEBSITES

American Association of Sexuality Educators, Counselors, and Therapists (AASECT). Certifies sex educators, counselors, and therapists and provides listings of local therapists dealing with sexual problems.

    http://www.aasect.org

American Congress of Obstetricians and Gynecologists (ACOG). Provides written materials relating to many aspects of preconception care, pregnancy, and childbirth.

    http://www.acog.org

American Society for Reproductive Medicine. Provides up-to-date information about all aspects of infertility.

http://www.asrm.org

Centers for Disease Control and Prevention, National Center on Birth Defects and Developmental Disabilities. Provides information about a variety of topics related to birth defects, including fetal alcohol syndrome and the importance of folic acid.

http://www.cdc.gov/ncbddd

Children Now: Talking with Kids. Provides advice for parents about talking with children about difficult issues, including sex, relationships, and STIs.

http://www.childrennow.org/index.php/learn/talking_with _kids/

Mayo Clinic Health Information. Good source of information on most aspects of health issues and care, including pregnancy.

http://www.mayoclinic.com

National Institute of Child Health and Human Development. Provides information about reproductive and genetic problems; sponsors the "Back to Sleep" campaign to fight SIDS.

http://www.nichd.nih.gov

http://www.nichd.nih.gov/sts (Safe to Sleep campaign)

Sexuality Information and Education Council of the United States (SIECUS). Provides information about many aspects of sexuality and has an extensive library and numerous publications.

http://www.siecus.org

The Kinsey Institute for Research in Sex, Gender, and Reproduction. One of the oldest and most respected institutions doing research on sexuality.

http://www.kinseyinstitute.org

SELECTED BIBLIOGRAPHY

American Diabetes Association. 2011. Diagnosis and classification of diabetes mellitus. *Diabetes Care* 34 (supp 1): S62-9.

American Psychological Association. 2012. *Answers to Your Questions about Transgender People, Gender Identity, and Gender Expression* (http://www.apa.org/topics/sexuality/transgender.aspx).

American Psychological Association. 2012. *Answers to Your Questions for a Better Understanding of Sexual Orientation & Homosexuality* (http://www.apa.org/topics/sexuality/orientation.aspx).

Baronciani, D., et al. 2011. Spreading and outcome of hematopoietic stem cell transplantation in beta thalassemia major. Data from EBMT registry. *Bone Marrow Transplantation* 46: S67.

Blanchette, H. 2011. The rising cesarean delivery rate in America: What are the consequences? *Obstetrics & Gynecology* 118(3): 687–690.

Brewer, G., and C. Hendrie. 2011. Evidence to suggest that copulatory vocalizations in women are not a reflexive consequence of orgasm. *Archives of Sexual Behavior* 40(3): 559–564.

Centers for Disease Control and Prevention. 2012. *Sexually Transmitted Disease Surveillance 2011.* Atlanta: U.S. Department of Health and Human Services.

Centers for Disease Control and Prevention. 2012. *Sudden Infant Death Syndrome (SIDS) and Sudden Unexpected Infant Death (SUID)* (http://www.cdc.gov/SIDS/index.htm).

Centers for Disease Control and Prevention. 2013. *CDC Fact Sheet: STDs and Pregnancy.* (http://www.cdc.gov/std/pregnancy/STDFact-Pregnancy.htm).

Centers for Disease Control and Prevention, American Society for Reproductive Medicine, and Society for Assisted Reproductive Technology. 2013. *2011 Assisted Reproductive Technology: Fertility Clinic Success Rates Report.* Atlanta : U.S. Department of Health and Human Services (http://www.cdc.gov/art/ART2011/PDFs/ART_2011_Clinic_Report-Full.pdf).

Centers for Disease Control and Prevention. 2014. *Youth Risk Behavior Surveillance System,* United States, 2013. *Morbidity and Mortality Weekly Report Surveillance Summaries* 63(4) (http://www.cdc.gov/HealthyYouth/yrbs/index.htm)

Centers for Disease Control and Prevention. 2009. *Healthy Youth—Sexual Risk Behaviors* (http://www.cdc.gov/HealthyYouth/sexualbehaviors/index.htm).

Centers for Disease Control and Prevention. 2013. *Human Papillomavirus* (http://www.cdc.gov/hpv/index.html).

Centers for Disease Control and Prevention. 2013. *Prostate Cancer* (http://www.cdc.gov/cancer/prostate/index.htm).

Chandra A., et al. 2011. Sexual behavior, sexual attraction, and sexual identity in the United States: Data from the 2006–2008 National Survey of Family Growth. *National Health Statistics Reports* No. 36. Hyattsville, MD: National Center for Health Statistics.

Chandra, A., C. E. Copen, and E. H. Stephen. 2013. Infertility and impaired fecundity in the United States, 1982–2010: Data from the National Survey of Family Growth. *National Health Statistics Reports,* no 67. Hyattsville, MD: National Center for Health Statistics.

Crooks, R., and K. Baur. 2014. *Our Sexuality.* Belmont, CA: Wadsworth /Cengage Learning.

Cystic Fibrosis Foundation Patient Registry. 2012. 2012 Annual Data Report. Bethesda, MD: Cystic Fibrosis Foundation (http://www.cff.org/UploadedFiles/research/ClinicalResearch/PatientRegistryReport/2012-CFF-Patient-Registry.pdf, accessed 4/14/2014).

European Union. 2014. "Denmark: Combining work and family life successfully." European Platform for Investing in Children. (http://europa.eu/epic/countries/denmark/index_en.htm)

Eyres, A., B. Bowie, J. Smithson, and S. Winslow. 2011. "Why Is Sex Fun?" *Curiosity.* Discovery Channel.

Fleischman, A. R., et al. 2010. Rethinking the definition of "term pregnancy." *Obstetrics and Gynecology* 116(1): 136–139.

Freeman, E. 2007. *Epidemiology and Etiology of Premenstrual Syndromes* (http://cme.medscape.com/viewarticle/553603).

Garcia-Falgueras, A., and D. Swaab. 2010. Sexual hormones and the brain: An essential alliance for sexual identity and sexual orientation. *Pediatric Endocrinology* 17: 22–35.

Goyal, D., et al. 2010. How much does low socioeconomic status increase the risk of prenatal and postpartum depressive symptoms in first-time mothers? *Women's Health Issues* 20(2): 96–104.

Hock, R. R. 2012. *Human Sexuality.* Upper Saddle River, NJ: Pearson.

Institute of Medicine of the National Academies. 2011. *The health of lesbian, gay, bisexual, and transgender people: Building a foundation for better understanding.* Consensus Report, March 31. Washington, DC: Institute of Medicine of the National Academies.(http://www.iom.edu/Reports/2011/The-Health-of-Lesbian-Gay-Bisexual-and-Transgender-People.aspx).

Ismail, S., et al. 2010. Screening, diagnosing and prevention of fetal alcohol syndrome: Is this syndrome treatable? *Developmental Neuroscience* 32(2): 91–100.

Joannides, P. 2013. *Guide to Getting It On.* Waldport, Oregon: Goofy Foot Press.

Koning, A. M., et al. 2010. Economic consequences of overweight and obesity in infertility: A framework for evaluating the costs and outcomes of fertility care. *Human Reproduction Update* 16(3): 246–254.

Labuski, C. 2013. Vulnerable vulvas: Female genital integrity in health and disease. *Feminist Studies* 39(1): 248–276.

Lavender, T., et al. 2006. Caesarean section for non-medical reasons at term. *Cochrane Database of Systematic Reviews* 19(3).

Lawn, J. E., et al. 2010. Global report on preterm birth and stillbirth (1 of 7): Definitions, description of the burden and opportunities to improve data. *BMC Pregnancy and Childbirth* 10(Suppl 1): S1.

Leguizamon, G. F., and N. P. Zeff. 2006. Hypertension and the pregnancy complicated by diabetes. *Current Diabetes Reports* 6(4): 297–304.

Lindau, S. T., and N. Gavrilova. 2010. Sex, health, and years of sexually active life gained due to good health. *British Medical Journal* 340: c810.

Lino, Mark. 2013. *Expenditures on Children by Families, 2012*. U.S. Department of Agriculture, Center for Nutrition Policy and Promotion. Miscellaneous Publication No. 1528–2012.

Livingston, G. 2013. Factank: "Among 38 nations, U.S. is the outlier when it comes to paid parental leave." *Fact Tank: News in the Numbers*, Pew Research Center.

Mayo Clinic. 2011. *Erectile Dysfunction* (http://www.mayoclinic.com /health /erectile-dysfunction/DS00162).

Mayo Clinic. 2011. *Premenstrual Syndrome* (http://www.mayoclinic.com /health/premenstrual-syndrome/DS00134/DSECTION=lifestyle-and home-remedies).

March of Dimes. 2012. *Postpartum Feelings* (http://www.marchofdimes .com/pregnancy/postpartum-depression.aspx, accessed 4/14/2014).

Melby, M. K., and M. Lampl. 2011. Menopause, a biocultural perspective. *Annual Review of Anthropology* 40: 53–70.

Merviel, P. et al. 2010. Predictive factors for pregnancy after intrauterine insemination (IUI): An analysis of 1038 cycles and a review of the literature. *Fertility and Sterility* 93(1): 79.

Meston, C., and D. Buss. 2007. Why humans have sex. *Archives of Sexual Behavior*, August.

Meston, C., and D. Buss. 2009. *Why Women Have Sex: Understanding Sexual Motivation*. New York: Henry Holt.

Muglia, L. J., and M. Katz. 2010. The enigma of spontaneous preterm birth. *New England Journal of Medicine* 362(6): 529–355.

National Cancer Institute at the National Institutes of Health. 2013. *Prostate Cancer* (http://www.cancer.gov/cancertopics/types/prostate).

National Center for Health Statistics. 2011. *Sexual behavior, sexual attraction, and sexual identity in the United States: Data from the 2006–2008 National Survey of Family Growth* (http://www.cdc.gov/nchs/data/nhsr /nhsr036.pdf).

National Center for Health Statistics. 2013. Births: Final data for 2012. *National Vital Statistics Reports* 62(9).

North American Menopause Society. 2010. *Estrogen and Progesterone Use in Post-Menopausal Women: 2010 Position Statement* (http://www .menopause .org/PSht10.pdf).

Reynolds, R. 2010. The effects of maternal labour analgesia on the fetus. *Best Practice & Research: Clinical Obstetrics & Gynaecology* 24(3): 289–302.

Rice, W., U. Friberg, and S. Gavrilets. 2013. Homosexuality via canalized sexual development: A testing protocol for a new epigenetic model. *BioEssays* 35(9): 764–770.

Sample, I. 2011. Female orgasm captured in series of brain scans. *The Guardian,* 14 November, 9.

Sibai, B. M. 2011. Disparity in the rate of eclampsia and adverse pregnancy outcome from eclampsia: A tale of two countries. *Obstetrics & Gynecology* 118(5): 976–977.

U.S. Department of Health and Human Services. 2011. *Aging Male Syndrome* (http://womenshealth.gov/mens-health/teens-fathers-minorities-older-men/older-men.cfm#ams).

U.S. Department of Agriculture, Center for Nutrition and Policy Promotion. 2013. *Expenditures on Children by Families, 2012.* Publication No. 1528–2012 (http://www.cnpp.usda.gov/publications/crc/crc2012.pdf).

U.S. Department of Health & Human Services, *Surgeon General's Family Health History Initiative* (http://www.hhs.gov/familyhistory/, accessed 4/14/2014).

World Health Organization. 2010. *Female Genital Mutilation* (http://www .who.int/mediacentre/factsheets/fs241/en/).

World Health Organization. 2012. *Male Circumcision for HIV Prevention: Publications.* (http://www.who.int/hiv/pub/malecircumcision/en/).

CHAPTER 6

Contraception and Abortion

CHAPTER OBJECTIVES

- Explain how contraceptives work
- List the most popular contraceptives and discuss their advantages, disadvantages, and effectiveness
- Choose a method of contraception based on the needs of the user and the safety and effectiveness of the method
- Differentiate between first- and second-trimester methods of abortion available in the United States
- Describe the current legal status of abortion in the United States
- Explain the current debate over abortion, including the main arguments of the pro-choice and pro-life points of view

---

For thousands of years, people have used **birth control** to manage **fertility** and prevent unwanted pregnancies. Records dating to the fourth century BCE describe foods, herbs, drugs, douches, and sponges used to prevent **conception**—the fusion of an ovum and sperm that creates a fertilized egg, or *zygote*. Early attempts at **contraception** (the act of blocking conception through a device, substance, or method) followed the same principle as many modern birth control methods.

Today women and men can choose from many different types of **contraceptives** to avoid unwanted pregnancies. Modern contraceptives take a wide variety of forms and work in different ways. Modern contraceptive methods are much more predictable and effective than in the past, and when it comes to making decisions about their sexual and contraceptive behavior, people in industrialized countries now have many options.

Still more than half of all pregnancies were unintended; of those, 40% ended in abortion.

In addition to preventing pregnancy, many contraceptive products—the "barrier methods"—play an important role in protecting against **sexually transmitted infections (STIs)**. (Note that this term has replaced the more familiar *sexually transmitted diseases*, or *STDs*.) Informing yourself about the realities and risks and making responsible decisions about sexual and contraceptive behavior are crucial components of lifelong wellness.

TERMS

birth control The practice of managing fertility and preventing unwanted pregnancies.

fertility The ability to reproduce.

conception The fusion of ovum and sperm, resulting in a fertilized egg, or *zygote*.

contraception The prevention of conception through the use of a device, substance, or method.

contraceptive Any agent or method that can prevent conception.

sexually transmitted infection (STI) Any of several contagious infections contracted through intimate sexual contact.

PRINCIPLES OF CONTRACEPTION

There are many effective approaches to contraception including the following:

• **Barrier methods** work by physically blocking the sperm from reaching the egg. Condoms are the most popular method based on this principle.

• **Hormonal methods,** such as oral contraceptives (birth control pills), alter the biochemistry of the woman's body, preventing ovulation (the release of the egg) and producing changes that make it more difficult for the sperm to reach the egg if ovulation does occur. *Intrauterine devices* prevent the sperm from reaching the egg through hormonal changes.

• **Natural methods** of contraception are based on the fact that the egg and the sperm have to be present at the same time for fertilization to occur; intercourse is avoided around the time of ovulation.

• **Surgical methods**—female and male sterilization—permanently prevent the union of sperm and eggs.

All contraceptive methods have advantages and disadvantages that make them appropriate for some people but not for others, and the best choice during one period of life may not be the best in another. Factors that affect the choice of method include effectiveness, convenience, cost, reversibility, side effects and risks, and protection against STIs. This chapter helps you sort through these factors to decide which contraceptive method is best for you.

Contraceptive effectiveness is partly determined by the reliability of the method itself—the failure rate if it were always used exactly as directed ("perfect use"). Effectiveness is also determined by characteristics of the user, including fertility of the individual, frequency of intercourse, and how consistently and correctly the method is used. This "typical use" **contraceptive failure rate** based on studies that directly measure the percentage of women experiencing an unintended pregnancy in the first year of contraceptive use. For example, the 9% failure rate of oral contraceptives means 9 out of 100 typical users will become pregnant in the first year. This failure rate is likely to be lower for women who are consistently careful in following instructions and higher for those who are frequently careless; the "perfect use" failure rate is 0.3%.

Another measure of effectiveness is the **continuation rate**—the percentage of people who continue to use the method after a specified period of time. This measure is important because many unintended pregnancies occur when a method is stopped and not immediately replaced with another. Thus a contraceptive with a high continuation rate would be more effective at preventing pregnancy than one with a low continuation rate. A high continuation rate also gives an indication of user satisfaction with a particular method.

Contraception is often divided into categories, or tiers, based on efficacy. There are four tiers: Tier 1 comprises the most effective forms of contraception and Tier 4 the least effective forms. Figure 6.1 offers a graphic depiction of these different tiers.

LONG-ACTING REVERSIBLE CONTRACEPTION

Long-acting reversible contraception (LARC) consists of intrauterine devices (IUDs) and implants. These methods of contraception give very high satisfaction rates and have been shown to decrease instances of unintended pregnancy and abortion more compared to other methods.

Intrauterine Devices (IUDs)

An **IUD** is a small plastic object placed in the uterus as a contraceptive. Three types of IUDs are now available in the United States: the Copper T-380A (also known as ParaGard), which provides protection for up to 10 years, and the Mirena and Skyla, both of which release small amounts of progestin and remain effective for up to three years.

> **QUICK STATS**
>
> About **400** eggs are released through ovulation during a woman's fertile life.
> —American College of Obstetricians and Gynecologists, 2012

> **TERMS**
>
> **barrier method**   A contraceptive that acts as a physical barrier, blocking sperm from uniting with an egg.
>
> **hormonal method**   A contraceptive that alters the biochemistry of a woman's body, preventing ovulation and making it more difficult for sperm to reach an egg if ovulation does occur.
>
> **natural method**   An approach to contraception that does not use drugs or devices; requires avoiding intercourse during the period of the woman's menstrual cycle when an egg is most likely to be present at the site of conception and the risk of pregnancy is greatest.
>
> **surgical method**   Sterilization of a male or female to permanently prevent the transport of sperm or eggs to the site of conception.
>
> **contraceptive failure rate**   The percentage of women using a particular contraceptive method who experience an unintended pregnancy in the first year of use.
>
> **continuation rate**   The percentage of people who continue to use a particular contraceptive after a specified period of time.
>
> **Long-acting reversible contraception (LARC)**   Intrauterine devices and implant methods of contraception, which earn high satisfaction rates and have been shown to decrease instances of unintended pregnancy and abortion compared to other methods.
>
> **Intrauterine device (IUD)**   A device inserted into the uterus as a contraceptive.

College tends to be a time of increased sexual activity for many young adults. Those who were sexually active in high school may have an increased number of partners or engage in riskier sexual behaviors once they enter college; those who abstained from intercourse during high school may begin to explore their sexuality once they enter this new environment. Surveys have shown that the majority of college students, up to 70%, engage in sexual activity, and some have more than one partner.

A large percentage of students report not using contraception during their most recent sexual activity. The study cited above found that only 56% of students used contraception during their most recent intercourse. Oral contraceptive pills were the most commonly used contraceptive, with about 60% of women using a contraceptive selecting this method; males who used a contraceptive at last intercourse reported having used the male condom approximately 66% of the time. Of note, the withdrawal method was used by 27% of respondents; this method does not protect against STIs and has a high failure rate.

Black and white college students differ somewhat in contraceptive use. Black students were more likely to have used a condom the last time they had vaginal intercourse compared with white students (63% of blacks versus 58% of whites). On the other hand, white students were far more likely to use hormonal contraception than black students (66% versus 42%). About 6% of black students reported using no contraception the last time they had vaginal intercourse, compared with fewer than 3% of white students. Unintended pregnancies were nearly four times higher among black college students compared with white students.

Although the oral contraceptive pill is a highly effective form of contraception when used as directed, and the male condom is effective at preventing the transmission of a wide variety of STIs, they must be used together to provide simultaneous protection against both pregnancy and STIs. This is particularly important for couples that are not in a long-term, mutually monogamous relationship. However, surveys show that college students use a male condom plus another form of contraception only about 45% of the time.

Around 2% of college women report having become pregnant in the prior year, many unintentionally. A disproportionate number of these pregnancies occur in students within community colleges; a 2007 survey found that 5.3% of attendees at community colleges reported a pregnancy during the year prior, whereas only 1.8% of students at four-year universities reported the same.

The consequences of pregnancy among college students can be significant. For example, one study found that 61% of women who became pregnant while attending community college subsequently dropped out. Those who continue their education face added expenses and stress. Given the importance of education in achieving long-term career and financial goals, the implementation of effective contraception during the college years can have a significant impact on the lives of young women. Unfortunately only 42% of students report being provided any information about pregnancy prevention by their college.

SOURCES: U.S. Department of Education, National Center for Education Statistics. 2002. *Short-Term Enrollment in Postsecondary Education: Student Background and Institutional Differences in Reasons for Early Departure, 1996–98*, NCES 2003–2153. Washington, DC: U.S. Department of Education; American College Health Association. 2011. *National College Health Assessment: Reference Group Executive Summary Spring 2011* (http://www.acha-ncha.org/docs/ACHA-NCHA-II_ReferenceGroup_ExecutiveSummary_Spring2011.pdf).

Current evidence suggests that ParaGard works primarily by preventing fertilization. Like ParaGard, Mirena and Skyla also work primarily by preventing fertilization. As a result of the slow release of very small amounts of progestin, the cervical mucus thickens and stops fertilization.

An IUD is threaded into a sterile inserter that is introduced through the cervix; a plunger pushes the IUD into the uterus. IUDs have two threads attached that protrude from the cervix into the vagina so a woman can feel them to make sure the device is in place. These threads are trimmed so that only 1–1½ inches remain in the upper vagina (Figure 6.2).

Advantages   Intrauterine devices are highly reliable and are simple and convenient to use, requiring no attention. IUDs have only local effects and tend to be very safe for all women, including those with complex medical problems. The long-term expense of using an IUD is also low. The main advantage is their excellent failure rate: Less than 1% of women using IUDs will get pregnant. In the absence of complication, they are also fully reversible, meaning that fertility is restored as soon as the IUD is removed.

Mirena has the added advantage of greatly decreasing blood flow during menstruation and is often used as a treatment for excessive bleeding. It has also been shown to prevent endometrial cancer and even reverse the endometrial changes that precede endometrial cancer. ParaGard has also been shown to decrease the risk of endometrial cancer, but the reasons for this are less clear.

Disadvantages   The IUD offers no protection against STIs. Most IUD side effects are limited to the genital tract. Side effects differ between the two types of IUD. Heavy menstrual flow and increased menstrual cramping sometimes occur with ParaGard, whereas Mirena causes a reduction in bleeding and cramping.

Effectiveness of Family Planning Methods

Most Effective	**Reversible**	**Permanent**	**How to make your method most effective**

Most Effective

Less than 1 pregnancy per 100 women in a year

Reversible

Implant	Intrauterine Device (IUD)	Male Sterilization (Vasectomy)	Female Sterilization (Abdominal, Laparoscopic, Hysteroscopic)
0.05 %*	LNG - 0.2 % Copper T - 0.8 %	0.15 %	0.5 %

How to make your method most effective

After procedure, little or nothing to do or remember.

Vasectomy and hysteroscopic sterilization: Use another method for first 3 months.

6-12 pregnancies per 100 women in a year

Injectable	Pill	Patch	Ring	Diaphragm
6 %	9 %	9 %	9 %	12 %

Injectable: Get repeat injections on time.

Pills: Take a pill each day.

Patch, Ring: Keep in place, change on time.

Diaphragm: Use correctly every time you have sex.

18 or more pregnancies per 100 women in a year

Male Condom	Female Condom	Withdrawal	Sponge
18 %	21 %	22 %	24 % parous women / 12 % nulliparous women

Fertility-Awareness Based Methods	Spermicide
24 %	28 %

Condoms, sponge, withdrawal, spermicides: Use correctly every time you have sex.

Fertility awareness-based methods: Abstain or use condoms on fertile days. Newest methods (Standard Days Method and TwoDay Method) may be the easiest to use and consequently more effective.

Least Effective

* The percentages indicate the number out of every 100 women who experienced an unintended pregnancy within the first year of typical use of each contraceptive method.

CS 242797

CONDOMS SHOULD ALWAYS BE USED TO REDUCE THE RISK OF SEXUALLY TRANSMITTED INFECTIONS.

Other Methods of Contraception

Lactational Amenorrhea Method: LAM is a highly effective, temporary method of contraception.

Emergency Contraception: Emergency contraceptive pills or a copper IUD after unprotected intercourse substantially reduces risk of pregnancy.

U.S. Department of Health and Human Services
Centers for Disease Control and Prevention

Adapted from World Health Organization (WHO) Department of Reproductive Health and Research, Johns Hopkins Bloomberg School of Public Health/Center for Communication Programs (CCP). Knowledge for health project. Family planning: a global handbook for providers (2011 update). Baltimore, MD; Geneva, Switzerland: CCP and WHO; 2011; and Trussell J. Contraceptive failure in the United States. Contraception 2011;83:397–404.

FIGURE 6.1   Categorization of contraceptives based on efficacy.

SOURCE: Centers for Disease Control and Prevention (http://www.cdc.gov/reproductivehealth/UnintendedPregnancy/PDF/Contraceptive_methods_508.pdf).

A serious but rare complication of IUD use is pelvic inflammatory disease (PID). Most pelvic infections among IUD users occur shortly after insertion, are relatively mild, and can be treated successfully with antibiotics.

IUDs are not suitable for women with suspected pregnancy, large tumors of the uterus, other anatomical abnormalities, or unexplained bleeding; Mirena is also not to be used in women with certain hormonally responsive cancers.

Because of the relatively high up-front costs associated with the IUDs, including the cost of the device as well as the practitioner's insertion fee, the IUD is typically most cost-effective for women who desire contraception for at least 6 months.

Effectiveness   The typical first-year failure rate of IUDs is 0.8% for ParaGard and 0.2% for Mirena. Effectiveness can be increased by periodically making sure that the device is in place and by using a backup method for the first week of IUD use. If pregnancy occurs, the IUD may need to be removed to safeguard the woman's health and to maintain the pregnancy; removal depends on the location of the IUD with respect to the pregnancy. If an IUD must be left in place during pregnancy, there is an increased risk of complications.

Contraceptive Implants

Contraceptive implants are placed under the skin of the upper arm and deliver a small but steady dose of progestin (a synthetic progesterone) over a period of years. One such implant, called Implanon/Nexplanon, is a single implant that is effective for three years and is considered to be one of the most effective forms of contraception (Figure 6.3). Contraceptive implants are best suited for women who wish to have continuous, highly effective, and long-term protection against pregnancy.

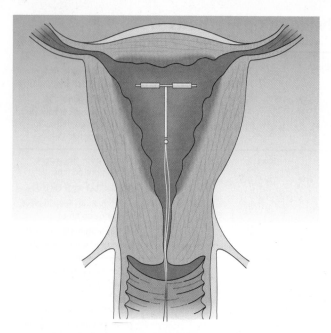

FIGURE 6.2   An IUD (Copper T-380A, or ParaGard) properly positioned in the uterus.

FIGURE 6.3   Placement of Contraceptive Implant. The Implanon/Nexplanon implant device has to be placed and removed by a trained medical professional.

Advantages   Contraceptive implants are highly effective, with a failure rate of less than 1%. After insertion of the implants, no further action is required; contraceptive effects are quickly reversed upon removal. Because implants contain no estrogen, they carry a lower risk of certain side effects, such as blood clots and other cardiovascular complications. Menstrual bleeding tends to decrease but becomes irregular. Women who are breastfeeding can use Nexplanon.

Disadvantages   An implant provides little to no protection against STIs. Although the implants are barely visible, their presence may bother some women. The up-front costs associated with the implant, including the cost of the device as well as the practitioner's fees, can be significant; therefore, the device is cost-effective only for users desiring more than 6 months of contraception.

Common side effects of contraceptive implants are menstrual irregularities, including longer menstrual periods, spotting between periods, or having no bleeding at all. The menstrual cycle usually becomes more regular after one year of use. Less common side effects include headaches, weight gain, breast tenderness, nausea, acne, and mood swings.

> Although they do not protect against STIs, **intrauterine devices and implants** are the most effective form of contraception.

Effectiveness   The overall failure rate for Nexplanon is estimated at about 0.05%. It is one of the most effective methods of contraception and also one of the most discreet.

SHORT-ACTING REVERSIBLE CONTRACEPTION

Oral Contraceptives: The Pill

About a century ago, a researcher noted that ovulation does not occur during pregnancy. Further research revealed the hormonal mechanism: During pregnancy, the corpus luteum secretes progesterone and estrogen in amounts high enough to suppress ovulation. **Oral contraceptives (OCs),** also known as *birth control pills* or "the pill," prevent ovulation by mimicking the hormonal activity of the corpus luteum. The active ingredients in OCs are estrogen and progestins, laboratory-made compounds that are closely related to progesterone. Today OCs are the most widely used form of contraception among unmarried women and are second only to sterilization among married women.

In addition to preventing ovulation, the birth control pill has other contraceptive effects. Its main mechanism of action is to inhibit the movement of sperm by thickening the cervical mucus, and in the rare event that ovulation does occur, it alters the rate of ovum transport by means of its hormonal effects on the fallopian tubes, and may prevent implantation by changing the lining of the uterus.

oral contraceptive (OC)   Hormone compounds (made of estrogen and progestins) in pill form that prevent conception by preventing ovulation; also called the *birth control pill* or "the pill".   TERMS

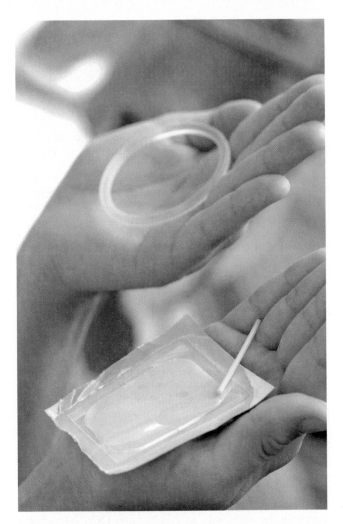

Reversible hormonal contraceptives are available in several forms. Shown here are the patch, the ring, and an implant.

Taking a few pills just prior to having sexual intercourse does not provide effective contraception. A backup contraceptive method is recommended during the first week and any subsequent cycle in which the woman forgets to take any pills.

Advantages   Oral contraceptives are fairly effective in preventing pregnancy. The majority of women who get pregnant while using the pill get pregnant because the pills were not taken as directed. The typical one-year failure rate is 9%. The pill is relatively simple to use and does not hinder sexual

Ask Yourself

QUESTIONS FOR CRITICAL THINKING AND REFLECTION

Prior to reading this section, how familiar were you with the principles of contraception? Did you know as much as you thought? Were you aware of the large number of contraceptive options that are currently available?

spontaneity. Most women also appreciate the predictable regularity of periods, as well as the reduction in cramps and blood loss. Women who have significant problems associated with menstruation may benefit from menstrual suppression with extended-cycle OCs. Finally, the pills are reversible and fertility returns shortly after stopping the pill.

Medical advantages include a decreased incidence of benign breast disease, acne, iron-deficiency anemia, ectopic pregnancy, colon and rectal cancer, endometrial cancer (in the lining of the uterus), and ovarian cancer.

OC use reduces dysmenorrhea (painful periods), endometriosis, and polycystic ovary syndrome.

Disadvantages   Although simple to ingest, remembering to take a pill every single day can be challenging. Furthermore, OCs do not protect against STIs. In some studies, OCs have been associated with increased risk of cervical chlamydia.

The majority of women do not experience any side effects associated with OC use. Among women who experience problems with OCs, the most common issue is bleeding during midcycle (called *breakthrough bleeding*), which is usually slight and tends to disappear after a few cycles. Symptoms of early pregnancy—such as morning nausea and swollen breasts—may appear during the first few months of OC use, although these side effects are uncommon with the low-dose pills in current widespread use. Other side effects can include depression, nervousness, changes in sex drive, dizziness, generalized headaches, migraine, and vaginal discharge.

Research shows that currently used low-dose OCs do not, on average, cause weight gain. Most women experience no change in their weight, while a small percentage lose weight, and about an equal percentage gain weight while taking OCs. The myth that OCs cause women to gain weight is actually dangerous because many unintended pregnancies have resulted when women avoided taking OCs due to unfounded fear of weight gain.

Another myth about OCs is that they can cause cancer. Actually, taking the pill greatly reduces a woman's risk for endometrial and ovarian cancers. OC use is associated with little, if any, increase in breast cancer and a slight increase in cervical cancer, but earlier detection and other variables (such as a woman's number of sexual partners) may account for much of this increase.

Serious OC side effects have been reported in a small number of women. These include blood clots, stroke, and heart attack, concentrated mostly in older women who smoke or have a history of circulatory disease. Recent studies have shown no increased risk of stroke or heart attack for healthy, young, nonsmoking women on lower-dosage pills. OC users may be slightly more prone to high blood pressure, gallbladder disease, and, very rarely, benign liver tumors.

Birth control pills are not recommended for women with a history of blood clots (or a close family member with unexplained blood clots at an early age), heart disease or stroke, migraines with changes in vision, any form of cancer or liver tumor, or impaired liver function. Women with certain other health conditions or behaviors, including migraines without changes in vision, high blood pressure, cigarette smoking, and sickle-cell disease, require close monitoring when taking the pill.

When deciding whether to use OCs, each woman needs to weigh the benefits against the risks. To make an informed decision, she should begin by getting advice from a health care professional. If you take the pill, you can take several steps to reduce the risks associated with OC use:

1. Request a low-dosage pill. (OCs recommended for most new users contain 20–35 micrograms of estrogen.)

2. Stop smoking.

3. Follow the directions carefully and consistently, making sure to take the pills at the same time every day.

4. Be alert to preliminary danger signals, which can be remembered by the word ACHES:

   Abdominal pain (severe).

   Chest pain (severe), cough, shortness of breath, or sharp pain on breathing in.

   Headaches (severe), dizziness, weakness, or numbness, especially if one-sided.

   Eye problems (vision loss or blurring) and/or speech problems.

   Severe leg pain (calf or thigh).

5. Make sure your health practitioner knows your personal and family medical history to help determine whether OCs may be unsafe for you.

6. Have regular **Pap tests,** pelvic exams, and breast exams as recommended by your health practitioner.

Overall, OC risks are generally very small unless you are over 35, are a smoker, or have specific medical problems. For the vast majority of young women, the known, directly associated risk of death from taking birth control pills is much, much lower than the risk of death from pregnancy (Table 6.1).

Effectiveness Oral contraceptive effectiveness varies substantially because it depends so much on individual factors. If taken as directed, the failure rate is as low as 0.3%. However, the typical user has a 9% failure rate. The continuation rate for OCs also varies; the average rate is 67% after one year. Besides forgetting to take the pill, another reason for OC failure is poor absorption of the drug due to vomiting or diarrhea, or to interactions with other medicines (including certain antibiotics, antiseizure medications, and the commonly used herb St. John's wort).

Pap test A scraping of cells from the cervix for examination under a microscope to detect cancer.

TERMS

Table 6.1	Risks of Contraception, Pregnancy, and Abortion

CONTRACEPTION	RISK OF DEATH
Oral contraceptives	
Nonsmoker	
Age 15–34	1 in 1,667,000
Age 35–44	1 in 33,300
Smoker	
Age 15–34	1 in 57,800
Age 35–44	1 in 5,200
IUDs	1 in 10,000,000
Barrier methods, spermicides	None
Fertility awareness–based methods	None
Tubal ligation	1 in 66,700
PREGNANCY	**RISK OF DEATH**
Pregnancy	1 in 6,900
ABORTION	**RISK OF DEATH**
Spontaneous abortion	1 in 142,900
Medical abortion	1 in 200,000
Surgical abortion	1 in 142,900

SOURCE: Hatcher, R. A., et al. *Contraceptive Technology,* 20th revised ed. Copyright © 2011 Ardent Media. Reprinted with permission.

Contraceptive Skin Patch

The contraceptive skin patch, Ortho Evra, is a thin, 1¾-inch square patch that slowly releases an estrogen and a progestin into the bloodstream. The contraceptive patch prevents pregnancy in the same way as combination OCs, following a similar schedule. Each patch is worn continuously for one week and is replaced on the same day of the week for three consecutive weeks. The fourth week is patch-free, allowing a woman to have her menstrual period.

The patch can be worn on the upper outer arm, abdomen, buttocks, or upper torso (excluding the breasts); it is designed to stick to skin even during bathing or swimming. If a patch should fall off for more than a day, the U.S. Food and Drug Administration (FDA) advises starting a new four-week cycle of patches and using a backup method of contraception for the first week. Patches should be discarded according to the manufacturer's directions to avoid leakage of hormones into the environment.

Advantages Because the patch provides the same combination of hormones as a combined birth control pill, the advantages are similar. The medical benefits of the patch include, but are not limited to, lighter, less painful menses; decreased risk of uterine and ovarian cancer; decreased anemia; and the ability to control your cycle. With both perfect and typical use, the patch is as effective as OCs in preventing pregnancy.

Disadvantages Like other hormonal contraceptives, the patch doesn't protect against STIs. Patch users should also use condoms for STI protection unless they are in a long-term monogamous relationship with an uninfected partner. Minor side effects are similar to those of OCs, although breast discomfort may be more common in patch users. Some women also experience skin irritation around the patch. More serious complications are thought to be similar to those of OCs, including an increased risk of side effects among women who smoke. However, because Ortho Evra exposes users to higher doses of estrogen than most OCs, patch use may further increase the risk of blood clots (venous thromboembolism). Recent studies show conflicting results regarding the risk of blood clots, but it is possible that the risk is slightly higher with the patch compared to low-dose OCs.

Effectiveness   With perfect use, the patch's failure rate is very low (0.3%) in the first year of use. The typical failure rate is approximately 9%, similar to that of the oral contraceptive pill.

Vaginal Contraceptive Ring

The NuvaRing is a vaginal ring that is molded with a mixture of progestin and estrogen. The two-inch ring slowly releases hormones and maintains blood hormone levels comparable to those found with OC use. The ring prevents pregnancy in the same way as OCs. A woman inserts the ring anytime during the first five days of her menstrual cycle and leaves it in place for three weeks. During the fourth week, when the ring is removed, her next menstrual cycle occurs. A new ring is then inserted 7 days later. Rings should be discarded according to the manufacturer's directions to avoid leakage of hormones into the environment. Backup contraception must be used for the first seven days of the first ring use or if the ring has been removed for more than three hours.

Advantages   The NuvaRing offers one month of protection with no daily or weekly action required. It does not require a fitting by a clinician, and exact placement in the vagina is not critical as it is with a diaphragm. The medical benefits of the patch include, but are not limited to, lighter, less painful menses; decreased risk of uterine and ovarian cancer; decreased anemia; and the ability to control your cycle.

Disadvantages   The NuvaRing provides no protection against STIs. Side effects are roughly comparable to those seen with OC use, except for a lower incidence of nausea and vomiting. Other side effects may include vaginal discharge, vaginitis, and vaginal irritation. Medical risks also are similar to those found with OC use.

Effectiveness   As with the pill and patch, the perfect use failure rate is around 0.3%. The ring's typical use failure rate is similar to the pill's at 9%.

Injectable Contraceptives

Hormonal contraceptive injections were first developed in the 1960s. The first injectable contraceptive approved for use in the United States was Depo-Provera, which uses long-acting progestins. Injected into the arm or buttocks, Depo-Provera is usually given every 12 weeks, although it may provide effective contraception for a few weeks beyond that. The product prevents pregnancy by inhibiting ovulation.

Advantages   Injectable contraceptives are highly effective and require little action on the part of the user. Because the injections leave no trace and involve no ongoing supplies, injectable contraceptives allow women almost total privacy in their decision to use contraception. Depo-Provera has no estrogen-related side effects.

Disadvantages   Injectable contraceptives provide no protection against STIs. A woman must visit a health care facility every three months to receive the injections. The side effects of Depo-Provera are similar to those of implants: Menstrual irregularities are the most common, and after one year of using Depo-Provera many women have no menstrual bleeding at all. Weight gain is a common side effect. After discontinuing the use of Depo-Provera, women may experience temporary infertility for up to 12 months.

Depo-Provera also has a unique risk: It can cause a reduction in bone density, especially in women who use it for an extended period. Although decreased bone density is a risk factor for osteoporosis and fractures, no studies have shown that this decreased density actually leads to increased fractures. Nonetheless, women who use Depo-Provera are advised to do weight-bearing exercise and ensure an adequate intake of dietary calcium. Multiple gynecologic associations believe that the benefits of this highly effective contraception outweigh the theoretical risks, and continuation should not be denied due to concerns regarding bone density.

Effectiveness   The perfect use failure rate is 0.2% for Depo-Provera. With typical use, the failure rate increases to 6% in the first year of use.

Male Condoms

The **male condom** is a thin sheath designed to cover the penis during sexual intercourse. Most brands available in the United States are made of latex, although condoms made of polyurethane and polyisoprene are also available. Condoms prevent sperm from entering the vagina and provide protection against most STIs. Condoms are the most widely used barrier method and the third most popular of all contraceptive methods used in the United States, after the pill and female sterilization.

The man or his partner must put the condom on the penis before it is inserted into the vagina because the small amounts of fluid that may be secreted unnoticed prior to

male condom   A thin sheath that covers the penis during sexual intercourse; used for contraception and to prevent STI transmission.

ejaculation often contain sperm capable of causing pregnancy. The rolled-up condom is placed over the head of the erect penis and unrolled down to the base of the penis, leaving a half-inch space (without air) at the tip to collect semen (Figure 6.4). Some brands of condoms have a reservoir tip designed for this purpose. Uncircumcised men must first pull back the foreskin of the penis. Partners must be careful not to damage the condom with fingernails, rings, or other rough objects.

Many condoms are prelubricated with water-based or silicone-based lubricants. These lubricants make the condom more comfortable and less likely to break. Many people find that using extra, non-oil-based lubricant can be helpful. Prelubricated condoms are also available containing the **spermicide** nonoxynol-9, the same agent found in many of the contraceptive creams that women use. However, spermicidal condoms are no more effective than condoms without spermicide. They cost more and have a shorter shelf life than most other condoms. Further, condoms with nonoxynol-9 have been

associated with urinary tract infections in women and, if they cause tissue irritation, an increased risk of HIV transmission. Planned Parenthood and many other public health agencies advise against the use of condoms lubricated with nonoxynol-9.

Water-based lubricants such as K-Y Brand Jelly or Astroglide can be used as needed. Any products that contain mineral or vegetable oil—including baby oil, many lotions, regular petroleum jelly, cooking oils (corn oil, shortening, butter, and so on), and some vaginal lubricants and antifungal or anti-itch creams—should not be used with latex condoms. Such products can cause latex to start disintegrating within 60 seconds, thus greatly increasing the chance of condom breakage. (Polyurethane is not affected by oil-based products.)

Advantages Condoms are easy to purchase and are available without prescription or medical supervision. In addition to being free of medical side effects (other than occasional allergic reactions), latex condoms help protect against STIs. A recent study determined that condoms may also protect women from human papillomavirus (HPV), which causes cervical cancer. Condoms made of polyurethane are appropriate for people who are allergic to latex. However, they are more likely to slip or break than latex condoms and therefore may give less protection against STIs and pregnancy. Polyisoprene condoms, marketed under the brand name SKYN, are safe for most people with latex allergies, stretchier, and less expensive than polyurethane condoms. Condoms made of lambskin are also available but permit the passage of HIV and other disease-causing organisms and are less effective for pregnancy prevention. Except for abstinence or intercourse within a monogamous relationship with an uninfected partner, the correct and consistent use of latex male condoms offers the most reliable available protection against the transmission of HIV.

Disadvantages The two most common complaints about condoms are that they diminish sensation and interfere with spontaneity. Although some people find these drawbacks serious, others consider them only minor distractions.

Effectiveness During the first year of typical condom use among 100 users, approximately 18 pregnancies will occur. And even with perfect use, the first-year failure rate is about 2%. At least some pregnancies happen because the condom is carelessly removed after ejaculation. Some may also occur because of breakage or slippage. Other contributing

FIGURE 6.4 Use of the male condom. (a) Place the rolled-up condom over the head of the erect penis. Hold the top half-inch of the condom (with air squeezed out) to leave room for semen. (b) While holding the tip, unroll the condom onto the penis. Gently smooth out any air bubbles. (c) Unroll the condom down to the base of the penis. (d) To avoid spilling semen after ejaculation, hold the condom around the base of the penis as the penis is withdrawn. Remove the condom away from your partner, taking care not to spill any semen.

ejaculation An abrupt discharge of semen from the penis during sexual stimulation.

spermicide A chemical agent that kills sperm.

TERMS

factors include poorly fitting condoms, insufficient lubrication (which increases the risk of breakage), excessively vigorous sex, and improper storage. (Because heat destroys rubber, latex condoms should not be stored for long periods in a wallet or a car's glove compartment.) To help ensure quality, condoms should not be used past their expiration date or more than five years past their date of manufacture (two years for those with spermicide).

If a condom breaks or is carelessly removed, a woman can reduce the risk of pregnancy somewhat by immediately taking an emergency contraceptive (discussed later in the chapter).

Female Condoms

The female condom is a clear, stretchy, disposable pouch with two rings that can be inserted into a woman's vagina. It was designed as an alternative to the male condom because the woman can control its use. It can be inserted up to eight hours before intercourse, so it need not interfere with the moment. It is about as effective in preventing pregnancy and the spread of STIs as the male condom.

The one-size-fits-all condom, called the FC2, consists of a soft, loose-fitting, nonlatex rubber sheath with two flexible rings. The ring at the closed end is inserted into the vagina and placed at the cervix much like a diaphragm. The ring at the open end remains outside the vagina. The female condom protects the inside of the vagina and part of the external genitalia.

The directions that accompany the FC2 should be followed closely. The manufacturer strongly recommends practicing inserting the female condom several times before actually using it for intercourse. Most women find that it is easy to use after they have practiced inserting the FC2 several times. The FC2 comes prelubricated with a silicone lubricant, but extra lubricant or a spermicide can be used if desired. As with male condoms, users need to take care not to tear the condom during insertion or removal. Following intercourse, the woman should remove the condom before standing up. By twisting and squeezing the outer ring, she can prevent the spilling of semen.

Advantages Female condoms can be inserted up to eight hours before sexual activity and are thus less disruptive than male condoms. Because the outer part of the condom covers the area around the vaginal opening as well as the base of the penis during intercourse, it offers potentially better protection against genital warts or herpes. The synthetic rubber pouch can be used by people who are allergic to latex. Because the material is thin and pliable, there is little loss of sensation. The FC2 is generously lubricated and the material conducts heat well, increasing comfort and natural feel during intercourse.

When used correctly, the female condom should theoretically provide protection against HIV transmission and STIs comparable to that of the latex male condom. However, in research involving typical users, the female condom was slightly less effective in preventing both pregnancy and STIs. Effectiveness improves with careful practice and instruction.

Disadvantages The female condom is unfamiliar to most people and requires practice to learn to use effectively. The outer ring of the female condom, which hangs visibly outside the vagina, may be bothersome to some couples during foreplay; if so, couples may choose to put the device in just before intercourse. During coitus, both partners must take care that the penis is inserted into the pouch, not outside it, and that the device does not slip inside the vagina. Female condoms, like male condoms, are made for one-time use. A single female condom costs about three to four times as much as a single male condom. Female condoms are harder to find than male condoms. Some pharmacies do not currently carry them, but this will likely change as the device becomes more popular. You can buy the FC2 at Planned Parenthood and online (see http://www.fc2.us.com/howto getfc2.html).

Effectiveness The typical first-year failure rate of the female condom is 21%. For women who follow instructions carefully and consistently, the failure rate is considerably lower—about 5%.

Diaphragm with Spermicide

The **diaphragm** is a dome-shaped cup of latex or silicone stretched over a collapsible metal ring. When correctly used with spermicidal cream or jelly, the diaphragm covers the cervix, blocking sperm from the uterus.

Diaphragms are available in the United States only by prescription. Because of individual anatomical differences among women, a diaphragm must be carefully fitted by a trained clinician to ensure both comfort and effectiveness. The fit should be checked with each routine annual medical examination, as well as after childbirth, abortion, abdominal or pelvic surgery, or a weight change of more than 10 pounds. However, a new "SILCS diaphragm" (a silicone device) has been approved in Europe and will hopefully soon be approved in the United States. The SILCS is one-size-fits-all and does not require a physician to insert the device.

A diaphragm should be used with spermicidal jelly or cream on the diaphragm before inserting it and checking its placement (Figure 6.5). If more than six hours elapse between the time of insertion and the time of intercourse, additional spermicide must be applied. The diaphragm must be left in place for at least six hours after the last act of coitus to give the spermicide enough time to kill all the sperm. With repeated intercourse, a condom should be used for additional protection.

diaphragm A contraceptive device consisting of a flexible, dome-shaped cup that covers the cervix and prevents sperm from entering the uterus.

TERMS

FIGURE 6.5 Use of the diaphragm. Wash your hands with soap and water before inserting the diaphragm. It can be inserted while squatting, lying down, or standing with one foot raised. (a) Place about a tablespoon of spermicidal jelly or cream in the concave side of the diaphragm, and spread it around the inside of the diaphragm and around the rim. (b) Squeeze the diaphragm into a long, narrow shape between the thumb and forefinger. Insert it into the vagina, and push it up along the back wall of the vagina as far as it will go. (c) Check its position to make sure the cervix is completely covered and that the front rim of the diaphragm is tucked behind the pubic bone.

To remove the diaphragm, the woman hooks the front rim down from the pubic bone with one finger and pulls it out. After each use, a diaphragm should be washed with mild soap and water, rinsed, patted dry, and examined for holes or cracks. Defects would most likely develop near the rim and can be spotted by looking at the diaphragm in front of a bright light. A diaphragm should be stored in its case.

Advantages Diaphragm use is less intrusive than male condom use because a diaphragm can be inserted up to six hours before intercourse. Its use can be limited to times of sexual activity only, and it allows for immediate and total reversibility. The diaphragm is free of medical side effects (other than rare allergic reactions) and increased risk of urinary tract infection.

Disadvantages Diaphragms must always be used with a spermicide, so a woman must keep both of these supplies with her whenever she anticipates sexual activity. Diaphragms require extra attention because they must be cleaned and stored with care to preserve their effectiveness. Some women cannot wear a diaphragm because of their vaginal or uterine anatomy.

Diaphragms have also been associated with a slightly increased risk of **toxic shock syndrome (TSS),** an occasionally fatal bacterial infection. To reduce the risk of TSS, a woman should wash her hands carefully with soap and water before inserting or removing the diaphragm, should not use the diaphragm during menstruation or when abnormal vaginal discharge is present, and should never leave the device in place for more than 24 hours.

Effectiveness The typical failure rates are 12% during the first year of use. The main causes of failure are incorrect insertion, inconsistent use, and inaccurate fitting. If a diaphragm slips during intercourse, a woman should use emergency contraception.

Cervical Cap

The **cervical cap,** another barrier device, is a small flexible cup that fits snugly over the cervix and is held in place by suction. This cervical cap is a clear silicone cup with a brim around the dome to hold spermicide and trap sperm, and a removal strap over the dome. It comes in three sizes and must be fitted by a trained clinician. It is used like a diaphragm, with a small amount of spermicide placed in the cup and on the brim before insertion. The cervical cap is reusable but must be replaced annually.

> **toxic shock syndrome (TSS)** A bacterial disease usually associated with tampon use, and sometimes diaphragm use; symptoms include fever, rash, nausea, headache, dizziness, confusion, fainting, sore throat, cough, and abdominal pain.
>
> **cervical cap** A small flexible cup that fits over the cervix; used with spermicide.
>
> TERMS

Many contraceptive methods work by blocking sperm from entering the cervix. Barrier methods pictured here are the diaphragm, the female condom, the male condom, the sponge, and the cervical cap.

which helps it fit snugly over the cervix. The sponge is made of polyurethane and is presaturated with the same spermicide used in contraceptive creams and foams. The sponge, which can be used only once, acts as a barrier and a spermicide and absorbs seminal fluid.

Advantages   The sponge offers advantages similar to those of the diaphragm and cervical cap. In addition, sponges can be obtained without a prescription or professional fitting, and they may be safely left in place for 24 hours without the addition of spermicide for repeated intercourse. Most women and men find the sponge to be comfortable and unobtrusive during sex.

Disadvantages   Reported disadvantages include difficulty with removal and an unpleasant odor if the sponge is left in place for more than 18 hours. Allergic reactions, such as irritation of the vagina, are more common with the sponge than with other spermicide products, probably because the overall dose of spermicide contained in each sponge is significantly higher than that used with other methods. If irritation of the vaginal lining occurs, the risk of yeast infections and STIs (including HIV) may increase. The sponge is a single-use device and must be thrown away after each use. Additionally, it cannot be used during menstruation. Because the sponge has also been associated with toxic shock syndrome, the same precautions must be taken as those described for diaphragm use.

Effectiveness   The typical effectiveness of the sponge is the same as that of the diaphragm (12% failure rate during the first year of use) for women who have never experienced childbirth. For women who have had a child, however, the failure rate rises to 24%.

Vaginal Spermicides

Spermicidal compounds developed for use with a diaphragm have been adapted for use without a diaphragm by combining them with a bulky base. Foams, creams, and jellies must be placed deep in the vagina near the cervical entrance and must be inserted no more than 60 minutes before intercourse. After an hour, their effectiveness is drastically reduced, and a new dose must be inserted.

The spermicidal suppository is small and easily inserted like a tampon. The vaginal contraceptive film (VCF) is a paper-thin two-inch square of film that contains spermicide. It is folded over one or two fingers and placed high in the vagina, as close to the cervix as possible.

Advantages   Advantages of the cervical cap are similar to those associated with diaphragm use. It is an alternative for women who cannot use a diaphragm because of anatomical reasons or recurrent urinary tract infections. The cap fits tightly, so it does not require backup condom use with repeated intercourse. It may be left in place for up to 48 hours.

Disadvantages   Along with most of the disadvantages associated with the diaphragm, difficulty with insertion and removal is more common for cervical cap users. Because there may be a slightly increased risk of toxic shock syndrome with prolonged use, the cap should not be left in place for more than 48 hours.

Effectiveness   Studies indicate that the average failure rate for the cervical cap is 16% for women who have never had a child and 32% for women who have had a child.

Contraceptive Sponge

The **contraceptive sponge** is a round, absorbent device about two inches in diameter with a polyester loop on one side (for removal) and a concave dimple on the other side,

contraceptive sponge   A contraceptive device   **TERMS** about two inches in diameter that fits over the cervix and acts as a barrier and spermicide and absorbs seminal fluid.

Advantages The use of vaginal spermicides is relatively simple and can be limited to times of sexual activity. They are readily available in most drugstores and do not require a prescription or a pelvic examination. Spermicides allow complete and immediate reversibility, and the only medical side effects are occasional allergic reactions.

Disadvantages When used alone, vaginal spermicides must be inserted shortly before intercourse, so their use may be seen as an annoying disruption. Some women find the slight increase in vaginal fluids after spermicide use unpleasant. Also, spermicides can alter the balance of bacteria in the vagina. Because this may increase the occurrence of yeast infections and urinary tract infections, women who are especially prone to these infections may want to avoid spermicides. Also, this contraception method does not protect against sexually transmitted infections such as gonorrhea, chlamydia, or HIV. Overuse of spermicides can irritate vaginal tissues; if this occurs, the risk of HIV transmission may increase.

Effectiveness Vaginal spermicides on their own are not very effective. The typical failure rate is about 28% during the first year of use. Spermicide is generally recommended only in combination with other barrier methods or as a backup to other contraceptives. Emergency contraceptives provide a better backup than spermicides, however.

Abstinence, Fertility Awareness, and Withdrawal

Millions of people worldwide do not use any of the contraceptive methods described earlier because of religious convictions, cultural prohibitions, poverty, or lack of information and supplies. If they use any method at all, they are likely to use one of the following relatively "natural" methods.

Abstinence The decision not to engage in sexual intercourse for a chosen period of time, or **abstinence,** has been practiced throughout history for a variety of reasons. Until relatively recently, many people abstained because they had no other contraceptive measures. Concern about possible contraceptive side effects, STIs, and unwanted pregnancy may be factors. For others, the most important reason for choosing abstinence is a moral one, based on cultural or religious beliefs or strongly held personal values.

> **QUICK STATS**
>
> **5.4%** of women who practice some sort of contraception rely on withdrawal as their birth control method.
>
> —National Survey on Family Growth, 2011

Fertility Awareness–Based Methods Women who practice a **fertility awareness–based method** of contraception abstain from intercourse during the fertile phase of their menstrual cycle. Ordinarily only one egg is released by the ovaries each month, and it lives about 24 hours unless it is fertilized. Sperm deposited in the vagina may be capable of fertilizing an egg for up to six or seven days, so conception can theoretically occur only during six to eight days of any menstrual cycle. However, predicting which eight days is difficult. Recent studies show that even in women who have regular menstrual cycles, it is possible to become pregnant at any time during the menstrual cycle. It is even more difficult to predict the fertile time of the cycle in women who have irregular menses—a situation that is very common, especially in teenagers and women who are approaching menopause.

Methods that attempt to predict the fertile times of a woman's cycle include calendar methods, temperature methods, and methods that rely on observation of the cyclical changes of the cervical mucus, as well as other characteristics of the cervix. Some women use a combination of methods to determine the time of ovulation.

Calendar methods are based on the idea that the average woman releases an egg 14–16 days before her period begins. To avoid pregnancy, she should abstain from intercourse for about eight days during her cycle, beginning several days before and during the time that ovulation is most likely to occur. However, in one recent study only about 10% of women with regular 28-day cycles actually ovulated 14 days before the next period. The situation is further complicated by the fact that many women have somewhat or very irregular cycles; calendar methods are extremely unreliable for these women.

Temperature methods are based on the knowledge that a woman's body temperature drops slightly just before ovulation and rises slightly after ovulation. A woman using the temperature method records her basal (resting) body temperature (BBT) every morning before getting out of bed and before eating or drinking anything. Once the temperature pattern is apparent (usually after about three months), the unsafe period for intercourse can be calculated as the interval from day 5 (day 1 is the first day of the period) until three days after the rise in BBT. To arrive at a shorter unsafe period, some women combine the calendar and temperature methods, calculating the first unsafe day from the shortest cycle of the calendar chart and the last unsafe day as the third day after a rise in BBT.

The *mucus method* (or Billings method) is based on changes in the cervical secretions throughout the menstrual cycle. During the estrogenic phase, cervical mucus increases and is clear and slippery. At the time of ovulation, some women can detect a slight change in the texture of the mucus and find that it is more likely to form an elastic thread when stretched between thumb and finger. After ovulation, these

---

> **TERMS**
>
> **abstinence** Avoidance of sexual intercourse; a method of contraception.
>
> **fertility awareness–based method** A method of preventing conception based on avoiding intercourse during the fertile phase of a woman's cycle.

secretions become cloudy and sticky and decrease in quantity. Infertile, safe days are likely to occur during the relatively dry days just before and after menstruation. These additional clues have been found to be helpful by some couples who rely on fertility awareness–based methods.

Any woman for whom pregnancy would be a serious problem should not rely on these methods alone because the failure rate is high—approximately 25% each year. Fertility awareness–based methods are not recommended for women who have very irregular cycles—about 15% of all menstruating women. Further, fertility awareness–based methods offer no protection against STIs. Some women use fertility awareness in combination with a barrier method to reduce their risk for unwanted pregnancy.

Withdrawal   In **withdrawal**, or *coitus interruptus*, the male removes his penis from the vagina just before he ejaculates. Withdrawal has a high failure rate because the male has to overcome a powerful biological urge. Further, because preejaculatory fluid may contain viable sperm, pregnancy can occur even if the man withdraws prior to ejaculation. Sexual pleasure is often affected because the man must remain in control and the sexual experience of both partners is interrupted.

The failure rate for typical use is about 22% in the first year. Withdrawal does not protect against STIs.

> Emergency contraceptives **do not result in an abortion** and do not interfere with an existing pregnancy.

Combining Methods

Couples can choose to combine the preceding methods in a variety of ways, both to add STI protection and to increase contraceptive effectiveness. For example, condoms are strongly recommended along with hormonal contraception whenever there is a risk of STIs (Table 6.2). For many couples, and especially for women, the added benefits far outweigh the extra effort and expense of using multiple methods. Table 6.3 summarizes the effectiveness of available contraceptive methods.

EMERGENCY CONTRACEPTION

Emergency contraception (EC) refers to postcoital methods—those used after unprotected sexual intercourse. An emergency contraceptive may be appropriate if a regularly used method has failed (for example, if a condom breaks) or if unprotected sex has occurred. Sometimes called the "morning-after pill," emergency contraceptives are designed only for emergency use and should not be relied on as a regular birth control method; other methods of birth control are more effective.

When emergency contraceptives were first approved by the FDA, opponents feared that they might act as an **abortifacient**—preventing implantation of a fertilized egg, theoretically causing abortion. However, recent evidence indicates that emergency contraceptives do not interrupt an established pregnancy. Next-day or after-sex pills work primarily by inhibiting or delaying ovulation and by blocking the transport of sperm and eggs.

Plan B, Plan B One-Step, Next Choice One Dose, and Ella are now in common use and are more effective, with fewer side effects,

TERMS

withdrawal   A method of contraception in which the man withdraws his penis from the vagina prior to ejaculation; also called *coitus interruptus*.

emergency contraception (EC)   A birth control method used after unprotected sexual intercourse has occurred.

abortifacient   An agent or substance that induces abortion.

Table 6.2	Contraceptive Methods and STI Protection

METHOD	LEVEL OF PROTECTION
Hormonal methods	Do not protect against HIV or STIs in lower reproductive tract; may increase risk of cervical chlamydia; provide some protection against PID.
IUD	Does not protect against STIs.
Latex, polyisoprene, or polyurethane male condom	Best method for protection against STIs (if used correctly); does not protect against infections from lesions that are not covered by the condom. (Lambskin condoms do not protect against STIs.)
Female condom	Reduction of STI risk similar to that of male condom; may provide extra protection for external genitalia.
Diaphragm, sponge, or cervical cap	Provides some protection against cervical infections and PID. Diaphragms, sponges, and cervical caps should not be relied on for protection against HIV.
Spermicide	Modestly reduces the risk of some vaginal and cervical STIs; does not reduce the risk of HIV, chlamydia, or gonorrhea. If vaginal irritation occurs, infection risk may increase.
Fertility awareness–based methods	Do not protect against STIs.
Sterilization	Does not protect against STIs.
Abstinence	Complete protection against STIs (as long as all activities that involve the exchange of body fluids are avoided).

Table 6.3 Contraceptives: From Most Effective to Least (Percentage of Women Experiencing Unintended Pregnancy within the First Year of Use)

METHOD REVERSIBLE METHODS	TYPICAL USE	PERFECT USE
Extremely effective:		
Complete abstinence		0.0%
Implant (Implanon)	0.05%	0.05%
Mirena IUD	0.2%	0.2%
ParaGard IUD	0.8%	0.6%
Injectable (3-month)	6.0%	0.2%
Very effective:		
Pill	9.0%	0.3%
Patch	9.0%	0.3%
Ring	9.0%	0.3%
Moderately effective:		
Male condom	18.0%	2.0%
Diaphragm	12.0%	6.0%
Sponge (if never had a child)	12.0%	9.0%
Cervical cap (if never had a child)	16.0%	9.0%
Female condom	21.0%	5.0%
Less effective:		
Periodic abstinence	24.0%	
Withdrawal	22.0%	4.0%
Spermicides	28.0%	18.0%
Sponge (if have had a child)	24.0%	20.0%
Cervical cap (if have had a child)	32.0%	26.0%
PERMANENT METHODS		
Vasectomy	0.15%	0.1%
Essure	0.2%	0.2%
Tubal sterilization	0.5%	0.5%
No method	85.0%	85.0%

SOURCE: Trussell, J. "Contraceptive Efficacy." In Hatcher, R. A., et al. *Contraceptive Technology,* 20th revised ed. Copyright © 2011 Ardent Media. Reprinted with permission.

stomach pain, headache, dizziness, and breast tenderness. If a woman is already pregnant, these pills will not interfere with the pregnancy. Current emergency contraceptives are considered very safe.

Plan B One-Step is available as an over-the-counter (OTC) drug (no prescription required) for everyone. Next Choice One Dose is available for persons 17 and older. To buy an emergency contraceptive, you need to ask for it at the pharmacy counter. It is recommended that you call ahead to make sure your pharmacy has EC on hand. The vast majority of pharmacies, especially the larger chains, currently carry emergency contraceptives.

Some clinicians advise women to keep a package of emergency contraceptives on hand in case their regular contraception method fails or they have unprotected intercourse. Research has found that ready access to emergency contraception improves the rate of use as well as decreasing the time to use. However, it does not lead to an increase in unprotected intercourse or STIs.

One reason why women fail to take emergency contraceptives even when they have them may be that they underestimate their risk of pregnancy. Many women still believe that they can't get pregnant from a single act of intercourse. Expense is also an issue for some women. EC is covered by some health plans as well as by Medicaid in many states. However, many women must pay directly for EC, which costs about $50.

To find out more about emergency contraception and how to obtain it in your area, visit the Emergency Contraception website at http://ec.princeton.edu. Planned Parenthood is a good source of information, as are most pharmacies. You can also call the Emergency Contraception Hotline (888-NOT-2-LATE) for more information about access.

Intrauterine devices can also be used for emergency contraception. If inserted within five days of unprotected intercourse, the Copper T ParaGard IUD (discussed earlier) is even more effective than pills for emergency contraception. It has the added benefit of providing up to 12 years of contraception.

than older methods of EC. Plan B One-Step, which replaced Plan B in 2009, contains a single progestin-only pill, whereas Next Choice One Dose has two pills that are taken 12 hours apart. The pills should be taken as soon as possible after inadequately protected sex. If taken within 24 hours after intercourse, emergency contraceptives may prevent as many as 75–95% of expected pregnancies. Overall they reduce pregnancy risk by about 89%. They are most effective if initiated in the first 12 hours, but they can be taken up to 120 hours after unprotected intercourse. Possible side effects include nausea,

PERMANENT CONTRACEPTION

Sterilization is permanent, and it is highly effective at preventing pregnancy. At present it is tied with the pill as the most commonly used contraceptive method in the United States

sterilization Surgically altering the reproductive system to prevent pregnancy. Vasectomy is the procedure in males; tubal sterilization or hysterectomy is the procedure in females. TERMS

Ask Yourself

QUESTIONS FOR CRITICAL THINKING AND REFLECTION

If you are sexually active, do you use any of the reversible methods described in the preceding sections? Based on the information given here, do you believe you are using your contraceptive perfectly, or in a way that increases your risk of an unintended pregnancy?

and is by far the most common method used worldwide. It is especially popular among couples who have been married 10 or more years and have had all the children they intend to have. Sterilization does not protect against STIs.

An important consideration in choosing sterilization is that, in most cases, it cannot be reversed. Although the chances of restoring fertility are being increased by modern surgical techniques, such operations are costly, and pregnancy can never be guaranteed.

Many studies indicate that male sterilization is preferable to female sterilization for a variety of reasons. The overall cost of a female procedure is about four times that of a male procedure, the surgery itself is more complex, and women are much more likely than men to experience complications following the operation. Further, feelings of regret seem to be more prevalent in women than in men after sterilization.

Male Sterilization: Vasectomy

The procedure for male sterilization, **vasectomy,** involves severing the vasa deferentia, two tiny ducts that transport sperm from the testes to the seminal vesicles. After surgery, the testes continue to produce sperm, but the sperm are absorbed into the body. Because the testes contribute only about 10% of the total seminal fluid, the actual quantity of ejaculate is only slightly reduced. Hormone production from the testes continues with very little change, and secondary sex characteristics are not altered.

Vasectomy is ordinarily performed in a physician's office and takes about 30 minutes. A local anesthetic is injected into the skin of the scrotum. Small incisions are made at the upper end of the scrotum where it joins the body, and the vas deferens on each side is exposed, severed, and tied off or sealed by electrocautery. Some doctors seal each of the vasa with a plastic clamp, which is the size of a grain of rice. The incisions are then closed with sutures, and a small dressing is applied. Pain and swelling are usually slight and can be relieved with ice compresses and a scrotal support. Bleeding and infection occasionally develop but are usually easily treated. After the procedure most men can return to work in two days.

Men can have sex after vasectomy as soon as they feel no discomfort, usually after about a week. Another method of contraception must be used for at least three months after vasectomy, however, because sperm produced before the operation may still be present in the semen.

Vasectomy is highly effective. In a small number of cases, a severed vas rejoins itself. The overall failure rate for vasectomy is 0.15%. About one-half of vasectomy reversals are successful, though this rate can vary significantly depending on the number of years since the initial surgery.

Female Sterilization

The most common method of female sterilization involves severing or blocking the oviducts, thereby preventing eggs from reaching the uterus, and sperm from entering the fallopian tubes. Ovulation and menstruation continue, but the unfertilized eggs are released into the abdominal cavity and absorbed. Hormone production by the ovaries and secondary sex characteristics are generally not affected.

Tubal sterilization (also called *tubal ligation*) is most commonly performed by a method called **laparoscopy.** A laparoscope, a camera containing a small light, is inserted through a small abdominal incision, and the surgeon looks through it to locate the fallopian tubes. Instruments are passed either through the laparoscope or through a second small incision, and the two fallopian tubes are sealed off with ties or staples or by electrocautery. General anesthesia is usually used. The operation takes about 30 minutes, and women can usually leave the hospital two to four hours after surgery. Tubal sterilization can also be performed shortly after a vaginal delivery through a small incision, or in the case of cesarean section during the same surgery.

Although tubal sterilization is riskier than vasectomy, with a rate of minor complications of about 6–11%, it is the more common procedure (see the box "Contraceptive Use among American Women"). Potential problems include bowel injury, wound infection, and bleeding. Serious complications are rare, and the death rate is low.

The failure rate for tubal sterilization is about 0.5%. When pregnancies occur, an increased percentage of them are ectopic (occurring outside the uterus). Ectopic pregnancy is dangerous and can even cause death, so any woman who suspects she might be pregnant after having tubal sterilization should seek medical help. Because successful reversal rates are low and the procedure is costly, female sterilization should be considered permanent.

A new form of incision-free female sterilization has also become available. This procedure can be performed with local anesthetic in a doctor's office and has a short recovery time. Called the Essure system, it consists of tiny springlike metallic implants that are inserted through the vagina and into the fallopian tubes, using a special catheter. Within 3 months, scar tissue forms over the implants, blocking the tubes.

Hysterectomy, removal of the uterus, is the preferred method of sterilization for only a small number of women, usually those with preexisting menstrual or other uterine problems.

---

vasectomy The surgical severing of the ducts that carry sperm to the ejaculatory duct. TERMS

tubal sterilization Severing or blocking the oviducts to prevent eggs from reaching the uterus; also called *tubal ligation.*

laparoscopy Examining the internal organs by inserting a small camera through an abdominal incision.

hysterectomy Total or partial surgical removal of the uterus.

DIVERSITY MATTERS
Contraceptive Use among American Women

Nearly all American women use contraceptives at some time during their lives. According to the National Center for Health Statistics, 99% of all U.S. women who have ever had intercourse have used a contraceptive.

About 62 million women in the United States are in their childbearing years (15–44) and thus face decisions about contraception. About 62% of these women currently use some form of contraception. Most of the remaining 38% are sterile, pregnant, trying to become pregnant, or not sexually active.

Only about 7% of American women are fertile, sexually active, not seeking pregnancy, and not using contraceptives. This small group, however, accounts for almost half of the 3 million unintended pregnancies that occur each year. The unintended pregnancies that occur among contraceptive users are usually the result of incorrect use of methods rather than the method itself failing. For example, one-third of barrier method users report not using their method every time they have intercourse.

Oral contraceptives and female sterilization are the two most popular methods among American women (see the accompanying table). However, choice of contraceptive method and consistency of use vary with age, marital status, and other factors:

- **Age:** Sterilization is much more common among older women, particularly those who are over 35 years of age or who have had children. Young women in their teens and twenties are more likely to use the pill or condoms. Older women, however, are more likely to use reversible methods consistently. They are less likely to miss pills and more likely to use barrier methods during every act of intercourse.

- **Marital status:** Women who are or were married have much higher rates of sterilization than women who have never been married. Those who have never been married have high rates of OC and condom usage.

- **Ethnicity:** Overall rates of contraceptive use as well as use of OCs are highest among white women. Female sterilization, implants, and injectable contraceptives are more often used by African American women and Latinas, and IUD use is highest among Latinas. Condom use is highest among Asian American women and is similar across other ethnic groups. Male sterilization is much more common among white men than among men of other ethnic groups.

- **Socioeconomic status and educational attainment:** Low socioeconomic status and low educational attainment are associated with high rates of female sterilization and low rates of pill and condom use. However, women who are poor or have low educational attainment and who use OCs have higher rates of consistent use than women who are wealthier or have more education. About 20% of women ages 15–44 lack adequate health insurance, increasing the cost and difficulty of obtaining contraceptives.

- **New trends:** About 10% of American women have used emergency contraception at least once, up from 4% in 2002. The percentage of women who have ever used the patch rose from 1% to 10% in the last six years. Rates of IUD use, especially among women who have already had at least one child, have also risen dramatically to nearly 8%.

Some trends in contraceptive use may also reflect the differing priorities and experiences of women and men. For example, female sterilization is more expensive and carries greater health risks than male sterilization—yet it is more than twice as common. (Worldwide, female sterilization is more than four times as common as male sterilization.) This pattern may reflect culturally defined gender roles and the fact that women are more directly affected by unintended pregnancy. In surveys, women rate pregnancy prevention as the single most important factor when choosing a contraceptive method; in contrast, men rate STI prevention as equally important.

METHOD	PERCENTAGE OF USERS
Pill	28.0
Tubal sterilization	27.1
Male condom	16.1
Vasectomy	9.9
IUD	5.5
Withdrawal	5.2
Three-month injectable (Depo-Provera)	3.2
Vaginal ring (Nuva-Ring)	2.4
Implant (Implanon), one month injectable (Lunelle), or patch (Ortho Evra)	1.1
Periodic abstinence (calendar method)	0.9
Other* (includes emergency contraception, sponge, cap, female condom)	0.4

SOURCES: Frost, L. J., et al. 2007. Factors associated with contraceptive use and nonuse, United States, 2004. *Perspectives on Sexual and Reproductive Health* 39(2): 90–99; Guttmacher Institute. 2010. *Facts in Brief: Facts on Contraceptive Use* (http://www.guttmacher.org/pubs/fb_contr_use.html); Mosher, W. D., and J. Jones. 2010. Use of contraception in the U.S.: 1982–2008. National Center for Health Statistics. *Vital Health Statistics* 23(29).

connect
ACTIVITY
DO IT ONLINE

Many people have a difficult time talking about contraception with a potential sex partner. How should you bring it up? And whose responsibility is it? Talking about the subject may be embarrassing at first, but imagine the possible consequences of not talking about it. An unintended pregnancy or a sexually transmitted infection could profoundly affect you for the rest of your life. Talking about contraception is one way of showing that you care about yourself, your partner, and your future.

Before you talk with your partner, explore your own thoughts and feelings. Find out the facts about different methods of contraception, and decide which one you think would be most appropriate for you. If you're nervous about having this discussion with your partner, it may help to practice with a friend.

Pick a good time to bring up the subject. It makes sense to have this discussion before you start having sex, but even if you've already had intercourse with your partner, it's important to be on the same page about contraception. A time when you're both feeling comfortable and relaxed will improve your chances of having a good discussion. Tell your partner what you know about contraception and how you feel about using it, and talk about what steps you both need to take to get and use a method you can live with. Listen to what your partner has to say, and try to understand his or her point of view. You may need to have more than one discussion, and it may take some time for both of you to feel comfortable with the subject.

If you want your partner to be involved but he or she isn't interested in talking about contraception, you may want to enlist the support of a friend, family member, or health care provider to help you make and implement decisions about contraception.

Ask Yourself

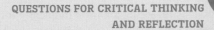

QUESTIONS FOR CRITICAL THINKING AND REFLECTION

Do you feel your sexual education up to this point in your life has been complete? Do you feel it has prepared you to have a healthy, safe, and responsible sexual life?

WHICH CONTRACEPTIVE METHOD IS RIGHT FOR YOU?

Each person must consider many variables in deciding which method is most acceptable and appropriate for her or him. Key considerations include those listed here:

1. *The implications of an unplanned pregnancy and the efficacy of the method.* Many teens and young adults fail to consider how their lives would be affected by an unexpected pregnancy. People who choose to be sexually active but would be negatively impacted by an unplanned pregnancy need to use an effective means of birth control and use it consistently.

2. *Health risks.* When considering any contraceptive method, determine whether it may pose a risk to your health. However, most women are candidates for most, if not all, methods of contraception. Remember that pregnancy carries significant health risks that are generally much greater than the risks of any method of contraception.

3. *STI risk.* STIs are another potential consequence of sex. In fact, several activities besides vaginal intercourse (such as oral and anal sex) can put you at risk for an STI. Condom use is of critical importance whenever any risk of STIs is present, even if you are using another contraceptive method to prevent pregnancy. This is especially true whenever you are not in an exclusive, long-term relationship.

4. *Convenience and comfort level.* The most convenient methods are the LARC methods (IUDs and implants) that do not require any work on the part of the person. Most women using hormonal methods also rank them high in convenience. If forgetting to take pills is a problem for you, a vaginal ring, contraceptive patch, implant, or injectable method may be a good alternative to the pill. For those who choose a barrier method, condoms are the most common. Some people think condom use disrupts spontaneity, but creative approaches to condom use can decrease these concerns. The diaphragm, cervical cap, contraceptive sponge, female condom, and spermicides can be inserted before intercourse begins, unlike condoms, which must be put on the erect penis.

5. *Type of relationship.* Barrier methods require more motivation and sense of responsibility from *each* partner than hormonal methods do. When the method depends on the cooperation of one's partner, assertiveness is necessary, no matter how difficult. This is especially true in new relationships, when condom use is most important.

6. *Ease and cost of obtaining and maintaining each method.* Investigate the costs of different methods. Under the Affordable Care Act, insurers (except for religious organizations) are required to cover the cost of contraception. On June 30, 2014, the Supreme Court ruled that closely held corporations with religious

objections may also opt out of the contraception coverage. Remember that your student health clinic probably provides family planning services, and most communities have low-cost family planning clinics, such as Planned Parenthood.

7. *Religious or philosophical beliefs.* For some people, abstinence and/or fertility awareness–based methods may be the only permissible contraceptive methods.

8. *Potential noncontraceptive benefits.* Women with dysmenorrhea, irregular periods, acne, endometriosis, severe premenstrual syndrome (PMS), and other medical problems may benefit from using a particular method of contraception. Be sure to discuss these issues with your health care provider so that you can take advantage of the noncontraceptive benefits associated with many methods of birth control.

Whatever your needs, circumstances, or beliefs, *do* make a choice about contraception. Not choosing anything is the one method known *not* to work. Contraception is an area in which taking charge of your health has immediate and profound implications for your future.

UNDERSTANDING ABORTION

Few issues are as complex and emotionally charged as abortion. In the United States, public attention has focused on the legal definition of abortion as well as on how and when abortion should be restricted. Although this debate is important, the most difficult aspects of abortion are personal.

The word **abortion,** generally refers to a pregnancy ending. A **spontaneous abortion,** also called a miscarriage, is a pregnancy that ends on its own. Twelve to fifteen percent of pregnant women experience spontaneous abortions, which occur most frequently during the first trimester. **Induced abortion,** or pregnancy termination, is a pregnancy that is deliberately ended. The rest of this chapter focuses on this latter type of abortion.

Personal Considerations for the Woman

For the pregnant woman who is considering abortion, the usual legal and moral arguments may sound meaningless, especially as she attempts to weigh the many short- and long-term ramifications for all those who are directly concerned. If she chooses abortion, can she accept the decision in terms of her own religious and moral beliefs? What are her long-term feelings likely to be regarding this decision? What are her partner's feelings regarding abortion, and how will she deal with his response? Does she know supportive people who will help her through the emotional adjustment? Which medical facility offering abortions would be most suitable for her? What about transportation and costs?

For the woman who decides against abortion and chooses instead to continue the pregnancy, there are other questions: If she decides to raise the child herself, will she have the resources to do it well? Is a supportive, lasting relationship with her partner likely? If not, how does she feel about being a single parent?

If the pregnant woman considers adoption, she will have to try to predict her emotional responses throughout the full-term pregnancy and the adoption process. What are her long-term feelings likely to be? What is the best setting for her during pregnancy? How can she best continue with her life and long-term goals? What type of adoption would be most appropriate?

Personal Considerations for the Man

Discussions regarding abortion frequently focus on a woman's role in the decision and the effects on her mental and physical health. Increasingly debated is the role the man should play in the decision to pursue an abortion. Multiple cases have been brought to the courts by men seeking the right to prevent an abortion. However, at this time, men do not have the legal right to prevent an abortion from occurring. The decision to pursue an abortion or not rests ultimately with the woman. Nevertheless, men are often involved in the decision-making process with their partners, and may experience a range of emotions similar to that felt by women. A small survey of men in the post-abortion period found that they experienced relief, a sense of responsibility, guilt, and grief in the months following an abortion.

Abortion Statistics

An unintended pregnancy is the reason that accounts for more than 95% of abortions. An **unintended pregnancy** includes pregnancies that are *mistimed* (i.e., a woman or couple wanted to become pregnant, but at a later date) or *unwanted* (a woman or a couple had not wanted to become pregnant at any time at all). More than half of women with unintended pregnancies continue their pregnancies and give birth. The remainder of women with unintended pregnancies have either an induced abortion or a miscarriage in relatively equal proportions.

Among American women, about 50% of all pregnancies are unintended; about 40% of such pregnancies end in abortion. About 22% of all pregnancies—wanted and

---

abortion A pregnancy ending.

TERMS

spontaneous abortion Also known as *miscarriage* or *pregnancy loss*; a pregnancy that ends on its own.

induced abortion A pregnancy that is deliberately ended; synonymous with pregnancy termination.

unintended pregnancy Mistimed (wrongly timed) or unwanted (not desired at all) pregnancy.

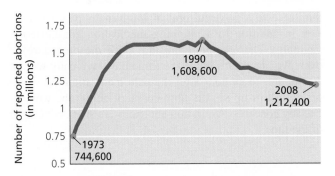

FIGURE 6.6 **Number of reported abortions in the United States, 1973–2008.**

SOURCE: Jones, R. K., et al. 2011. Abortion incidence and access to services in the United States, 2008. *Perspectives on Sexual and Reproductive Health* 43(1): 41–50.

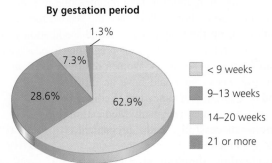

FIGURE 6.7 **Distribution of abortions by the woman's age and by the weeks of gestation: 2008.**

SOURCES: Jones, R. K., L. B. Finer, and S. Singh. 2010. *Characteristics of U.S. Abortion Patients, 2008.* New York: Guttmacher Institute; Centers for Disease Control and Prevention. 2012. Abortion surveillance, United States—2008. *Morbidity and Mortality Weekly Report* 60(SS15): 1–41.

unwanted—end in abortion, not including those that end in miscarriage. From 1973 through 2008, approximately 50 million legal abortions were performed in the United States.

After the U.S. Supreme Court's ruling in *Roe v. Wade,* the number of abortions rapidly increased (Figure 6.6). According to the Guttmacher Institute (a private organization that tracks statistics on reproductive health issues, including contraception and abortion), nearly 750,000 abortions occurred in 1973; the number rose each year after that until 1990, when it peaked at 1.6 million. Since then, the number reported has steadily declined; between 2001 and 2008, the most recent year with complete data, around 1.2 million abortions were performed each year.

The number of late-term abortions has dropped over time, as well. Most women have abortions early in pregnancy: 90% take place within the first trimester (see Figure 6.7).

Lifestyle Indicators Several lifestyle indicators frequently given as reasons for terminating a pregnancy include lack of financial resources; interference with the woman's work, educational aspirations, or ability to care for dependents; reluctance to become a single mother; or problems in a relationship. Planned Parenthood estimates that about one out of three American women will have an abortion by age 45.

Women who choose to have an abortion vary widely; they represent various ages, religions, races, and levels of education. Poverty has been identified as a key factor leading to an abortion. In 2008, 42% of women undergoing an abortion were poor by federal standards.

Fetal and Maternal Indicators Women or couples with an intended pregnancy may ultimately decide to end the pregnancy if they learn that the fetus has a life-threatening genetic abnormality or a severe developmental anomaly. The pregnant woman's illnesses such as severe high blood pressure or kidney disease, can also motivate the decision for abortion. If she knows that her health is at risk,

Ask Yourself

QUESTIONS FOR CRITICAL THINKING AND REFLECTION

Suppose you are in the position of supporting a friend who has gone through an abortion. What sort of physical or emotional signals would you look for? What kind of support would you be willing to offer?

ending the pregnancy before the fetus becomes **viable** (able to survive outside the womb) may prevent a life-threatening problem.

METHODS OF ABORTION

The way a pregnancy is ended depends on how far along a woman is in her pregnancy. Ultrasound (a device that shows an image of the developing fetus) is the most accurate way to determine this. If an ultrasound is not available, the date of the woman's last period provides an estimate.

viable Able to survive outside the uterus. TERMS

First-Trimester Abortion

As noted earlier, 90% of abortions in the United States take place in the first trimester. Women who are about 2 months pregnant (less than or equal to 9 weeks) can choose between medication and aspiration abortion. In 2008, medication abortion accounted for about one-quarter of these abortions.

Medication abortion entails taking two different medications to end an already existing pregnancy. Women who have a medication abortion take mifepristone in a doctor's office and then go home. They take the second medication, misoprostol, on their own. This second medication causes period-like cramps and causes the pregnancy to pass usually within 4 but up to 48 hours. Women return to see their provider 1–2 weeks later and have an ultrasound or a serum pregnancy test to confirm they are no longer pregnant. Medication abortion successfully ends pregnancies 95–97% of the time.

Aspiration abortion also known as "suction abortion" or dilation and curettage (D&C) can be used for women who are more than 9 weeks pregnant and as far along as 14 weeks (slightly into the early second trimester). This procedure is performed in a medical facility (usually in the outpatient setting and rarely in a hospital) by trained providers. The procedure is done through the vagina exclusively. It requires use of an instrument called a **suction curettage** that opens the cervix (opening to the uterus); the straw-shaped tube is attached to a vacuum device that removes the pregnancy. The procedure may cause strong cramps and usually takes fewer than 10 minutes. Women undergoing the procedure receive a powerful oral or intravenous pain medication in addition to a numbing medication administered vaginally. The cramping subsides once the procedure is over. Women return home the same day—typically within 30 minutes to an hour after the pain medication has worn off. A follow-up visit is not necessary unless the woman has any concerns. Aspiration abortions are successful 98% of the time.

Second-Trimester Abortion

About 10% of abortions take place in the second trimester (greater than 4 months or 12 weeks of pregnancy). Women who are this far along in their pregnancy or farther (6 months or 18 weeks) can choose from two different procedures: dilation and evacuation (D&E) or induction abortion.

As the pregnancy advances into its 4th month, the preferred procedure to end the pregnancy is called **dilation and evacuation (D&E).** This, too, is a safe procedure and usually takes about 20 minutes. However, unlike aspiration abortion, a D&E is more involved, frequently requiring two separate visits—one to prepare for the procedure and the second to have the procedure itself. The preparation involves the use of dilators in the cervix to help slowly open it up. This dilation process makes the next day's evacuation procedure safe. Like aspiration abortion, the evacuation part is performed vaginally; the combined use of suction and other instruments is used to remove the pregnancy. Women are either asleep during the procedure or they receive pain medication intravenously. Once the medication from the procedure wears off, women can go home—usually the same day. Most procedures can be performed in an outpatient setting, depending on the type of medication and support staff available.

Another technique used is **induction abortion**, also known as *labor induction* or *induction termination.* To stimulate uterine contractions and opening of the cervix, women are given a combination of mifepristone/misoprostol. A woman goes into labor and delivers the fetus in 6–24 hours. Women are also administered strong pain medications either intravenously or through an epidural.

The types of complications associated with a D&E are similar to aspiration abortion and other surgical procedures. A woman's body changes dramatically as pregnancy progresses, and abortion techniques become more technically difficult. Thus, the chance of having a complication in the second trimester is higher than in the first, but overall lower than having a complication related to birth. The most dangerous but very rare complication resulting from D&E is called **uterine perforation,** where the uterus is injured and may cause injury to internal organs; additional surgery may be needed for repair.

TERMS

medication abortion An abortion procedure typically done during the first trimester of pregnancy and involves the ingestion of two drugs: mifepristone and misoprostol; the most effective regimen to date.

aspiration abortion A vaginal procedure that involves the removal of the pregnancy through suction; also known as *suction abortion* or *dilation and curettage.*

suction curettage A suction instrument used for removal of the embryo or fetus through dilation and curettage.

dilation and evacuation (D&E) The method of abortion most commonly used between 13 and 24 weeks of pregnancy. Following dilation of the cervix, both vacuum aspiration and curettage instruments are used as needed.

induction abortion An infrequently used method of late-term abortion, in which chemicals or medications are used to induce abortion and labor.

uterine perforation A rare complication resulting from D&E in which the uterus is injured and may also cause injury to internal organs.

PHYSICAL AND PSYCHOLOGICAL EFFECTS OF ABORTION

Abortion does not cause infertility, jeopardize a woman's ability to have children in the future, compromise her reproductive organs, or increase her chances of cancer in any way. Furthermore, the recovery is rapid, usually lasting just a few days. Still, many people have concerns about possible aftereffects.

The incidence of immediate physical problems following an abortion (infection, bleeding, trauma to the cervix or uterus, and incomplete abortion requiring repeat curettage) varies widely. The potential for problems is significantly reduced by a woman's good health, early timing of the abortion, use of the suction method, performance by a well-trained clinician, and the availability and use of prompt follow-up care.

Problems related to infection can be minimized through preabortion testing and treatment for gonorrhea, chlamydia, and other infections. Some clinicians routinely give antibiotics after an abortion, whereas others treat only those women who have a history or current symptoms of pelvic infection.

Relief, guilt, regret, loss, or anger are often felt by many women after an abortion. Some go through a period of depression while making the decision to proceed with an abortion or shortly after it is performed. When a woman feels she was pressured into sexual intercourse or into the abortion, she may feel bitter. If she had strongly believed abortion to be immoral, she may wonder if she is still a good person. Many of these feelings are strongest immediately after the abortion.

Between 2008 and 2010, the Turnaway Study recruited women seeking abortions across the United States, some of whom succeeded in undergoing the procedure and others who were "turned away" because their pregnancies were too far along. Researchers found that a person's feelings toward an unintended pregnancy and feelings toward having an abortion are mixed—many women felt regret about an unwanted pregnancy and felt that the decision to have an abortion was the right decision for them.

Rates of mental health problems do not appear higher in those who had an abortion compared to those who gave birth or vice versa, suggesting that women are resilient despite their difficult circumstances. The most profound measurable effect observed in the group of women denied an abortion is that they were three times more likely to end up below the federal poverty line two years later compared to women who had abortions, though before the unintended pregnancy they had similar socioeconomic status. As many women predict when making a decision to have an abortion, having a child strains their resources to a significant degree.

QUICK STATS

More than one in three American women have an abortion before they turn 45.
—Planned Parenthood, 2012

CURRENT LEGAL STATUS

In 1973 in the landmark case of *Roe v. Wade,* the U.S. Supreme Court made abortion legal. To replace the restrictions most states still imposed at that time, the justices devised new standards to govern abortion decisions. They divided pregnancy into three parts, or *trimesters*, giving a woman less choice about abortion as her pregnancy advances toward full term. According to *Roe v. Wade,* in the first trimester, the abortion decision must be left to the judgment of the pregnant woman and her physician. During the second trimester, similar rights remain up to the point when the fetus becomes viable. Today most clinicians define this point as 24 weeks of gestation. When the fetus is considered viable, a state may regulate and even bar all abortions except those considered necessary to preserve the mother's life or health.

Although abortion remains legal throughout the United States, subsequent rulings by the Supreme Court have allowed states to regulate abortion throughout pregnancy as long as no "undue burden" is imposed on women seeking this treatment. As a result, states have passed multiple laws every year that regulate access to abortions. Some states have passed laws that limit access to abortion, whereas other states have passed laws that preserve the right to abortion. Examples of restrictive laws include: (http://www.guttmacher.org/statecenter/spibs/spib_OAL.pdf)

- *Physician and hospital requirements*
- *State-mandated counseling*
- *Waiting periods*
- *Parental Involvement*

Since the passing of the Hyde Amendment in 1976, Congress has barred the use of federal Medicaid funds to pay for abortions, except when a woman's life is in danger or in cases of rape or incest. The Affordable Care Act (2010) explicitly permits states to dictate the circumstances under which abortions may be performed or insured. Currently 17 states provide nonfederal public money to assist some poor women seeking medically necessary abortions. Concerns have been raised that a two-tiered system has been created—one for women with means to pay for an abortion and another for those without.

THE PUBLIC DEBATE ABOUT ABORTION

Abortion is one of the most polarized and politicized issues of our times and has been since the 1960s. Although the most vocal groups in the abortion debate tend to paint a black-and-white picture, most Americans view abortion as a complex issue without any easy answers.

Pro-life groups oppose abortion on the basis of their belief that life begins at conception. They believe that the fertilized egg must be afforded the same rights as a human being. Many pro-life supporters do not consider the availability of legal abortion as essential to women's well-being but view it instead as having an overall destructive effect on our traditional morals and values. *Pro-choice groups* support the view that the decision to end or continue a pregnancy is a personal matter. The pro-choice viewpoint holds that distinctions must be made between the stages of fetal development and that preserving the fetus early in pregnancy (or *gestation*) is not always the ultimate moral concern. Members of this group maintain that women must have the freedom to decide whether and when to have children.

Pro-choice groups believe that the decision to end or continue a pregnancy is a personal matter. Pro-life groups oppose abortion based on a belief that life begins at conception.

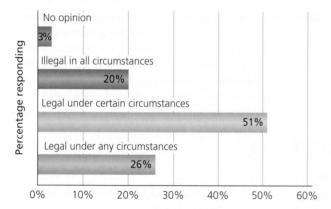

FIGURE 6.8   Public opinion about abortion.

SOURCE: Gallup Inc. 2012. *Public Opinion about Abortion* (http://www.gallup.com /poll/1576/abortion.aspx). Copyright 2012 Gallup Inc. All rights reserved. The content is used with permission; however, Gallup retains all rights of republication.

Opinions about abortion have remained constant over time. Although nearly half of Americans feel that abortion is morally wrong, an overwhelming majority supports legal availability of abortion services in some circumstances. Most Americans oppose governmental regulation of women's reproductive decisions and also feel that paying for an abortion should be an individual's responsibility. Most do not support the use of public funds to help poor women obtain abortions; they also do not support inclusion of abortion benefits in a national basic health care plan. (See Figure 6.8.)

TIPS FOR TODAY AND THE FUTURE

Your decisions about contraception are among the most important you will make in your life. You may never have to face an unintended pregnancy, but you should know what choices you would have, as well as where you stand on the issue of abortion.

RIGHT NOW YOU CAN:

- If you're sexually active, consider whether you are confident that you're doing everything possible to prevent an unwanted pregnancy.
- If you're sexually active, discuss your contraceptive method with your partner. Make sure you are using the method that works best for you.
- Work with your partner to choose a backup contraceptive method to use in case your primary method isn't effective enough. Consider keeping an emergency contraceptive on hand in case of a slip-up.
- Examine your feelings about the possibility of becoming a parent, especially if it were to happen unintentionally.
- Consider your views on the morality of abortion, and whether it is acceptable under certain circumstances.

IN THE FUTURE YOU CAN:

- Talk to your physician about contraception and get his or her advice on choosing the best method.
- Occasionally discuss your contraceptive method with your partner to make sure it continues to meet your needs. A change in health status or lifestyle may make a different form of contraception preferable in the future.
- If you are sexually active or plan to become sexually active, talk to your partner about abortion. Do you share similar views and feelings, or are they different? How would you resolve conflicts about this issue?
- If you are sexually active, reexamine your contraceptive method and make sure you have made the right choice. Remember that, aside from abstinence, no method of contraception is 100% effective.

Connect to Your Choices

Have you ever thought about why you choose the contraceptive methods you use—or choose not to use? Have you ever thought about where you get your ideas and beliefs about abortion? Many factors can influence the choices we make and the views we have, some not as obvious as others. Do you choose what's readily available in pharmacies or use a method your health care provider recommended, even though you don't like it? Do you go along with your partner's preferences because it's easier than saying what you would like? Do you identify with your parents' views on abortion, or with the views of a political party?

What are the external factors that influence your choices about contraception or views on abortion? What are your inner motivations and core values, and how do they affect your choices? Based on what you learned in this chapter, will you make some different choices in the future? If so, what will they be?

Go online to Connect to complete this activity: www.mcgraw-hillconnect.com

SUMMARY

• The choice of contraceptive method depends on effectiveness, convenience, cost, reversibility, side effects and risk factors, protection against STIs, and noncontraceptive benefits. Measures of effectiveness include failure rate and continuation rate.

• Hormonal methods may include a combination of estrogen and progestins, or progestins alone. Hormones may be delivered via pills, patch, vaginal ring, IUD, implants, or injections. Hormonal methods prevent ovulation, inhibit the movement of sperm, and affect the uterine lining so that implantation is prevented.

• IUDs can provide very effective long-term (3–12 years) contraception and are especially useful for women who want contraception for at least 6 months.

• Male condoms are simple to use, are immediately reversible, and provide STI protection; female condoms can be inserted hours before intercourse.

• The diaphragm, cervical cap, and contraceptive sponge cover the cervix and block sperm from entering; all need to be used with or contain spermicide.

• Vaginal spermicides come in the form of foams, creams, jellies, suppositories, and film.

• So-called natural methods include abstinence, withdrawal, and fertility awareness–based methods.

• Combining methods can increase contraceptive effectiveness and help protect against STIs. The most common combination is a hormonal method, such as the birth control pill, combined with condoms.

• The most commonly used emergency contraceptive, Plan B One-Step, is available without a prescription.

• Vasectomy—male sterilization—involves severing the vasa deferentia. Female sterilization involves severing or blocking the oviducts so that the egg cannot reach the uterus.

• Issues to be considered in choosing a contraceptive include the individual health risks of each method, the implications of an unplanned pregnancy, STI risk, convenience and comfort level, type of relationship, the cost and ease of obtaining and maintaining each method, and religious or philosophical beliefs.

• In medical terms there are two distinct types of abortion: *spontaneous abortion* and *induced abortion*. A spontaneous abortion is a pregnancy that ends on its own and is referred to as "miscarriage" or "pregnancy loss." Induced abortion is a pregnancy that is deliberately ended.

• First-trimester abortion methods include medication abortion, which involves administering a combination of drugs very early in pregnancy; drugs used include mifepristone and misoprostol. Aspiration abortion, also known as suction curettage or D & C, involves the use of an electric pump to remove the uterine contents.

• The most common second-trimester abortion methods are dilation and evacuation (D & E) and induction abortion, also known as labor induction or induction termination. In both procedures the uterus is emptied using aspiration and surgical instruments.

• Physical complications following abortion can be minimized by overall good patient health, early timing, use of the suction method, a well-trained physician, and follow-up care. Psychological aftereffects of abortion vary with the individual; the strongest feelings usually occur immediately after the abortion. Having a supportive partner, friend, or family member can be helpful.

• The 1973 *Roe v. Wade* Supreme Court case devised new standards to govern abortion decisions; based on the trimesters of pregnancy, it limited a woman's choices as her pregnancy advanced. Although the Supreme Court continues to uphold its 1973 decision, later rulings gave states further power to regulate abortion.

• The controversy between pro-life and pro-choice viewpoints focuses on the issue of when life begins. Pro-life groups believe that a fertilized egg is a human life from the moment of conception. Pro-choice groups distinguish between stages of fetal development and argue that a woman should make the final decision regarding her pregnancy.

• Overall public opinion in the United States supports legal abortion in at least some circumstances and opposes overturning *Roe v. Wade*. Opinion changes according to individual situations.

BOOKS

Adamec, C. A., and L. C. Miller. 2006. *The Encyclopedia of Adoption* (Facts on File Library of Health and Living), 3rd ed. New York: Facts on File, Inc. *Covers a wide range of adoption-related issues, such as gay/lesbian adoptions, the rights of birth fathers, transracial adoptions, and international adoptions.*

Alters, S. M., ed. 2010. *Abortion: An Eternal Social and Moral Issue* (Information Plus Reference Series). Farmington Hills, MI: Gale Cengage. *A brief reference outlining legal, political, and ethical issues.*

Boston Women's Health Book Collective. 2011. *Our Bodies, Ourselves.* New York: Simon & Schuster. *Broad coverage of many women's health concerns, with extensive coverage of contraception.*

Davenport, D. 2006. *The Complete Book of International Adoption.* New York: Broadway Books. *A detailed look at the process of adopting children from different countries.*

Glasier, A., and B. Winikoff. 2009. *Fast Facts: Contraception,* 3rd ed. Oxford: Health Press. *Basic facts and figures related to contraceptive methods. Succinct and easy to read.*

Hatcher, R. A., et al. 2011. *Contraceptive Technology,* 20th ed. New York: Bridging the Gap Foundation. *A reliable source of up-to-date information on contraception.*

National Abortion and Reproductive Rights Action League Foundation. 2012. *Who Decides? A State-by-State Review of Abortion and Reproductive Rights.* Washington, DC: NARAL Foundation. *An in-depth annual review of the legal status of reproductive rights in the United States.*

Nolan, K. G. 2010. *Abortion: Legislative and Legal Issues.* New York: Nova Science Publishers. *An examination of the legal history of abortion in the United States.*

Zieman, M., et al. 2010. *A Pocket Guide to Managing Contraception,* 2010–2012 ed. Tiger, GA: Ardent Media. *An easy-to-use, reliable source of contraceptive information.*

ORGANIZATIONS, HOTLINES, AND W EBSITES

Association of Reproductive Health Professionals. Offers educational materials about family planning, contraception, and other reproductive health issues; the website includes an interactive questionnaire to help people choose contraceptive methods.

http://www.arhp.org

Bedsider.Org Provides information on all methods of contraception. Describes how to use a method, typical side effects, cost, and how to get the method.

Emergency Contraception Hotline. Provides information and referrals.

888-NOT-2-LATE

Emergency Contraception website. Provides extensive information about emergency contraception; sponsored by the Office of Population Research at Princeton University.

http://ec.princeton.edu

Guttmacher Institute. A nonprofit institute for reproductive health research, policy analysis, and public education.

http://www.guttmacher.org

It's Your Sex Life. Provides information about sexuality, relationships, contraceptives, and STDs; geared toward teenagers and young adults. Provided by the Kaiser Family Foundation and MTV.

http://www.itsyoursexlife.com

Kaiser Family Foundation: Women's Health Policy: Contraception. Provides information and reports focused on how policies impact reproductive health care and access to contraceptives.

http://kff.org/other/womens-health-policy-contraception/

Managing Contraception. Provides brief descriptions and tips for using many forms of contraception. Features a detailed survey to help with contraceptive choices.

http://www.managingcontraception.com

MedlinePlus: Abortion. Managed by the U.S. National Library of Medicine and the National Institutes of Health, this site provides a list of informational resources about various aspects of abortion.

http://www.nlm.nih.gov/medlineplus/abortion.html

National Abortion and Reproductive Rights Action League. Provides information about the politics of the pro-choice movement. Also provides information about the abortion laws and politics in each state.

http://www.prochoiceamerica.org

National Abortion Federation. Provides information and resources on the medical and political issues relating to abortion; managed by health care providers.

http://www.prochoice.org

National Adoption Center. A national agency focused on finding adoptive homes for children with special needs or who are currently in foster care.

http://www.adopt.org

National Right to Life Committee. Provides information about alternatives to abortion and the politics of the pro-life movement.

http://www.nrlc.org

Planned Parenthood Federation of America. Provides information on family planning, contraception, and abortion and offers counseling services.

http://www.plannedparenthood.org

The following are some of the many organizations focusing on family planning and reproductive health issues worldwide:

International Planned Parenthood Federation

http://www.ippf.org

United Nations Population Fund

http://www.unfpa.org

SELECTED BIBLIOGRAPHY

Advancing New Standards in Reproductive Health. Turnaway Study [Internet]. www.ansirh.org. [cited 2014 Jan 3]. Available from: http://www.ansirh.org/research/turnaway.php.

American College of Obstetricians and Gynecologists. 2010. Noncontraceptive uses of hormonal contraceptives. *Obstetrics and Gynecology* 115(1): 206–218.

American College of Obstetricians and Gynecologists. 2011. *Contraceptives* (http://www.acog.org/~/media/For%20Patients/faq021.pdf?dmc1&ts20120301T1336161249).

Biggs M., H. Gould, and D. Foster. 2013. Understanding why women seek abortions in the U.S. *BMC Women's Health* 13(1): 29.

Bitzer, J., and J. A. Simon. 2011. Current issues and available options in hormonal contraception. *Contraception* 84(4): 342–356.

Boonstra, H., et al. 2006. *Abortion in Women's Lives.* New York: Guttmacher Institute.

Burke, A. E. 2011. The state of hormonal contraception today: Benefits and risks of hormonal contraceptives: Progestin-only contraceptives. *American Journal of Obstetrics and Gynecology* 205(4): S14–S17.

Castellsague, X., et al. 2011. Intrauterine device use, cervical infection with human papillomavirus, and risk of cervical cancer: A pooled analysis of 26 epidemiologic studies. *Lancet Oncology* 11(12): 1023–1031.

Centers for Disease Control and Prevention. 2012. Abortion surveillance—United States, 2008. *Morbidity and Mortality Weekly Report* 60(SS15): 1–41.

Charles, V. E., et al. 2008. Abortion and long-term mental health outcomes: A systematic review of the evidence. *Contraception* 78(6): 436–450.

Cohen, S. A.2007. New data on abortion incidence, safety illuminate key aspects of worldwide abortion debate. *Guttmacher Policy Review* 10(4): 2–5.

Cremer, M., and R. Masch. 2010. Emergency contraception: past, present and future. *Minerva Ginecologica* 62(4): 361–371.

Dehlendorf, C., et al. 2011. Race, ethnicity and differences in contraception among low-income women. *Perspectives on Sexual and Reproductive Health* 43(3): 181–187.

Diedrich, J., et al. 2010. Induction of fetal demise before abortion. *Contraception* 81(6): 462–473.

Ely, G. E., and C. N. Dulmus.2010. Disparities in access to reproductive health options for female adolescents. *Social Work in Public Health* 25(3): 341–351.

Fine, Paul, et al. 2010. Ulipristal acetate taken 48–120 hours after intercourse for emergency contraception. *Obstetrics and Gynecology* 115: 257–263.

Finer, L. B., and K. Kost. 2011. Unintended pregnancy rates at the state level. *Perspectives on Sexual and Reproductive Health* 43(2): 78–87.

Finer, L. B., and M. R. Zolna. 2011. Unintended pregnancy in the United States: Incidence and disparities, 2006. *Contraception* 84(5): 478–485.

Fritz, M. A., and L. Speroff, eds. 2010. *Clinical Gynecologic Endocrinology and Infertility,* 8th ed. Philadelphia: Lippincott Williams & Wilkins.

Guttmacher Institute. 2012. *Facts on American Teens' Sexual and Reproductive Health* (http://www.guttmacher.org/pubs/FB-ATSRH.html).

Guttmacher Institute. 2012 Update. *U.S. Teenage Pregnancies, Births and Abortions: National and State Trends and Trends by Race and Ethnicity* (www.guttmacher.org/pubs/USTPtrends.pdf).

Guttmacher Institute. 2012. *Facts on Unintended Pregnancy in the United States* [Internet]. www.guttmacher.org. [cited 2013 Aug 12]. pp. 1–4. Available from: http://www.guttmacher.org/pubs/FB-Unintended-Pregnancy-US.pdf.

Guttmacher Institute. 2012. *State Policies in Brief: An Overview of Abortion Laws* (http://www.guttmacher.org/statecenter/spibs/spib_OAL.pdf).

Guttmacher Institute. 2013. *Facts on Induced Abortion in the United States* (http://www.guttmacher.org/pubs/fb_induced_abortion.html).

Guttmacher Institute. 2014. *State Funding of Abortion under Medicaid* [Internet]. www.guttmacher.org. [cited 2014 Jan 7]. pp. 1–3. Available from: http://www.guttmacher.org/statecenter/spibs/spib_SFAM.pdf.

Hannaford, P. C., et al. 2010. Mortality among contraceptive pill users: Cohort evidence from Royal College of General Practitioners' Oral Contraception Study. *British Medical Journal* DOI: 10.1136/bmj.c927.

Hyde Amendment Codification Act. S. 1488, 112th Cong. (2011).

Jick, S. S., et al. 2010. Postmarketing study of Ortho Evra and levonorgestesterol oral contraceptives containing hormonal contraceptives with 30 mcg of ethinyl estradiol in relation to nonfatal venous thromboembolism. *Contraception* 81(1): 16–21.

Jones, R. K., and L. B. Finer. 2012. Who has second-trimester abortions in the United States? *Contraception* 85(6): 544–51.

Jones, R. K., and M. L. Kavanaugh. 2011. Changes in abortion rates between 2000 and 2008 and lifetime incidence of abortion. *Obstetrics and Gynecology* 117(6): 1358–1366.

Kossler, K., et al. 2011. Perceived racial, socioeconomic and gender discrimination and its impact on contraceptive choice. *Contraception* 84(3): 273–279.

Kulier, R., et al. 2011. Medical methods for first trimester abortion. *Cochrane Database Systematic Review* 11:CD002885.

Leung et al. 2010. Mechanisms of action of hormonal emergency contraceptives. *Pharmacotherapy* 30(2): 158–168.

Lopez, L. M., et al. 2011. Hormonal contraceptives for contraception in overweight or obese women. *Obstetrics and Gynecology* 116(5): 1206–1207.

Lopez, L. M., et al. 2011. Steroidal contraceptives: Effect on bone fractures in women. *Cochrane Database of Systematic Reviews*, 6 July (7): CD006033.

Lynd, K., et al. 2013. Simplified medical abortion using a semi-quantitative pregnancy test for home-based follow-up. *International Journal of Gynecology & Obstetrics* 121(2): 144–148.

Lyus, R., et al. 2011. Use of the Mirena LNG-IUS and ParaGard CuT380A intrauterine devices in nulliparous women. *Contraception* 81(5): 367–371.

Macaluso, M., et al. 2007. Efficacy of the male latex condom and of the female polyurethane condom as barriers to semen during intercourse: A randomized clinical trial. *American Journal of Epidemiology* 166(1): 88–96.

Mansour, D., et al. 2011. Fertility after discontinuation of contraception: A comprehensive review of the literature. *Contraception* 84(5): 465–477.

Meyer, J. L., et al. 2011. Advance provision of emergency contraception among adolescent and young adult women: A systematic review of the literature. *Journal of Pediatric and Adolescent Gynecology* 24(1): 2–9.

Michielsen, D., and R. Beerthuizen. 2010. State-of-the-art of non-hormonal methods of contraception: IV. Male sterilization. *European Journal of Contraception and Reproductive Health Care* 15(2): 136–149.

Mohamad, A. M., et al. 2011. Combined contraceptive ring versus combined oral contraceptive. *International Journal of Gynecology and Obstetrics* 114(2): 145–148.

Moore, A. M., L. Frohwirth, and N. Blades. 2011. What women want from abortion counseling in the United States: A qualitative study of abortion patients in 2008. *Social Work in Health Care* 50(6): 424–442.

Norris, A., et al. 2011. Abortion stigma: A reconceptualization of constituents, causes, and consequences. *Women's Health Issues* 21(3): S49–S54.

Ramasamy, R., and P. N. Schlegel. 2011. Vasectomy and vasectomy reversal: An update. *Indian Journal of Urology* 27(1): 92–97, (http://www.ncbi.nlm.nih.gov/pmc/articles/PMC3114592/).

Raymond, E. G., and D. A. Grimes. 2012. The comparative safety of legal induced abortion and childbirth in the United States. *Obstetrics and Gynecology* 119(2.1): 215–219.

Richardson, A. R., and F. N. Maltz. 2011. Ulipristal acetate: Review of the efficacy and safety of a newly approved agent for emergency contraception. *Clinical Therapeutics*, Dec. 7 (online first: http://dx.doi.org/10.1016/j.clinthera.2011.11.012).

Shellenberg, K. M., and A. O. Tsui. 2012. Correlates of perceived and internalized stigma among abortion patients in the USA: An exploration by race and Hispanic ethnicity. *International Journal of Gynecology & Obstetrics* 118(Suppl 2):S152–9.

Sedgh G, et al. 2012. Induced abortion: Incidence and trends worldwide from 1995 to 2008. Lancet 379(9816):625–32.

Singh, S., et al. 2010. Unintended pregnancy: Worldwide levels, trends, and outcomes. *Studies in Family Planning* 41(4): 241–250.

Stålhandske, M. L., M. Ekstrand, and T. Tydén. 2011. Women's existential experiences within Swedish abortion care. *Journal of Psychosomatic Obstetrics and Gynecology* 32(1): 35–41.

SteelFisher, G. K., and J. M. Benson. 2010. "Attitudes about Abortion." Blendon, R. M., et al., eds. *American Public Opinion and Health Care.* Washington, DC: CQ Press, 264–91.

Stoll, B. J., et al. 2010. Neonatal outcomes of extremely preterm infants from the NICHD Neonatal Research Network. *Pediatrics* 126(3): 443–56.

Taylor D., et al. 2013. Multiple determinants of the abortion care experience: From the patient's perspective. *American Journal of Medical Quality.* April 14.

Upadhyay, U. D., et al. 2013. Denial of abortion because of provider gestational age limits in the United States. American Journal of Public Health [epub first before 15 August print version], e1–e8.

Van Vliet, H. A., et al. 2011. Triphasic versus monophasic oral contraceptives for contraception. *Cochrane Database of Systematic Reviews,* 9 November (11): CD:003553.

Ventura, S. J., et al. 2014. Estimated pregnancy rates and rates of pregnancy outcomes for the United States, 1990–2008. National Vital Statistics Report 60(7): 1–22.

Weitz, T. A. 2010. Rethinking the mantra that abortion should be "safe, legal, and rare." *Journal of Women's History.* 22(3): 161–72.

Winner, B., et al. 2012. Effectiveness of long-acting reversible contraception. *New England Journal of Medicine* 366(21) 1998–2007.

World Health Organization. 2011. Unsafe abortion: Global and regional estimates of the incidence of unsafe abortion and associated mortality in 2008 [Internet]. 6th ed. [cited 2013 Aug 12]. pp. 1–67. Available from: http://whqlibdoc.who.int/publications/2011/9789241501118_eng.pdf.

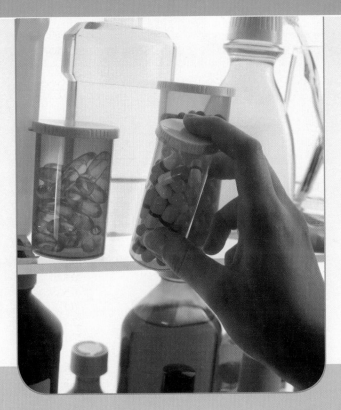

CHAPTER OBJECTIVES

- Define and discuss the concepts of addictive behavior, substance misuse, and substance dependence

- Explain factors contributing to drug misuse and addiction

- List the major categories of psychoactive drugs and describe their effects, methods of use, and potential for addiction and dependence

- Discuss social issues related to drug misuse and its prevention and treatment

- Evaluate the role of drugs and other addictive behaviors in your life and identify your risk factors for addiction or substance use disorder

Drug Misuse and Addiction

The use of **drugs** for both medical and social purposes is widespread in America (Table 7.1). Many Americans believe that every problem has or should have a chemical solution. For fatigue, many turn to caffeine; for insomnia, sleeping pills; for anxiety or boredom, prescription medication or alcohol or other recreational drugs. Advertisements, social pressures, and the human desire for quick solutions to difficult problems all contribute to the prevailing attitude that drugs can ease all pain. But benefits often come with the risk of harmful consequences, and drug use can—and in many cases does—pose serious or even life-threatening risks.

The most serious risks are addiction and impairment of daily activities. The drugs most often associated with addiction and impairment are **psychoactive drugs**—those that alter a person's experiences or consciousness. In the short term, psychoactive drugs can cause **intoxication,** a state in which sometimes unpredictable physical and emotional changes occur. A person who is intoxicated may experience potentially serious changes in physical functioning. His or her emotions and judgment may be affected in ways that lead to uncharacteristic and unsafe behavior. Recurrent drug use can have profound physical, emotional, and social effects.

ADDICTIVE BEHAVIOR

Although addiction is most often associated with drug use, many experts now extend the concept of addiction to other behaviors. **Addictive behaviors** are habits that have gotten out of control, with resulting negative effects on a person's health. The American Society of Addiction Medicine says that **addiction** is a chronic disease that disrupts brain systems

TERMS

drug Any chemical other than food intended to affect the structure or function of the body.

psychoactive drug A drug that can alter a person's consciousness or experience.

intoxication The state of being mentally affected by a chemical (literally, a state of being poisoned).

addictive behavior Compulsive behavior associated with craving and pursuit of physical or psychological reward that interferes with family, school, work, and recreational activities.

addiction A chronic disease that disrupts the brain's system of motivation and reward, characterized by a compulsive desire and increasing need for a substance or behavior, and by harm to the individual and/or society.

Table 7.1	Nonmedical Drug Use among Americans, 2012 (Percent using in past month)		
	YOUNG ADULTS AGED 18–25	YOUTHS AGED 12–17	ALL AMERICANS AGED 12 AND OLDER
ILLICIT DRUGS	21.3	9.5	9.2
Marijuana* and hashish	18.7	7.2	7.3
Cocaine	1.1	0.1	0.6
Heroin	0.2		0.2
Methamphetamine	0.2		0.1
Hallucinogens	1.7	0.9	0.4
Ecstasy	1.0	0.5	0.3
Inhalants	0.4	1.1	0.7
NONMEDICAL USE OF PSYCHOTHERAPEUTICS	5.3	3.0	2.6
Pain relievers	3.8	N/A	1.9
Oxycontin	0.4		0.2
Tranquilizers	1.7	N/A	0.8
Stimulants	1.1		0.5
Sedatives	0.3		0.1
TOBACCO (ALL FORMS)	40.8	10.7	27.4
Cigarettes	31.8	6.6	22.1
Smokeless tobacco	6.4	2.3	3.5
Cigars	11.2		5.2
Pipe tobacco	1.8		0.8
ALCOHOL	60.2	12.9	52.1
Binge alcohol use	40.6	7.8	23.0
Heavy alcohol use	13.6	1.7	6.5

*See section below ("Marijuana and Other Cannabis Products") for information about the legal status of marijuana.

SOURCE: Substance Abuse and Mental Health Services Administration. 2013. *Results from the 2012 National Survey on Drug Use and Health: Summary of National Findings*, NSDUH Series H-46, HHS Publication No. (SMA) 13-4795. Rockville, MD: Substance Abuse and Mental Health Services Administration.

that regulate motivation and reward. The most characteristic feature of addiction is behavioral—a nearly uncontrollable pursuit of physical or psychological reward and/or relief through substance use or behaviors such as gambling. Addiction involves craving and the inability to recognize neither significant risk nor other problems with behaviors, interpersonal relationships, and emotional response. Like other chronic diseases, addiction often involves cycles of relapse and remission. Without treatment, addiction is progressive and can result in disabling or deadly health consequences.

What Is Addiction?

Historically the term *addiction* was applied only when the habitual use of a drug produced chemical changes in the user's body. Now, physiological and psychological effects are both criteria in the American Psychiatric Association's (APA) descriptions of addictive behavior.

tolerance Lower sensitivity to a drug so that a given dose no longer exerts the usual effect and larger doses are needed.

Though experts now agree that addiction is more fully defined by behavioral characteristics, they also agree that changes in the brain underlie addiction. One such change is **tolerance,** in which the body adapts to a drug so that the initial dose no longer produces the original emotional or psychological effects. This process means the user has to take larger and larger doses of a drug to achieve the same high. The concept of addiction as a disease process, one based in identifiable changes to brain cells and brain chemistry rather than a moral failing, has led to many advances in the understanding and treatment of drug addiction.

Some scientists think that other behaviors may share some of the chemistry of drug addiction. They suggest that activities like gambling, eating, exercising, and sex release brain chemicals that cause a pleasurable rush in much the same way that psychoactive drugs do. The brain's own chemicals thus become the "drug" that can cause addiction. These theorists suggest that all addictions—whether to drugs or to pleasurable activities—have a common mechanism in the brain. In this view, addiction is partly the result of our own natural wiring.

The view that addiction is based in our brain chemistry does *not* imply that people are not responsible for their addictive behavior. All addictions involve an initial voluntary step, and other factors such as lifestyle and personality traits play key roles in the development of addiction.

Diagnostic and Statistical Manual of Mental Disorders (DSM-5)

In 2013, the APA released the 5th edition of the *Diagnostic and Statistical Manual of Mental Disorders* (*DSM-5*). The APA defines addiction as compulsive, drug-seeking behavior, which falls on one end of a continuum of a **substance use disorder**. The term substance use disorder combines a distinction in the DSM's previous editions of dependence and abuse. **Dependence** involves normal responses, such as tolerance and withdrawal, to prescribed medications; **abuse** or addiction is a psychological or physical dependence on a substance or behavior. Dependence can occur without a physical component, based solely on compulsive use.

There are 11 DSM-5 criteria for a substance use disorder, including developing tolerance to the substance; experiencing **withdrawal**—when concentrations of the addictive substance in the body drop and causes unpleasant physical and cognitive symptoms as a result; taking the substance in larger than necessary amounts and for longer than necessary; spending a great deal of time getting and using the substance and recovering from its effects; and giving up all forms of social and professional activities and responsibilities.

In terms of severity, meeting

- 2–3 criteria indicate a mild disorder
- 4–5 criteria point to a moderate disorder
- 6 or more criteria are evidence of a severe disorder

The Development of Addiction

An addiction often starts when a person does something to bring pleasure or avoid pain. The activity may be drinking beer, using the Internet, playing the lottery, or shopping. If it works, the person is likely to repeat it. Reinforcement leads to an increasing dependence on the behavior. Tolerance develops, and the person needs more of the substance or behavior to feel the expected effect. Eventually the behavior becomes a central focus of the person's life, and other areas such as school performance or relationships deteriorate. The behavior no longer brings pleasure, but repeating it is necessary to avoid withdrawal.

Although many common behaviors are potentially addictive, most people who engage in them do not develop problems. The reason lies in the combination of factors that are involved in the development of addiction, including personality, lifestyle, heredity, the social and physical environment, and the nature of the substance or behavior in question.

Characteristics of People with Addictions

The causes and course of an addiction are extremely varied, but people with addictions (commonly referred to as *addicts*) seem to share some characteristics. Many use a substance or activity as a substitute for healthier coping strategies. People vary in their ability to manage their lives, and those who have trouble dealing with stress and painful emotions may be susceptible to addiction.

Some people may have a genetic predisposition to addiction to a particular substance based on a variation in brain chemistry. People with addictive disorders usually have a distinct preference for a particular addictive behavior. They also often have problems with impulse control and self-regulation and tend to be risk takers.

Examples of Addictive Behaviors

Behaviors that are not related to drugs can become addictive for some people. Such behaviors can include eating, gambling, and playing video games. Any substance or activity that becomes the focus of a person's life at the expense of other needs and interests can be damaging to health. Like addiction to drugs, behavioral or nondrug addiction involves symptoms such as craving, loss of control over the behavior, tolerance, withdrawal, and a repeating pattern of recovery and relapse. These symptoms suggest that nondrug addictions promote changes in the brain regions and systems associated with misuse and addiction to alcohol, nicotine, or other drugs.

Compulsive Gambling Compulsive gamblers cannot control the urge to gamble, even in the face of ruin. The consequences of compulsive gambling are not just financial; the suicide rate of compulsive gamblers is 20 times higher than that of the general population. About 1% of adult Americans are compulsive (pathological) gamblers, and another 2% are "problem

TERMS

substance misuse or abuse The use of any substance despite adverse social, psychological, or medical consequences; the use may be intermittent and with or without tolerance and physical dependence.

substance use disorder Cluster of symptoms involving cognitive, bodily and social impairment related to the continued use of a substance. A single disorder measured on a continuum from mild to severe.

dependence The result of physiological or psychological adaptation that occurs in response to frequent use of a substance (which includes behaviors such as gambling); typically associated with tolerance and withdrawal.

abuse a psychological or physical dependence on a substance or behavior

withdrawal Physical and psychological symptoms that follow the interrupted use of a drug on which a user is physically dependent; symptoms may be mild or life threatening.

gamblers." This addiction is currently viewed by the APA to be as serious as substance disorder. Some 42% of college students gamble at least once in a year, and about 3% gamble at least once a week. Sixty-five percent of pathological gamblers commit crimes to support their gambling habit.

The APA recognizes pathological gambling as a mental disorder associated with 10 characteristic behaviors, including preoccupation with gambling, unsuccessful efforts to quit, using gambling to escape problems, and lying to family members to conceal the extent of gambling. These characteristics have much in common with the behavioral dysfunctions used to describe addiction. Many compulsive gamblers also have drug and alcohol misuse problems.

Compulsive Exercising Compulsive exercising is now recognized as a serious departure from normal behavior. Compulsive exercising is often accompanied by more severe psychiatric disorders such as anorexia nervosa and bulimia. Traits often associated with compulsive exercising include an excessive preoccupation and dissatisfaction with body image, use of laxatives or vomiting to lose weight, and development of other obsessive-compulsive symptoms.

Work Addiction People who are excessively preoccupied with work are often called *workaholics*. Work addiction, however, is actually based on a set of specific symptoms, including an intense work schedule; the inability to limit your own work schedule; the inability to relax, even when away from work; and failed attempts at curtailing the intensity of work (in some cases).

Work addiction typically coincides with a well-known risk factor for cardiovascular disease—the Type A personality. Traits associated with Type A personality include competitiveness, ambition, drive, time urgency, restlessness, hyper alertness, and hostility.

Sex and Love Addiction Behaviors associated with sex addiction include an extreme preoccupation with sex, a compulsion to have sex repeatedly in a given period of time, spending a great deal of time and energy looking for partners or having sex, using sex as a means of relieving painful feelings, and suffering negative emotional, personal, and professional consequences as a result of sexual activities.

Even therapists who challenge the concept of sex addiction recognize that some people become overly preoccupied with sex, cannot seem to control their sex drive, and act in potentially harmful ways.

Compulsive Buying or Shopping A compulsive buyer repeatedly gives in to the impulse to buy more than he or she needs or can afford. Compulsive spenders usually buy

luxury items rather than daily necessities, even though they are usually distressed by their behavior and its social, personal, and financial consequences. Some experts link compulsive shopping with neglect or abuse during childhood; it also seems to be associated with eating disorders, depression, and bipolar disorder.

Internet Addiction In the nearly 20 years since the Internet became widely available, millions of Americans have become compulsive Internet users—as many as 1 out of 8 people; college students approximate 1 out of 7. To spend more time online, Internet addicts skip other important activities. Despite negative financial, social, or academic consequences, compulsive Internet users don't feel able to stop. As with other addictive behaviors, online addicts may be using their behavior to alleviate stress or avoid painful emotions.

THE EVOLUTION OF DRUG USE

Using drugs to alter consciousness is an ancient and universal pursuit. People have used alcohol for celebration and intoxication for thousands of years. People in all parts of the world have exploited the psychoactive properties of plants, such as the coca plant in South America and the opium poppy in the Far East. But many drugs have addictive properties and change the chemistry of the brain; their use can open the door to the problems of misuse and dependence.

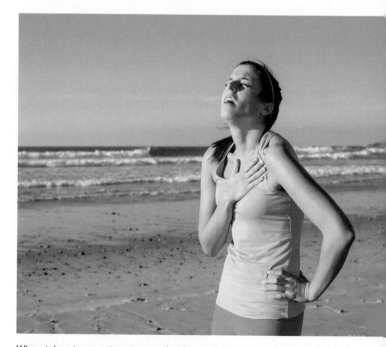

When taken to an extreme, even healthy activities such as exercise can become addictive.

Have you ever repeatedly or compulsively engaged in a behavior that had negative consequences? What was the behavior, and why did you continue? Did you ever worry that you were losing control? Were you able to bring the behavior under control?

Who Misuses Drugs Today?

Drug misuse and addiction occur at all income and education levels, among all ethnic groups, and across all age groups (see the box "Drug Use among College Students"). Society is concerned with the casual or recreational use of illegal drugs because it is not possible to know when it will lead to addiction. Some casual users develop substance-related problems; others do not. Some drugs are more likely than others to lead to addiction (Table 7.2), but even some heroin or cocaine users do not meet the APA's criteria for substance use disorder.

It isn't possible to accurately predict who will misuse drugs or become addicted, but young people at a high risk of *trying* drugs—the first step toward misuse—share certain characteristics. They tend to be the following:

- **Male.** Males are twice as likely as females to misuse drugs.

- **A troubled adolescent.** Teens are more likely to try drugs if they have poor self-image or self-control, use tobacco, or suffer from certain mental or emotional problems.

- **A thrill-seeker.** A sense of invincibility is a factor in drug experimentation.

- **In a dysfunctional family.** A chaotic home life or parental abuse increases the risk of drug use. The same is true for children from a single-parent home or whose parents didn't complete high school.

> **QUICK STATS**
>
> In 2012 an estimated **23.9 million** Americans aged 12 or older were illicit drug users.
>
> —National Survey on
> Drug Use and Health, 2013

- **In a peer group that accepts drug use.** Young people who are uninterested in school and earn poor grades are more likely to try drugs.

- **Poor.** Young people who live in disadvantaged areas are more likely to be around drugs at a young age.

- **A girl dating an older boy.** Adolescent girls who date boys two or more years older than themselves are more likely to use drugs.

What about people who *don't* use drugs? As a group, non-users also share some characteristics. Not surprisingly, people who perceive drug use as risky and who disapprove of it are less likely to use drugs than those who believe otherwise. Drug use is also less common among people who have positive self-esteem and self-concept and who are assertive, independent thinkers who are not controlled by peer pressure. Self-control, social competence, optimism, academic achievement, and regular church attendance are also linked to lower rates of drug use.

Home environments are also influential Young people who communicate openly with and feel supported by their parents are also less likely to use drugs.

Why Do People Use Drugs?

Young people may be drawn to drugs by the allure of the exciting and illegal. They may be curious, rebellious, or vulnerable to peer pressure. Young people may want to imitate adult models in their lives or in the movies. Most people who take illicit drugs do so experimentally, typically trying a drug one or more times but not continuing. The main factors in the initial choice of a drug are whether it is available and whether peers are using it.

Although some people use drugs because they have a desire to alter their mood or are seeking a spiritual experience, others are motivated by a desire to escape boredom, anxiety, depression, feelings of worthlessness, or other distressing symptoms of psychological problems. They use drugs as a way to cope with the difficulties they experience in life. For people living in poverty, many of these reasons for using drugs are magnified. The problems are more devastating, the need for escape more compelling. Further, the buying and selling of drugs provide access to an unofficial alternative economy that may seem like an opportunity for success.

Risk Factors for Misuse and Addiction

Research indicates that some people may be born with a brain chemistry or metabolism that makes them more vulnerable to addiction.

Research also shows that about one-third of people with psychological disorders also have a substance use disorder; about one-third of those have another mental disorder.

Table 7.2	Psychoactive Drugs and Their Potential for Substance Disorder and Addiction
Very high	Amphetamine, cocaine, nicotine, heroin, and other opiates
High	Caffeine, PCP
Moderate	Alcohol, marijuana, benzodiazepines
Low	Psychedelics, steroids
Very low	Antidepressant, antimanic, and antipsychotic medications

SOURCE: Adapted from Miller, William R, et al. 2011. *Treating Addiction: A Guide for Professionals*. New York: Guilford Press.

Drug use in college has long been recognized as a significant health problem that affects many students. By some measures of substance misuse, double-digit prevalence is still the defining characteristic of drug use on college campuses for certain drugs.

According to the most recent survey data from the Substance Abuse and Mental Health Services Administration (SAMHSA), 21.3% of young adults aged 18–25 reported using an illicit drug in the past 30 days (refer to Table 7.1). This number represents a slight increase from 2008 (19.7%), driven largely by an increase in marijuana use from 16.6% in 2008 to 18.7% in 2012. Other surveys show that recreational drug use is fairly common among college students. According to the 2011 American College Health Association–National College Health Assessment, 16.7% of college students reported using marijuana at least once in the past 30 days. Another 12.9% said they had used some other drug at least once in the past 30 days.

Drug use on college campuses has been examined extensively, and many experts believe that no single factor can explain the widespread impact of this phenomenon. Family history, peer pressure, depression, anxiety, low self-esteem, and the dynamics of college life (for example, the drive to compete and a distorted perception of drug use among peers) have been suggested as potential explanations for college-age drug use.

Excessive alcohol use often accompanies illicit drug use and the risk of combining drugs and alcohol increases with the number of drinks a young adult consumes during a single session. In 2012, among the 17.0 million heavy drinkers aged 12 or older, 31.0% were illicit drug users. Persons who were not current alcohol users were less likely to have used illicit drugs in the past month (4.2%) than those who reported (a) current use of alcohol but no binge or heavy use (7.1%), (b) binge use but no heavy use (18.5%), or (c) heavy use of alcohol (31.0%). The term *AOD* (alcohol and other drug) has been coined to refer to this type of substance use among college students. Further, AOD use and depression and/or anxiety are generally recognized as coexisting conditions that require a comprehensive approach to prevention and treatment. Despite the growing awareness among college counselors and other health professionals who work with college students, it is not entirely clear whether anxiety and depression precede the onset of alcohol and drug use or whether early precollege exposure to alcohol and drug use exacerbates more serious psychiatric disorders by the time a student enters college. A third line of research suggests that AOD use, depression, and anxiety share common causes such as genetic predisposition and family history.

However, one aspect of drug use among college students remains clear: AOD use has dramatic consequences for the educational, family, and community lives of students. Poor academic performance has been linked with AOD use. Further, driving while intoxicated remains one of the most dangerous outcomes associated with AOD use affecting families and communities.

connect™
ACTIVITY
DO IT ONLINE

Diagnosing psychological problems among people with substance use disorders can be difficult because drug intoxication and withdrawal can mimic the symptoms of a mental illness.

Social factors can influence drug dependence. These factors include growing up with a family member who uses drugs, belonging to a peer group that emphasizes or encourages drug use, and living in poverty.

Other Risks of Drug Misuse

Addiction is not the only serious potential consequence of drug misuse. In 2011 nearly 2.5 million emergency department visits were related to drug misuse or abuse.

Intoxication   People who are under the influence of drugs—intoxicated—may act in uncharacteristic and unsafe ways because both their physical and mental functioning are impaired. They are more likely to be injured from a variety of causes, to have unsafe sex, and to be involved in incidents of aggression and violence.

Unexpected Side Effects   Psychoactive drugs have many physical and psychological effects beyond the alteration of consciousness. These effects range from nausea and constipation to paranoia, depression, and heart failure. Some drugs also carry the risk of fatal overdose.

Unknown Drug Constituents   There is no quality control in the illegal drug market, so the composition, dosage, and toxicity of street drugs are highly variable. Studies indicate that half of all street drugs don't contain their promised primary ingredient. In some cases, a drug may be present in unsafe dosages or mixed with other drugs to boost its effects. Makers of street drugs aren't held to any safety standards, so illicit drugs can be contaminated or even poisonous.

Risks Associated with Injection Drug Use   Many injection drug users (IDUs) share or reuse needles, syringes, and other injection supplies, which can easily become contaminated with the user's blood. Small amounts of blood can carry enough human immunodeficiency virus (HIV) and hepatitis C virus (HCV) to be infectious. In 2010, 13% of new diagnoses of HIV infection in men were due to injection drug use and another 7% to male-to-male sexual contact and injection drug use. Injection drug use also accounts for nearly half of new HCV infections.

The surest way to prevent diseases related to injection drug use is to never inject drugs. Syringe exchange programs (SEPs)—where IDUs can trade a used syringe for a new one—have been advocated to help slow the spread of HIV and reduce the rates and cost of other health problems associated with injection drug use. Getting people off drugs is clearly the best solution, but there are far more IDUs than treatment facilities can currently handle.

Legal Consequences Many psychoactive drugs are illegal, so possessing them can result in large fines and imprisonment. According to the FBI, the highest arrest counts for all types of crimes were for drug use violations (estimated at 1.5 million out of 12.2 million total arrests in 2012).

HOW DRUGS AFFECT THE BODY

The drugs discussed in this chapter have complex and variable effects, many of which can be traced to changes in brain chemistry. However, the same drug may affect different people differently or the same person in different ways under different circumstances. Beyond a fairly predictable general change in brain chemistry, the effects of a drug may vary depending on drug factors, user factors, and social factors.

Changes in Brain Chemistry

Once a psychoactive drug reaches the brain, it acts on one or more **neurotransmitters,** either increasing or decreasing their concentration

and actions. Cocaine, for example, affects dopamine, a neurotransmitter thought to play a key role in the process of reinforcement—the brain's way of telling itself "That's good; do the same thing again." When a neurotransmitter is released by one neuron, it travels across a gap, called a *synapse,* to signal another neuron.

The duration of a drug's effect depends on many factors and may range from 5 minutes (crack cocaine) to 12 or more hours (LSD). As drugs circulate through the body, they are metabolized by the liver and eventually excreted by the kidneys in urine. Small amounts may also be eliminated in other ways, including in sweat, in breast milk, and via the lungs.

Factors That Influence a Drug's Effect

When different drugs or dosages produce different effects, the differences are usually caused by one or more of five different drug factors:

1. The **pharmacological properties** of a drug are its effects on a person's body chemistry, behavior, and psychology. Pharmacological properties also include the amount of a drug required to exert various effects, the time course of the effects, and other characteristics such as a drug's chemical composition.

2. The **dose-response function** is the relationship between the amount of drug taken and the type and intensity of its effects. Many psychological effects of drugs reach a plateau in the dose-response function, so that increasing the dose does not increase the effect any further. With LSD, for example, the maximum changes in perception occur at a certain dose, and no further changes in perception take place if higher doses are taken. However, all drugs have more than one effect, and the dose-response functions usually are different for different effects. This means that increasing the dose of any drug may begin to result in additional effects, which are likely to be more unpleasant or dangerous at high doses.

> Psychoactive drugs work by **affecting one or more neurotransmitters in the brain.**

neurotransmitter A brain chemical that transmits nerve impulses.   TERMS

pharmacological properties The overall effects of a drug on a person's behavior, psychology, and chemistry.

dose-response function The relationship between the amount of a drug taken and the intensity and type of the resulting effect.

3. The **time-action function** is the relationship between the time elapsed since a drug was taken and the intensity of its effect. A drug's effects are greatest when its concentrations in body tissues are changing fastest, especially if they are increasing.

4. The person's *drug use history* may influence the effects of a drug. A given amount of alcohol, for example, will affect a habitual drinker less than an occasional drinker. Tolerance to some drugs builds rapidly. To experience the same effect, a user has to abstain from the drug for a period of time before that dosage will again exert its original effects.

5. The *method of drug use* directly affects the strength of the response. Methods of use include ingestion, inhalation, injection, and absorption through the skin or tissue linings. Drugs are usually injected in one of three ways: intravenously (IV, or mainlining), intramuscularly (IM), or subcutaneously (SC, or skin popping).

Physical Factors

Certain physical and psychological characteristics help determine how a person will respond to a drug. Body mass is one variable: The effects of a certain dose of a drug on a 150-pound person will be greater than its effect on a 200-pound person. Other variables include general health and genetic factors. For example, some people have an inherited ability to rapidly metabolize a cough suppressant called dextromethorphan, which also has psychoactive properties. These people must take a higher-than-normal dose to get a given cough suppressant effect.

If a person's biochemical state is already altered by another drug, this too can make a difference. Some drugs intensify the effects of other drugs, as is the case with alcohol and sedatives. Some drugs block the effects of other drugs, such as when a tranquilizer is used to relieve anxiety caused by cocaine. Interactions between drugs, including many prescription and over-the-counter (OTC) medications, can be unpredictable and dangerous.

One physical condition that requires special precautions is pregnancy. It can be risky for a woman to use any drugs at all during pregnancy, including alcohol and common OTC products like cough medicine. The risks are greatest during the first trimester, when the fetus's body is rapidly forming and even small biochemical alterations in the mother can have a devastating effect on fetal development.

Even later, the fetus is more susceptible than the mother to the adverse effects of any drugs she takes. The fetus may even become physically dependent on a drug being taken by the mother and suffer withdrawal symptoms after birth.

Psychological Factors

Sometimes a person's response to a drug is strongly influenced by the user's expectations about how he or she will react (the psychological *set*). With large doses, the drug's chemical properties seem to have the strongest effect on the user's response. But with small doses, psychological (and social) factors are often more important. When people strongly believe that a given drug will affect them a certain way, they are likely to experience those effects regardless of the drug's pharmacological properties. In one study, regular users of marijuana reported a moderate level of intoxication (**high**) after using a cigarette that smelled and tasted like marijuana but contained no THC, the active ingredient in marijuana. This is an example of the **placebo effect**—when a person receives an inert substance yet responds as if it were an active drug. In other studies, subjects who smoked low doses of real marijuana that they believed to be a placebo experienced no effects from the drug. Clearly the user's expectations had a greater effect on the smokers than the drug itself.

Social Factors

The *setting* is the physical and social environment surrounding the drug use. If a person uses marijuana at home with trusted friends and pleasant music, the effects are likely to be different from the effects if the same dose is taken in an austere experimental laboratory with an impassive research technician. Similarly, a dose of alcohol that produces mild euphoria and stimulation at a noisy, active cocktail party might induce sleepiness and slight depression when taken at home while alone.

REPRESENTATIVE PSYCHOACTIVE DRUGS

The following sections and Figure 7.1 introduce six representative groups of psychoactive drugs: opioids, central nervous system (CNS) depressants, central nervous system stimulants,

---

time-action function The relationship between the time elapsed since a drug was taken and the intensity of its effect.

TERMS

high The subjectively pleasing effects of a drug, usually felt quite soon after the drug is taken.

placebo effect A response to an inert or innocuous substance given in place of an active drug.

Ask Yourself

QUESTIONS FOR CRITICAL THINKING AND REFLECTION

Has an over-the-counter medication (such as a decongestant) ever made you feel strange, drowsy, or even high? Did you expect to react to the medication that way? Do such reactions influence the way you use over-the-counter drugs?

marijuana and other cannabis products, hallucinogens, and inhalants. Some of these drugs are classified according to how they affect the body. Others—the opioids and the cannabis products—are classified according to their chemical makeup.

Opioids

Also called *narcotics,* **opioids** are natural or synthetic (laboratory-made) drugs that relieve pain, cause drowsiness, and induce **euphoria.** Natural opioid-like hormones released by the brain called endorphins can inhibit pain and induce euphoria. Opium, morphine, heroin, methadone, codeine, hydrocodone, oxycodone, meperidine, and fentanyl are opioids. When taken at prescribed doses, opioids have beneficial medical uses, including pain relief and cough suppression. Opioids tend to reduce anxiety and produce lethargy, apathy, and an inability to concentrate.

Although the euphoria associated with opioids is an important factor in their misuse, many people experience a feeling of uneasiness when they first use these drugs. Even so, the misuse of opioids often results in addiction. Tolerance can develop rapidly and be pronounced. Withdrawal symptoms include cramps, chills, sweating, nausea, tremors, irritability, and feelings of panic.

According to the Substance Abuse and Mental Health Services Administration (SAMHSA), heroin use has been rising since 2007, increasing from 373,000 yearly users to 669,000 in 2012. Heroin overdose deaths have also spiked, increasing 45% from 2006 to 2010. The potentially high but variable purity of street heroin poses a risk of unintentional overdose. Symptoms of overdose include respiratory depression, coma, and constriction of the pupils; death can result.

When taken as prescribed in tablet form, these drugs treat moderate to severe chronic pain and do not typically lead to misuse. However, as is the case with other opioids, use of prescription painkillers can lead to misuse and addiction. When taken in large doses or combined with other drugs, oxycodone and hydrocodone can cause fatal respiratory depression.

Central Nervous System Depressants

Central nervous system **depressants,** also known as **sedative-hypnotics,** depress the **central nervous system (CNS).** The result can range from mild **sedation** to death. See Figure 7.1.

Types The various types of barbiturates are similar in chemical composition and action, but they differ in how quickly and how long they act.

Antianxiety agents, also called sedatives or **tranquilizers,** include the benzodiazepines such as Xanax, Valium, Librium, clonazepam (Klonopin), and flunitrazepam (Rohypnol, also called roofies). Other CNS depressants include methaqualone (Quaalude), ethchlorvynol (Placidyl), chloral hydrate, and gamma hydroxybutyrate (GHB).

Effects CNS depressants reduce anxiety and cause mood changes, impaired muscular coordination, slurring of speech, and drowsiness or sleep. Mental functioning is also affected, but the degree varies from person to person and also depends on the kind of task the person is trying to do. Most people become drowsy with small doses, although a few become more active.

From Use to Misuse People are usually introduced to CNS depressants either through a medical prescription or through drug-using peers. The use of Rohypnol and GHB

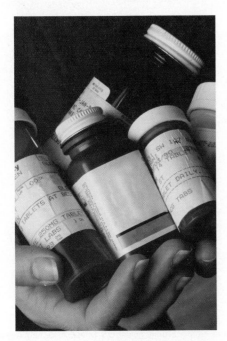

Prescription painkillers such as oxycodone and hydrocodone are opioids that can have serious consequences such as fatal respiratory depression. The recreational use of these drugs is reported to be about 2% of the population aged 12 and over.

opioid Any of several natural or synthetic drugs that relieve pain and cause drowsiness and/or euphoria; examples are opium, morphine, and heroin; also called a *narcotic.* TERMS

euphoria An exaggerated feeling of well-being.

depressant, sedative-hypnotic A drug that decreases nervous or muscular activity, causing drowsiness or sleep.

central nervous system (CNS) The brain and spinal cord.

sedation The induction of a calm, relaxed, often sleepy state.

tranquilizer A central nervous system (CNS) depressant that reduces tension and anxiety.

Category	Representative drugs	Street names	Appearance	Methods of use	Short-term effects
Opioids	Heroin	Dope, H, junk, brown sugar, smack	White/dark brown powder; dark tar or coal-like substance	Injected, smoked, snorted	Relief of anxiety and pain; euphoria; lethargy, apathy, drowsiness, confusion, inability to concentrate; nausea, constipation, respiratory depression
	Opium	Big O, black stuff, hop	Dark brown or black chunks	Swallowed, smoked	
	Morphine	M, Miss Emma, monkey, white stuff	White crystals, liquid solution	Injected, swallowed, smoked	
	Oxycodone, codeine, hydrocodone	Oxy, O.C., killer, Captain Cody, schoolboy, vike	Tablets, powder made from crushing tablets	Swallowed, injected, snorted	
Central nervous system depressants	Barbiturates	Barbs, reds, red birds, yellows, yellow jackets	Colored capsules	Swallowed, injected	Reduced anxiety, mood changes, lowered inhibitions, impaired muscle coordination, reduced pulse rate, drowsiness, loss of consciousness, respiratory depression
	Benzodiazepines (e.g., Valium, Xanax, Rohypnol)	Candy, downers, tranks, roofies, forget-me pill	Tablets	Swallowed, injected	
	Methaqualone	Ludes, quad, quay	Tablets	Injected, swallowed	
	Gamma hydroxy butyrate (GHB)	G, Georgia home boy, grievous bodily harm	Clear liquid, white powder	Swallowed	
Central nervous system stimulants	Amphetamine, methamphet-amine	Bennies, speed, black beauties, uppers, chalk, crank, crystal, ice, meth	Tablets, capsules, white powder, clear crystals	Injected, swallowed, smoked, snorted	Increased and irregular heart rate, blood pressure, metabolism; increased mental alertness and energy; nervousness, insomnia, impulsive behavior; reduced appetite
	Cocaine, crack cocaine	Blow, C, candy, coke, flake, rock, toot, snow	White powder, beige pellets or rocks	Injected, smoked, snorted	
	Ritalin	JIF, MPH, R-ball, Skippy	Tablets	Injected, swallowed, snorted	
Marijuana and other cannabis products	Marijuana	Dope, grass, joints, Mary Jane, reefer, skunk, weed, pot	Dried leaves and stems	Smoked, swallowed	Euphoria, slowed thinking and reaction time, confusion, anxiety, impaired balance and coordination, increased heart rate
	Hashish	Hash, hemp, boom, gangster	Dark, resin-like compound formed into rocks or blocks	Smoked, swallowed	
Hallucinogens	LSD	Acid, boomers, blotter, yellow sunshines	Blotter paper, liquid, gelatin tabs, pills	Swallowed, absorbed through mouth tissues	Altered states of perception and feeling; nausea; increased heart rate, blood pressure; delirium; impaired motor function; numbness, weakness
	Mescaline (peyote)	Buttons, cactus, mesc	Brown buttons, liquid	Swallowed, smoked	
	Psilocybin	Shrooms, magic mushrooms	Dried mushrooms	Swallowed	
	Ketamine	K, special K, cat valium, vitamin K	Clear liquid, white or beige powder	Injected, snorted, smoked	
	PCP	Angel dust, hog, love boat, peace pill	White to brown powder, tablets	Injected, swallowed, smoked, snorted	
	MDMA (ecstasy)	X, peace, clarity, Adam, Molly	Tablets	Swallowed	
Inhalants	Solvents, aerosols, nitrites, anesthetics	Laughing gas, poppers, snappers, whippets	Household products, sprays, glues, paint thinner, petroleum products	Inhaled through nose or mouth	Stimulation, loss of inhibition, slurred speech, loss of motor coordination, loss of consciousness

FIGURE 7.1 Commonly misused drugs and their effects.

SOURCES: The Partnership for a Drug-Free America. 2014. *Drug Guide by Name* (http://www.drugfree.org/portal/drug_guide); U.S. Drug Enforcement Agency. 2011. *Drug Information* (http://www.justice.gov/dea/concern/concern.htm); National Institute on Drug Abuse. 2011. *Commonly Abused Drugs* (http://www.drugabuse.gov/DrugPages/DrugsofAbuse.html).

(discussed in greater detail later in this chapter) is often associated with dance clubs and raves. The misuse of CNS depressants by a medical patient may begin with repeated use for insomnia and progress to dependence through increasingly larger doses at night, coupled with doses during stressful times during the day.

Most CNS depressants, including alcohol, can lead to addiction. Tolerance, sometimes for up to 15 times the usual dose, can develop with repeated use. Tranquilizers can produce physical dependence even at ordinary prescribed doses. Withdrawal symptoms can be more severe than those accompanying opioid addiction and are similar to the DTs of alcoholism. They may begin as anxiety, shaking, and weakness but may turn into convulsions and possibly cardiovascular collapse and death.

While intoxicated, people on depressants cannot function well. They are confused and are frequently obstinate, irritable, and abusive. Long-term use of depressants like alcohol can lead to serious physical effects including brain damage, with impaired ability to reason and make judgments.

Overdosing with CNS Depressants   Too much depression of the central nervous system slows respiration and may stop it entirely. CNS depressants are particularly dangerous in combination with another depressant, such as alcohol.

Club Drugs   Some people refer to club drugs as soft drugs because they see them as recreational—for the casual, weekend user—rather than as addictive. But club drugs have many potential negative effects and are particularly potent and unpredictable when mixed with alcohol. Substitute drugs are often sold in place of club drugs, putting users at risk for taking dangerous combinations of unknown drugs.

Rohypnol (flunitrazepam) is a sedative that is 10 times more potent than Valium. Its effects, which are magnified by alcohol, include reduced blood pressure, dizziness, confusion, gastrointestinal disturbances, and loss of consciousness. Users of Rohypnol may develop physical and psychological dependence on the drug. Rohypnol has never been approved for medical use by the U.S. Food and Drug Administration (FDA); along with some other club drugs, it is used as a "date rape drug." Because they can be added to beverages surreptitiously, these drugs may be unknowingly consumed by intended rape victims. In addition to depressant effects, some drugs also cause *anterograde amnesia*—the loss of memory of things occurring while under the influence of the drug. Rohypnol can be fatal if combined with alcohol.

GHB (gamma hydroxybutyrate) can be produced in clear liquid, white powder, tablet, and capsule form. GHB is a CNS depressant that in large doses or when taken in combination with alcohol or other depressants can cause sedation, loss of consciousness, respiratory arrest, and death. GHB may cause prolonged and potentially life-threatening withdrawal symptoms. GHB is often produced clandestinely, resulting in widely varying degrees of purity; it has been responsible for many poisonings and deaths.

Central Nervous System Stimulants

Central nervous system **stimulants** speed up the activity of the nervous or muscular system. Under their influence, the heart rate accelerates, blood pressure rises, blood vessels constrict, the pupils and bronchial tubes dilate, and gastric and adrenal secretions increase. There is greater muscular tension and sometimes an increase in motor activity. Small doses usually make people feel more awake and alert, and less fatigued and bored. The most common CNS stimulants are cocaine, amphetamines, nicotine, ephedrine, and caffeine.

Cocaine   Usually derived from the leaves of coca shrubs that grow high in the Andes in South America, cocaine is a potent CNS stimulant. It is usually snorted and absorbed through the nasal mucosa or injected intravenously, providing rapid increases of the drug's concentration in the blood and therefore fast, intense effects. Another method of use involves processing cocaine with baking soda and water, yielding the ready-to-smoke form of cocaine known as crack. Crack is typically available as small beads or pellets smokable in glass pipes.

EFFECTS   The effects of cocaine are usually intense but short-lived. The euphoria lasts from 5 to 20 minutes and ends abruptly, to be replaced by irritability, anxiety, or slight depression. When cocaine is absorbed via the lungs by either smoking or inhalation, it reaches the brain in about 10 seconds, and the effects are particularly intense. This is part of the appeal of smoking crack. The effects from IV injections occur almost as quickly—in about 20 seconds. Since the mucous membranes in the nose briefly slow absorption, the onset of effects from snorting takes 2–3 minutes. Heavy users may inject cocaine intravenously every 10–20 minutes to maintain the effects.

The larger the cocaine dose and the more rapidly it is absorbed into the bloodstream, the greater the immediate— and sometimes lethal—effects. Sudden death from cocaine is most commonly the result of excessive CNS stimulation that causes convulsions and respiratory collapse, irregular heartbeat, extremely high blood pressure, blood clots, and possibly heart attack or stroke. Although rare, fatalities can occur in healthy young people; among people aged 18–59, cocaine users are seven times more likely than nonusers to have a heart attack. Chronic cocaine use produces inflammation of the nasal mucosa, which can lead to persistent bleeding and ulceration of the septum between

---

Rohypnol   (flunitrazepam) A sedative that is 10 times more potent than Valium; used as a "date-rape" drug.   TERMS

GHB   (gamma hydroxybutyrate) A central nervous system depressant that can be produced in clear liquid, white powder, tablet, and capsule form.

stimulant   A drug that increases nervous or muscular activity.

the nostrils. The use of cocaine may also cause paranoia and aggressiveness. When steady cocaine users stop taking the drug, they experience a sudden "crash" characterized by depression, agitation, and fatigue, followed by a period of withdrawal.

COCAINE USE DURING PREGNANCY Cocaine rapidly passes from the mother's bloodstream into the placenta and can have serious effects on the fetus. A woman who uses cocaine during pregnancy is at higher risk for miscarriage, premature labor, and stillbirth. She is more likely to deliver a low-birth-weight baby who has a small head circumference. Her infant may be at increased risk for defects of the genitourinary tract, cardiovascular system, central nervous system, and extremities. It is difficult to pinpoint the effects of cocaine because many women who use cocaine also use tobacco and alcohol.

Infants whose mothers use cocaine may also be born intoxicated. Cocaine also passes into breast milk and can intoxicate a breastfeeding infant.

Amphetamines
Amphetamines (uppers) are a group of synthetic chemicals that are potent CNS stimulants. Some common drugs in this family are amphetamine (Benzedrine), dextroamphetamine (Dexedrine), and methamphetamine (Methedrine). Crystal methamphetamine (also called ice) is a smokable, high-potency form of methamphetamine, or meth.

EFFECTS Small doses of amphetamines usually make people feel more alert. Amphetamines generally increase motor activity but do not measurably alter a normal, rested person's ability to perform tasks calling for challenging motor skills or complex thinking. When amphetamines improve performance, it is primarily by counteracting fatigue and boredom. In small doses, amphetamines increase heart rate and blood pressure and change sleep patterns.

Amphetamines are sometimes used to curb appetite, but after a few weeks the user develops tolerance and higher doses are necessary. When people stop taking the drug, their appetite usually returns, and they gain back the weight they lost.

MISUSE AND ADDICTION Much amphetamine misuse begins as an attempt to cope with a temporary situation. A student cramming for an exam or an exhausted long-haul truck driver can go a little longer by taking amphetamines, but the results can be disastrous. The likelihood of making bad judgments significantly increases. The stimulating effects may also wear off suddenly, and the user may precipitously feel exhausted or fall asleep ("crash").

> **state dependence** A situation in which information learned in a drug-induced state is difficult to recall when the effect of the drug wears off.
>
> **psychosis** A severe mental disorder characterized by a distortion of reality; symptoms might include delusions or hallucinations.
>
> TERMS

Another problem is **state dependence,** the phenomenon whereby information learned in a certain drug-induced state is difficult to recall when the drug wears off. Performance may deteriorate when students use drugs to study and then take tests in their normal, nondrug state. Repeated use of amphetamines, even in moderate doses, often leads to tolerance and the need for increasingly larger doses. The result can be severe disturbances in behavior, including a temporary state of paranoid **psychosis,** with delusions of persecution and episodes of unprovoked violence.

Methamphetamine is more addictive than other forms of amphetamine. It also is more dangerous because it is more toxic and its effects last longer. In the short term, meth can cause rapid breathing, increased body temperature, insomnia, tremors, anxiety, and convulsions. Meth use has been linked to high-risk sexual behavior and increased rates of STIs, including HIV infection. In the long term, the effects of meth can include weight loss, severe acne, hallucinations, paranoia, violence, and psychosis. Meth use causes extensive tooth decay and tooth loss, a condition referred to as "meth mouth." Meth takes a toll on the user's heart and can cause heart attack and stroke. Methamphetamine users have signs of brain damage similar to those seen in Parkinson's disease patients that appear to persist even after drug use ceases, causing impaired memory and motor coordination. Withdrawal from meth causes symptoms that may include muscle aches and tremors, profound fatigue, deep depression, despair, and apathy. Addiction to methamphetamine is associated with pronounced psychological cravings and obsessive drug-seeking behavior.

Women who use amphetamines during pregnancy risk premature birth, stillbirth, low birth weight, and early infant death. Babies born to amphetamine-using mothers have a higher incidence of cleft palate, cleft lip, and deformed limbs. They may also experience symptoms of withdrawal.

Ritalin
A stimulant with amphetamine-like effects, Ritalin (methylphenidate) is used to treat attention-deficit/hyperactivity disorder (ADHD). When taken orally at

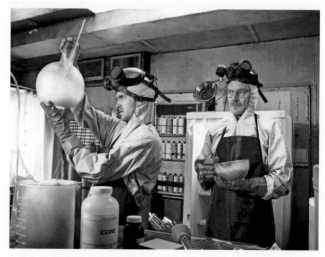

Crystal meth is often manufactured in small, in-home "laboratories," like the one featured in the RV of the popular TV series "Breaking Bad."

Table 7.3	Caffeine Content of Popular Beverages		
COFFEE	SERVING SIZE (OZ.)	TYPICAL CAFFEINE LEVEL (MG)*	
Regular coffee, brewed	8	95	
Regular coffee, instant	8	93	
Espresso	1	64	
Decaffeinated coffee, brewed	8	5	
Decaffeinated coffee, instant	8	2	
TEA			
Regular tea, brewed	8	47	
Decaffeinated tea, brewed	8	2	
Green tea, brewed	8	Varies	
SODA			
Code Red Mountain Dew	12	54	
Mello Yello	12	53	
Diet Coke	12	47	
Dr. Pepper, Diet Dr. Pepper	12	41	
Sunkist Orange Soda	12	41	
Pepsi	12	38	
Coca-Cola Classic, Diet Pepsi	12	35	
ENERGY DRINKS			
No Name	8.4	280	
SoBe No Fear	16	174	
Monster Energy, Rockstar	16	160	
SoBe Adrenaline Rush	16	152	
Full Throttle, Full Throttle Fury	16	144	
AMP Energy Drink	16	143	
Red Bull	8.3	76	
Vault	8	47	

*Caffeine levels vary greatly by brand of product, manner of preparation, and amount consumed. The amounts shown here are averages based on tests conducted by a variety of organizations. The U.S. Food and Drug Administration limits the amount of caffeine in cola and pepper soft drinks to 71 milligrams per 12-ounce serving. To find the exact amount of caffeine in any product, check that product's label.

SOURCES: Center for Science in the Public Interest. 2007. *Caffeine Content of Food & Drugs* (http://www.cspinet.org/new/cafchart.htm); Mayo Clinic. 2008. *Caffeine Content in Tea, Soda, and More* (http://www.mayoclinic.com /health/caffeine/AN01211); U.S. Department of Agriculture, Agricultural Research Service. 2009. *USDA National Nutrient Database for Standard Reference, Release 22* (http://www.ars .usda.gov/ba/bhnrc/ndl).

prescribed levels, it has little potential for misuse. When injected or snorted, however, dependence and tolerance can rapidly result.

Caffeine Caffeine is probably the most popular psychoactive drug and also one of the most ancient. It is found in coffee, tea, cocoa, soft drinks, headache remedies, and OTC preparations like NoDoz. (Table 7.3 lists typical levels of caffeine in several popular beverages.) In ordinary doses, caffeine produces greater alertness and a sense of well-being. It also decreases feelings of fatigue or boredom, so using caffeine may enable a person to keep at physically tiring or repetitive tasks longer. Such use is usually followed, however, by a sudden letdown. Caffeine does not noticeably influence a person's ability to perform complex mental tasks unless fatigue, boredom, or other factors have already affected normal performance.

Caffeine mildly stimulates the heart and respiratory system, increases muscular tremor, and enhances gastric secretion. Higher doses may cause nervousness, anxiety, irritability, headache, disturbed sleep, and gastric irritation or peptic ulcers. In people with high blood pressure, caffeine can cause blood pressure to rise even further above normal; in people with type 2 diabetes, caffeine may cause glucose and insulin levels to rise after meals.

Drinks containing caffeine are rarely harmful for most people, but some tolerance develops, and withdrawal symptoms of irritability, headaches, and even mild depression occur. People can usually avoid problems by simply decreasing their daily intake of caffeine.

ENERGY "SHOTS" The popularity of small (1.5- to 3- ounce) energy drinks has increased dramatically in recent years. Worldwide sales of products such as 5-Hour Energy reached $9 billion in 2011. Because these products are sold as dietary supplements rather than food, their caffeine content is not regulated by the Food and Drug Administration. Each 2- ounce "shot" typically contains the same amount (roughly 100 mg) of caffeine as a regular-size cup of coffee.

Marijuana and Other Cannabis Products

With 17.4 million current users, marijuana is the most widely used illegal drug in the United States. This status may be changing as more states (21 at the time of writing) legalize medical marijuana as well as regulated nonmedical usage (so far 2 states—Colorado and Washington). THC (tetrahydrocannabinol) is the main active ingredient in marijuana. Marijuana plants that grow wild often have less than 1% THC in their leaves. When selected strains are cultivated by separation of male and female plants (*sinsemilla*), the bud leaves from the flowering tops may contain 7–8% THC. Hashish, a potent preparation made from the thick resin that exudes from the marijuana leaves, may contain up to 14% THC.

These various preparations have all been known and used for centuries, so the frequently heard claim that today's marijuana is more potent than the marijuana of the 1970s is not strictly true. However, because a greater proportion of the marijuana sold today is the higher-potency (and more expensive) sinsemilla, the average potency of street marijuana has increased.

Short-Term Effects and Uses At low doses, marijuana users typically experience euphoria, a heightening of subjective sensory experiences, a slowing down of the perception of passing time, and a relaxed attitude. With moderate doses, marijuana's effects become stronger, and the user can also expect to have impaired memory function, disturbed thought patterns, lapses of attention, and feelings of **depersonalization,** in which the mind seems to be separated from the body.

Very high doses produce feelings of depersonalization, marked sensory distortion, and changes in body image (such as a feeling that the body is very light). Inexperienced users sometimes think these sensations mean they are going crazy and become anxious or even panicky.

Physiologically, marijuana increases heart rate and dilates certain blood vessels in the eyes, which creates the characteristic bloodshot eyes. Because THC affects parts of the brain controlling balance, coordination, and reaction time, marijuana use impairs driving performance. The combination of alcohol and marijuana significantly impairs driving performance and increases crash risk.

Both Colorado and Washington permit the recreational use of marijuana. The Supreme Court has held that state laws permitting medical marijuana use cannot supersede federal law. Thus, anyone using marijuana can still be prosecuted under federal drug laws, although the Obama administration indicated that it would not pursue such prosecutions.

Long-Term Effects The most probable long-term effect of smoking marijuana is respiratory damage, including impaired lung function and chronic bronchial irritation. Although no evidence links marijuana use to lung cancer, it may cause changes in lung tissue that promote cancer growth. Marijuana users may be at increased risk for emphysema and cancer of the head and neck, and among people with chronic conditions like cancer and AIDS, marijuana use is associated with increased risk of fatal lung infections. (These are key reasons why the Institute of Medicine has recommended the development of alternative methods of delivering the potentially beneficial compounds in marijuana.) Heavy users may experience learning problems, as well as subtle impairments of attention and memory that may or may not be reversible following long-term abstinence.

---

depersonalization A state in which a person loses the sense of his or her reality or perceives his or her body as unreal.

hallucinogen Any of several drugs that alter perception, feelings, or thoughts; examples are LSD, mescaline, and PCP.

synesthesia A condition in which a stimulus evokes not only the sensation appropriate to it but also another sensation of a different character, such as when a color evokes a specific smell.

flashback A perceptual distortion or bizarre thought that recurs after the chemical effects of a drug have worn off.

TERMS

Long-term use may also decrease testosterone levels and sperm counts and increase sperm abnormalities.

Heavy marijuana use during pregnancy may cause impaired fetal growth and development, low birth weight, and increased risk of ectopic pregnancy. Marijuana may act synergistically with alcohol to increase the damaging effects of alcohol on the fetus. THC rapidly enters breast milk and may impair an infant's early motor development.

Hallucinogens

As shown in Figure 7.1, **hallucinogens** are a group of drugs whose predominant pharmacological effect is to alter the user's perceptions, feelings, and thoughts.

LSD LSD (lysergic acid diethylamide) is one of the most powerful psychoactive drugs. Tiny doses will produce noticeable effects in most people, such as an altered sense of time, visual disturbances, and an improved sense of hearing, mood changes, and distortions in how people perceive their bodies. Dilation of the pupils and slight dizziness, weakness, and nausea may also occur. With larger doses, users may experience a phenomenon known as **synesthesia:** feelings of depersonalization and other alterations in the perceived relationship between the self and external reality.

A severe panic reaction, which can be terrifying in the extreme, can result from taking any dose of LSD. Even after the drug's chemical effects have worn off, spontaneous **flashbacks** and other psychological disturbances can occur.

MDMA MDMA (methylenedioxymethamphetamine), and variants called ecstasy (MDMA with a stimulant such as caffeine added) and molly (a powder said to be "purer" than ecstasy), may be classified as a hallucinogen or a stimulant. Users may experience euphoria, increased energy, and a heightened sense of belonging. Using MDMA can produce dangerously high body temperature and potentially fatal dehydration. Some users experience confusion, depression, anxiety, paranoia, muscle tension, involuntary teeth clenching, blurred vision, nausea, and seizures. Even low doses can affect concentration, judgment, and driving ability. Tolerance can develop, leading users to take the drug more frequently, to use higher doses, or to combine MDMA with other drugs to enhance the drug's effects.

Other Hallucinogens Most other hallucinogens have the same general effects as LSD, but there are some variations. For example, a DMT (dimethyltryptamine) or ketamine high does not last as long as an LSD high; an STP (4-methyl-2,5-dimethoxyamphetamine) high lasts longer. MDMA has both hallucinogenic and amphetamine-like properties. Tolerance to MDMA develops quickly, and high doses can cause anxiety, delusions, and paranoia.

PCP (phencyclidine) reduces and distorts sensory input, especially proprioception—the sensation of body position and movement—and creates a state of sensory deprivation.

PCP was initially used as an anesthetic but was unsatisfactory because it caused agitation, confusion, and delirium (loss of contact with reality). Because it can be easily made, PCP is often available illegally and is sometimes used as an inexpensive replacement for other psychoactive drugs.

Mescaline, derived from the peyote cactus, is the ceremonial drug of the Native American Church. It causes effects similar to LSD, including altered perception and feeling; increased body temperature, heart rate, and blood pressure; weakness and trembling; and sleeplessness. Mescaline is expensive, so most street mescaline is diluted LSD or a mixture of other drugs. Hallucinogenic effects can be obtained from certain mushrooms (*Psilocybe mexicana,* or "magic mushrooms"), certain morning glory seeds, nutmeg, jimsonweed, and other botanical products, but unpleasant side effects, such as dizziness, have limited the popularity of these products.

Inhalants

Inhaling certain chemicals can produce effects ranging from heightened pleasure to delirium and death. Inhalants fall into several major groups: (1) volatile solvents, which are found in products such as paint thinner, glue, and gasoline; (2) aerosols, which are sprays that contain propellants and solvents; (3) nitrites, such as butyl nitrite and amyl nitrite; (4) anesthetics, which include nitrous oxide (laughing gas).

Inhalant use tends to be highest among younger adolescents and declines with age. Inhalant use is difficult to control because inhalants are easy to obtain. They are present in a variety of seemingly harmless products, from dessert-topping sprays to underarm deodorants, that are both inexpensive and legal. Using the drugs also requires no illegal or suspicious paraphernalia. Inhalant users get high by sniffing, snorting, "bagging" (inhaling fumes from a plastic bag), or "huffing" (placing an inhalant-soaked rag in the mouth).

Although different in makeup, nearly all inhalants produce effects similar to those of anesthetics, which slow down body functions. Low doses may cause users to feel slightly stimulated; at higher doses, users may feel less

inhibited and less in control. Sniffing high concentrations of the chemicals in solvents or aerosol sprays can cause a loss of consciousness, heart failure, and death. High concentrations of any inhalant can also cause death from suffocation by displacing oxygen in the lungs and central nervous system. Deliberately inhaling from a bag or in a closed area greatly increases the chances of suffocation. Other possible effects of the excessive or long-term use of inhalants include damage to the nervous system; hearing loss; increased risk of cancer; and damage to the liver, kidneys, and bone marrow.

Prescription Drug Misuse

The National Institute on Drug Abuse (NIDA) describes prescription drug misuse as the use of a medication without a prescription, in a way other than as prescribed, or for the experience or feelings elicited. National surveys show that prescription medications—such as those used to treat pain, attention deficit disorders, and anxiety—are being abused at a rate second only to marijuana and alcohol among Americans age 14 and older.

Among high school seniors, nonmedical use within the past year of Adderall—the prescription form of amphetamine used to treat ADHD—has increased from 5.8% in 2009 to 7.4% in 2013. More than one in five seniors (21.5%) have used at least one prescription medication without a doctor's orders at least once; 15% report use in the past year. A study of college students found that almost two-thirds (61.8%) were offered prescription stimulants for nonmedical use by their senior year and 31% used. Studying was the predominant motive, and the most common source was a friend with a prescription.

Synthetic Recreational Drugs

In recent years herbal or synthetic recreational drugs have become increasingly available. These "designer drugs" are intended to have pharmacological effects similar to those of illicit drugs but to be chemically distinct from them and therefore either legal or impossible to detect in drug screening. The drugs fall into two main groups. One group is marketed as synthetic marijuana and sold as "herbal incense," or "herbal highs" with names such as Spice, K2, Genie, and Mr. Nice Guy. The other group is marketed as stimulants with properties like those of cocaine or amphetamine and sold as "bath salts" with names such as Zoom, Ivory Wave, and White Rush.

Spice and other synthetic mimics of THC are distributed in the form of dried leaves or powder. They are typically smoked, using a pipe or by rolling in a cigarette paper, but can also be ingested as an infusion such as tea, or inhaled. The active ingredients in Spice and similar products are synthetic cannabinoids that act on brain cells to produce effects similar to those of THC, such as physical relaxation, changes in perception, elevated mood, and mild euphoria. These drugs may seem new to adults, but more than 1 in 10 American high school seniors (11.3%) report using synthetic marijuana in 2012, according to the "Monitoring the Future" survey conducted by the University of Michigan. The level of use dropped sharply (to 7.9% among 12th graders) in 2013, but is roughly three times the rate reported for inhalants or cocaine and six times the rate for methamphetamine.

In 2012, synthetic marijuana was the second-most widely used illicit drug among 10th and 12th graders (after marijuana), and the third-most widely used among 8th graders (after marijuana and inhalants). Spice and similar products have not been included in any wide-scale animal or human studies, and little information is available in international medical databases. The blends of ingredients vary widely, but these products typically contain more than a dozen different plant-derived compounds, which give rise to a wide variety of drug combinations. Calls to poison control centers for exposure to synthetic marijuana doubled between 2010 and 2011, with patients describing symptoms that include rapid heart rate, vomiting, agitation, confusion, and hallucinations. In March 2011 the U.S. Drug Enforcement Administration (DEA) banned five synthetic cannabinoids used in Spice and similar products.

"Bath salts," marketed as cocaine or methamphetamine substitutes, are widely available on the Internet. They contain the synthetic stimulants mephedrone, methylone, or methylenedioxypyrovalerone (MDPV). Similar in effect to MDMA ("ecstasy"), MDPV is a synthetic version of the active ingredient found in the stimulant khat, which is widely used in countries of the Middle East. The products are sold in small packets of salt-like crystals with warnings like "novelty only" and "not for human consumption." Bath salts can be ingested by smoking, eating, or injecting the bath salts or by crushing them and snorting the powder. The speed of onset is up to 15 minutes depending on how the drug is ingested, and the effects may last as long as six hours. The effects of bath salts can be severe and include combative violent behavior, extreme agitation, confusion, hallucinations, hypertension, chest pain, and suicidal thoughts. In 2010 poison centers in the United States received 304 calls about reactions to bath salts; the number rose to 6,138 calls in 2011. In September 2011 the DEA banned three of the drugs found in bath salts; possession or sale of the chemicals or products that contain them is now illegal. Since then, poison center calls have dropped by more than half and overall use of synthetic recreational drugs has declined among young Americans.

DRUG USE: THE DECADES AHEAD

Although the use of some drugs, both legal and illegal, has declined dramatically since the 1970s, the use of others has held steady or increased. Mounting public concern has led to great debate and a wide range of opinions about what should be done. Efforts to combat the problem include workplace drug testing, tougher law enforcement and prosecution, and treatment and education. With drugs entering the country on a massive scale from South America, Southeast Asia, and elsewhere, and being distributed through tightly controlled drug-smuggling organizations and street gangs, the success of any program is uncertain.

Drugs, Society, and Families

According to the Department of Justice, National Drug Intelligence Center, and Institute on Drug Abuse, the cost to society of illicit drug use alone is $193 billion annually. That figure is higher than the cost of many major health problems, including diabetes, obesity, and smoking. But the costs are more than just financial—they are also paid in human pain and suffering.

The criminal justice system is inundated with people accused of crimes related to drug possession, sale, or use. The FBI reports that roughly 1.5 arrests are made annually for drug violations. In 2009, the most recent year for which data are available, 18% of state prison inmates (252,000) were serving time for drug offenses. In 2010 about half of federal inmates (107,000) were in prison because of drug offenses.

The Bureau of Justice Statistics reports that about half of all state and federal prisoners—roughly 850,000 men and women—meet diagnostic criteria for drug misuse or addiction. Many assaults and murders are committed when people try to acquire or protect drug territories, settle disputes about drugs, or steal from dealers. Violence and gun use are common in neighborhoods where drug trafficking is prevalent. Addicts commit more robberies and burglaries than criminals not on drugs. People under the influence of drugs, especially alcohol, are more likely to commit violent crimes like rape and murder than people who do not use drugs.

To what extent is drug misuse also a health care issue for society? In the United States, illegal drug use leads to more than 800,000 emergency department admissions and nearly 20,000 deaths annually. Although it is in the best interest of society to treat addicts who want help, there is not nearly enough space in treatment facilities to help the millions of Americans who need immediate treatment.

Drug misuse also takes a toll on individuals and families. Children born to women who use drugs such as alcohol, tobacco, or cocaine may have long-term health problems.

> Many American businesses **require workers to take drug tests;** some employers offer counseling and treatment support for workers who test positive.

atmosphere. Administered by ex-addicts, these programs use confrontation, strict discipline, and unrelenting peer pressure to attempt to resocialize the addict with a different set of values. Halfway houses, which are transitional settings between a 24-hour-a-day program and independent living, are an important phase of treatment for some people.

Groups and Peer Counseling Groups such as Alcoholics Anonymous (AA) and Narcotics Anonymous (NA) have helped many people. People treated in drug substitution programs or substance use treatment centers are often urged or required to join a self-help group as part of their recovery. These groups follow a 12-step program. Group members' first step is to acknowledge that they have a problem over which they have no control. Peer support is a critical ingredient of these programs, and members usually meet at least once a week. Each member is paired with a sponsor to call on for advice and support if the temptation to relapse becomes overwhelming. Chapters of AA and NA meet on some college campuses; community-based chapters are listed in the phone book, in local newspapers, and online.

Many colleges also have peer counseling programs, in which students are trained to help other students who have drug problems. A peer counselor's role may be as limited as referring a student to a professional with expertise in substance dependence for an evaluation or as involved as helping arrange a leave of absence from school for participation in a drug treatment program (see the box "If Someone You Know Has a Drug Problem . . .").

Harm Reduction Strategies Because many attempts at treatment are at first unsuccessful, some experts advocate the use of harm reduction strategies. The goal of harm reduction is to minimize the negative effects of drug use and misuse: A common example is the use of designated drivers to reduce alcohol-related motor vehicle crashes. Drug substitution programs such as methadone maintenance are a form of harm reduction—although participants remain drug dependent, the negative individual and social consequences of their drug use are reduced. Syringe exchange programs, designed to reduce transmission of HIV and hepatitis C, are another harm reduction approach. Some experts have also suggested free testing of street drugs for purity and potency to help users avoid unintentional toxicity or overdose.

Codependency Many treatment programs also offer counseling for those who are close to drug abusers. Drug misuse takes a toll on friends and family members, and counseling can help people work through painful feelings of guilt and powerlessness. **Codependency,** in which a person close to the drug abuser is controlled by the abuser's behavior, sometimes develops. Codependent people may come to believe that love, approval, and security are contingent on their taking care of the abuser. People can become codependent naturally because they want to help when someone they love becomes dependent on a drug. They may assume that their good intentions will persuade the drug user to stop.

Codependent people often engage in behaviors that remove or soften the effects of drug use on the user—so-called *enabling* behaviors. The habit of enabling can inhibit a drug abuser's recovery because the person never has to experience the consequences of his or her behavior. For this reason, many treatment programs involve the whole family.

Have you ever been an enabler in a relationship? You may have if you've ever done any of the following:

- Given someone one more chance to stop abusing drugs, then another, and another
- Made excuses or lied for someone to his or her friends, teachers, or employer
- Joined someone in drug use and blamed others for your behavior
- Lent money to someone to continue drug use
- Stayed up late waiting for or gone out searching for someone who uses drugs
- Felt embarrassed or angry about the actions of someone who uses drugs
- Ignored the drug use because the person got defensive when you brought it up
- Avoided confronting a friend or relative who was obviously intoxicated or high on a drug

If you come from a codependent family or see yourself developing codependency relationships or engaging in enabling behaviors, consider acting now to make changes in your patterns of interaction. Remember, you cannot cause or cure drug addiction in another person.

Preventing Drug Misuse

The best solution to drug misuse is prevention. Government attempts at controlling the drug problem have historically focused on stopping the production, importation, and distribution of illegal drugs. A new national drug policy announced in 2010, however, redirects federal funding and efforts into stopping the demand for drugs. Developing persuasive antidrug educational programs may offer the best hope for solving the drug problem in the future. Indirect approaches to prevention involve building young people's self-esteem, improving their academic skills, and increasing their recreational opportunities. Direct approaches involve providing information about the adverse effects of drugs and teaching tactics that help students resist peer pressure to use drugs in various situations. Developing strategies for resisting peer pressure is one of the more effective techniques.

codependency A relationship in which a non–substance-abusing partner or family member is controlled by the abuser's behavior; codependent people frequently engage in enabling behaviors.

TERMS

TAKE CHARGE
If Someone You Know Has a Drug Problem . . .

Changes in behavior and mood in someone you know may signal a growing dependence on drugs. Signs that a person's life is beginning to focus on drugs include the following:

- Sudden withdrawal or emotional distance

- Rebellious or unusually irritable behavior

- A loss of interest in usual activities or hobbies

- A decline in school performance

- A sudden change in the chosen group of friends

- Changes in sleeping or eating habits

- Frequent borrowing of money or stealing

- Secretive behavior about personal possessions, such as a backpack or the contents of a drawer

- Deterioration of physical appearance

If you believe a family member or friend has a drug problem, locate information about drug treatment resources available on campus or in your community. Communicate your concern, provide him or her with information about treatment options, and offer your support during treatment. If the person continues to deny having a problem, talk with an experienced counselor about setting up an intervention—a formal, structured confrontation designed to end denial by having family, friends, and other caring people present their concerns to the drug user. Participants in an intervention would indicate the ways in which the individual is hurting others as well as himself or herself. If your friend or family member agrees to treatment, encourage him or her to attend a support group such as Narcotics Anonymous or Alcoholics Anonymous.

And finally, examine your relationship with the abuser for signs of codependency. If necessary, get help for yourself; friends and family of drug users can often benefit from counseling.

Connect to Your Choices

connect™

Have you ever thought about why you make the choices you do about drugs? Many factors can influence the drug-related choices we make, some not as obvious as others. If you use drugs—or if you don't—have you been influenced by attitudes toward drug use in your family or peer group? Do you take drugs when they're offered at parties because it's easier than saying no? Are you influenced by the lyrics of songs that make drug use sound glamorous?

What are the external factors that influence your drug-related choices? What are your inner motivations and core values, and how do they affect your choices? Based on what you learned in this chapter, will you make some different choices in the future? If so, what will they be?

Go online to Connect to complete this activity: www.mcgraw-hillconnect.com

Ask Yourself

QUESTIONS FOR CRITICAL THINKING AND REFLECTION

Do you know someone who may have a drug problem? What steps, if any, have you taken to help that person? If you were using drugs and felt that things had gone out of control, what would you want your friends to do for you?

TIPS FOR TODAY AND THE FUTURE

RIGHT NOW YOU CAN:

- If you are a regular caffeine user, look for ways to cut back.
- Consider whether you or someone you know might benefit from drug counseling. Find out what types of services are available on campus or in your area.

IN THE FUTURE YOU CAN:

- Think about the drug-related attitudes of people you know. For example, talk to two older adults and two fellow students about their attitudes toward legalizing marijuana. What are the differences in their opinions, and how do they account for them?
- Analyze media portrayals of drug use. As you watch TV shows and movies, note the way they depict drug use among people of different ages and backgrounds. How realistic are the portrayals, in your view? Think about the influence they have on you and your peers.

Prevention efforts need to focus on the different motivations individuals have for using and abusing specific drugs at different ages. For example, adolescents in junior or senior high school are often more responsive to peer counselors. Many young adults tend to be influenced by efforts that focus on health education. For all ages, it is important to provide nondrug alternatives—such as recreational facilities, counseling, greater opportunities for leisure activities, and places to socialize—that speak to the individual's or group's specific reasons for using drugs. Reminding young people that most people, no matter what age, are *not* users of illegal drugs is a critical part of preventing substance misuse.

SUMMARY

- Addictive behaviors are self-reinforcing. Addicts experience a strong compulsion for the behavior and a loss of control over it; an escalating pattern of misuse with serious negative consequences may result.

- The sources or causes of addiction include heredity, personality, lifestyle, and environmental factors. People may use an addictive behavior as a means of alleviating stress or painful emotions.

- Some common behaviors are potentially addictive, including gambling, shopping, sexual activity, Internet use, eating, and working.

- Drug misuse is a maladaptive pattern of drug use that persists despite adverse social, psychological, or medical consequences.

- Drug addiction involves taking a drug compulsively, which includes neglecting constructive activities because of it and continuing to use it despite experiencing adverse effects resulting from its use. Tolerance and withdrawal symptoms are often present.

- Reasons for using drugs include the lure of the illicit; curiosity; rebellion; peer pressure; and the desire to alter your mood or escape boredom, anxiety, depression, or other psychological problems.

- Psychoactive drugs affect the mind and body by altering brain chemistry. The effect of a drug depends on its properties and on how it's used (drug factors), the physical and psychological characteristics of the user (user factors), and the physical and social environment surrounding the drug use (social factors).

- Opioids relieve pain, cause drowsiness, and induce euphoria; they reduce anxiety and produce lethargy, apathy, and an inability to concentrate.

- CNS depressants slow down the overall activity of the central nervous system; they reduce anxiety and cause mood changes, impaired muscular coordination, slurring of speech, and drowsiness or sleep.

- CNS stimulants speed up the activity of the central nervous system, causing acceleration of the heart rate, a rise in blood pressure, dilation of the pupils and bronchial tubes, and an increase in gastric and adrenal secretions.

- Marijuana usually causes euphoria and a relaxed attitude at low doses; very high doses produce feelings of depersonalization and sensory distortion. The long-term effects may include chronic bronchitis and cancer; use during pregnancy may impair fetal growth.

- Hallucinogens alter perception, feelings, and thoughts and may cause an altered sense of time, visual disturbances, and mood changes.

- Inhalants are present in a variety of everyday products; they can cause delirium. Their use can lead to loss of consciousness, heart failure, suffocation, and death.

- Economic and social costs of drug misuse include the financial costs of law enforcement, treatment, and health care and the social costs of crime, violence, and family problems. Drug testing and drug legalization have been proposed to address some of the problems related to drug use.

- Approaches to treatment include medication, treatment centers, self-help groups, and peer counseling; many programs also offer counseling to family members.

FOR MORE INFORMATION

BOOKS

Hanson, G. R., et al. 2008. *Drugs and Society,* 10th ed. Boston: Jones & Bartlett. *Discusses the impact of drug misuse on individuals' lives and on the broader society.*

Ksir, C., C. L. Hart, and O. S. Ray. 2010. *Drugs, Society, and Human Behavior,* 14th ed. New York: McGraw-Hill. *Examines drugs and behavior from behavioral, pharmacological, historical, social, legal, and clinical perspectives.*

Reding, N. 2010 *Methland: The Death and Life of an American Small Town.* New York: Bloomsbury USA. *The author chronicles the epidemic of meth production and addiction that overtook rural America—and one tiny Iowa town—as small farms and businesses declined in the wake of globalization.*

Rosen Publishing. 2009. *Drug Abuse and Society Series.* New York: Rosen Publishing. *A series of short books, each exploring a different type of drugs—from prescription medicine to club drugs—and their use and misuse.*

Young, K , and C. Nabuco, eds. 2011. *Internet Addiction: A Handbook and Guide to Evaluation and Treatment.* Hoboken, NJ: John Wiley & Sons, Inc.

ORGANIZATIONS, HOTLINES, AND WEBSITES

CASAColumbia (Center on Addiction and Substance Abuse at Columbia University). Provides information about the costs of substance abuse to individuals and society.

http://www.casacolumbia.org

Club Drugs. Provides information about drugs commonly classified as "club drugs."

http://www.drugabuse.gov/drugs-abuse/club-drugs

DAWN (Drug Abuse Warning Network). Public health surveillance system that monitors drug-related hospital emergency departments (EDs) and drug-related deaths.

http://www.samhsa.gov/data/DAWN.aspx

Drug Enforcement Administration: Drug Information. Provides basic facts about major drugs of abuse, including penalties for drug trafficking.

http://www.justice.gov/dea/concern/concern.htm

Gamblers Anonymous. Includes questions to help diagnose gambling problems and resources for getting help.

http://www.gamblersanonymous.org/ga/

Go Ask Alice. An Internet health question-and-answer resource produced by Alice! Health Promotion at Columbia University. See "Alcohol and Other Drugs" in the Q&A library.

http://goaskalice.columbia.edu

Higher Education Center for Alcohol and Other Drug Abuse and Violence Prevention. Gives information about alcohol and drug abuse on campus and links to related sites.

http://www.higheredcenter.org

National Council on Problem Gambling. Provides information and help for people with gambling problems and their families, including a searchable directory of counselors.

http://www.ncpgambling.org

National Drug Information, Treatment, and Referral Hotlines. Sponsored by the SAMHSA Center for Substance Abuse Treatment, these hotlines provide information on drug abuse and on HIV infection as it relates to substance abuse; referrals to support groups and treatment programs are available.

800-662-HELP

800-729-6686 (Spanish)

800-487-4889 (TDD for hearing impaired)

National Institute on Drug Abuse. Develops and supports research on drug abuse prevention programs.

http://www.drugabuse.gov

Substance Abuse and Mental Health Services Administration (SAMHSA). Provides statistics, information, and other resources related to substance abuse prevention and treatment.

http://www.samhsa.gov

See also the listings for Chapter 8.

SELECTED BIBLIOGRAPHY

American College Health Association. 2013. *American College Health Association—National College Health Assessment II: Reference Group Undergraduates Executive Summary Spring 2013.* Hanover, MD: American College Health Association.

American Psychiatric Association. 2013. *Diagnostic and Statistical Manual of Mental Disorders,* 5th ed. *(DSM-5).* Washington, DC: American Psychiatric Publishing.

Centers for Disease Control and Prevention. 2012. *HIV Surveillance Report, 2011; vol. 23* (http://www.cdc.gov/hiv/pdf/statistics_2011 _HIV_Surveillance_Report_vol_23.pdf).

Drug Enforcement Administration, U.S. Department of Justice. 2011. *Drugs of Abuse: A DEA Resource Guide, 2011 Edition* (http://www .justice.gov/dea /pubs/drugs_of_abuse.pdf).

Garnier-Dykstra, L. M., et al. 2012. Nonmedical use of prescription stimulants during college: Four- year trends in exposure opportunity, use, motives, and sources. *Journal of American College Health* 60(3): 226–234.

Giles, G. E., et al., 2012. Differential cognitive effects of energy drink ingredients: Caffeine, taurine, and glucose. *Pharamcology, Biochemistry, and Behavior* 102(4): 569–577.

Johnston, L. D., et al. 2013. "American teens more cautious about using synthetic drugs." Ann Arbor, MI: University of Michigan News Service, 18 December (http://www.monitoringthefuture.org).

Koester, P., et al. 2012. Cortical thinning in amphetamine –type stimulant users. Neuroscience 221: 182–192.

Lucas, P. Cannabis as an adjunct to or substitute for opiates in the treatment of chronic pain. *Journal of Psychoactive Drugs* 44(2): 125–133.

National Council on Problem Gambling. 2010. *What Is Problem Gambling?* (http://www.ncpgambling.org/i4a/pages/index.cfm?pageid=1).

Office of National Drug Control Policy. 2012. *2010 National Strategy* (http://www.http://www.whitehouse.gov/ondcp/2012-national -drug-control-strategy/).

Patrick, M. E., et al. 2012. HIV/AIDS risk behaviors and substance use by young adults in the United States. *Prevention Science* 13(5): 532–538.

Porter, R. S., et. al. 2011. *The Merck Manual of Diagnosis and Therapy,* 19th ed. New York: Wiley.

Reith, G. 2012. Beyond addiction and compulsion: The continuing role of environment in the case of pathological gambling. *Addiction* 107(10): 1736–1737.

Rugani, G. 2012. Symptomatological features of patients with and without Ecstasy use during their first psychotic episode. *International Journal of Environmental Research and Public Health* 9(7): 2283–2292.

Singer, L. T., et al. 2012. One-year outcomes of prenatal exposure to MDMA and other recreational drugs. *Pediatrics* 130(3): 407–413.

Substance Abuse and Mental Health Services Administration. 2013. *Results from the 2012 National Survey on Drug Use and Health: Summary of National Findings,* NSDUH Series H-46, HHS Publication No. (SMA) 13-4795. Rockville, MD: SAMHSA.

Tashkin, D. P., M.S. Simmons, and C. H. Tseng. 2012. Impact of changes in regular use of marijuana and/or tobacco on chronic bronchitis. *COPD* 9(4): 367–374.

U.S. Department of Justice, Federal Bureau of Investigation. 2013. *Crime in the United States: 2012* (http://www.fbi.gov/about-us/cjis/ucr /crime-in-the-u.s/2012/crime-in-the-u.s.-2012).

Van Ryzin, M.J., G. M. Fosco, and T. J. Dishion. 2012. Family and peer predictors of substance use from early adolescence to early adulthood: An 11-year prospective analysis. *Addictive Behaviors* 37(12): 1314–1324.

CHAPTER OBJECTIVES

- Explain how alcohol is absorbed and metabolized by the body
- Describe the immediate and long-term effects of drinking alcohol
- Describe different forms of alcohol misuse and their consequences
- List the reasons why people start using tobacco and why they continue to use it
- Explain the short- and long-term health risks associated with tobacco use
- Describe strategies for using alcohol responsibly, and develop plans for quitting tobacco use and avoiding environmental tobacco smoke.

CHAPTER **8**

Alcohol and Tobacco

Despite numerous prohibitions against it throughout history, alcohol has been the most popular psychoactive drug in the Western world. Alcohol plays contradictory roles in human behavior. Used in moderation, alcohol can enhance social occasions by loosening inhibitions and creating pleasant feelings of relaxation. But alcohol use can also be unhealthful. Like other drugs, alcohol produces physiological effects that can impair functioning in the short term while causing devastating damage in the long term. For some people, alcohol use can fuel an addiction, leading to a lifetime of recovery or, for a few, to debilitation and death.

This chapter discusses the complexities of alcohol and tobacco use and provides information that will help you make choices that are right for you. The term *abuse* has been replaced by **misuse** or **excessive use,** following the publication of a new edition of the *Diagnostic and Statistical Manual of Mental Disorders* (DSM-5, 2013).

THE NATURE OF ALCOHOL

If you are ever around people who are drinking, you probably notice that alcohol seems to affect different people in different ways. One person may seem to get drunk after just a drink or two, while another appears to tolerate a great deal of alcohol without becoming intoxicated. These differences make alcohol's effects on the body seem mysterious and help explain why many misconceptions have evolved about alcohol use. The following sections explain how alcohol works in the body.

Alcoholic Beverages

Technically speaking, there are many kinds of **alcohol**, and each is an organic compound. In this book, however, the term *alcohol* refers only to ethyl alcohol (or ethanol, often

---

misuse or excessive use Drinking alcohol to the point of slurring words and engaging in risky behavior such as drunk driving.

alcohol The intoxicating ingredient in fermented or distilled beverages; a colorless, pungent liquid.

TERMS

abbreviated as ETOH). Other kinds of alcohol, such as methanol (wood alcohol) and isopropyl alcohol (rubbing alcohol) are highly toxic and can cause death if consumed.

Common Alcoholic Beverages

There are several basic types of alcoholic beverages. Ethanol is the psychoactive ingredient in each of them:

- Beer is a mild intoxicant brewed from a mixture of grains. By volume, beer usually contains 3–6% alcohol.

- Ales and malt liquors, which also have grain bases and are similar to beer in their processing, typically contain 6–8% alcohol by volume.

- Wines are made by fermenting the juices of grapes or other fruits. During *fermentation*, sugars from the fruit react with yeast to create ethanol and other by-products. In table wines, the concentration of alcohol is about 9–14%. A more potent type of wine, *fortified wine*, is called this because extra alcohol is added during its production. Fortified wines—such as sherry, port, and Madeira—contain about 20% alcohol.

- Hard liquor—such as gin, whiskey, rum, tequila, vodka, and liqueur—is made by *distilling* brewed or fermented grains or other plant products. Hard liquors usually contain 35–50% alcohol.

The concentration of alcohol in a beverage is indicated by its **proof value,** which amounts to two times the percentage concentration. For example, if a beverage is 100 proof, it contains 50% alcohol by volume. Two ounces of 100-proof whiskey contain one ounce of pure alcohol. The proof value of hard liquor can usually be found on the bottle's label.

"Standard Drinks" versus Actual Servings

When discussing alcohol consumption, the term **one drink** or (*a standard drink*) refers to the amount of a beverage that typically contains about 0.6 ounce of alcohol. A 12-ounce bottle of beer, a 5-ounce glass of wine, and a 1.5-ounce shot of hard liquor are all considered one drink.

A typical serving of most alcoholic beverages is larger (sometimes significantly larger) than a single standard drink.

This is particularly true of mixed drinks, which often include more than one type of hard liquor.

Caloric Content

Alcohol provides 7 calories per gram, and the alcohol in one drink (14–17 grams) supplies about 100–120 calories. Most alcoholic beverages also contain some carbohydrate; for example, one beer provides about 150 total calories. The "light" in light beer refers to calories; a light beer typically has close to the same alcohol content as a regular beer and about 100 calories. A 5-ounce glass of red wine has 100 calories; white wine has 96. A 3-ounce margarita supplies 157 calories, a 6-ounce cosmopolitan has 143 calories, and a 6-ounce rum and Coke contains about 180 calories.

Absorption

When a person ingests alcohol, the bloodstream rapidly absorbs about 20% of it from the stomach. About 75% is absorbed from the stomach through the upper part of the small intestine. Any remaining alcohol enters the bloodstream farther along the gastrointestinal (GI) tract. Once in the bloodstream, alcohol produces sensations of intoxication.

The rate of absorption is affected by a variety of factors. For example, the carbonation in a beverage like champagne increases the rate of alcohol absorption. Artificial sweeteners (commonly used in drink mixers) have the same effect. Food in the stomach slows the rate of absorption, as does the drinking of highly concentrated alcoholic beverages such as hard liquor.

Metabolism and Excretion

Because alcohol easily moves through most biological membranes, it is rapidly distributed throughout most body tissues. Alcohol **metabolizes,** transforms into usable parts and waste, mainly in the liver, though a small amount of alcohol is metabolized in the stomach. (See the box "Metabolizing Alcohol: Our Bodies Work Differently.")

About 2–10% of ingested alcohol is not metabolized in the liver or other tissues but is excreted unchanged by the lungs, kidneys, and sweat glands. Excreted alcohol causes the telltale smell on a drinker's breath and is the basis of breath and urine analyses for alcohol levels.

Alcohol readily enters the human brain, affecting neurotransmitters, the chemicals that carry messages between brain cells. These changes are temporary, creating many of the immediate effects of drinking alcohol. With chronic heavy use, however, alcohol's disruptive effects can become permanent, resulting in loss of brain function and changes in brain structure.

Alcohol Intake and Blood Alcohol Concentration

Blood alcohol concentration (BAC) is the ratio of alcohol in a person's blood by weight, expressed as the percentage of alcohol measured in a deciliter of blood. BAC is affected by

Do you and your friends react differently to alcohol? If so, your reactions may be affected by genetic differences in alcohol metabolism. Alcohol is metabolized mainly in the liver, where an enzyme, alcohol dehydrogenase, converts the alcohol into a toxic substance called acetaldehyde. Acetaldehyde causes many of alcohol's noxious effects. Ideally it is quickly broken down to a less active by-product, acetate, by another enzyme, acetaldehyde dehydrogenase (ALDH). Acetate can then separate into water and carbon dioxide and easily be eliminated. But people vary in the length of time it takes to break down the toxins in alcohol and in how efficiently they can process them. Some differences in metabolism are associated with ethnicity.

Some people, primarily those of Asian descent, inherit ineffective or inactive variations of that latter enzyme, acetaldehyde dehydrogenase. Others, including some of African and Jewish descent, have forms of alcohol dehydrogenase that metabolize alcohol to acetaldehyde very quickly. Either way, toxic acetaldehyde builds up when these people drink alcohol. They experience a reaction called *flushing syndrome*. Their skin feels hot, their heart and respiration rates increase, and they may get a headache, vomit, or break out in hives. The severity of their reactions is affected by the inherited form of their alcohol-metabolizing enzymes. Drinking makes some people so uncomfortable that they are unlikely to develop alcohol addiction.

The body's response to acetaldehyde is the basis for treating alcohol misuse with the drug disulfiram (Antabuse), which inhibits the action of acetaldehyde dehydrogenase. When a person taking disulfiram ingests alcohol, acetaldehyde levels increase rapidly, and he or she develops an intense flushing reaction along with weakness, nausea, vomiting, and other disagreeable symptoms.

How people behave in relation to alcohol is influenced in complex ways by a wide range of factors, including liver size, body mass, and social and cultural influences. But individual choices and behavior are strongly influenced by specific genetic characteristics.

connect ACTIVITY DO IT ONLINE

BAC Zones:	90–109 lb								110–129 lb								130–149 lb								150–169 lb								170–189 lb								190–209 lb								210 lb & Over							
Time from First Drink	Total Drinks								Total Drinks								Total Drinks								Total Drinks								Total Drinks								Total Drinks								Total Drinks							
	1	2	3	4	5	6	7	8	1	2	3	4	5	6	7	8	1	2	3	4	5	6	7	8	1	2	3	4	5	6	7	8	1	2	3	4	5	6	7	8	1	2	3	4	5	6	7	8	1	2	3	4	5	6	7	8
1 hr																																																								
2 hr																																																								
3 hr																																																								
4 hr																																																								

☐ (0.00%) Not impaired ☐ (0.05–0.07%) Usually impaired

☐ (0.01–0.04%) Sometimes impaired ☐ (0.08% and up) Always impaired

FIGURE 8.1 Approximate blood alcohol concentration and body weight. This chart illustrates the BAC an average person of a given weight would reach after drinking the specified number of drinks in the time shown. The federal legal limit for BAC for drivers is 0.08%; for drivers under 21 years of age, many states have zero-tolerance laws that set BAC limits of 0.01% or 0.02%.

the amount of alcohol consumed in a given amount of time and by individual factors:

- *Body weight:* In most cases, a smaller person develops a higher BAC than a larger person after drinking the same amount of alcohol (Figure 8.1). A smaller person has less overall body tissue into which alcohol can be distributed.

- *Percentage of body fat:* A person with a higher percentage of body fat will usually develop a higher BAC than a more muscular person of the same weight. Alcohol does not concentrate as much in fatty tissue as in muscle and most other tissues, in part because fat has fewer blood vessels.

- *Sex:* Women metabolize less alcohol in the stomach than men do because the stomach enzyme that breaks down alcohol before it enters the bloodstream is four times more active in men than in women, thus releasing more unmetabolized alcohol into the bloodstream in women. Hormonal fluctuations may also affect the rate of alcohol metabolism, making a woman more susceptible to high BACs at certain times during her menstrual cycle.

BAC also depends on the balance between the rate of alcohol absorption and the rate of alcohol metabolism. A man who weighs 150 pounds and has normal liver function metabolizes about 0.3 ounce of alcohol per hour, the equivalent of about half a 12-ounce bottle of beer or half a 5-ounce glass of wine.

The rate of alcohol metabolism varies among individuals and is largely determined by genetic factors and drinking behavior. Chronic drinking activates enzymes that metabolize alcohol in the liver, so people who drink frequently metabolize alcohol at a more rapid rate than nondrinkers. Although the rate of alcohol absorption can be slowed by factors like food, the metabolic rate *cannot* be influenced by exercise, breathing deeply, eating, drinking coffee, or taking other drugs. Whether a person is asleep or awake, the rate of alcohol metabolism is the same.

If a person absorbs slightly less alcohol each hour than he or she can metabolize in an hour, the BAC remains low. People can drink large amounts of alcohol this way over a long period of time without becoming noticeably intoxicated. Even so, they run the risk of long-term health problems (described later in the chapter). If a person drinks alcohol more quickly than it can be metabolized, the BAC will steadily increase, and he or she will become more and more drunk.

ALCOHOL AND HEALTH

The effects of alcohol consumption on health depend on the individual, the circumstances, and the amount of alcohol consumed.

The Immediate Effects of Alcohol

Alcohol depresses the central nervous system (CNS), and its effects vary with the BAC. But in general, alcohol slows reactions, impairs coordination and judgment, and, eventually, sedates to inactivity. The senses become less acute. In men, alcohol reduces erection response.

The effects of alcohol are more pronounced when the BAC is rapidly increasing than when it is slowly increasing, steady, or decreasing. They are also more pronounced when a person drinks on an empty stomach because alcohol is absorbed more quickly and the BAC rises more quickly.

Low Concentrations of Alcohol   The effects of alcohol can first be felt at a BAC of about 0.03–0.05%. These effects may include lightheadedness, relaxation, and a release of inhibitions. Most drinkers experience mild euphoria and become more sociable. When people drink in social settings, alcohol often seems to act as a stimulant, enhancing conviviality or assertiveness. This apparent stimulation occurs because alcohol depresses inhibitory centers in the brain.

Higher Concentrations of Alcohol   At higher concentrations, the pleasant effects tend to be replaced by more negative ones: interference with motor coordination, verbal performance, and intellectual functions. The drinker often becomes irritable and may be easily angered or given to crying. When the BAC reaches 0.1%, most sensory and motor functioning is reduced, and many people become sleepy.

Vision, smell, taste, and hearing become less acute. At 0.2% most drinkers are completely unable to function, either physically or psychologically, because of the pronounced depression of the central nervous system, muscles, and other body systems. Coma usually occurs at a BAC of 0.35%, and any higher level can be fatal.

Alcohol Hangover   The symptoms of a hangover include headache, shakiness, nausea, diarrhea, fatigue, and impaired mental functioning. During a hangover, heart rate and blood pressure increase, making some individuals more vulnerable to heart attacks. Electroencephalography (brain wave measurement) shows diffuse slowing of brain waves for up to 16 hours after BAC drops to 0.0%. Studies of pilots, drivers, and skiers all indicate that coordination and cognition are impaired in a person with a hangover, increasing the risk of injury. A hangover is probably caused by a combination of the toxic products of alcohol breakdown, dehydration, and hormonal effects.

Alcohol Poisoning   Drinking large amounts of alcohol in a short time can rapidly raise the BAC into the lethal range. Death from alcohol poisoning may be caused either by central nervous system and respiratory depression or by inhaling fluid or vomit into the lungs. The amount of alcohol that renders a person unconscious is dangerously close to a fatal dose. Although passing out may prevent someone from drinking more, BAC can keep rising during unconsciousness because the body continues to absorb ingested alcohol into the bloodstream. Special care should be taken to ensure the safety of anyone who has been drinking heavily, especially if he or she passes out (see the box "Dealing with an Alcohol Emergency").

Using Alcohol with Other Drugs   Alcohol-drug combinations are a leading cause of drug-related deaths. Using alcohol while taking a medication that depresses the CNS

Ask Yourself

QUESTIONS FOR CRITICAL THINKING AND REFLECTION

Have you ever had a hangover or watched someone else suffer through one? Did the experience affect your attitude about drinking? In what way?

Being very drunk is potentially life-threatening. Helping a drunken friend could save a life.

- If the person is unconscious, don't assume she is just "sleeping it off." Place her on her side with her knees up. This position helps prevent choking if she vomits.

- Monitor airway, breathing, and circulation (check pulse).

- Stay with the person. You need to be ready to help if she vomits or stops breathing.

- Don't try to give the person anything to eat or drink, including coffee or other drugs. Don't give cold showers or try to make her walk around. None of these things help anyone to sober up, and they can be dangerous.

Call 911 immediately in any of the following instances:

- You can't wake the person even with shouting or shaking.

- The person is taking fewer than eight breaths per minute, or her breathing seems shallow or irregular.

- You think the person took other drugs with alcohol.

- The person has had an injury, especially a blow to the head.

- The person drank a large amount of alcohol in a short period of time and then became unconscious. Death caused by alcohol poisoning most often occurs when the blood alcohol level rises very quickly due to rapid ingestion of alcohol.

If you aren't sure what to do, call 911. You may save a life.

increases the effects of both drugs, potentially leading to coma, respiratory depression, and death. Such drugs include barbiturates, Valium-like drugs, narcotics such as codeine, and OTC antihistamines such as Benadryl. For people who consume three or more drinks per day, use of OTC pain relievers like aspirin, ibuprofen, or acetaminophen increases the risk of stomach bleeding and liver damage. Some antibiotics and diabetes medications can also interact dangerously with alcohol.

Many illegal drugs are especially dangerous when combined with alcohol. Life-threatening overdoses occur at much lower doses when heroin and other narcotics are combined with alcohol. When cocaine and alcohol are used together, they form a toxic substance called cocaethylene, which is responsible for more than half of all cocaine-related deaths. A recent trend among young drinkers is mixing alcoholic beverages with caffeinated ones, especially highly caffeinated energy drinks (see the box "Alcoholic Energy Drinks: The Dangers of Being 'Drunk and Wide Awake'").

Alcohol-Related Injuries and Violence   The combination of impaired judgment, weakened sensory perception, reduced inhibitions, impaired motor coordination, and increased aggressiveness and hostility that characterizes alcohol intoxication can be dangerous. Through homicide, suicide, automobile crashes, and other traumatic incidents, alcohol use is linked to more than 88,000 American deaths each year. The majority of people who attempt suicide have been drinking. Among successful suicides, alcohol use is common as well; a recent analysis of 5,550 suicide deaths found that one-third involved alcohol. Alcohol use more than triples the risk of fatal injuries during leisure activities such as swimming and boating. More than 50% of fatal falls and serious burns happen to people who have been drinking.

Alcohol and Aggression   In 2012 more than 2.2 million arrests were made for alcohol-related offenses (driving under the influence of alcohol, public drunkenness, and liquor law violations). Alcohol use contributes to over 50% of all murders, assaults, and rapes. It is frequently found in the bloodstream of victims as well as perpetrators. Some people become violent under alcohol's influence; such individuals may be predisposed to aggressive, impulsive behavior that tends to get exacerbated by alcohol.

Alcohol misuse can wreak havoc on home life. Marital discord and domestic violence often exist in the presence of excess alcohol. Heavy drinking by parents is associated with abuse of their children, typically emotional or psychological abuse.

Alcohol and Sexual Decision Making   Alcohol seriously impairs a person's ability to make wise decisions about sex. Heavy drinkers are also more likely to have multiple sex partners and to engage in other forms of high-risk sexual behavior. Rates of sexually transmitted infections (including HIV) and unwanted pregnancy are higher among people who drink heavily than among people who drink moderately or not at all.

Drinking and Driving

In 2009, 10,839 Americans were killed in accidents involving drivers with a BAC of 0.08% or higher—close to one-third of all traffic fatalities for the year. Each year more than 275,000 people are injured in alcohol-related car crashes—an average of one person injured every two minutes. In the 2010 National Survey on Drug Use and Health, 15.1% of Americans aged 18–20 admitted driving under the influence of alcohol at least once.

People who drink are unable to drive safely because their judgment is impaired, their reaction time is slower, and their coordination is reduced. Some driving skills are affected at BACs of 0.02% and lower.

Alcoholic Energy Drinks: The Dangers of Being "Drunk and Wide Awake"

Over the past decade, the practice of blending alcoholic beverages with highly caffeinated energy drinks has grown increasingly popular, particularly among young adults and underage drinkers. According to the Centers for Disease Control and Prevention (CDC), 31% of 12- to 17-year-olds and 34% of 18- to 24-year-olds regularly drink caffeinated alcoholic beverages (CABs), also known as alcoholic energy drinks (AEDs). The caffeine in a CAB masks the depressant effects of the alcohol, producing a "drunk and wide awake" state of alert intoxication, potentially leading the drinker to consume more alcohol than he or she would otherwise. Caffeine does nothing to speed the metabolism of the alcohol by the liver.

More than 13,000 emergency department (ED) visits related to the highly caffeinated drinks were reported in 2009, according to researchers from the U.S. Substance Abuse and Mental Health Services Administration (SAMHSA). Nearly half the emergencies occurred after the beverages were mixed with alcohol or other drugs, and young adults aged 18 to 25 accounted for more than half of those cases, the researchers found.

Commercial CABs are typically malt- or distilled-spirits-based and have higher alcohol content than beer (5–12% alcohol by volume compared to 6–8% for beer). The amount of caffeine and other stimulants in a CAB is usually not reported by the manufacturer. Health officials are concerned that many CABs contain much higher levels of caffeine than are found in soft drinks, which are limited by the U.S. Food and Drug Administration (FDA) to 200 parts per million—the amount that meets the criteria for being "generally regarded as safe (GRAS)" for human consumption. However, SAMHSA researchers found some energy drinks that contained as much as 500 mg of caffeine—four to five times the amount in a cup of coffee.

A growing body of evidence highlights the risks associated with the use of caffeinated alcoholic beverages. For example, studies cited by the CDC have reported the following:

- Being in a "drunk/awake" state can lead to risky behaviors such as drunk driving, unplanned sex or sexual assault, and aggression.

- CAB drinkers are three times as likely as non-CAB drinkers to binge-drink.

- CAB drinkers are about twice as likely as non-CAB drinkers to report being taken advantage of sexually, taking advantage of someone sexually, or riding with a driver who was under the influence of alcohol.

- Emerging evidence indicates that CAB use, especially by adolescents, may lead to an increased risk of alcohol or drug dependence later in life.

These concerns and others led the FDA to launch an investigation into the safety, and even the legality, of commercial CABs. Prior to this investigation, two manufacturers of CABs voluntarily removed their products from the market and committed to discontinuing production of such beverages permanently. In light of this development, and skepticism among scientists that CABs can be proven safe, the CAB market may start to shrink—if not disappear altogether—in the near future.

SOURCES: Arria, A. M., et al. 2009. *Letter to the FDA Regarding the Use of Caffeine in Alcoholic Beverages* (http://www.fda.gov/downloads/food/foodingredientspackaging/ucm190372.pdf); Centers for Disease Control and Prevention. 2010. *Alcohol and Public Health: Caffeinated Alcoholic Beverages* (http://www.cdc.gov/alcohol/fact-sheets/cab.htm); U.S. Food and Drug Administration. 2010. Caffeinated Alcoholic Beverages (http://www.fda.gov/food/foodingredientspackaging/ucm190366.htm); U.S. Substance Abuse and Mental Health Services Administration, Center for Behavioral Health Statistics and Quality. 2011. *The DAWN Report: Emergency Department Visits Involving Energy Drinks.* Rockville, MD: SAMHSA (http://www.samhsa.gov/data/2k11/web_dawn_089/web_dawn_089_html.pdf).

The *dose-response function* is the relationship between the amount of alcohol or drug consumed and the type and intensity of the resulting effect. Higher doses of alcohol are associated with a much greater probability of automobile crashes (Figure 8.2). A person driving with a BAC of 0.14% is over 40 times more likely to be involved in a crash than someone with no alcohol in his or her blood.

In addition to an increased risk of injury and death, driving while intoxicated can have serious legal consequences. Drunk driving is against the law. The legal limit for BAC is 0.08% in all states, the District of Columbia, and Puerto Rico. Stiff penalties for drunk driving include fines, loss of license, confiscation of vehicle, and jail time. Under current zero-tolerance laws in many states, drivers under age 21 who have consumed *any* alcohol may have their licenses suspended.

If you are out of your home and drinking, find alternative transportation or appoint a *designated driver* who doesn't drink and can provide safe transportation home.

It's more difficult to protect yourself against someone else who drinks and drives. Learn to be alert to the erratic driving that signals an impaired driver. Warning signs include wide, abrupt, and illegal turns; straddling the center line or lane marker; driving against traffic; driving on the shoulder; weaving, swerving, or nearly striking objects or other vehicles; following too closely; erratic speed; driving with headlights off at night; and driving with the windows down in very cold weather. If you see any of these signs in another driver, avoid that vehicle by pulling off the road or turning at the nearest intersection. Report the driver to the police.

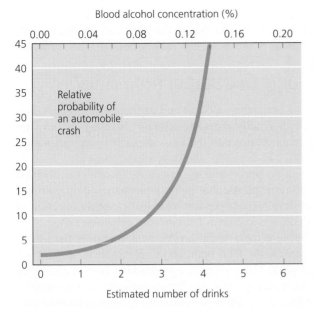

FIGURE 8.2 **The dose-response relationship between BAC and automobile crashes.**

The graph shows:
- Top axis: Blood alcohol concentration (%), ranging from 0.00, 0.04, 0.08, 0.12, 0.16, 0.20
- Y-axis: Relative probability of an automobile crash, ranging from 0 to 45
- Bottom axis: Estimated number of drinks, ranging from 0 to 6

The Long-Term Effects of Chronic Misuse

Because alcohol is distributed throughout most of the body, it affects many different organs and tissues (Figure 8.3).

The Digestive System Even in the short term, alcohol can alter the functioning of the liver. Within just a few days of heavy alcohol consumption, fat begins to accumulate in liver cells, resulting in the development of "fatty liver." If drinking continues, inflammation of the liver can occur, resulting in alcoholic hepatitis, a frequent cause of hospitalization and death in alcoholics. Both fatty liver and alcoholic hepatitis are potentially reversible if the person stops drinking. With continued alcohol use, however, liver cells are progressively damaged and then destroyed. The destroyed cells are replaced by fibrous scar tissue, a condition known as **cirrhosis.** People with cirrhosis who continue to drink have only a 50% chance of surviving five or more years.

> **cirrhosis** A disease in which the liver is severely damaged by alcohol, other toxins, or infection.
>
> **TERMS**

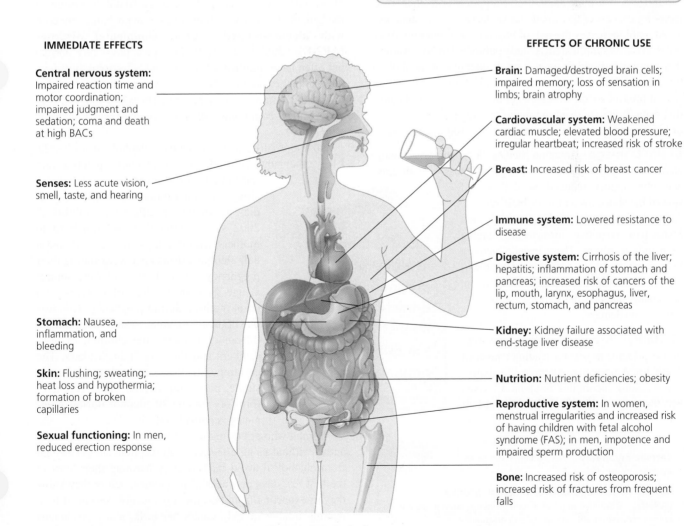

IMMEDIATE EFFECTS

Central nervous system: Impaired reaction time and motor coordination; impaired judgment and sedation; coma and death at high BACs

Senses: Less acute vision, smell, taste, and hearing

Stomach: Nausea, inflammation, and bleeding

Skin: Flushing; sweating; heat loss and hypothermia; formation of broken capillaries

Sexual functioning: In men, reduced erection response

EFFECTS OF CHRONIC USE

Brain: Damaged/destroyed brain cells; impaired memory; loss of sensation in limbs; brain atrophy

Cardiovascular system: Weakened cardiac muscle; elevated blood pressure; irregular heartbeat; increased risk of stroke

Breast: Increased risk of breast cancer

Immune system: Lowered resistance to disease

Digestive system: Cirrhosis of the liver; hepatitis; inflammation of stomach and pancreas; increased risk of cancers of the lip, mouth, larynx, esophagus, liver, rectum, stomach, and pancreas

Kidney: Kidney failure associated with end-stage liver disease

Nutrition: Nutrient deficiencies; obesity

Reproductive system: In women, menstrual irregularities and increased risk of having children with fetal alcohol syndrome (FAS); in men, impotence and impaired sperm production

Bone: Increased risk of osteoporosis; increased risk of fractures from frequent falls

FIGURE 8.3 **The immediate and long-term effects of alcohol misuse.**

Alcohol can inflame the pancreas, causing nausea, vomiting, abnormal digestion, and severe pain. Unlike cirrhosis, which usually occurs after years of heavy alcohol use, pancreatitis can occur after one or two severe binge-drinking episodes. Acute pancreatitis is often fatal; in survivors it can become a chronic condition.

The Cardiovascular System   The effects of alcohol on the cardiovascular system depend on the amount of alcohol consumed. Moderate doses of alcohol—one drink or less a day for women and one to two drinks a day for men—may reduce the risk of heart disease and heart attack in some people. (The possible health benefits of alcohol are discussed later in this chapter.) However, higher doses of alcohol harm the cardiovascular system. In some people, more than two drinks a day will elevate blood pressure, making stroke and heart attack more likely. Some alcoholics show a weakening of the heart muscle, a condition known as **cardiac myopathy.** Binge drinking can cause "holiday heart," a syndrome characterized by serious abnormal heart rhythms, which usually appear within 24 hours of a binge episode.

Cancer   In 2000 the U.S. Department of Health and Human Services added alcoholic beverages to its list of known human carcinogens. Chronic alcohol consumption is a clear risk factor for cancers of the mouth, throat, larynx, and esophagus.

Alcohol increases the risk of breast cancer, but quantifying the risk is complicated. A study published in 2011 shows that regularly drinking even a small quantity of alcohol—three to six drinks a week—could significantly increase the risk of breast cancer. Research conducted in 2009 indicates that even moderate drinking may encourage the recurrence of breast cancer in women who have survived the disease.

Brain Damage   Imaging studies document that many alcoholics experience brain shrinkage with loss of both gray and white matter, reduced blood flow, and slowed metabolic rates in some brain regions. About half of the alcoholics in the United States have cognitive impairments, ranging from mild to severe. These include memory loss, dementia, and compromised problem-solving and reasoning abilities. Malnutrition, particularly thiamine deficiency, contributes to severe brain damage.

Mortality   Excessive alcohol consumption is a factor in several leading causes of death for Americans. Average life expectancy among alcoholics is about 15 years less than among nonalcoholics. About half

the deaths caused by alcohol are due to chronic conditions such as cirrhosis and cancer; the other half are due to acute conditions or events such as car crashes, falls, and suicide.

Alcohol Use during Pregnancy

During pregnancy, alcohol and its metabolic product acetaldehyde readily cross the placenta, harming the developing fetus. Damage to the fetus depends on the amount of alcohol consumed and the stage of the pregnancy. Early in pregnancy, heavy drinking can cause spontaneous abortion or miscarriage. Alcohol in early pregnancy, during critical fetal development periods, can also cause a collection of birth defects known as *fetal alcohol syndrome (FAS)*.

Because rapid brain development continues throughout pregnancy, the fetal brain stays vulnerable to alcohol use until birth. Although effects of drinking later in pregnancy do not typically cause the characteristic physical deformities of FAS, getting drunk just once during the final three months of pregnancy can damage a fetal brain.

FAS is a permanent, incurable condition that causes life-long disability; it is among the most common preventable causes of intellectual disability in the Western world. Full-blown FAS occurs in up to 15 of every 10,000 live births in the United States. About three times as many babies are born with **alcohol-related neurodevelopmental disorder (ARND).** Children with ARND appear physically normal but often have significant learning and behavioral disorders. As adults, they are more likely to develop substance use disorders and to have criminal records. The whole range of FAS and ARND is commonly called *fetal alcohol spectrum disorder (FASD)*.

No one is sure exactly how much alcohol causes FASD. Like other untoward effects of alcohol, genetics and individual differences in metabolism, along with environmental factors such as diet, are thought to affect vulnerability. A 2002 study found that children born to mothers who drank as little as one and a half alcoholic drinks per week during their pregnancy weighed less and were shorter at age 14 than children of mothers who drank nothing during pregnancy. This was one of the first studies to show a significant difference between the children of non-drinkers and those of light drinkers. The children's smaller size may be a marker for subtle, persistent alcohol damage. Therefore, no amount of alcohol during pregnancy is considered safe.

Women who are trying to conceive, or who are sexually active without using effective contraception, should abstain from alcohol to avoid inadvertently harming their fetus in the first few days or weeks of pregnancy, before they know they're expecting. And because any alcohol consumed by a nursing mother quickly enters her milk, many physicians advise nursing mothers to abstain from drinking alcohol.

> QUICK STATS
>
> **12.2%** (about one in eight) of pregnant women drink alcohol, and almost **2%** (about 1 in 50) are binge drinkers.
>
> —CDC, 2012

cardiac myopathy   Weakening of the heart muscle through disease.   TERMS

alcohol-related neurodevelopmental disorder (ARND)   Cognitive and behavioral problems seen in people whose mothers drank alcohol during pregnancy.

Have you ever witnessed or been involved in an alcohol emergency? Did you think the situation was urgent at the time? What were the circumstances surrounding the event? How did the people involved deal with it?

Possible Health Benefits of Alcohol

Numerous studies have shown that, on average, light to moderate drinkers (no more than one drink per day for women, and two drinks per day for men) live longer than either abstainers or heavy drinkers.

The benefits of drinking alcohol relate to heart health. Young adults who drink *any* amount of alcohol are more likely to die than nondrinkers of the same age. By contrast, alcohol consumption appears to confer health benefits primarily to older individuals. The clearest evidence of benefit relates to coronary heart disease (CHD). The lowest rates of CHD deaths occur with moderate alcohol use, which in studies show a positive effect on both healthy people and individuals at risk for CHD. In a 2006 study of men age 50 and over, those who drank moderately each day reduced their risk of CHD by about 40% compared to men who never drank. The difference was not as great in women. Moderate drinking may improve heart health by raising blood levels of HDL (the beneficial form of cholesterol), by thinning the blood, and by reducing inflammation and the risk of dangerous blood clots, all of which can contribute to the risk of a heart attack. Some evidence also suggests that moderate drinkers may be less likely to develop or better able to manage a variety of other conditions, including diabetes, high blood pressure, strokes, arterial blockages in the legs, cognitive decline (including Alzheimer's disease), and benign prostrate enlargement.

EXCESSIVE USE OF ALCOHOL

The *DSM-5* is refocusing general understanding of excessive alcohol use. It diagnoses behavior based on a continuum of mild, moderate, severe, and extreme. Rather than using the terms "alcoholic" or "nonalcoholic," the *DSM-5* prefers **alcoholic use disorder.** If a person meets two of the following criteria, s/he has at least a mild disorder. Greater than four criteria indicate alcoholism or a severe alcohol use disorder:

1. Alcohol is often consumed in large amounts over a long period.
2. Unsuccessful efforts to control alcohol use.
3. Excessive time spent in using alcohol or recovering from its effects.
4. A strong desire or craving to use alcohol.
5. Persistent alcohol use causing a failure to fulfill obligations at work, school, or home.
6. Continued alcohol use despite recurrent physical or psychological problems caused by the effects of alcohol.
7. Important social or recreational activities reduced because of alcohol use.
8. Persistent alcohol use in situations that are physically risky.
9. A need for increased amounts of alcohol to achieve a desired effect (increased tolerance).
10. Symptoms of withdrawal, such as sweating, increased pulse rate, hand tremor, insomnia, nausea, and anxiety.

According to the National Survey on Drug Abuse and Health for 2012 almost 7% of Americans were classified as heavy alcohol users. Excessive alcohol use is responsible for 80,000 deaths per year among Americans and is the third leading lifestyle-related cause of death.

Alcohol Use Disorder: From Mild to Extreme

Severe *alcohol use disorder,* or **alcoholism,** involves more extensive problems with alcohol use, usually involving physical tolerance and withdrawal.

How can you tell if you or someone you know has serious problems with alcohol? Look for the following warning signs:

- Drinking alone or secretively
- Using alcohol deliberately and repeatedly to perform or get through difficult situations
- Using alcohol as a way to "self-medicate" in order to dull strong emotions or negative feelings
- Feeling uncomfortable on certain occasions when alcohol is not available
- Escalating alcohol consumption beyond an already established drinking pattern
- Consuming alcohol heavily in risky situations, such as before driving
- Getting drunk regularly or more frequently than in the past
- Drinking in the morning

---

alcoholic use disorder   Misuse of alcohol that leads to clinically significant impairment.

alcoholism   A pathological use of alcohol or impairment in functioning due to alcohol; characterized by tolerance of alcohol and withdrawal symptoms.

TERMS

Binge Drinking

Binge drinking is a pattern of rapid, periodic drinking that brings a person's blood alcohol concentration up to 0.08% or higher, typically with five or fewer drinks for men, or four drinks for women, typically within about two hours.

Among Americans under 21 years old, most drinking occurs in the form of bingeing, and over 90% of the alcohol they drink is consumed while binge drinking. Over half the alcohol consumed by all adults in the United States is downed during binge drinking.

Binge drinking profoundly affects students' lives (see the box "College Binge Drinking"). Frequent binge drinkers are three to seven times more likely than non–binge drinkers to engage in unplanned or unprotected sex, to drive after drinking, and to get hurt or injured (Table 8.1). Binge drinkers are also more likely to miss classes, fall behind in schoolwork, and argue with friends. The more frequent the binges, the more problems these students encounter.

Alcoholism

Alcoholism (or alcohol dependence) is usually characterized by tolerance to alcohol and withdrawal symptoms when consumption stops.

Patterns and Prevalence   Alcoholism occurs among people of all ethnic groups and at all socioeconomic levels.

There are different patterns of excessive alcohol misuse, including these four common ones:

- Regular daily intake of large amounts.
- Regular heavy drinking limited to weekends.
- Long periods of sobriety interspersed with binges of daily heavy drinking lasting for weeks or months.
- Heavy drinking limited to periods of stress.

Once established, alcoholism often exhibits a pattern of exacerbations and remissions. Alcoholism is not hopeless, however; many alcoholics achieve permanent abstinence.

Health Effects   *Tolerance* means that a drinker needs more alcohol to achieve intoxication or the desired effect, that the effects of continued use of the same amount of alcohol are diminished, or that the drinker can function adequately at doses or a BAC that would produce significant impairment in a casual user. Heavy users of alcohol may need to consume about 50% more than they originally needed in order to experience the same degree of intoxication.

Withdrawal symptoms include trembling hands (shakes or jitters), a rapid pulse and accelerated breathing rate, insomnia, nightmares, anxiety, and gastrointestinal upset.

More severe withdrawal symptoms occur in about 5% of alcoholics. These include seizures (sometimes called "rum fits"), confusion, and **hallucinations** such as seeing visions or hearing voices. Still less common is **delirium tremens (the DTs)**, a medical emergency characterized by severe disorientation, confusion, epileptic-like seizures, and vivid hallucinations, often of vermin and small animals. The mortality rate from DTs can be as high as 15%.

Alcoholics face all the physical health risks associated with intoxication and chronic drinking described earlier in the chapter. Some damage is compounded by nutritional deficiencies that often accompany alcoholism. A mental problem associated with alcohol use is profound memory gaps (commonly known as blackouts).

VITAL STATISTICS		
Table 8.1	**The Effects of Binge Drinking on College Students**	

	PERCENTAGE OF STUDENTS EXPERIENCING PROBLEMS	
ALCOHOL-RELATED PROBLEM	NON-BINGE DRINKERS	FREQUENT BINGE DRINKERS
Drove after drinking alcohol	18	58
Did something they regretted	17	62
Argued with friends	10	43
Engaged in unplanned sex	9	41
Missed a class	9	60
Got behind in schoolwork	9	42
Had unprotected sex	4	21
Got hurt or injured	4	28
Got into trouble with police	2	14
Had five or more of these problems since school year began	4	48

SOURCE: Wechsler, H., and B. Wuethrich. 2003. *Dying to Drink: Confronting Binge Drinking on College Campuses*, reprint ed. Emmaus, PA: Rodale.

binge drinking   Periodically drinking alcohol to **TERMS** the point of severe intoxication: about four drinks (for women) and five drinks (for men) consumed within a period of about two hours.

hallucination   A false perception that does not correspond to external reality, such as seeing visions or hearing voices that are not there.

delirium tremens (the DTs)   A state of confusion brought on by the reduction of alcohol intake in an alcohol-dependent person; other symptoms are sweating, trembling, anxiety, hallucinations, and seizures.

Although college binge drinking has been a serious problem for decades, it has recently come under a harsh spotlight due largely to highly publicized alcohol-related tragedies on campus. Deaths from alcohol overdose, alcohol-related injuries (including those from motor vehicle crashes), violent crimes, student riots, and serious vandalism have all drawn attention to the epidemic of heavy drinking on college campuses.

Drinking on campus is pervasive. Approximately 61% of college students report having drunk alcohol at least once in the past month. According to the 2008 National Survey on Drug Use and Health, nearly 41% of college students reported binge drinking at least once in the past month, and 16% reported being heavy drinkers.

Every year, more than 1,800 college students aged 18–24 die from alcohol-related injuries. Another 600,000 sustain unintentional alcohol-related injuries, 700,000 are assaulted by other students who have been drinking, and 100,000 are victims of alcohol-related date rape or sexual assault.

These statistics have shocked many students, administrators, and parents into demanding changes in college attitudes and policies regarding alcohol. In response, the Task Force of the National Advisory Council on Alcohol Abuse and Alcoholism was formed. Its report documents the extent of the alcohol problem and is a call to action for colleges and their surrounding communities to reexamine their alcohol policies and overhaul the campus drinking culture. These efforts, according to the Task Force, must focus on three levels:

1. Ultimately *each student* is accountable and must take responsibility for his or her own behavior. Programs that encourage and support development of healthy attitudes toward alcohol are needed. These programs should target students at increased risk of developing alcohol problems: first-year students, Greek organization members, and athletes. Treatment should be readily available for problem drinkers.

2. The *student body as a whole* must work to discourage

alcohol abuse. These efforts include promoting alcohol-free activities, reducing availability of alcohol, and avoiding social and commercial promotion of alcohol on campus. There should be an environment of acceptance of students who choose to abstain, and disapproval of students who drink to excess. Fraternities, sororities, eating clubs, and other campus organizations should be held accountable for inappropriate alcohol use, especially involving underage students, that takes place on their premises.

3. *Colleges and surrounding communities* must cooperate to discourage excessive drinking. College administrators, law enforcement, bar and liquor store owners, residents who live near campus, and the court system must all do their part to reduce the availability of cheap alcohol and to enforce existing laws. Those who enable students to drink irresponsibly must be held accountable.

In 2007 the U.S. Surgeon General's Call to Action to Prevent and Reduce Underage Drinking suggested (1) eliminating alcohol sponsorship of athletic events and other social activities; (2) implementing responsible alcohol policies; and (3) possibly restricting sale of alcohol at campus facilities such as sports stadiums, campus pubs, and concert halls.

Some schools have attempted to shift classes to Fridays and even Saturdays after it was found that binge drinking increases when students don't have Friday classes. Increasingly, incoming students are required to take a three-hour online class about alcohol. And there is stricter punishment for underage drinking and public drunkenness on some campuses, with the likelihood of suspension for repeat offenders.

Many colleges ban ads for alcoholic drinks in college newspapers and during broadcasts of college athletic events. Flyers, posters, and other promotions for cheap drinks, such as two-for-one specials, happy hours, all you can drink, and ladies' night, are banned on many campuses. In these college communities, bars and restaurants that cater to students are discouraged from offering cheap alcohol incentives.

Social and Psychological Effects Alcohol use causes more serious social and psychological problems than all other forms of drug abuse combined. For every person who is an alcoholic, another three or four people are directly affected.

Alcoholics frequently suffer mental disorders in addition to their substance dependence. Alcoholics are much more likely than nonalcoholics to suffer from clinical depression, panic disorder, schizophrenia, borderline personality disorder, and antisocial personality disorders. People with anxiety or panic attacks may try to use alcohol to lessen their anxiety, even though alcohol often makes these disorders worse. Alcoholics also often have other substance misuse problems.

Causes of Alcoholism The precise causes of alcoholism are unknown, but many factors are probably involved. Some studies suggest that as much as 50–60% of a person's risk for alcoholism is determined by genetic factors. Not all children of alcoholics become alcoholic, however, and it is clear that other factors are involved. A person's risk of developing alcoholism may be increased by having certain personality disorders, having grown up in a violent or otherwise troubled household, and imitating the alcohol abuse of peers and other role models. People who begin drinking excessively in their teens are especially prone to binge drinking and alcoholism later in life.

Treatment Some alcoholics recover without professional help. How often this occurs is unknown, but possibly as many as one-third stop drinking on their own or reduce their drinking enough to eliminate problems.

Most alcoholics, however, require a treatment program of some kind in order to stop drinking. Many different kinds of programs exist. No single treatment works for everyone, so a person may have to try different programs before finding the right one.

One of the oldest and best-known recovery programs is Alcoholics Anonymous (AA). In many communities AA consists of self-help groups that meet several times each week and follow a 12-step program. Important steps for people in these programs include recognizing that they are "powerless over alcohol" and must seek help from a "higher power" to regain control of their lives. By verbalizing these steps, the alcoholic directly addresses the denial that is often prominent in alcoholism and other addictions. Many AA members have a sponsor of their choosing who is available by phone 24-hours a day for individual support and crisis intervention.

Other recovery approaches are available. Some, like Rational Recovery and Women for Sobriety, deliberately avoid any emphasis on higher spiritual powers. A more controversial approach to problem drinking is offered by the group Moderation Management, which encourages people to manage their drinking behavior by limiting intake or abstaining.

Al-Anon and Alateen are companion programs to AA for families and friends of alcoholics. In Al-Anon, spouses and others explore how they enable the alcoholic to drink by denying, rationalizing, or covering up his or her drinking and how they can change this codependent behavior.

Inpatient hospital rehabilitation is useful for some alcoholics, especially if they have serious medical or mental problems or if life stressors threaten to overwhelm them.

There are also several medical treatments for alcoholism.

• *Disulfiram* (Antabuse) inhibits the metabolic breakdown of acetaldehyde and causes patients to flush and feel ill when they drink, thus theoretically inhibiting impulse drinking.

> Alcohol treatment programs **achieve extended sobriety for about 50% of alcoholics** who participate.

• *Naltrexone* (ReVia, Depade) binds to a brain pleasure center that reduces the craving for alcohol and decreases its pleasant, reinforcing effects.

• *Injectable naltrexone* (Vivtrol) is a single monthly shot administered by a health professional.

• *Acamprosate* (Campral) helps people maintain abstinence after they have stopped drinking.

Alcohol treatment programs are successful in achieving an extended period of sobriety for about half of those who participate. Success rates of conventional treatment programs are about the same for men and women and for people from different ethnic groups. AA remains the mainstay of treatment for most people and is often a component of even the most expensive treatment programs.

Gender and Ethnic Differences

Alcohol misusers come from all socioeconomic levels and cultural groups, but notable differences appear in drinking patterns between men and women and among different ethnic groups (Table 8.2).

	VITAL STATISTICS
Table 8.2	Users and Abusers of Alcohol in the United States by Demographic Characteristics: 2010

	PAST YEAR PREVALENCE (PERCENTAGE)	
	ALCOHOL USE	ALCOHOL ABUSE OR DEPENDENCE
Gender		
Male	69.4	9.5
Female	63.5	4.7
Ethnicity		
White	70.8	7.4
Black or African American	57.8	5.7
American Indian and Alaska Native	51.2	14.0
Native Hawaiian/Pacific Islander	N/A*	5.0
Asian American	55.6	3.2
Hispanic or Latino	58.8	7.6
Two or more races	62.8	7.4
Total Population	**66.4**	**7.0**

*N/A = Not available

SOURCE: Substance Abuse and Mental Health Services Administration. 2011. *Results from the 2010 National Survey on Drug Use and Health: Summary of National Findings*, NSDUH Series H-41, HHS Publication No. (SMA) 11-4658. Rockville, MD: SAMHSA.

Men   Men are more likely than women to drink alcohol, to misuse alcohol, and to develop an alcohol use disorder. Among white American men, excessive drinking often begins in the teens or 20s and progresses gradually through the 30s until the man is clearly identifiable as an alcoholic by the time he is in his late 30s or early 40s. Other men may remain controlled drinkers until later in life, sometimes becoming alcoholic in association with retirement, the loss of friends and loved ones, boredom, illness, or psychological disorders.

Women   Women tend to become alcoholic at later ages and with fewer years of heavy drinking. It is not unusual for women in their 40s or 50s to succumb to alcoholism after years of controlled drinking.

Women alcoholics develop cirrhosis and other medical complications more often and after a shorter period of heavier drinking than men, and have higher death rates—including deaths from cirrhosis—than male alcoholics. Female alcoholics are less likely to seek early treatment for drinking problems, possibly because of the social stigma attached to problem drinking. In addition, women may have an inherently greater biological risk for drinking alcohol.

African Americans   As a group, African Americans use less alcohol than most other groups (including European Americans), but they face disproportionately high levels of alcohol-related birth defects, cirrhosis, cancer, hypertension, and other medical problems. In addition, African Americans are more likely than members of other ethnic groups to be victims of alcohol-related homicides, criminal assaults, and injuries. African American women are more likely to abstain from alcohol use than white women, but among black women who drink there is a higher percentage of heavy drinkers.

AA groups of predominantly African Americans are effective, perhaps because essential elements of AA—sharing common experiences, mutual acceptance of one another as human beings, and trusting a higher power—are already a part of African American culture.

Latinos   Drinking patterns among Latinos vary significantly, depending on their specific cultural background and how long they and their families have lived in the United States. Drunk driving and cirrhosis are the most common causes of alcohol-related death and injury among Hispanic men. Hispanic women are more likely to abstain from alcohol than white or black women, but those who drink are at special risk for problems. Treating the entire family as a unit is an important part of treatment because family pride, solidarity, and support are important aspects of Latino culture.

Asian Americans   As a group, Asian Americans have lower-than-average rates of alcohol misuse. However, acculturation may somewhat weaken the generally strong Asian taboos and community sanctions against alcohol use. For many Asian Americans, though, the genetically based physiological aversion to alcohol remains a deterrent to misuse. Ethnic agencies, health care professionals, and ministers seem to be the most effective sources of treatment for members of this group, when needed.

Native Americans and Native Alaskans   Alcohol misuse is one of the most widespread and severe health problems among Native Americans and Native Alaskans, especially for adolescents and young adults. Excessive drinking varies from tribe to tribe but is generally high in both men and women. The rate of alcoholism among Native Americans is twice that of the general population, and the death rate from alcohol-related causes is about eight times higher. Treatment may be more effective if it reflects tribal values.

Helping Someone with an Alcohol Problem

Helping a friend or relative with an alcohol problem requires skill and tact. Start by making sure you are not enabling someone to continue excessively using alcohol. Enabling takes many forms, such as making excuses for the alcohol abuser—for example, saying "he has the flu" when it is really a hangover. Another important step is open, honest labeling—"I think you have a problem with alcohol." Such explicit statements usually elicit emotional rebuttals and may endanger a relationship. However, you are not helping your friends by allowing them to deny their problems with alcohol or other drugs. Taking action shows that you care. Even when problems are acknowledged, there is usually reluctance to get help. You can't cure a friend's drinking problem, but you can guide him or her to appropriate help. Your best role might be to obtain information about the available resources and persistently encourage their use.

WHO USES TOBACCO?

Rates of smoking vary based on gender, age, ethnicity, and education level (Table 8.3). According to the CDC National Health Interview Survey, 17.5% of Americans 18 and older were cigarette smokers in 2013. Young adults aged 18 to 25 had the highest rate of current tobacco product use (38.1%).

Table 8.3 — Who Smokes?

| | PERCENTAGE OF SMOKERS | | |
	MEN	WOMEN	TOTAL
Ethnic Group (Age ≥ 18)			
White	22.5	18.8	20.6
Black	24.2	15.5	19.4
Asian	14.9	5.5	9.9
American Indian/ Alaskan Native	34.4	29.1	31.5
Latino	17.0	8.6	12.9
Education (Age ≥ 25)			
≤ 8 years	20.0	9.9	15.0
9–11 years	40.3	29.2	34.6
12 years (no diploma)	29.4	20.9	25.1
GED	47.0	43.2	45.3
High school graduate	27.9	20.0	23.8
Associate degree	21.4	17.5	19.3
Undergraduate degree	9.8	8.7	9.3
Graduate degree	5.2	4.8	5.0
Total	**21.6**	**16.5**	**19.0**

SOURCE: Centers for Disease Control and Prevention. 2012. Vital signs: Current cigarette smoking among adults—United States, 2011. *Morbidity and Mortality Weekly Report* 61(44): 889–894.

Ask Yourself

QUESTIONS FOR CRITICAL THINKING AND REFLECTION

Do any of your friends or family members smoke or use smokeless tobacco? What effect has it had on their health and relationships? Have you ever discussed their tobacco use with them? Why or why not?

About 21.6% of men and 16.5% of women reported that they currently smoked cigarettes. Adults with less than a 12th-grade education were much more likely to smoke cigarettes than those with a college degree.

WHY PEOPLE USE TOBACCO

Although people start smoking for a variety of reasons, they usually become long-term smokers after becoming addicted to nicotine—the key psychoactive ingredient in tobacco smoke.

Nicotine Addiction

The primary reason why people continue to use **tobacco** is that they have become addicted to a powerful psychoactive drug: **nicotine.** Many researchers consider nicotine to be the most physically addictive of all the psychoactive drugs, including cocaine and heroin.

Some neurological studies indicate that nicotine acts on the brain in much the same way as cocaine and heroin. Nicotine reaches the brain via the bloodstream seconds after it is inhaled or, in the case of spit tobacco, absorbed through membranes of the mouth or nose. It triggers the release of powerful chemical messengers in the brain, including epinephrine, norepinephrine, and dopamine. But unlike street drugs, most of which are used to achieve a high, nicotine's primary attraction seems to lie in its ability to modulate everyday emotions.

At low doses, nicotine acts as a stimulant. It increases heart rate and blood pressure. In adults, nicotine can enhance alertness, concentration, information processing, memory, and learning. The opposite effect, however, occurs in teens who smoke; they show impairment in memory and other cognitive functions.

Loss of Control   About 69% of smokers say they want to quit completely, and about 52.4% of smokers try to quit each year. Regular tobacco users live according to a rigid cycle of need and gratification. On average, they can go no more than 40 minutes between doses of nicotine; otherwise they begin feeling edgy and irritable and have trouble concentrating. Tobacco users may plan their daily schedule around opportunities to satisfy their nicotine cravings; this loss of control and personal freedom can affect all the dimensions of wellness.

> **Spit tobacco users** maintain blood nicotine levels as high as those of cigarette smokers.

Tolerance and Withdrawal   Tobacco users build up tolerance to nicotine—a condition in which higher doses of nicotine are required to produce the same initial effect. Whereas one cigarette may make a beginning smoker nauseated and dizzy, a long-term smoker may have to chain-smoke a pack or more to experience the same effects. For most regular tobacco users, sudden abstinence from nicotine produces predictable withdrawal symptoms. These symptoms, which come on several hours after the last dose of nicotine, can include severe cravings, insomnia, confusion, tremors, difficulty concentrating, fatigue, muscle pains, headache, nausea, irritability, anger, and depression. Although most of these symptoms of physical dependence pass in two or three days, the craving associated with addiction persists. Even years after quitting, many ex-smokers report intermittent, intense urges to smoke.

Social and Psychological Factors

Social and psychological forces combine with physiological addiction to maintain the tobacco habit. Many people, for example, have established habits of smoking while doing

tobacco   The leaves of cultivated tobacco plants prepared for smoking, chewing, or use as snuff.

nicotine   A poisonous, addictive substance found in tobacco and responsible for many of the effects of tobacco.

TERMS

something else—while talking, working, drinking, and so on. The spit tobacco habit is also associated with certain situations—studying, drinking coffee, or playing sports. These associations can make it more difficult for users to break their habits because the activities they associate with tobacco use continue to trigger their urge.

Why Start in the First Place?

In the United States, nearly 90% of all adult smokers report that they started smoking before age 18. The average age for starting smokers and smokeless tobacco users is around 15. The earlier people begin smoking, the more likely they are to become heavy smokers—and to die of tobacco-related disease.

Young people start using tobacco for a variety of reasons. Many young, white, male athletes, for example, begin using spit tobacco to emulate professional athletes. Young women commonly take up smoking because they think it will help them lose weight or stay thin. Most often, however, young people start smoking simply because their peers are already doing it; smoking gives them a way to fit in with a crowd.

Rationalizing the Dangers Making the decision to smoke requires minimizing or denying the health risks of tobacco use. A sense of invincibility, characteristic of many adolescents and young adults, also contributes to the decision to use tobacco.

Many teenagers believe they can stop smoking when they want. In fact, adolescents are more vulnerable to nicotine than are older tobacco users. Compared with older smokers, adolescents become heavy smokers and develop dependence after fewer cigarettes. Nicotine addiction can start within a few days of smoking and after just a few cigarettes. In polls, about 75% of smoking teens state they wish they had never started.

Emulating Smoking in the Media
Both the Institute of Medicine and the National Cancer Institute have identified media portrayals of smoking as a key influence on young people who start smoking. In fact, studies by the National Cancer Institute have concluded that a direct causal relationship exists between media portrayals of smoking and actual smoking initiation by young moviegoers.

In general, the portrayal of smoking in films and television does not reflect U.S. patterns of tobacco use. The prevalence of smoking among lead characters is three to four times that among comparable Americans. Films typically show smokers as white, male, well educated, successful, and

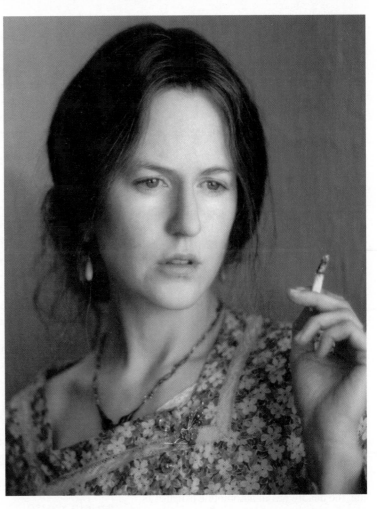

Films that feature actors such as Nicole Kidman smoking successfully advertise for the tobacco industry.

> After just a few cigarettes, nicotine addiction can start within a few days of smoking.

attractive. In reality, smokers tend to be poor and to have less education. Public campaigns to reduce images of smoking in movies have succeeded to an extent; smoking is shown less often in film and television shows now than even just a few years ago. Still, antismoking advocates say that films are still a critical and highly successful form of advertising for the tobacco industry.

HEALTH HAZARDS

Tobacco adversely affects nearly every part of the body, including the brain, stomach, mouth, and reproductive organs.

Tobacco Smoke: A Toxic Mix

Tobacco smoke contains thousands of chemical substances, several hundred of which are known to be harmful to humans, including acetone (nail polish remover), ammonia, hexamine (lighter fluid), and toluene (industrial solvent).

QUESTIONS FOR CRITICAL THINKING
AND REFLECTION

What has influenced your decision to smoke, not to smoke, or to quit smoking? Have you ever felt that images or messages in the media were encouraging you to use tobacco? How do you react to such messages?

Smoke from a typical unfiltered cigarette contains about 5 billion particles per cubic millimeter—50,000 times as many as are found in an equal volume of smoggy urban air. These particles, when condensed, form a brown, sticky mass called **cigarette tar.**

Carcinogens and Poisons   At least 69 chemicals in tobacco smoke are linked to the development of cancer. Some, such as benzo(a)pyrene and urethane, are **carcinogens**—that is, they directly cause cancer. Other chemicals, such as formaldehyde, are **cocarcinogens;** they do not themselves cause cancer but combine with other chemicals to stimulate the growth of certain cancers, at least in laboratory animals. Tobacco also contains poisonous substances, including arsenic and hydrogen cyanide. In addition to being an addictive psychoactive drug, nicotine is a poison that can be fatal in high doses.

Cigarette smoke contains carbon monoxide, the deadly gas in automobile exhaust, in concentrations 400 times greater than is considered safe in industrial workplaces. Carbon monoxide displaces oxygen in red blood cells, depleting the body's supply of oxygen needed for extra work. Carbon monoxide also impairs visual acuity, especially at night.

Additives   Tobacco manufacturers use additives to manipulate the taste and effect of cigarettes and other tobacco products. Additives account for roughly 10%, by weight, of a cigarette, and include sugars and other flavoring agents, humectants (compounds that keep tobacco from drying out), and chemicals that enhance the addicting properties of nicotine.

> **cigarette tar**   A brown, sticky mass created when the chemical particles in tobacco smoke condense.
>
> **carcinogen**   Any substance that causes cancer.
>
> **cocarcinogen**   A substance that works with a carcinogen to cause cancer.
>
> **sidestream smoke**   The uninhaled smoke from a burning cigarette.
>
> **cerebral cortex**   The outer layer of the brain, which controls complex behavior and mental activity.

TERMS

Other flavor components, such as theobromine and glycyrrhizin, act as bronchodilators, opening the lungs' airways and making it easier for nicotine to get into the bloodstream.

Some additives are intended to make **sidestream smoke** (the uninhaled smoke from a burning cigarette) less obvious and objectionable. Nearly 600 chemicals, approved as safe when used as food additives, but may form carcinogens when heated or burned."

"Reduced Harm" Cigarettes   Some smokers choose low-tar, low-nicotine, or filtered cigarettes because they believe them to be less dangerous alternatives. The tobacco industry has long promoted such products as "reduced harm" cigarettes, but there is no such thing as a safe cigarette. Smokers who switch to a low-nicotine brand often compensate by smoking more cigarettes, inhaling more deeply, taking larger or more frequent puffs, or blocking ventilation holes with lips or fingers to offset the effects of filters. In 2010 the use of terms like "light," "mild," or "low" on cigarette labels was banned by federal law.

Menthol Cigarettes   About 70% of African American smokers smoke menthol cigarettes, as compared to 30% of whites. Studies have found that African Americans absorb more nicotine than other groups and metabolize it more slowly; they also have lower rates of successful quitting. The anesthetizing effect of menthol, which may allow smokers to inhale more deeply and hold smoke in their lungs for a longer period, may be partly responsible for these differences.

> Federal law prohibits the use of terms such as "light" and "mild" on cigarette packaging.

The Immediate Effects of Smoking

The beginning smoker often has symptoms of mild nicotine poisoning, including the following: dizziness; faintness; rapid pulse; cold, clammy skin; nausea; vomiting and diarrhea.

The effects of nicotine on smokers vary, depending greatly on the size of the nicotine dose and how much tolerance one has built up through previous smoking. Nicotine can either excite or tranquilize the nervous system, depending on dosage.

Nicotine has many other immediate effects. It stimulates the part of the brain called the **cerebral cortex.** It also stimulates the adrenal glands to discharge adrenaline. Nicotine inhibits the formation of urine; constricts the blood vessels, especially in the skin; accelerates the heart rate; and elevates blood pressure. Smoking depresses hunger sensations and dulls the taste buds.

The Long-Term Effects of Smoking

Smoking is linked to many deadly and disabling diseases. Research indicates that the total amount of tobacco smoke inhaled is a key factor contributing to disease. People who smoke more cigarettes per day, inhale deeply, puff frequently, smoke cigarettes down to the butts, or begin smoking at early ages run a greater risk of disease than do those who smoke more moderately or who do not smoke at all.

Cardiovascular Disease Although lung cancer tends to receive the most publicity, one form of cardiovascular disease, **coronary heart disease (CHD),** is actually the most widespread single cause of death for cigarette smokers. CHD often results when the arteries that supply the heart muscle with blood develop **atherosclerosis.** In atherosclerosis, fatty deposits called **plaques** form on the inner walls of arteries, causing them to narrow and stiffen. Smoking and exposure to environmental tobacco smoke (ETS) permanently accelerate the rate of plaque accumulation in the coronary arteries—50% for smokers, 25% for ex-smokers, and 20% for people regularly exposed to ETS. The plaque completely blocks the flow of blood to a portion of the heart resulting in a type of heart attack called a **myocardial infarction.**

CHD can also interfere with the heart's electrical activity, resulting in disturbances of the normal heartbeat rhythm.

Smokers have a death rate from CHD that is 70% higher than that of nonsmokers. The risks of CHD decrease rapidly when a person stops smoking. This is particularly true for younger smokers, whose coronary arteries have not yet been extensively damaged. Cigarette smoking has been linked to other cardiovascular diseases, including the following:

• *Stroke:* a sudden interference with the circulation of blood in a part of the brain, resulting in the destruction of brain cells.

• *Aortic aneurysm:* a bulge in the aorta caused by a weakening in its walls.

• *Pulmonary heart disease:* a disorder of the right side of the heart, caused by changes in the blood vessels of the lungs.

Lung Cancer and Other Cancers Cigarette smoking is the primary cause of lung cancer. Those who smoke two or more packs of cigarettes a day have lung cancer death rates 12–25 times greater than those of nonsmokers. The dramatic rise in lung cancer rates among women in the past 40 years clearly parallels the increase of smoking in this group; lung cancer now exceeds breast cancer as the leading cause of cancer deaths among women. The risk of developing lung cancer increases with the number of cigarettes smoked each day and the number of years of smoking. Evidence suggests that after 1 year without smoking, the risk of lung cancer decreases substantially. After 10 years, the risk of lung cancer among ex-smokers is 50% lower than that of continuing smokers.

QUICK STATS

Smoking accounts for at least 30% of cancer deaths and 87% of all lung cancer deaths.
—American Cancer Society, 2013

Research has also linked smoking to cancers of the trachea, mouth, pharynx, esophagus, larynx, pancreas, bladder, kidney, breast, cervix, stomach, liver, colon, and skin.

Chronic Obstructive Pulmonary Disease A smoker's lungs are constantly exposed to dangerous chemicals and irritants, so they must work harder to function adequately. The stresses placed on the lungs by smoking can permanently damage lung function and lead t o *chronic obstructive pulmonary disease (COPD),* also known as chronic obstructive lung disease or chronic lower respiratory disease. COPD was the third leading cause of death in the United States in 2010 (the most recent year for which complete data are available). This progressive and disabling disorder consists of several different but related diseases; emphysema and chronic bronchitis are two of the most common.

Smoking is the primary cause of **emphysema,** a disabling condition in which the air sacs in the walls of the lungs lose their elasticity and are gradually destroyed. The lungs' ability to take in oxygen and expel carbon dioxide is impaired. A person with emphysema is often breathless, gasps for air, and has the feeling of drowning. The heart must pump harder and may become enlarged. People with emphysema often die from a damaged heart. There is no known way to reverse this disease.

Persistent, recurrent inflammation of the bronchial tubes characterizes **chronic bronchitis.** When the cell lining of the bronchial tubes is irritated, it secretes excess mucus. Bronchial congestion is followed by a chronic cough, which makes breathing more and more difficult. If smokers have chronic bronchitis, they face a greater risk of lung cancer, no matter how old they are or how many cigarettes they smoke. Chronic bronchitis seems to be a shortcut to lung cancer.

Even when the smoker shows no signs of lung impairment or disease, cigarette smoking damages the respiratory system. Normally the cells lining the bronchial tubes secrete *mucus*, a sticky fluid that collects particles of soot, dust, and other

TERMS

coronary heart disease (CHD) Cardiovascular disease caused by hardening of the arteries that supply oxygen to the heart muscle; also called *coronary artery disease.*

atherosclerosis Cardiovascular disease caused by the deposit of fatty substances (called *plaque*) in the walls of the arteries.

plaque A deposit on the inner wall of blood vessels; blood can coagulate around plaque and form a clot.

myocardial infarction A heart attack caused by the complete blockage of a main coronary artery.

emphysema A disease characterized by a loss of lung tissue elasticity and destruction of the air sacs, impairing the lungs' ability to take in oxygen and expel carbon dioxide.

chronic bronchitis Recurrent, persistent inflammation of the bronchial tubes.

substances in inhaled air. Mucus is carried up to the mouth by the continuous motion of *cilia*, which are hairlike structures that protrude from the inner surface of the bronchial tubes. If the cilia are destroyed or impaired, or if inhaled air contains more pollutants than the system can remove, the protection provided by cilia is lost.

Cigarette smoke first slows and then stops the action of the cilia. Eventually it destroys them, leaving delicate membranes exposed to injury from substances inhaled in cigarette smoke or from the polluted air. This interference with the functioning of the respiratory system often leads rapidly to the conditions known as *smoker's throat* and *smoker's cough,* as well as to shortness of breath. Even smokers of high school age show impaired respiratory function compared with nonsmokers of the sa me age. Other respiratory effects of smoking include a worsening of allergy and asthma symptoms and an increase in the smoker's susceptibility to colds.

Additional Health, Cosmetic, and Economic Concerns

People who smoke are more likely to develop peptic ulcers because smoking impairs the body's healing ability. Smoking also increases the risk of gastroesophageal reflux, which causes heartburn. Smoking affects blood flow in the veins and arteries of the penis and is an independent risk factor for erectile dysfunction. Smoking is linked to reduced fertility in both men and women. Smokers are at increased risk for tooth decay and gum and periodontal diseases, with symptoms appearing by the mid-20s. Smoking dulls the senses of taste and smell. Over time it increases the risk of hearing loss and of blindness. Smokers have higher rates of motor vehicle crashes, fire-related injuries, and back pain. Smoking can cause premature skin wrinkling, premature baldness, stained teeth, discolored fingers, and a persistent tobacco odor in clothes and hair. Smoking contributes to osteoporosis, increases the risk of complications from diabetes, and accelerates the course of multiple sclerosis. In September 2011 the average per-pack price of cigarettes was $5.62. A pack-a-day habit cost more than $2000 per year for cigarettes alone.

Cumulative Effects The cumulative effects of tobacco use fall into two general categories. The first category is reduced life expectancy. A male who takes up smoking before age 15 and continues to smoke is only half as likely to live to age 75 as a male who never smokes. Females who have similar smoking habits also have a reduced life expectancy.

The second category involves quality of life. A national health survey begun in 1964 shows that smokers spend one-third more time away from their jobs because of illness than nonsmokers.

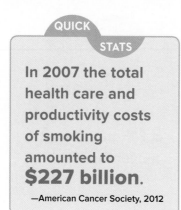

Both male and female smokers show a greater rate of acute and chronic disease than people who have never smoked. Smokers become disabled at younger ages than nonsmokers and have more years of unhealthy life as well as shorter life spans.

Gender Differences in Health Hazards As the rate of smoking among women approaches that of men (Figure 8.4), so do rates of tobacco-related illness and death. Although overall risks of tobacco-related illness are similar for women and men, sex appears to make a difference in some diseases. Women, for example, are more at risk for smoking-related blood clots and strokes than are men, and the risk is even greater for women using oral contraceptives. Among men and women with the same smoking history, the odds for developing three major types of cancer, including lung cancer, is 1.2–1.7 times higher in women than in men. Women who smoke have higher rates of osteoporosis (a bone-thinning disease that can lead to fractures), thyroid-related diseases, and depression than women who don't smoke.

Women who smoke also have risks associated with reproduction and the reproductive organs. Smoking is associated with greater menstrual bleeding, greater duration of painful menstrual cramps, and more variability in menstrual cycle length. Smokers have a more difficult time becoming pregnant, and when they do become pregnant, they face increased chances of miscarriage or placental disorders that lead to bleeding and premature delivery; rates of ectopic pregnancy, preeclampsia, and stillbirth are also higher among women who smoke. In addition, smoking is a risk factor for cervical cancer.

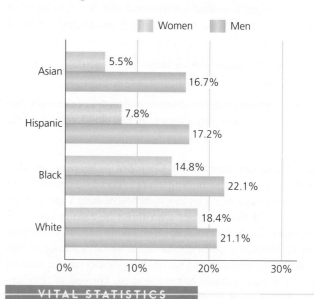

VITAL STATISTICS

FIGURE 8.4 Differences in smoking prevalence between American men and women by ethnicity/race, in 2012.

SOURCE: Agaku, I. T. 2014. Current cigarette smoking among adults—United States, 2005–2012. *Morbidity and Mortality Weekly Report* 63(02): 29–34, Centers for Disease Control and Prevention.

Other Forms of Tobacco Use

Many smokers have switched from cigarettes to other forms of tobacco, such as spit (smokeless) tobacco, cigars, pipes, clove cigarettes, bidis, hookahs, and e-cigarettes. These alternatives, however, are far from safe.

Spit (Smokeless) Tobacco   More than 8.2 million adults and about 7.7% of all high school students are current spit tobacco users, with a higher prevalence of current smokeless tobacco use among male (12.8%) than female (2.5%) students. About 80% of users start by the ninth grade.

Spit tobacco comes in two major forms: snuff and chewing tobacco (chew). In snuff, the tobacco leaf is processed into a coarse, moist powder and mixed with flavorings. Snuff is usually sold in small tins. Users place a wad of tobacco in their mouth and then chew or suck it to release the nicotine. All types of smokeless tobacco cause an increase in saliva production, and the resulting tobacco juice is spit out or swallowed.

The nicotine in spit tobacco—along with flavorings and additives—is absorbed through the gums and lining of the mouth. Holding an average-size dip in the mouth for 30 minutes delivers about the same amount of nicotine as two or three cigarettes. Because of its nicotine content, spit tobacco is highly addictive. Some users keep it in their mouth even while sleeping.

Although not as dangerous as smoking cigarettes, the use of spit tobacco carries many health risks. Gums and lips become dried and irritated and may bleed. White or red patches may appear inside the mouth; this condition, known as *leukoplakia,* can lead to oral cancer. About 25% of regular spit tobacco users have *gingivitis* (inflammation) and recession of the gums and bone loss around the teeth, especially where the tobacco is usually placed. The senses of taste and smell are usually dulled.

One of the most serious effects of spit tobacco is an increased risk of oral cancer—cancers of the lip, tongue, cheek, throat, gums, roof and floor of the mouth, and larynx. Spit tobacco contains at least 28 chemicals known to cause cancer, and long-term snuff use may increase the risk of oral cancer by as much as 50 times. Surgery to treat oral cancer is often disfiguring and may involve removing parts of the face, tongue, cheek, or lip.

Cigars and Pipes   Cigar smoking has increased steadily since the early 1990s. Cigars are most popular among white males aged 18–44 with higher-than-average income and education, but women are also smok ing cigars in record numbers. Cigar use is also growing among young people: In government surveys, 13% of American high school students reported having smoked at least one cigar in the previous month. Fewer than 1% of Americans, mostly males who also smoke cigarettes, are pipe smokers.

> A large cigar may contain **as much tobacco as a whole pack of cigarettes**.

Because cigar and pipe smoke is more alkaline than cigarette smoke, users of cigars and pipes do not need to inhale in order to ingest nicotine; instead they absorb nicotine through the gums and lining of the mouth. Cigars contain more tobacco than cigarettes and so contain more nicotine and produce more tar when smoked. Large cigars may contain as much tobacco as a whole pack of cigarettes and may take one or two hours to smoke.

The health risks of cigars depend on the number of cigars smoked and whether the smoker inhales. Because most cigar and pipe users do not inhale, they have a lower risk of cancer and cardiovascular and respiratory diseases than cigarette smokers. However, their risks are substantially higher than those of nonsmokers. For example, compared to nonsmokers, people who smoke one or two cigars per day without inhaling have 6 times the risk of cancer of the larynx. The risks are much higher for cigar smokers who inhale: They have 27 times the risk of oral cancer and 53 times the risk of cancer of the larynx compared to nonsmokers, and their risk of heart and lung diseases approaches that of cigarette smokers. Smoking a cigar immediately impairs the ability of blood vessels to dilate, reducing the amount of oxygen delivered to tissues, including the heart muscle, especially during stress. Pipe and cigar smoking are also risk factors for pancreatic cancer, which is almost always fatal.

Nicotine addiction is another concern. The recent rise in cigar use among teens has raised concerns because nicotine addiction almost always develops in the teen or young adult years. More research is needed to determine if cigar use by teens will develop into nicotine addiction and frequent use of either cigarettes or spit tobacco.

Clove Cigarettes and Bidis   Clove cigarettes, also called *kreteks* or *chicartas,* are made of tobacco mixed with chopped cloves; they are imported primarily from Indonesia and Pakistan. Clove cigarettes contain almost twice as much tar, nicotine, and carbon monoxide as conventional cigarettes and so present all the same health hazards. Some chemical constituents of cloves may also be dangerous. There have been a number of serious respiratory injuries and deaths from the use of clove cigarettes.

Bidis, or "beadies," are small cigarettes imported from India that contain species of tobacco different from those used by U.S. cigarette manufacturers. The tobacco in bidis is hand-rolled in Indian ebony leaves (tendu) and then often flavored; clove, mint, chocolate, and fruit varieties are available. Bidis contain up to four times more nicotine than U.S. cigarettes and twice as much tar.

Hookah   Hookahs—sometimes called water pipes or *shisha*—are pipes use for smoking specially flavored tobacco (e.g., apple, mint, cherry). The hookah has four main parts: the head, body, hose, and water urn. As the smoke is inhaled through the mouthpiece attached to the hose that passes through the water urn, the water cools the smoke and emits it as vapor.

Although cigarette smoking has decreased among high school and college students, hookah smoking has increased.

Although it originated in ancient Persia and India, hookah use has gained popularity around the globe in recent years. In 2006 an estimated 300 hookah bars operated in the United States; since then the number has grown and continues to grow.

The 2014 Monitoring the Future Survey among 12th grade students found that 21.4% of high school seniors in the United States had used hookahs in 2013, up significantly from 17.1% in 2010. Hookah smoking increased also among college students in the United States, ranging from 22% to 40% of students.

> **environmental tobacco smoke (ETS)** Smoke that enters the atmosphere from the burning end of a cigarette, cigar, or pipe, as well as smoke that is exhaled by smokers; also called *secondhand smoke*.
>
> **TERMS**

Hookah smoking carries many of the same health risks as cigarette smoking; it is therefore *not* a safe alternative. In fact, due to the mode of smoking (inhalation), hookah smokers may absorb higher concentrations of the toxins commonly found in cigarette smoke. One hour of hookah smoking involves 200 puffs, whereas an average cigarette involves 20 puffs. The volume of smoke inhaled during a typical hookah session is about 90,000 milliliters (ml), compared with 500–600 ml inhaled when smoking a cigarette.

E-Cigarettes The electronic cigarette, also known as an *e-cig,* is a battery-powered device that resembles a real cigarette. Instead of containing tobacco, the device uses a changeable filter that contains one or more chemicals, such as nicotine, flavorings, and other compounds. The user "smokes" an e-cig by sucking the filtered end; the device's battery heats the chemicals to create an inhalable vapor. During use, the device's tip even glows like the burning end of a real cigarette.

Although electronic cigarettes have been advertised as a way to help smokers quit smoking, no evidence submitted to the Food and Drug Administration (FDA) supports this claim. In fact, according to scientists from the Roswell Park Cancer Institute, electronic cigarettes get hot enough to produce carcinogens and other toxic chemicals like formaldehyde, also found in traditional cigarettes, or diethylene glycol, which is a toxic chemical in antifreeze.

Marketers of e-cigs have claimed that the devices deliver only nicotine, making them a safe cigarette that does not cause cancer and can serve as an alternative to other nicotine replacement products such as gum and patches. According to the FDA, however, not all e-cigs actually contain nicotine. Further, the FDA has warned that some varieties of e-cigs are flavored, apparently to make them appeal to teenagers and other first-time smokers. The products do not carry the same types of warnings required on tobacco products. Eight senators have called on the FDA to focus on the harmful vapors that e-cigs produce as well as the ingredients they contain. New York City, Chicago, and Los Angeles have recently banned e-cigarettes from some private and public places.

THE EFFECTS OF SMOKING ON THE NONSMOKER

Tobacco users aren't the only ones who suffer ill effects. Tens of thousands of nonsmokers die each year because of exposure to secondhand smoke. Further, the medical and societal costs of tobacco use are enormous.

Environmental Tobacco Smoke

The U.S. Environmental Protection Agency (EPA) has designated **environmental tobacco smoke (ETS)**—more commonly called *secondhand smoke*—a Class A carcinogen. The Surgeon General has concluded that there is no safe level of exposure to ETS; even brief exposure can cause serious harm.

What antismoking ordinances are in effect in your community? Does your school prohibit smoking on campus? Do you think these rules have been effective in reducing smoking or exposure to ETS? Do you support such regulations? Why or why not?

Millions of American infants and children are regularly exposed to environmental tobacco smoke.

Environmental tobacco smoke consists of mainstream smoke and sidestream smoke. Smoke exhaled by smokers is referred to as **mainstream smoke.** Sidestream smoke enters the atmosphere from the burning end of a cigarette, cigar, or pipe. Nearly 85% of the smoke in a room where someone is smoking comes from sidestream smoke. Undiluted sidestream smoke, because it is not filtered through either a cigarette filter or a smoker's lungs, has twice as much tar and nicotine, three times as much benzo(a)pyrene, almost three times as much carbon monoxide, and three times as much ammonia.

In rooms where people are smoking, levels of carbon monoxide can exceed those permitted by Federal Air Quality Standards for outside air. In a typical home with the windows closed, it takes about six hours for 95% of the airborne cigarette smoke particles to clear. The carcinogens in the secondhand smoke from a single cigar exceed those of three cigarettes, and cigar smoke contains up to 30 times more carbon monoxide.

ETS Effects Nonsmokers subjected to ETS frequently develop coughs, headaches, nasal discomfort, and eye irritation. Other symptoms range from breathlessness to sinus problems. People with allergies tend to suffer the most.

ETS causes 3400 lung cancer deaths and about 46,000 deaths from heart disease each year in people who do not smoke. ETS aggravates asthma and increases the risk for breast and cervical cancers.

Scientists have been able to measure changes that contribute to lung tissue damage and potential tumor promotion in the bloodstreams of healthy young test subjects who spend just three hours in a smoke-filled room. After just 30 minutes of exposure to ETS, the function in the coronary arteries of healthy nonsmokers is reduced to the same level as that of smokers.

Infants, Children, and ETS Infants and children are perhaps the most vulnerable group to the harmful effects of ETS. Recent studies have shown that infants exposed to smoke from more than 21 cigarettes a day are more than *23 times* more likely to die of sudden infant death syndrome (SIDS) than are babies not exposed to ETS. Chemicals in

> According to the U.S. Surgeon General, **there is no safe level of exposure to secondhand smoke.**

tobacco smoke also show up in breast milk, and breastfeeding may pass more chemicals to the infant of a smoking mother than direct exposure to ETS.

ETS triggers bronchitis, pneumonia, and other respiratory infections in infants and toddlers up to age 18 months, resulting in as many as 15,000 hospitalizations each year.

Older children suffer, too. ETS is a risk factor for asthma and aggravates the symptoms of children who already have asthma. ETS is also linked to reduced lung function and fluid buildup in the middle ear, a contributing factor in middle-ear infections, a leading reason for childhood surgery. Children and teens exposed to ETS score lower on tests of reading and reasoning. Later in life, people exposed to ETS as children are at increased risk for lung cancer, emphysema, and chronic bronchitis.

Smoking and Pregnancy

Smoking almost doubles a pregnant woman's chance of having a miscarriage, and it significantly increases her risk of ectopic pregnancy. Maternal smoking causes hundreds of infant deaths in the United States each year, primarily due to premature delivery and smoking-related problems with the placenta. Maternal smoking is a major factor in low birth weight, which puts newborns at high risk for infections and other serious problems. If a nonsmoking mother is regularly exposed to ETS, her infant is also at greater risk for low birth weight.

mainstream smoke Smoke that is inhaled by a smoker and then exhaled into the atmosphere. **TERMS**

Babies born to mothers who smoke more than two packs a day perform poorly on developmental tests in the first hours after birth, compared to babies of nonsmoking mothers. Later in life, obesity, hyperactivity, short attention span, and lower scores on spelling and reading tests all occur more frequently in children whose mothers smoked during pregnancy than in those born to nonsmoking mothers. Prenatal tobacco exposure has also been associated with behavioral problems in children.

WHAT CAN BE DONE?

There are many ways to act against this public health threat.

Action at Many Levels

Thousands of local ordinances across the nation now restrict or ban smoking in restaurants, stores, workplaces, and even public outdoor spaces. An assessment made in 2010 found that nearly 80% of Americans live in municipalities that restrict or ban smoking in public buildings, workplaces, restaurants, and bars. Hundreds of colleges and universities now have totally smoke-free campuses or prohibit smoking in residential buildings. As local nonsmoking laws proliferate, evidence mounts that environmental restrictions are effective in encouraging smokers to quit.

At the state level, many tough antitobacco laws have been passed. As of January 2012, comprehensive smoke-free air laws were in effect in 35 states, the District of Columbia, and Puerto Rico. California has one of the most aggressive—and successful—tobacco control programs, combining taxes on cigarettes, graphic advertisements, and bans on smoking in bars and restaurants.

Regulation of Tobacco

Until 2009, the U.S. FDA did not have the power to regulate tobacco products. That changed when Congress passed the Family Smoking Prevention and Tobacco Control Act, which gives the agency the power to dictate how much nicotine is included in tobacco products. Under this law the FDA can eliminate or control levels of the thousands of chemical additives used to make tobacco more appealing and addictive. In addition, the legislation strengthens health warnings and places even greater limits on tobacco advertising, both of which have had a significant impact on smoking prevalence. In Canada, larger graphic warnings on cigarette labels have resulted in an estimated 12–20% reduction in smoking rates between 2000 and 2009.

The World Health Organization has taken the lead in international anti-tobacco efforts by sponsoring the Framework Convention on Tobacco Control. Another international activity is the annual commemoration of World No Tobacco Day (May 31), on which smokers are encouraged to stop smoking for one day.

Such local, state, national, and international efforts represent progress, but health activists warn that tobacco industry influence remains strong. The tobacco industry contributes heavily to sympathetic legislative officeholders and candidates, spending millions on federal lobbying activities. The tobacco industry has also focused increasing attention on the developing world, exporting its products to countries where there are few or no consumer protection laws in place.

Individual Action

Nonsmokers have the right not only to breathe clean air but also to take action to help solve one of society's most serious public health threats. Here are a few actions you can take. When a smoker violates a no-smoking designation, complain. If your favorite restaurant or shop doesn't have a nonsmoking policy, ask the manager to adopt one. If you see children buying tobacco, report this illegal activity to the facility manager or the police. Learn more about addiction and tobacco cessation so you can better support the tobacco users you know. Vote for candidates who support antitobacco measures; contact local, state, and national representatives to express your views.

HOW A TOBACCO USER CAN QUIT

Giving up tobacco is a long-term, intricate process. Research shows that tobacco users move through predictable stages—from being uninterested in stopping, to thinking about change, to making a serious effort to stop, to finally maintaining abstinence. But most attempt to quit several times before they finally succeed. Relapse is a normal part of the process.

The Benefits of Quitting

Giving up tobacco provides immediate health benefits to men and women of all ages (Table 8.4). The younger people are when they stop smoking, the more pronounced the health improvements. And these improvements gradually but invariably increase as the period of nonsmoking lengthens. It's never too late to quit, though. According to a Surgeon General's report, people who quit smoking, regardless of age, live longer than people who continue to smoke.

Options for Quitting

Most tobacco users—69% in a recent survey—want to quit, and half of those who want to quit will make an attempt this year. What are their options? No single method works for everyone, but each does work for some people some of the time.

Table 8.4	Benefits of Quitting Smoking

Within 20 minutes of your last cigarette:
- You stop polluting the air
- Blood pressure drops to normal
- Pulse rate drops to normal
- Temperature of hands and feet increases to normal

8 hours:
- Carbon monoxide level in blood drops to normal
- Oxygen level in blood increases to normal

24 hours:
- Chance of heart attack decreases

48 hours:
- Nerve endings start regrowing
- Ability to smell and taste is enhanced

2–3 months:
- Circulation improves
- Walking becomes easier
- Lung function increases up to 30%

1–9 months:
- Coughing, sinus congestion, fatigue, and shortness of breath all decrease

1 year:
- Heart disease death rate is half that of a smoker

5 years:
- Stroke risk drops nearly to the risk for nonsmokers

10 years:
- Lung cancer death rate drops to 50% of that of continuing smokers
- Incidence of other cancers (mouth, throat, larynx, esophagus, bladder, kidney, and pancreas) decreases
- Risk of ulcer decreases

15 years:
- Risk of lung cancer is about 25% of that of continuing smokers
- Risks of heart disease and death are close to those of nonsmokers

Behavior Strategies Choosing to quit requires developing a strategy for success. Some people quit cold turkey, whereas others taper off slowly. There are over-the-counter and prescription products that help many people. Behavioral factors that have been shown to increase the chances of a smoker's permanent smoking cessation are support from others and regular exercise. Support can come from friends and family and/or formal group programs sponsored by organizations such as the American Cancer Society and the American Lung Association, or by your college health center or community hospital. Programs that combine group support with nicotine replacement therapy have rates of continued abstention as high as 35% after one year.

Most smokers in the process of quitting experience both physical and psychological effects of nicotine withdrawal, and exercise can help with both. For many smokers, tobacco use is associated with certain times and places—following a meal, for example. Resolving to walk after dinner instead of lighting up provides a distraction from cravings and eliminates the cues that trigger a desire to smoke. In addition, many people worry about weight gain associated with quitting. Although most ex-smokers do gain a few pounds, at least temporarily, incorporating exercise into a new tobacco-free routine lays the foundation for healthy weight management. The health risks of adding a few pounds are minimal compared to the risks of continued smoking.

Free telephone quitlines are emerging as a popular and effective strategy to help stop smoking. Quitlines are staffed by trained counselors who help each caller plan a personal quitting strategy, usually including a combination of nicotine replacement therapy, changes in daily habits, and emotional support.

HHS has a national toll-free number, 1-800-QUITNOW (1-800-784-8669), to serve as a single access point for smokers seeking information and assistance in quitting. As with any significant change in health-related behavior, giving up tobacco requires planning, sustained effort, and support. It is an ongoing process, not a one-time event.

Smoking Cessation Products Each year millions of Americans visit their doctors in the hope of finding a drug that can help them stop smoking. Although pharmacological options are limited, the few available drugs have proved successful.

CHANTIX (VARINICLINE) The newest smoking cessation drug, marketed under the name Chantix, works in two ways: It reduces nicotine cravings, easing the withdrawal process, and it blocks the pleasant effects of nicotine. The drug acts on neurotransmitter receptors in the brain.

Unlike most smoking cessation products currently on the market, Chantix is not a nicotine replacement. For this reason, smokers may be advised to continue smoking for the first few days of treatment to avoid withdrawal and to allow the drug to build up in their bodies. The approved course of treatment is 12 weeks, but the duration and recommended dosage depend on several factors, including the smoker's general health and the length and severity of his or her nicotine addiction.

Side effects reported with Chantix include nausea, headaches, vomiting, sleep disruptions, and changes in taste perception. People with kidney problems or who take certain medications should not take Chantix, and it is not recommended for women who are pregnant or nursing. In 2008 the FDA issued a public health advisory warning that some Chantix users suffered adverse reactions, such as behavioral changes, agitation, depression, suicidal thoughts, and attempted suicide. Anyone taking Chantix should immediately notify his or her doctor of any sudden change in mood or behavior.

ZYBAN (BUPROPION) Bupropion is an antidepressant (prescribed under the name Wellbutrin) as well as a smoking cessation aid (prescribed under the name Zyban).

> **It's never too late to stop smoking,** and smokers have a variety of options for quitting.

As a smoking cessation aid, bupropion eases the symptoms of nicotine withdrawal and reduces the urge to smoke. Like Chantix, it acts on neurotransmitter receptors in the brain.

Bupropion users have reported an array of side effects, but they are rare. Side effects may be reduced by changing the dosage, taking the medicine at a different time of day, or taking it with or without food. Bupropion is not recommended for people with specific physical conditions or who take certain drugs. Zyban and Wellbutrin should not be taken together.

NICOTINE REPLACEMENT PRODUCTS The most widely used smoking cessation products replace the nicotine that the user would normally get from tobacco. The user continues to get nicotine, so withdrawal symptoms and cravings are reduced. Although still harmful, nicotine replacement products provide a cleaner form of nicotine without the thousands of poisons and tars produced by burning tobacco. Less of the product is used over time as the need for nicotine decreases.

Nicotine replacement products come in several forms, including patches, gum, lozenges, nasal sprays, and inhalers. They are available in a variety of strengths and can be worked into many different smoking cessation strategies. Most are available without a prescription.

The nicotine patch is popular because it can be applied and forgotten until it needs to be removed or changed, usually every 16 or 24 hours. Placed on the upper arm or torso, it releases a steady stream of nicotine, which is absorbed through the skin. The main side effects are skin irritation and redness. Nicotine gum and nicotine lozenges have the advantage of allowing the smoker to use them whenever he or she craves nicotine. Side effects of nicotine gum include

TIPS FOR TODAY AND THE FUTURE

The responsible use of alcohol means drinking in moderation or not at all. The best approach to tobacco use is never to start.

RIGHT NOW YOU CAN:

- Consider whether there is a history of alcohol misuse or dependence in your family.
- Think about your current drinking habits. For example, count the number of parties you attended in the past month and how many drinks you had at each one.
- Take stock of the number of alcoholic beverages in your home. Does there always seem to be a lot on hand? Do you find yourself purchasing alcohol frequently? What do your purchasing habits say about your drinking?
- If you smoke, think about the next time you'll want a cigarette, such as while talking on the phone this afternoon or relaxing after dinner tonight. Visualize yourself enjoying this activity without smoking.

IN THE FUTURE YOU CAN:

- Think about the next party you plan to attend. Decide how much you will drink at the party, and how you will get home afterward.
- Watch your friends' behavior at events where drinking is involved. Do any of them show signs of a drinking problem? If so, consider what you can do to help.
- If you smoke, resolve to quit. Research your options for quitting and choose the one you think will work best for you.
- Recruit a friend or family member to help you quit smoking. Arrange to talk to this person whenever you feel the urge to smoke.

mouth sores and headaches; nicotine lozenges can cause nausea and heartburn. Nicotine nasal sprays and inhalers are available only by prescription.

Although all these products have proved to be effective in helping users stop smoking, experts recommend them only as one part of a complete smoking cessation program. Such a program should include regular professional counseling and physician monitoring.

SUMMARY

- Alcohol is a CNS depressant. At low doses, it tends to make people feel relaxed.

- Alcohol use increases the risk of injury and violence; drinking before driving is particularly dangerous, even at low doses.

- Chronic alcohol use has negative effects on the digestive and cardiovascular systems and increases cancer risk and overall mortality.

- Pregnant women who drink risk giving birth to children with a cluster of birth defects known as fetal alcohol syndrome (FAS). Even occasional drinking during pregnancy can cause brain injury in the fetus.

- Alcohol misuse involves drinking in dangerous situations or drinking to a degree that causes academic, professional, interpersonal, or legal difficulties.

- Alcoholism is characterized by more extensive problems with alcohol, usually involving tolerance and withdrawal.

- Binge drinking is a common form of alcohol misuse on college campuses that has negative effects on both drinking and nondrinking students.

- Physical consequences of alcoholism include the direct effects of tolerance and withdrawal, as well as all the problems associated with chronic drinking. Psychological problems include memory loss and additional mental disorders such as depression.

- Smoking is the largest preventable cause of ill health and death in the United States. Nevertheless, millions of Americans use tobacco.

- People who begin smoking are usually imitating others or responding to seductive advertising. Smoking is associated with low education level and the use of other drugs.

- Tobacco smoke is made up of hundreds of different chemicals, including some that are carcinogenic or poisonous or that damage the respiratory system.

- Nicotine acts on the nervous system as a stimulant or a depressant. It can cause blood pressure and heart rate to increase, straining the heart.

- Cardiovascular disease is the most widespread cause of death for cigarette smokers. Cigarette smoking is the primary cause of lung cancer and is linked to many other cancers and respiratory diseases.

- The use of spit tobacco leads to nicotine addiction and is linked to a variety of cancers of the head and neck.

- Cigars, pipes, clove cigarettes, bidis, hookahs, and e-cigarettes are not safe alternatives to cigarettes. Using them results in lung, lip, larynx, and pancreatic cancers, COPD, and emphysema, among other conditions.

- Environmental tobacco smoke (ETS) contains high concentrations of toxic chemicals and can cause headaches, eye and nasal irritation, and sinus problems. Long-term exposure to ETS causes cancer and heart disease.

- Smoking during pregnancy increases the risk of miscarriage, stillbirth, congenital abnormalities, premature birth, and low birth weight. SIDS, behavior problems, and long-term impairments in development are also risks.

- Giving up smoking is a difficult and long-term process. Although most ex-smokers quit on their own, some smokers benefit from stop-smoking programs, OTC and prescription medications, and support groups.

FOR MORE INFORMATION

BOOKS

American Lung Association. 2004. *How to Quit Smoking without Gaining Weight.* New York: American Lung Association. *Provides methods for smokers who want to quit but are afraid they'll gain weight as a result.*

Carr, A. 2010. *The Easy Way to Stop Smoking.* New York: Sterling. *A best-selling self-help book for smokers who want to stop.*

Dean, M. 2007. *Empty Cribs: The Impact of Smoking on Child Health.* New York: Arts & Sciences Publishing. *Examines the effects of smoking on children, before and after birth.*

Doyle, R., and J. Nowinski, J. 2012. *Alost Alcoholic: Is My (or My Loved One's) Drinking a Problem?* Center City, MN: Hazelden, Harvard Health Books. *Provides tools to assess patterns of alcohol use; evaluate its impact on relationships, work, and personal well-being; develop strategies for changing; and make informed decisions about your next steps.*

Kinney, J. 2011. *Loosening the Grip: A Handbook of Alcohol Information,* 10th ed. New York: McGraw-Hill. *An authoritative source of information on alcohol use and its impact on families and societies.*

Lu, K. 2006. *Media and College Binge-Drinking: Direct and Indirect Media Influences on Drinking Norms.* Ann Arbor: ProQuest/UMI. *A quantitative review of the effect of the media on students' perceptions about drinking.*

Seaman, B. 2006. *Binge: Campus Life in an Age of Disconnection and Excess.* New York: Wiley. *An exploration of campus life at 12 residential colleges and universities, with discussions on the effects of student isolation, peer pressure, and drinking on today's students.*

Vaknin, J. 2007. *Smoke Signals: 100 Years of Tobacco Advertising.* London: Middlesex University Press. *An exploration of the many ways tobacco products have been marketed to consumers.*

ORGANIZATIONS, HOTLINES, AND WEBSITES

Action on Smoking and Health (ASH). An advocacy group that provides statistics, news briefs, and other information.
   http://ash.org

Al-Anon Family Group Headquarters. Provides information and referrals to local Al-Anon and Alateen groups. The website includes a self-quiz to determine if you are affected by someone's drinking.
   http://www.al-anon.alateen.org

Alcoholics Anonymous (AA) World Services. Provides general information about AA, literature about alcoholism, and information about AA meetings and related 12-step organizations.
   http://www.aa.org

AlcoholScreening.Org. Provides information about alcohol and health, referrals for treatment and support groups, and a drinking self-assessment.
   http://www.alcoholscreening.org

Alcohol Treatment Referral Hotline. Provides referrals to local intervention and treatment providers.
   800-ALCOHOL

American Cancer Society (ACS). Sponsor of the annual Great American Smokeout; provides information about the dangers of tobacco, as well as tools for prevention and cessation for both smokers and users of spit tobacco.

http://www.cancer.org

American Lung Association. Provides information about lung diseases, tobacco control, and environmental health.

http://www.lungusa.org

Bacchus Network. An association of college- and university-based peer education programs that focus on prevention of alcohol abuse and promotion of campus health safety.

http://www.bacchusnetwork.org

CDC's Tobacco Information and Prevention Source (TIPS). Provides research results, educational materials, and tips on how to quit smoking; website includes special sections for kids and teens.

http://www.cdc.gov/tobacco

The College Alcohol Study. Harvard School of Public Health. Provides information about and results from the recent studies of binge drinking on college campuses.

http://www.hsph.harvard.edu/news/magazine
/winter09bingingproblems/

Environmental Protection Agency Indoor Air Quality/ETS. Provides information and links about secondhand smoke.

http://www.epa.gov/smokefree

Mothers Against Drunk Driving (MADD). Supports efforts to develop solutions to the problems of drunk driving and underage drinking and provides news, information, and brochures about many topics, including a guide for giving a safe party.

http://www.madd.org

National Association for Children of Alcoholics (NACoA). Provides information and support for children of alcoholics.

888-554-COAS

http://www.nacoa.org

National Council on Alcoholism and Drug Dependence (NCADD). Provides information and counseling referrals.

212-269-7797; 800-NCA-CALL (24-hour Hope Line)

http://www.ncadd.org

National Institute on Alcohol Abuse and Alcoholism (NIAAA). Provides booklets and other publications on a variety of alcohol-related topics, including fetal alcohol syndrome, alcoholism treatment, and alcohol use and minorities.

http://www.niaaa.nih.gov

Nicotine Anonymous. A 12-step program for tobacco users.

http://www.nicotine-anonymous.org

Rational Recovery. A free self-help program that offers an alternative to 12-step programs; the emphasis is on learning the skill of abstinence.

http://www.rational.org

Smokefree.Gov. Provides step-by-step strategies for quitting as well as expert support via telephone or instant messaging.

http://www.smokefree.gov

Substance Abuse and Mental Health Services Administration. Provides statistics and information about alcohol abuse, including

resources for people who want to help friends and family members overcome alcohol abuse problems.

http://store.samhsa.gov/home

World Health Organization Tobacco Free Initiative. Promotes the goal of a tobacco-free world.

http://www.who.int/tobacco/en

World No Tobacco Day (WNTD). Provides information about the annual worldwide event to encourage people to quit smoking; includes general information about tobacco use and testimonials of ex-smokers.

http://www.who.int/tobacco/wntd/2012/announcement/en/index.html

SELECTED BIBLIOGRAPHY

Alcoholism and alcohol abuse: Medications. 2013 *New York Times,* 8 March. (http://www.nytimes.com/health/guides/disease/alcoholism/medications.html, reviewed excerpt of In-Depth Report.)

American Cancer Society. 2013. *Cancer Facts and Figures, 2013.* Atlanta: American Cancer Society.

American Lung Association. 2011. *Trends in Tobacco Use* (http://www.lungusa.org/finding-cures/our-research/trend-reports/Tobacco-Trend-Report.pdf).

American Lung Association. 2012. *State of Tobacco Control 2012* (http://www.stateoftobaccocontrol.org/SOTC_2012.pdf).

American Psychiatric Association. 2013. *Diagnostic and Statistical Manual of Mental Disorders,* 5th ed. *(DSM-5).* Washington, DC: American Psychiatric Publishing.

Campaign for Tobacco-Free Kids. 2011. *State Cigarette Excise Tax Rates and Rankings.* Washington, DC: Campaign for Tobacco-Free Kids.

Centers for Disease Control and Prevention. 2009. Cigarette smoking among adults and trends in smoking cessation—United States, 2008. *Morbidity and Mortality Weekly Report* 58(44): 1227–1232.

Centers for Disease Control and Prevention. 2010. Vital signs: Nonsmokers' exposure to secondhand smoke—United States, 1999–2009. *Morbidity and Mortality Weekly Report* 59(35): 1141–1146.

Centers for Disease Control and Prevention. 2011. Quitting smoking among adults—United States, 2001–2010. *Morbidity and Mortality Weekly Report* 60(44).

Centers for Disease Control and Prevention. 2012. Vital signs: Current cigarette smoking among adults—United States, 2011. *Morbidity and Mortality Weekly Report* 61(44): 889–894.

Centers for Disease Control and Prevention. 2014. *Smoking and Tobacco Use Fact Sheet: Tobacco-Related Mortality* (http://www.cdc.gov/tobacco/data_statistics/fact_sheets/health_effects/tobacco_related_mortality).

Centers for Disease Control and Prevention. 2012. *Alcohol and Public Health* (http://www.cdc.gov/alcohol/index.htm).

Centers for Disease Control and Prevention. 2012. Alcohol use and binge drinking among women of childbearing age—United States, 2006–2010. *Morbidity and Mortality Weekly Report Weekly* 61(28): 534–538. (http://www.cdc.gov/mmwr/preview/mmwrhtml/mm6128a4.htm?s_cid=mm6128a4_w)

Chen, Wendy Y., et al. Moderate alcohol consumption during adult life, drinking patterns, and breast cancer risk. *Journal of the American Medical Association* 306(17): 1884–1890.

College Drinking Prevention. 2013. *A Snapshot of Annual High-Risk College Drinking Consequences* (http://www.collegedrinkingprevention.gov/StatsSummaries/snapshot.aspx).

Collins, G. B., et al. 2006. Drug adjuncts for treating alcohol dependence. *Cleveland Clinic Journal of Medicine* 73(7): 641–644.

Costello, R. M. 2006. Long-term mortality from alcoholism: A descriptive analysis. *Journal of Studies on Alcohol and Drugs* 67(5): 694–699.

Division of Reproductive Health, National Center for Chronic Disease Prevention and Health Promotion. 2013. *Tobacco Use and Pregnancy* (http://www.cdc.gov/reproductivehealth/TobaccoUsePregnancy/index.htm).

Federal Trade Commission. 2013. *Federal Trade Commission Cigarette Report for 2011*. Washington, DC: FTC.

Huang, J., F. J. Chalupka, and G. T. Fong. 2013. Cigarette graphic warning labels and smoking prevalence in Canada: A critical examination and reformulation of the FDA regulatory impact analysis. *Tobacco Control* (online first, doi:10.1136/tobaccocontrol-2013-051170).

Jha, P., et al. 2013. 21st century hazards of smoking and benefits of cessation in the United States. *New England Journal of Medicine 368*: 341–50.

Johnston, L. D., et al. 2014. *Monitoring the Future National Results on Adolescent Drug Use: Overview of Key Findings, 2013*. Ann Arbor, MI: Institute for Social Research, University of Michigan.

Johnston, L. D., et al. 2013. "Teen smoking continues to decline in 2013." University of Michigan News Service: Ann Arbor, MI, 18 December (http://www.monitoringthefuture.org).

Mallett, K. A., et al. 2013. An update of research examining college student alcohol-related consequences: New perspectives and implications for interventions. *Alcoholism: Clinical and Experimental Research* 37(5): 709–16.

National Center for Health Statistics. 2010. National hospital ambulatory medical care survey: 2007 emergency department summary. *National Health Statistics Reports* 26. Hyattsville, MD: National Center for Health Statistics.

National Center for Health Statistics. 2011. Deaths: Final data for 2008. *National Vital Statistics Reports* 59(10).

National Center for Health Statistics. 2012. Summary health statistics for U.S. adults: National Health Interview Survey, 2011. *National Vital Statistics* 10(256).

National Highway Traffic Safety Administration. 2009. *Traffic Safety Facts 2008: Alcohol-Impaired Driving*. Washington, DC: National Highway Traffic Safety Administration, DOT Pub. 811–155.

Parker-Pope, T. 2012. *America's Drinking Binge* (http://well.blogs.nytimes.com/2012/01/11/americas-drinking-binge).

Penn State. 2012. Early intervention may curb dangerous college drinking. *Science Daily* (http://www.sciencedaily.com/releases/2012/01/120130131204.htm).

Perrone, M. 2014. Senators warn of carcinogen risk with e-cigarettes. *Associated Press, SFGate*, 8 May.

Substance Abuse and Mental Health Services Administration. 2011. *Results from the 2010 National Survey on Drug Use and Health: Summary of National Findings*. NSDUH Series H-41, HHS Publication No. (SMA) 11-4658. Rockville, MD: SAMHSA.

Substance Abuse and Mental Health Services Administration. 2012. *Nearly Half of College Student Treatment Admissions Were for Primary Alcohol Abuse* (http://www.samhsa.gov/data/spotlight/Spotlight054College2012.pdf).

Substance Abuse and Mental Health Services Administration. 2013. *Results from the 2012 National Survey on Drug Use and Health: Summary of National Findings*. Rockville, MD: Office of Applied Studies, NSDUH Series H-46, HHS Publication No. (SMA) 13-4795.

Titus-Ernstoff, L., et al. 2008. Longitudinal study of viewing smoking in movies and initiation of smoking by children. *Pediatrics* 121(1): 15–21.

U.S. Department of Health and Human Services. 2014. *The Health Consequences of Smoking—50 Years of Progress: A Report of the Surgeon General*. Atlanta: HHS, Centers for Disease Control and Prevention, National Center for Chronic Disease Prevention and Health Promotion, Office on Smoking and Health.

U.S. Department of Justice, Federal Bureau of Investigation. 2013. *Crime in the United States: 2012* (http://http://www.fbi.gov/about-us/cjis/ucr/crime-in-the-u.s/2012/crime-in-the-u.s.-2012/tables/29tabledatadecpdf).

U.S. Food and Drug Administration Center for Tobacco Products. 2010. *2009–2010: Inaugural Year in Review*. Washington, DC: FDA.

Ward, B. W., et al. 2014. "Current Cigarette Smoking." Early release of selected estimates based on data from the January–September 2013 National Health Interview Survey. Hyattsville, MD: National Center for Health Statistics (http://www.cdc.gov/nchs/data/nhis/earlyrelease/earlyrelease201403.pdf).

Zhang, J., et al. 2014. Comparison of clinical features between non-smokers with COPD and smokers with COPD: A retrospective observational study. *International Journal of Chronic Obstructive Pulmonary Disease* 9: 57–63.

BEHAVIOR CHANGE STRATEGY
Kicking the Tobacco Habit

You can look forward to a longer and healthier life if you join the 48 million Americans who have quit using tobacco. The steps for quitting described here are discussed in terms of the most popular tobacco product in the United States—cigarettes—but they can be adapted for all forms of tobacco.

Gather Information

Start with:

- Which of the following smoke: Family, friends, and acquaintances. *Please circle one or more.*

- Do family members *encourage* or *discourage* you from stopping smoking? *Please circle one.*

- How interested are you in stopping smoking? Strongly, somewhat, a little, not much, not at all. *Please circle one.*

- If you decide to quit smoking, how confident are you that you will succeed? Strongly, somewhat, a little, not much, not at all. *Please circle one.*

Keep a detailed journal about your personal smoking behavior. Write down the time you smoke each cigarette of the day, the situation you are in, how you feel, where you smoke, and how strong your craving for the cigarette is, plus any other information that seems relevant. Part of the job is to identify patterns of smoking that are connected with routine situations (for example, the after-dinner cigarette, the coffee break smoke, the tension-reduction cigarette). Use this information to discover the behavior patterns involved in your smoking habit.

Make the Decision to Quit

Choose a date in the near future when you expect to be relatively stress-free and can give quitting the energy and attention it will require. Don't choose a date right before or during finals week, for instance. Consider making quitting a gift: Choose your birthday as your quit date, for example, or make quitting a Father's Day or Mother's Day present.

You might also want to coordinate your quit date with a buddy—a fellow tobacco user who wants to quit or a nonsmoker who wants to give up another bad habit or begin an exercise program. Tell your friends and family when you plan to quit. Ask them to offer encouragement and help hold you to your goal.

Decide what approach to quitting will work best for you. Will you go cold turkey, or will you taper off? Will you use nicotine patches or gum? Will you join a support group or enlist the help of a buddy? Prepare a contract for quitting, as discussed in Chapter 1. Set firm dates and rewards, and sign the contract. Post it in a prominent place.

Prepare to Quit

One of the most important things you can do to prepare to quit is to develop and practice nonsmoking relaxation techniques. Many smokers find that they use cigarettes to help them unwind in tense situations or to relax at other times. If this is true for you, you'll need to find and develop effective substitutes. It takes time to become proficient at relaxation techniques, so begin practicing before your quit date. Refer to the detailed discussion of relaxation techniques in Chapter 2.

Other things you can do to help prepare for quitting include the following:

- Make an appointment to see your physician. Ask about OTC and prescription aids for tobacco cessation and whether one or more might be appropriate for you.

- Make a dentist's appointment to have your teeth cleaned the day after your target quit date.

- Start an easy exercise program if you're not exercising regularly already.

- Buy some sugarless gum. Stock your kitchen with low-calorie snacks.

- Clean and air out your car, and air out your house. Wash all your clothes and linens, and dry clean any nonwashable clothes.

- Throw away all your cigarette-related paraphernalia (ashtrays, lighters, and so on).

- The night before your quit day, get rid of all your cigarettes. Have fun with this—get your friends or family to help you tear them up.

- Make your last few days of smoking inconvenient: Smoke only outdoors and when alone. Don't do anything else while you smoke.

Quitting

Your first few days without cigarettes will probably be the most difficult. It's hard to give up such a strongly ingrained habit, but remember that millions of Americans have done it—and you can, too. Plan and rehearse the steps you will take when you experience a powerful craving. Avoid or control situations that you know from your journal are powerfully associated with your smoking (see the accompanying table). If your hands feel empty without a cigarette, try holding or fiddling with a small object such as a paper clip, pencil, or small toy.

Social support can also be a big help. Arrange with a buddy to help you with your weak moments, and call him or her whenever you feel overwhelmed by an urge to smoke. Tell people you've just quit. You may discover many inspiring former smokers who can encourage you and reassure you that it's possible to quit and lead a happier, healthier life. Find a formal support group to join if you think it will help.

Maintaining Nonsmoking

The smoking urges that linger once you've quit should be carefully tracked and controlled because they can cause relapses if left unattended. Keep track of these urges in your journal to help you deal with them. If certain situations still trigger the urge for a cigarette, change something about those situations to break past associations. If stress or boredom causes strong smoking urges, use a relaxation technique, take a brisk walk, have a stick of gum, or substitute some other activity for smoking.

Don't set yourself up for a relapse. If you allow yourself to get overwhelmed at school or work or to gain weight, it will be easier to convince yourself that now isn't the right time to quit. This *is* the right time. Continue to practice time management and relaxation techniques. Exercise regularly, eat sensibly, and get enough sleep. These habits not only will ensure your success at remaining tobacco-free but also will serve you well in stressful times throughout your life. In fact, former smokers who have quit for at least three months report reduced stress levels, probably because quitting smoking lowers overall arousal.

Watch out for patterns of thinking that can make not smoking more difficult. Focus on the positive aspects of not smoking, and give yourself lots of praise—you deserve it. Stick with the schedule of rewards you developed for your contract.

Keep track of the emerging benefits that come from having quit. Items that might appear on your list include improved stamina, an increased sense of pride at having kicked a strong addiction, a sharper sense of taste and smell, no more smoker's cough, and so on. Keep track of the money you're saving by not smoking, and spend it on things you really enjoy. And if you do lapse, be gentle with yourself. Lapses are a normal part of quitting. Forgive yourself, and pick up where you left off.

STRATEGIES FOR DEALING WITH HIGH-RISK SMOKING SITUATIONS

Cues and High-Risk Situations	Suggested Strategies
Awakening in the morning	Brush your teeth as soon as you wake up. Take a shower or bath.
Drinking coffee	Do something else with your hands. Drink tea or another beverage instead.
Eating meals	Sit in nonsmoking sections of restaurants. Get up from the table right after eating, and start another activity. Brush your teeth right after eating.
Driving a car	Clean the car thoroughly and air it out when you quit smoking. Chew sugarless gum or eat a low-calorie snack. Take public transportation or ride your bike. Turn on the radio and sing along.
Socializing with friends who smoke	Suggest nonsmoking events (movies, theater, shopping). Tell friends you've quit and ask them not to smoke around you, offer you cigarettes, or give you cigarettes if you ask for them.
Drinking at a bar, restaurant, or party	Try to take a nonsmoker with you, or associate with nonsmokers. Let friends know you've just quit. Moderate your intake of alcohol (it can weaken your resolve).
Encountering stressful situations	Practice relaxation techniques. Take some deep breaths. Get out of your room or house. Go somewhere that doesn't allow smoking. Take a shower, chew gum, call a friend, or exercise.

SOURCE: Adapted from Kraner, S. E., and K. E. Graham. 1991. Helping your patients who smoke quit for good: A quick and easy approach. *Postgraduate Medicine* 90(1): 233–248. Copyright 1991, with permission from JTE MULTIMEDIA.

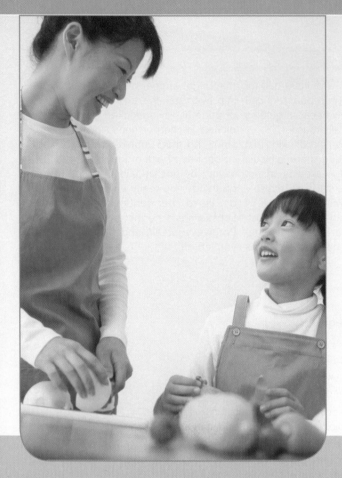

CHAPTER 9

CHAPTER OBJECTIVES

- Describe MyPlate, a food guidance system to help people apply the Dietary Guidelines for Americans to their own diets
- List the essential nutrients, and describe the functions they perform in the body
- Describe the guidelines that have been developed to help people choose a healthy diet, avoid nutritional deficiencies, and reduce their risk of diet-related chronic diseases
- Discuss nutritional guidelines for vegetarians and for special population groups
- Explain how to use food labels and other consumer tools to make informed choices about foods
- Put together a personal nutrition plan based on affordable foods that you enjoy and that promote wellness, today as well as in the future

Nutrition Basics

C hoosing foods that provide the nutrients you need while limiting the substances linked to disease should be an important part of your daily life. Your diet changes as you go through different life stages, and it is guided by current energy needs, daily nutrient requirements, locally available foods, foods that you will choose to eat, and your health condition. When actively involved in sports, for example, your energy needs will be higher than when you are inactive, even if your age and body size remained the same. Similarly, energy needs for lactating mothers are higher than those of nonlactating mothers of corresponding body size and physical activity levels.

nutrition The science of food and dietary supplements, and how the body uses them in health and disease.

TERMS

This chapter explores how the U.S. food system and global nutrition transitions influence the type and amount of food we eat, as well as examines the role of personal dietary choices and the basic principles of **nutrition.** It introduces the six classes of essential nutrients and explains their roles in health and disease. It also provides guidelines for designing a healthy diet plan.

NUTRITIONAL REQUIREMENTS: COMPONENTS OF A HEALTHY DIET

You probably think about your diet in terms of the foods you like to eat. More important for your health, though, are the nutrients contained in those foods. Your body requires proteins, fats, carbohydrates, vitamins, minerals, and

Touring Lifestyle Behaviors

Alcohol Use: Stages of Intoxication

Tobacco Use: Immediate Effects and Long-Term Health Risks

Exercise: Immediate Effects and Long-Term Health Benefits

The Greenhouse Effect, Climate Change, and You

GOALS OF THE TOUR

1. **Alcohol Use.** Describe the stages of intoxication and the effects experienced in each stage.

2. **Tobacco Use.** Identify and describe the immediate effects and long-term health risks of tobacco use.

3. **Exercise.** Identify and describe the immediate effects and long-term health benefits of exercise.

4. **The Greenhouse Effect.** Explain the greenhouse effect and describe actions individuals can take to reduce their carbon footprint.

Alcohol Use: Stages of Intoxication

1 Describe the stages of intoxication and the effects experienced at each stage.

Blood alcohol concentration (BAC) rises quickly with alcohol consumption, but alcohol is metabolized at a relatively slow rate—about 1 drink per hour. Note that rate of alcohol metabolism varies widely depending on sex, body weight, ethnicity, age, food in the stomach, genetics, and other factors—so the effects at different BACs also vary.

One drink =

a 12-ounce beer

or

a 1.5-ounce shot

or

a 5-ounce glass of wine

Number of drinks in 1 hour before the legal BAC limit of 0.08 is reached

Weight in pounds	Drinks in 1 hour
90–109	1
110–129	1
130–149	2
150–169	2
170–189	2
190–200+	3

150 lbs
130 lbs
180 lbs
170 lbs
102 lbs
200 lbs

BAC
0.00
0.02   0.05   0.08   **0.10**   0.15

effects

BAC: 0.01–0.05
Relaxation; mild euphoria; reduced inhibition; decreased alertness; impaired motor coordination and judgment.
Approximate time to metabolize: 2–3 hours

BAC: 0.10–0.15
Mood swings; aggression; staggering gait; impaired balance; slurred speech.
Approximate time to metabolize: 7–10 hours

BAC: 0.05–0.10
Emotional instability; exaggerated feelings and behaviors; impaired reasoning, judgment, and visual tracking; slowed information processing, reflexes, and reaction time; sleepiness; nausea. Legally intoxicated at 0.08% in all 50 states.
Approximate time to metabolize: 3–6 hours

Tobacco Use: Immediate Effects and Long-Term Health Risks

Identify and describe the immediate effects and long-term health risks of tobacco use.

2

Immediate Effects

Brain
- Nicotine triggers release of sedating and stimulating chemicals in brain

Skin
- Nicotine constricts blood vessels, reducing blood flow to skin

Heart
- Nicotine increases heart rate, elevates blood pressure
- Heart must work harder to deliver oxygen to cells

Lungs, bronchi
- Smoke is absorbed into bloodstream and carried throughout the body
- Oxygen delivery to cells is impaired

Liver
- Nicotine causes liver to convert glycogen to glucose and release it into bloodstream, raising blood sugar levels

Adrenal glands
- Nicotine triggers release of adrenaline, causing stimulating effects throughout the body and reduced body temperature in extremities

Kidneys
- Nicotine inhibits production of urine

Digestive system
- Nicotine depresses appetite and hunger contractions

Reproductive system
- In pregnant women, nicotine and chemicals are passed to fetus

Exercise: Immediate Effects and Long-Term Health Benefits

3 Identify and describe the immediate effects and long-term health benefits of exercise.

Immediate Effects

Brain
- Increased oxygen and nutrients to brain
- Increased levels of neurotransmitters

Heart
- Increased heart rate
- Greater volume of blood pumped to body

Lungs
- Increased breathing rate
- Increased oxygen consumption

Stomach
- Reduced blood flow to digestive system

Muscles
- Increased blood flow to muscles
- Increased energy production in muscles

Skin
- Increased blood flow to skin
- Increased sweating to maintain safe body temperature

The Greenhouse Effect, Climate Change, and You

Explain the greenhouse effect and describe actions individuals can take to reduce their carbon footprint.

4

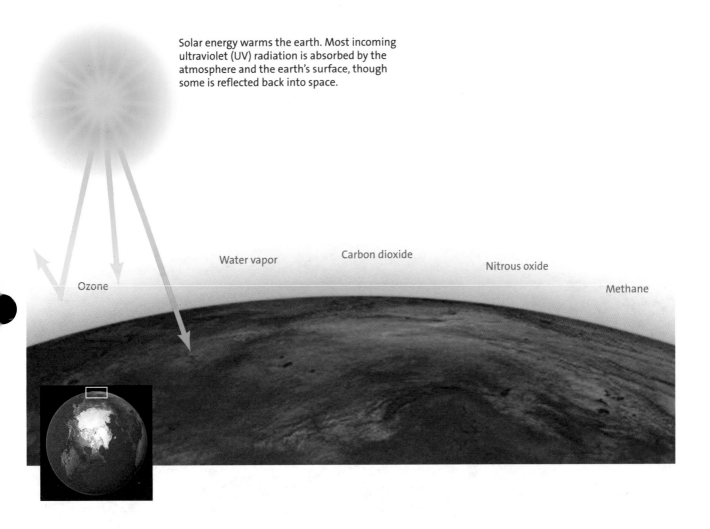

Solar energy warms the earth. Most incoming ultraviolet (UV) radiation is absorbed by the atmosphere and the earth's surface, though some is reflected back into space.

Water vapor

Carbon dioxide

Nitrous oxide

Ozone

Methane

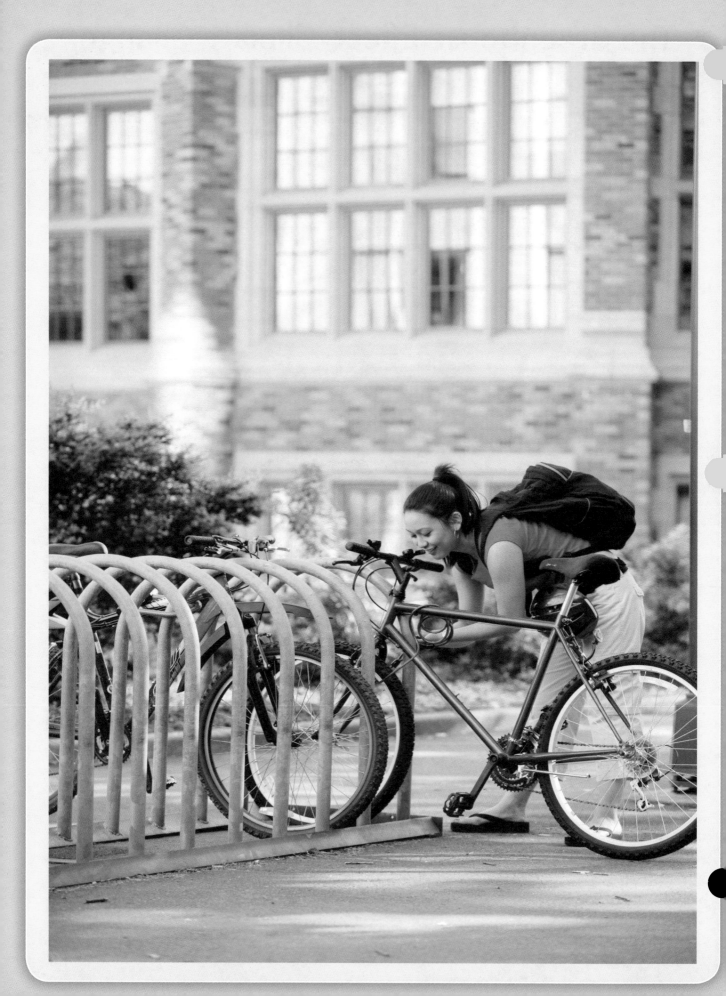

water—about 45 **essential nutrients.** In this context, the word *essential* means that you must get these substances from food because your body is unable to manufacture them or make an adequate amount to meet your physiological needs. The body needs some essential nutrients in relatively large amounts; these **macronutrients** include protein, fat, carbohydrate, and water. **Micronutrients,** such as vitamins and minerals, are required in much smaller amounts.

Most nutrients become available to the body through the process of **digestion,** in which the foods eaten are broken down into compounds the gastrointestinal tract can absorb and for the body to process further and use for normal body functions (Figure 9.1). An adequate diet must provide enough essential nutrients and energy to support and regulate various vital body functions.

The amount of energy in foods is expressed as **kilocalories (kcal).** One kilocalorie represents the amount of heat required to raise the temperature of 1 liter of water by 1°C. An average person needs about 2000 kilocalories per day to meet his or her energy needs. In common usage, people usually refer to kilocalories as *calories,* which is technically inaccurate, but this text uses the familiar word *calorie* to stand for the larger energy unit; you'll also find the word *calorie* used on food labels. What's the difference between "energy" and "calorie?" **Energy** is the capacity to do work. Calories are used to measure energy. The energy in food is chemical energy, which the body converts to mechanical, electrical, or heat energy.

Of the six broad classes of nutrients, fat supplies the most energy per gram (9 calories) followed by protein and carbohydrate, which supply 4 calories per gram.

Alcohol, though not an important component of the diet, also supplies energy, providing 7 calories per gram. (One gram equals a little less than 0.04 ounce.) The high energy content of fat is one reason why high fat consumption is not recommended. Moreover, carbohydrate, protein, or alcohol consumed in excess of your energy needs may be converted into fat that is then stored in the body.

Proteins—The Basis of Body Structure

Proteins form important parts of the body's main structural components: muscles and bones. Proteins also form important parts of blood, enzymes, some hormones, and cell membranes. When consumed, proteins also provide energy (4 calories per gram) for the body.

Amino Acids   The building blocks of proteins are called **amino acids.** Twenty common amino acids are found in food proteins. Nine of these amino acids are essential (or indispensable). As long as foods supply certain nutrients, the body can produce the other 11 amino acids.

Complete and Incomplete Proteins   Individual protein sources are considered *complete* if they supply all the essential amino acids in adequate amounts and *incomplete* if

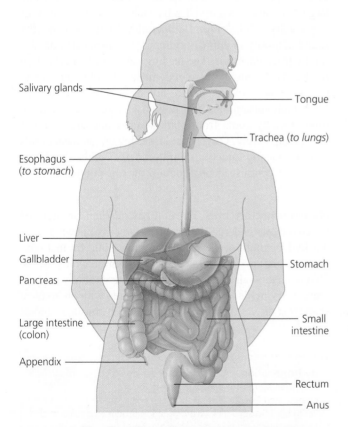

FIGURE 9.1   The digestive system. Food is partially broken down by being chewed and mixed with saliva in the mouth. After traveling to the stomach via the esophagus, food is broken down further by stomach acids and other secretions. As food moves through the digestive tract, it is mixed by muscular contractions to facilitate further digestion and absorption. Most absorption of nutrients occurs via the lining of the small intestine. The large intestine reabsorbs excess water; the remaining solid wastes are collected in the rectum and excreted through the anus.

Salivary glands

Tongue

Trachea (*to lungs*)

Esophagus
(*to stomach*)

Liver

Gallbladder

Pancreas

Stomach

Large intestine
(colon)

Small
intestine

Appendix

Rectum

Anus

TERMS

essential nutrients   Dietary components the body must get from foods or supplements because it cannot manufacture them to meet its needs.

macronutrient   An important nutrient required by the body in relatively large amounts.

micronutrient   An important nutrient required by the body in minute amounts.

digestion   The process of breaking down foods into compounds the gastrointestinal tract can absorb and the body can use.

kilocalorie   A measure of energy content in food; 1 kilocalorie represents the amount of heat needed to raise the temperature of 1 liter of water 1°C; commonly referred to as a *calorie.*

energy   The capacity to do work, measured by calories. We get energy from certain nutrients in food.

protein   An essential nutrient that forms important parts of the body's main structures (muscles and bones) as well as blood, enzymes, hormones, and cell membranes; also provides energy.

amino acid   One of the building blocks of proteins; 20 common amino acids are found in foods.

they do not. Meat, fish, poultry, eggs, milk, cheese, and soy provide complete proteins. Incomplete proteins, which come from other plant sources such as legumes and nuts, are good sources of most essential amino acids but are usually low in one or more.

Certain combinations of vegetable proteins, such as grains and legumes, for example, wheat and peanuts in a peanut butter sandwich, allow each vegetable protein to make up for the amino acids missing in the other protein. The combination yields a complete protein. Many traditional food pairings, such as beans and rice or corn and beans, have emerged as dietary staples because they are complementary proteins.

Recommended Protein Intake Adequate daily intake of protein for adults is 0.8 gram per kilogram (0.36 gram per pound) of body weight, corresponding to 50 grams of protein per day for someone who weighs 140 pounds and 65 grams of protein for someone who weighs 180 pounds.

Most Americans meet or exceed the protein intake needed for adequate nutrition. If you consume substantially more protein than your body needs, the extra energy from protein is synthesized into fat for storage or burned for energy requirements. A little extra protein is not harmful, but it can contribute excess energy and fat to the diet because protein-rich foods, especially those from animal sources, can be high in fat.

Recommendations for how much protein (and other nutrients) to consume as a percentage of total daily energy intake have been published by the Food and Nutrition Board of the Institute of Medicine. These recommendations, called Acceptable Macronutrient Distribution Ranges (AMDRs), aim to ensure adequate intake of essential nutrients and also reduce the risk of chronic diseases. The AMDR for protein is 10–35% of total daily calorie intake, depending on the individual's age, and the range of proteins should be fairly broad. Because most people in the United States meet the recommendations for protein, the 2010 Dietary Guidelines for Americans emphasize a variety of low-fat protein choices to encourage people to reduce energy intake.

Fats—Essential in Small Amounts

At 9 calories per gram, fats, also known as *lipids,* are the most concentrated source of energy. The fats stored in your body represent usable energy, help insulate your body, and support and cushion your organs. Fats in the diet help your body to absorb fat-soluble vitamins, and they add important flavor and texture to foods. Fats are the major fuel for the body during rest and light activity. Two fats, linoleic acid and alpha-linolenic acid, are essential components of the diet.

> A 2014 study analysis has challenged the widely accepted hypothesis that saturated fat causes coronary heart disease.

Types and Sources of Fats Called *triglycerides,* most of the fats in foods are fairly similar in composition, generally including a molecule of glycerol (an alcohol) with three fatty acid chains attached to it. Animal fat, for example, is made primarily of triglycerides.

Within a triglyceride, differences in the fatty acid structure result in different types of fats. Depending on this structure, a fat may be saturated or unsaturated, monounsaturated or polyunsaturated, depending on how many double bonds exist in the structure of the fatty acid chains. The essential fatty acids linoleic acid and alpha-linolenic acid are both polyunsaturated (they have two or more double bonds). Although different types of fatty acids have different characteristics, their varied effects on health have been challenged by a recent study (see the box "Rethinking Butter: New Research on Saturated Fats."

Food fats are usually composed of both saturated and unsaturated fatty acids. The dominant type of fatty acid determines the fat's characteristics. Food fats containing large amounts of saturated fatty acids or trans fatty acids are usually solid at room temperature; they are generally found naturally in animal products or in products containing hydrogenated oils. The leading sources of saturated fat in the American diet are red meats (hamburger, steak, roasts), whole milk, cheese, hot dogs, and lunchmeats. Most monounsaturated and polyunsaturated fatty acids in foods usually come from plant sources and are liquid at room temperature. Olive, canola, safflower, and peanut oils contain mostly monounsaturated fatty acids. Soybean, corn, and cottonseed oils contain mostly polyunsaturated fatty acids.

Hydrogenation and Trans Fats When unsaturated vegetable oils undergo the chemical process known as partial **hydrogenation,** the result is a more solid fat that contains a mixture of saturated and unsaturated fatty acids. Hydrogenation also changes some unsaturated fatty acids to **trans fatty acids**—unsaturated fatty acids with an atypical shape that affects their behavior in the body. In some studies

---

hydrogenation A chemical process by which hydrogen atoms are added to molecules of unsaturated fats, increasing the degree of saturation and turning liquid oils into solid fats. Hydrogenation produces a mixture of saturated fatty acids, and *cis* (standard) and *trans* forms of unsaturated fatty acids.

trans fatty acid A type of unsaturated fatty acid produced during the process of hydrogenation; trans fats have an atypical shape that affects their chemical activity. Trans fats are associated with an increase in LDL-cholesterol and a lowering of HDL-cholesterol, attributes that are associated with risk of heart disease.

TERMS

A 2014 analysis published in *Annals of Internal Medicine* has challenged the widely accepted saturated fat hypothesis that butter and other sources of saturated fat cause coronary heart disease. A Cambridge University analysis looked at 27 prior clinical trials and 49 observational studies, consisting of more than 600,000 participants. It concluded "current evidence does not clearly support cardiovascular guidelines that encourage high consumption of polyunsaturated fatty acids and low consumption of total saturated fats." Even findings on omega-3 fatty acids did not confirm past assumptions that they are "heart-healthy." Also, the effects of trans fats, which have been considered particularly deadly, are not clear. The analysis found little evidence for a relationship between eating different types of fat and heart disease. These results are similar to another analysis, published in the *American Journal of Clinical Nutrition* in 2010, which found "no significant evidence . . . that dietary saturated fat is associated with an increased risk of coronary heart disease."

Commenting on the new Cambridge study, Professor Tom Sanders, Department of Nutrition and Dietetics at King's College, London, suggests that these results do not give permission to load up on lots of fat.

Current guidelines restrict the intake of both saturated and trans fats. Health experts are particularly concerned about trans fats because of their double-negative effect on heart health—they both raise LDL and lower HDL. Consuming trans fats appears to increase the risk of both cardiovascular disease and type 2 diabetes. In recent years, as awareness of these health risks has grown, cities and states have banned the use of trans fats in restaurants and food prepared for retail sale, and food manufacturers have reduced the amount of trans fats they use. According to the Center for Science in the Public Interest, the amount of trans fat added to our food supply has declined by more than 50% since 2005. Reduction in consumption of trans fatty acids has also been documented by the CDC. By federal regulation, the trans fat content of packaged food items is listed on their labels. Consumers can also check for the presence of trans fats by examining the ingredient list of a food for partially hydrogenated oil or vegetable shortening. As of January 2014, the Food and Drug Administration is in the process of removing trans fatty acids from the category of food additives generally regarded as safe. These approaches are expected to substantially further reduce trans fat consumption in the US.

Dietary fat affects health in other ways besides heart disease risk. Diets high in fatty red meat are associated with an increased risk of certain forms of cancer, especially colon cancer. A high-fat diet can also make weight management more difficult, because fat is a concentrated source of calories.

Although more research is needed on the precise effects of different types and amounts of fat on overall health, a great deal of evidence points to the fact that most people benefit from keeping their overall fat intake at recommended levels.

---

trans fats are associated with an increase in **low-density lipoprotein cholesterol (LDL-C)**, or "bad" cholesterol, and a lowering of **high-density lipoprotein cholesterol (HDL-C)**, or "good" cholesterol. These attributes are thought to be part of a dietary pattern that correlates with heart disease. (See Table 9.1.)

Food manufacturers use hydrogenation to increase the stability of an oil so it can be reused for deep frying, to improve the texture of certain foods (to make pie crusts flakier, for example), and to extend the shelf life of foods made with oil. Hydrogenation is also used to transform liquid oil into margarine or vegetable shortening.

Hydrogenated vegetable oils are not the only plant fats that contain high amounts of saturated fats. Palm and coconut oils, although derived from plants, are also highly saturated.

Recommended Fat Intake

To meet the body's demand for essential fats, adult men need about 17 grams per day of linoleic acid and 1.6 grams per day of alpha-linolenic acid; adult women need 12 grams of linoleic acid and 1.1 grams of alpha-linolenic acid. It takes only 3–4 teaspoons (15–20 grams) of vegetable oil per day incorporated into your diet to supply these essential fats. Most Americans consume sufficient amounts of the essential fats; limiting unhealthy fats is a much greater health concern.

Limits for total fat, saturated fat, and trans fat intake have been set by a number of government and research organizations. As with protein, a range of levels of fat consumption is associated with good health. The AMDR for total fat is 20–35% of total daily calories. Although more difficult for consumers to monitor, AMDRs have also been set for omega-6 fatty acids (5–10% of total calories) and omega-3 fatty acids (0.6–1.2% of total calories) as part of total daily fat intake.

> **TERMS**
>
> **cholesterol**   A waxy substance in the blood and cells, needed for synthesis of cell membranes, vitamin D, and hormones.
>
> **low-density lipoprotein (LDL)**   Blood fat that transports cholesterol to organs and tissues; excess amounts result in the accumulation of deposits in artery walls, causing hardening of the arteries and potential cardiovascular disease.
>
> **high-density lipoprotein (HDL)**   Blood fat that helps transport cholesterol out of the arteries, thereby protecting against cardiovascular disease.

Table 9.1 Types of Fatty Acids

TYPE OF FATTY ACID	FOUND IN*
Saturated	• Animal fats (especially fatty meats and poultry fat and skin) • Butter, cheese, and other high-fat dairy products • Palm and coconut oils
Trans	• Some frozen pizza • Some types of popcorn • Deep-fried fast foods • Stick margarines, shortening • Packaged cookies and crackers • Processed snacks and sweets
Monounsaturated	• Olive, canola, and safflower oils • Avocados, olives • Peanut butter (without added fat) • Many nuts, including almonds, cashews, pecans, and pistachios
Polyunsaturated—Omega-3[†]	• Fatty fish, including salmon, white albacore tuna, mackerel, anchovies, and sardines • Compared to fish, lesser amounts are found in walnut, flaxseed, canola, and soybean oils; tofu; walnuts; flaxseeds; and dark green leafy vegetables
Polyunsaturated—Omega-6[†]	• Corn, soybean, and cottonseed oils (often used in margarine, mayonnaise, and salad dressings)

*Food fats contain a combination of types of fatty acids in various proportions. For example, canola oil is composed mainly of monounsaturated fatty acids (62%) but also contains polyunsaturated (32%) and saturated (6%) fatty acids.

[†]The essential fatty acids are polyunsaturated: linoleic acid is an omega-6 fatty acid and alpha-linolenic acid is an omega-3 fatty acid.

For advice on setting individual intake goals, see the box "Setting Intake Goals for Protein, Fat, and Carbohydrate." To determine how close you are to meeting your personal intake goals for fat, keep a running total over the course of the day. For prepared foods, food labels list the numbers of grams of fat, protein, and carbohydrate. Nutrition information is also available in many grocery stores, in inexpensive published nutrition guides, and online (see "For More Information" at the end of the chapter). By checking these resources, you can keep track of the total grams of fat, protein, and carbohydrate you eat and assess your current diet.

Carbohydrates—An Ideal Source of Energy

Carbohydrates are needed in the diet primarily to supply energy for body cells. Some cells, such as those found in the brain and other parts of the nervous system and in blood, use only the carbohydrate glucose for fuel. During high-intensity exercise, muscles also use energy from carbohydrates as their primary fuel source.

TERMS

carbohydrate   An essential nutrient, required for energy for cells; sugars, starches, and dietary fiber are all carbohydrates.

glucose   A simple sugar that is the body's basic fuel.

glycogen   A starch stored in the liver and muscles.

Simple and Complex Carbohydrates   Carbohydrates are classified into two groups: simple and complex. *Simple carbohydrates* include single sugar molecules (monosaccharides) and double sugar molecules (disaccharides). The monosaccharides are glucose, fructose, and galactose. The disaccharides are pairs of single sugars; they include sucrose or table sugar (fructose + glucose), maltose or malt sugar (glucose + glucose), and lactose. Simple carbohydrates add sweetness to foods; they are found naturally in fruits and milk and are added to soft drinks, fruit drinks, candy, and sweet desserts. There is no evidence that any type of simple carbohydrate is more nutritious than any others.

Complex carbohydrates include starches and most types of dietary fiber. Starches are found in a variety of plants, especially grains (wheat, rye, rice, oats, barley, millet), legumes (dry beans, peas, and lentils), and tubers (potatoes and yams). Most other vegetables contain a mixture of complex and simple carbohydrates.

During digestion, your body breaks down carbohydrates into simple sugar molecules, such as **glucose,** for absorption. Once glucose is in the bloodstream, the pancreas releases the hormone insulin, which allows cells to take up glucose and use it for energy. The liver and muscles take up glucose to provide carbohydrate storage in the form of a starch called **glycogen.** Some people have problems controlling blood glucose levels, a disorder called *diabetes mellitus.*

Refined Carbohydrates versus Whole Grains
Complex carbohydrates can be further divided into refined, or processed, carbohydrates and unrefined carbohydrates, or

The Food and Nutrition Board has established goals to help ensure adequate intake of the essential amino acids, fatty acids, and carbohydrates. The daily goals for adults follow:

	MEN	WOMEN
Protein	56 grams	46 grams
Fat: Linoleic acid	17 grams	12 grams
Fat: Alpha-linolenic acid	1.6 grams	1.1 grams
Carbohydrate	130 grams	130 grams

Recommended protein intake in grams per day can be calculated more specifically by multiplying your body weight in kilograms by 0.8 or your body weight in pounds by 0.36. (Refer to the "Nutrition Resources" section in the Behavior Change Strategy box at the end of the chapter for information for specific age groups and life stages.)

To meet your daily energy needs, you need to consume more than the minimally adequate amounts of the energy-providing nutrients listed here, which alone supply only about 800–900 calories.

The Food and Nutrition Board provides additional guidance in the form of Acceptable Macronutrient Distribution Ranges (AMDRs), as noted in the text. The ranges can help you balance your intake of the energy-providing nutrients in ways that ensure adequate intake while reducing the risk of chronic disease. The AMDRs for protein, total fat, and carbohydrate follow:

Protein	10–35% of total daily calories
Total fat	20–35% of total daily calories
Carbohydrate	45–65% of total daily calories

To set individual goals, begin by estimating your total daily energy (calorie) needs. If your weight is stable, your current energy intake is the number of calories needed to maintain your weight at your current activity level. Next select percentage goals for protein, fat, and carbohydrate. You can allocate your total daily energy intake among the three classes of macronutrients to suit your preferences, but make sure that the three percentages you select total 100% and that you meet the minimum intake goals listed.

To translate your own percentage goals into daily intake goals expressed in calories and grams, multiply the appropriate percentages by total daily energy intake and then divide the results by the corresponding calories per gram. For example, a fat limit of 35% applied to a 2200-calorie diet would be calculated as follows: $0.35 \times 2200 = 770$ calories of total fat; $770 \div 9$ calories per gram $= 86$ grams of total fat. (Remember that fat has 9 calories per gram and that protein and carbohydrate have 4 calories per gram.)

whole grains. Before they are processed, all grains are **whole grains,** consisting of an inner layer, the germ; a middle layer, the endosperm; and an outer layer, the bran. During processing, the germ and bran are often removed, leaving just the starchy endosperm. The refinement of whole grains transforms whole-wheat flour into white flour, brown rice into white rice, and so on.

Refined carbohydrates usually retain all the calories of their unrefined counterparts, but they tend to be much lower in fiber, vitamins, minerals, and other beneficial compounds. Unrefined carbohydrates tend to take longer to chew and digest than refined ones; they also enter the bloodstream more slowly. This slower digestive pace tends to make people feel full sooner and for a longer period. Also, a slower rise in blood glucose levels following the consumption of complex carbohydrates may help in the management of diabetes. Whole grains are also high in dietary fiber and so have all the benefits of fiber (discussed later).

Consumption of whole grains has been linked to a reduced risk of heart disease, diabetes, and cancer and plays an important role in gastrointestinal health and body weight management. For all these reasons, whole grains are recommended over those that have been refined. (See the box "Choosing More Whole-Grain Foods.")

Glycemic Index   Insulin and glucose levels rise and fall following a meal or snack containing any type of carbohydrate. Some foods cause a quick and dramatic rise in glucose and insulin levels, whereas others have a slower, more moderate effect. A food that has a rapid effect on blood glucose levels is said to have a high **glycemic index.** The glycemic index of a food indicates the type of carbohydrate in that food.

Attempting to base food choices on glycemic index is a difficult task. For people with particular health concerns, such as diabetes, glycemic index may be an important consideration in choosing foods. But for most people, the best bet is to choose a variety of vegetables daily and to limit foods that are high in added sugars and low in other nutrients.

> **TERMS**
>
> **whole grain**   The entire edible portion of a grain (such as wheat, rice, or oats), consisting of the germ, endosperm, and bran; processing removes parts of the grain, often leaving just the endosperm.
>
> **glycemic index**   A measure of how a particular food affects blood glucose levels.

TAKE CHARGE
Choosing More Whole-Grain Foods

Because whole-grain foods offer so many health benefits, federal dietary guidelines recommend six or more servings of grain products every day, with at least half of those servings from whole grains. Currently, however, Americans average less than one serving of whole grains per day.

What Are Whole Grains?

The first step in increasing your intake of whole grains is to correctly identify them. The following are whole grains:

Whole wheat	Whole-grain corn
Whole rye	Popcorn
Whole oats	Brown rice
Oatmeal	Whole-grain barley

More unusual choices include bulgur (cracked wheat), millet, kasha (roasted buckwheat kernels), quinoa, wheat and rye berries, amaranth, wild rice, graham flour, whole-grain kamut, whole-grain spelt, and whole-grain triticale.

Wheat flour, unbleached flour, enriched flour, and degerminated corn meal are not whole grains. Wheat germ and wheat bran are also not whole grains, but they are the constituents of wheat typically left out when wheat is processed and so are healthier choices than regular wheat flour, which typically contains just the grain's endosperm.

Checking Packages for Whole Grains

To find packaged foods, read the list of ingredients and check for special health claims related to whole grains. The *first* item on the list of ingredients should be one of the whole grains in the preceding list.

The U.S. Food and Drug Administration (FDA) allows manufacturers to include special health claims for foods that contain 51% or more whole-grain ingredients. Such products may display a statement such as the following on their packaging: "Rich in whole grain." "Made with 100% whole grain." "Diets rich in whole-grain foods may help reduce the risk of heart disease and certain cancers." However, many whole-grain products do not carry such claims. This is one more reason to check the ingredient list to make sure you're buying a product made from one or more whole grains.

Recommended Carbohydrate Intake On average, Americans consume 200–300 grams of carbohydrate per day—well above the 130 grams needed to meet the body's requirement for essential carbohydrate. A range of intakes is associated with good health; the AMDR for carbohydrates is 45–65% of total daily calories. That's about 225–325 grams of carbohydrate for someone who consumes 2000 calories per day. The focus should be on consuming a variety of foods rich in complex carbohydrates, especially whole grains. Athletes in training can especially benefit from high-carbohydrate diets (60–70% of total daily calories), which enhance the amount of carbohydrates stored in their muscles and therefore provide more fuel for use during endurance events or long workouts. Added sugars include the white and brown sugar and high-fructose corn syrup added to foods like candy, baked goods, and sodas and other sugar-sweetened beverages. Currently, added sugars contribute 16% of the total calories in the typical American diet. Foods high in added sugars are generally high in calories and low in nutrients and fiber, thus providing "empty calories." The U.S. Department of Agriculture's (USDA) Food Patterns recommendations (based on the Dietary Guidelines for Americans) are designed so that people can meet nutrient needs and have no more than 5–15% of their daily energy intake from solid fats *and* added sugars together. To reduce your intake of added sugars, limit soft drinks, candy, desserts, and sweetened fruit drinks. The sugars in your diet should come mainly from fruits, which are excellent sources of vitamins and minerals, and from low-fat or fat-free milk and other dairy products, which are high in protein and calcium.

Fiber—A Closer Look

Fiber is the term given to nondigestible carbohydrates provided by plants. Instead of being digested, like starch, fiber moves through the intestinal tract and provides bulk for feces in the large intestine, which in turn facilitates elimination. In the large intestine, bacteria break down some types of fiber into acids and gases, which explains why consuming too much fiber can lead to intestinal gas. Even though humans don't digest fiber, it is necessary for good health.

Types of Fiber The Food and Nutrition Board has defined two types of fiber:

• **Dietary fiber** refers to the nondigestible carbohydrates (and the noncarbohydrate substance *lignin*) that are naturally present in plants such as grains, fruits, legumes, and vegetables. There are two types of dietary fiber: soluble and insoluble. Both types are important for health. **Soluble (viscous) fiber** such as that found in oat bran or legumes can delay stomach emptying, slow the movement of glucose into the blood after eating, and reduce absorption of cholesterol. **Insoluble fiber,** such as that found in wheat bran or psyllium seed, increases fecal bulk and helps prevent constipation, hemorrhoids, and other digestive disorders.

- **Functional fiber** refers to nondigestible carbohydrates that have been either isolated from natural sources or synthesized in a laboratory and then added to a food product or dietary supplement.

- **Total fiber** is the sum of dietary and functional fiber in your diet.

A high-fiber diet can help reduce the risk of type 2 diabetes, heart disease, and pulmonary disease, as well as improve gastrointestinal health and aid in the management of metabolic syndrome and body weight. Some studies have linked high-fiber diets with a reduced risk of colon and rectal cancer. Other studies have suggested that other characteristics of diets rich in fruits, vegetables, and whole grains may be responsible for this reduction in risk.

Sources of Fiber All plant foods contain some dietary fiber. Fruits, legumes, oats (especially oat bran), and barley all contain the viscous types of fiber that help lower blood glucose and cholesterol levels. Wheat (especially wheat bran), other grains and cereals, and vegetables are good sources of cellulose and other fibers that help prevent constipation. Psyllium, which is often added to cereals or used in fiber supplements and laxatives, improves intestinal health and also helps control glucose and cholesterol levels. The processing of packaged foods can remove fiber, so it is important to rely on fresh fruits and vegetables and foods made from whole grains as your main sources of fiber.

Recommended Fiber Intake To reduce the risk of chronic disease and maintain intestinal health, the Food and Nutrition Board recommends a daily fiber intake of 38 grams for adult men and 25 grams for adult women. Americans currently consume about half this amount. Fiber should come from foods, not supplements, which should be used only under medical supervision.

Vitamins—Organic Micronutrients

Vitamins are organic (carbon-containing) substances required in small amounts to regulate various processes within living cells (Table 9.2). Humans need 13 vitamins; of these, 4 are fat-soluble (A, D, E, and K), and 9 are water-soluble (C, and the B-complex vitamins thiamin, riboflavin, niacin, vitamin B-6, folate, vitamin B-12, biotin, and pantothenic acid).

> Even though we don't digest fiber, **it is necessary for good health.**

Functions of Vitamins Many vitamins help chemical reactions take place. They provide no energy to the body directly but help unleash the energy stored in carbohydrates, proteins, and fats. Other vitamins are critical in the production of red blood cells and the maintenance of the nervous, skeletal, and immune systems. Some vitamins act as **antioxidants,** which help preserve the health of cells.

Sources of Vitamins The human body does not manufacture most of the vitamins it requires and must obtain them from foods. Vitamins are abundant in fruits, vegetables, and grains. In addition, many processed foods, such as flour and breakfast cereals, contain added vitamins. A few vitamins are made in certain parts of the body: The skin makes vitamin D when it is exposed to sunlight, and intestinal bacteria make vitamin K. Table 9.2 lists good food sources of vitamins.

Vitamin Deficiencies If your diet lacks a particular vitamin, characteristic symptoms of deficiency can develop (see Table 9.2). Physicians have known about some common deficiency-related ailments for generations. For example, *scurvy* is a potentially fatal illness caused by a long-term lack of vitamin C. Children who do not get enough vitamin D can develop *rickets,* which leads to potentially disabling bone deformations. Vitamin A deficiency may cause blindness, and anemia can develop in people whose diet lacks vitamin B-12, folate, or B-6. Although the data are not conclusive, low levels of folate and vitamins B-6 and B-12 have been linked to an increased risk of heart disease and stroke.

New research is tying vitamin deficiencies with other health risks, as well. For example, experts once thought that vitamin D was the only vitamin that played a role in bone health. Now scientists know that vitamins C and K, as well as several B vitamins, are also important in the prevention of

---

TERMS

insoluble fiber Fiber that does not dissolve in water and is not broken down by bacteria in the large intestine.

functional fiber Nondigestible carbohydrates either isolated from natural sources or synthesized; these may be added to foods and dietary supplements.

total fiber The total amount of dietary fiber and functional fiber in the diet.

vitamins Carbon-containing substances needed in small amounts to help promote and regulate chemical reactions and processes in the body.

antioxidant A substance that can reduce the breakdown of food or body constituents by free radicals; the actions of antioxidants include binding oxygen, donating electrons to free radicals, and repairing damage to molecules.

| Table 9.2 | Facts about Vitamins | | | |

VITAMIN	IMPORTANT DIETARY SOURCES	MAJOR FUNCTIONS	SIGNS OF PROLONGED DEFICIENCY	TOXIC EFFECTS OF MEGADOSES
Fat-soluble				
Vitamin A	Liver, milk, butter, cheese, fortified margarine, carrots, spinach, orange and deep-green vegetables and fruits	Immune function and maintenance of vision, skin, linings of the nose, mouth, digestive and urinary tracts	Night blindness, scaling skin, increased susceptibility to infection, loss of appetite, anemia, kidney stones	Liver damage, miscarriage, birth defects, headache, vomiting, diarrhea, vertigo, double vision, bone abnormalities
Vitamin D	Fortified milk and margarine, fish oils, butter, egg yolks (sunlight on skin also produces vitamin D)	Development and maintenance of bones and teeth, promotion of calcium absorption	Rickets (bone deformities) in children; bone softening, loss, and fractures in adults	Kidney damage, calcium deposits in soft tissues, depression, death
Vitamin E	Vegetable oils, whole grains, nuts and seeds, green leafy vegetables, asparagus, peaches	Protection and maintenance of cellular membranes	Red blood cell breakage and anemia, weakness, neurological problems, muscle cramps	Relatively nontoxic, but may cause excess bleeding or formation of blood clots
Vitamin K	Green leafy vegetables; smaller amounts widespread in other foods	Production of factors essential for blood clotting and bone metabolism	Hemorrhaging	None reported
Water-soluble				
Biotin	Cereals, yeast, egg yolks, soy flour, liver; widespread in foods	Synthesis of fats, glycogen, and amino acids	Rash, nausea, vomiting, weight loss, depression, fatigue, hair loss	None reported
Folate	Green leafy vegetables, yeast, oranges, whole grains, legumes, liver	Amino acid metabolism, synthesis of RNA and DNA, new cell synthesis	Anemia, weakness, fatigue, irritability, shortness of breath, swollen tongue	Masking of vitamin B-12 deficiency
Niacin	Eggs, poultry, fish, milk, whole grains, nuts, enriched breads and cereals, meats, legumes	Conversion of carbohydrates, fats, and proteins into usable forms of energy	Pellagra (symptoms include diarrhea, dermatitis, inflammation of mucous membranes, dementia)	Flushing of the skin, nausea, vomiting, diarrhea, liver dysfunction, glucose intolerance
Pantothenic acid	Animal foods, whole grains, broccoli, potatoes; widespread in foods	Metabolism of fats, carbohydrates, and proteins	Fatigue, numbness and tingling of hands and feet, gastrointestinal disturbances	None reported
Riboflavin	Dairy products, enriched breads and cereals, lean meats, poultry, fish, green vegetables	Energy metabolism; maintenance of skin, mucous membranes, and nervous system structures	Cracks at corners of mouth, sore throat, skin rash, hypersensitivity to light, purple tongue	None reported
Thiamin	Whole-grain and enriched breads and cereals, organ meats, lean pork, nuts, legumes	Conversion of carbohydrates into usable forms of energy, maintenance of appetite and nervous system function	Beriberi (symptoms include muscle wasting, mental confusion, anorexia, enlarged heart, nerve changes)	None reported
Vitamin B-6	Eggs, poultry, fish, whole grains, nuts, soybeans, liver, kidney, pork	Metabolism of amino acids and glycogen	Anemia, convulsions, cracks at corners of mouth, dermatitis, nausea, confusion	Neurological abnormalities and damage
Vitamin B-12	Meat, fish, poultry, fortified cereals	Synthesis of blood cells, other metabolic reactions	Anemia, fatigue, nervous system damage, sore tongue	None reported
Vitamin C	Peppers, broccoli, spinach, brussels sprouts, citrus fruits, strawberries, tomatoes, potatoes, cabbage, other fruits and vegetables	Maintenance and repair of connective tissue, bones, teeth, and cartilage; promotion of healing; absorption of iron	Scurvy, anemia, reduced resistance to infection, loosened teeth, joint pain, poor wound healing, hair loss, poor iron absorption	Urinary stones in some people, acid stomach from ingesting supplements in pill form, nausea, diarrhea, headache, fatigue

SOURCES: Food and Nutrition Board, Institute of Medicine. 2006. *Dietary Reference Intakes: The Essential Guide to Nutrient Requirements.* Washington, DC: The National Academies Press (http://www.nap.edu/openbook.php?record_id=11537&page1); Shils, M. E., et al., eds. 2005. *Modern Nutrition in Health and Disease,* 10th ed. Baltimore: Lippincott Williams & Wilkins.

osteoporosis. A great deal of recent research has focused on vitamin D, with inconsistent results for conditions such as cardiovascular disease and cancers.

Overall, vitamin deficiency diseases are common in rural areas of developing countries; they are relatively rare in the United States because vitamins are readily available from our fortified food supply. Still, many Americans consume lower-than-recommended amounts of several vitamins. Even in the face of new findings, there is not enough evidence to suggest that the majority of the population begin taking vitamin supplements. Supplementation is discussed in detail later in this chapter.

Vitamin Excesses   Extra vitamins in the diet can also be harmful, especially when taken as supplements for an extended period of time. Megadoses of fat-soluble vitamins are particularly dangerous because the excess is stored in the body rather than excreted, increasing the risk of toxicity. Even when vitamins are not taken in excess, relying on supplements for an adequate intake of vitamins can be a problem because many health benefits from other, nonvitamin ingredients in foods are likely to be missed.

Minerals—Inorganic Micronutrients

Minerals are inorganic (noncarbon-containing) elements you need in relatively small amounts to help regulate body functions, aid in the growth and maintenance of body tissues, and help release energy (Table 9.3). There are about 17 essential minerals. The major minerals, which the body needs in amounts exceeding 100 milligrams per day, include calcium, phosphorus, magnesium, sodium, potassium, and chloride. The essential trace minerals, which you need in minute amounts, include copper, fluoride, iodide, iron, selenium, and zinc.

Characteristic symptoms develop if an essential mineral is consumed in a quantity too small or too large for good health. The minerals commonly lacking in the American diet are iron, calcium, potassium, and magnesium. Iron-deficiency **anemia** is a problem in many age groups, but particularly among menstruating women and among women who have had multiple pregnancies. Researchers fear that poor calcium intakes in childhood are sowing the seeds for future **osteoporosis,** especially in women. (see the box "Eating for Healthy Bones").

Water—Vital but Often Ignored

Water is the major component in both foods and the human body: we are composed of about 50–60% water. Our need for other nutrients, in terms of weight, is much less than our need for water. We can live up to 50 days without food but only a few days without water.

Water is distributed all over the body, among lean and other tissues and in blood and other body fluids. Water is used in the digestion and absorption of food and is the medium in which most of the chemical reactions take place within the body. Some water-based fluids, like blood, transport substances around the body, whereas other fluids serve as lubricants or cushions. Water also helps regulate body temperature.

Water is contained in almost all foods, particularly in liquids, fruits, and vegetables. The foods and beverages you consume provide 80–90% of your daily water intake; the remainder is generated through metabolism. You lose water each day in urine, feces, and sweat and through evaporation from your lungs.

Most people can maintain a healthy water balance by consuming beverages at meals and drinking fluids in response to thirst. The Food and Nutrition Board has set levels of adequate water intake to maintain hydration. All fluids, including those containing caffeine, can count toward your total daily fluid intake. Under these guidelines, men need about 3.7 total liters of water daily, with 3.0 liters (about 13 cups) coming from beverages; women need 2.7 total liters, with 2.2 liters (about 9 cups) coming from beverages. If you exercise vigorously or live in a hot climate, you need to consume additional fluids to maintain a balance between water consumed and water lost. Severe dehydration causes weakness and can lead to death.

Other Substances in Food

Many substances in food are not essential nutrients but may influence health.

Antioxidants   When the body uses oxygen or breaks down certain fats or proteins as a normal part of metabolism, it gives rise to substances called **free radicals.**

Table 9.3 — Facts about Selected Minerals

MINERAL	IMPORTANT DIETARY SOURCES	MAJOR FUNCTIONS	SIGNS OF PROLONGED DEFICIENCY	TOXIC EFFECTS OF MEGADOSES
Calcium	Milk and milk products, tofu, fortified orange juice and bread, green leafy vegetables, bones in fish	Formation of bones and teeth, control of nerve impulses, muscle contraction, blood clotting	Stunted growth in children, bone mineral loss in adults, urinary stones	Kidney stones, calcium deposits in soft tissues, inhibition of mineral absorption, constipation
Fluoride	Fluoridated water, tea, marine fish eaten with bones	Maintenance of tooth and bone structure	Higher frequency of tooth decay	Increased bone density, mottling of teeth, impaired kidney function
Iodine	Iodized salt, seafood, processed foods	Essential part of thyroid hormones, regulation of body metabolism	Goiter (enlarged thyroid), cretinism (birth defect)	Depression of thyroid activity, hyperthyroidism in susceptible people
Iron	Meat and poultry, fortified grain products, dark green vegetables, dried fruit	Component of hemoglobin, myoglobin, and enzymes	Iron-deficiency anemia, weakness, impaired immune function, gastrointestinal distress	Nausea, diarrhea, liver and kidney damage, joint pains, sterility, disruption of cardiac function, death
Magnesium	Widespread in foods and water (except soft water); especially found in grains, legumes, nuts, seeds, green vegetables, milk	Transmission of nerve impulses, energy transfer, activation of many enzymes	Neurological disturbances, cardiovascular problems, kidney disorders, nausea, growth failure in children	Nausea, vomiting, diarrhea, central nervous system depression, coma; death in people with impaired kidney function
Phosphorus	Present in nearly all foods, especially milk, cereal, peas, eggs, meat	Bone growth and maintenance, energy transfer in cells	Impaired growth, weakness, kidney disorders, cardiorespiratory and nervous system dysfunction	Drop in blood calcium levels, calcium deposits in soft tissues, bone loss
Potassium	Meats, milk, fruits, vegetables, grains, legumes	Nerve function, body water balance	Muscular weakness, nausea, drowsiness, paralysis, confusion, disruption of cardiac rhythm	Cardiac arrest
Selenium	Seafood, meat, eggs, whole grains	Defense against oxidative stress, regulation of thyroid hormone action	Muscle pain and weakness, heart disorders	Hair and nail loss, nausea and vomiting, weakness, irritability
Sodium	Salt, soy sauce, salted foods, tomato juice	Body water balance, acid–base balance, nerve function	Muscle weakness, loss of appetite, nausea, vomiting; deficiency is rarely seen	Edema (excess fluid buildup), hypertension in sensitive people
Zinc	Whole grains, meat, eggs, liver, seafood (especially oysters)	Synthesis of proteins, RNA, and DNA; wound healing; immune response; ability to taste	Growth failure, loss of appetite, impaired taste acuity, skin rash, impaired immune function, poor wound healing	Vomiting, impaired immune function, decline in blood HDL levels, impaired copper absorption

SOURCES: Food and Nutrition Board, Institute of Medicine. 2006. *Dietary Reference Intakes: The Essential Guide to Nutrient Requirements.* Washington, DC: The National Academies Press (http://www.nap.edu/openbook.php?record_id=11537&page1); Shils, M. E., et al., eds. 2005. *Modern Nutrition in Health and Disease,* 10th ed. Baltimore: Lippincott Williams & Wilkins.

Environmental factors such as cigarette smoke, exhaust fumes, radiation, excessive sunlight, certain drugs, and stress can increase free radical production. A free radical is a chemically unstable molecule that reacts with fats, proteins, and DNA, damaging cell membranes and mutating genes. Free radicals have been implicated in aging, cancer, cardiovascular disease, and other degenerative diseases like arthritis.

Antioxidants found in foods can help protect the body from damage by free radicals in several ways. Some prevent or reduce the formation of free radicals; others remove free radicals from the body; still others repair some types of free

Ask Yourself

QUESTIONS FOR CRITICAL THINKING AND REFLECTION

Experts say that two of the most important factors in a healthy diet are eating the "right" kinds of carbohydrates and eating the "right" kinds of fats. Based on what you've read so far in this chapter, which are the "right" carbohydrates and fats? How would you say your own diet stacks up when it comes to carbohydrates and fats?

Osteoporosis is a condition in which the bones become dangerously thin and fragile over time. In 2014, the National Osteoporosis Foundation estimated the prevalence of osteoporosis in the United States to be at 10.2 million, and an additional 43.4 million adults over age 50 have low bone mass. Women account for about 80% of osteoporosis cases. Most of our adult bone mass is built by age 18 in girls and age 20 in boys. After bone density peaks between ages 25 and 35, bone mass is lost slowly over time and then at an increasing rate after menopause. To prevent osteoporosis, the best strategy is to build as much bone as possible during your youth and do everything you can to maintain it as you age. Up to 50% of bone loss is determined by controllable lifestyle factors such as resistance training and diet. Key nutrients for bone health include the following:

- **Calcium.** Getting enough calcium is important throughout life to build and maintain bone mass. Milk, yogurt, and calcium-fortified orange juice, bread, and cereals are all good sources.

- **Vitamin D.** Vitamin D is necessary for bones to absorb calcium. The Institute of Medicine recommends a daily intake of 600–800 IU of vitamin D for most people. The National Osteoporosis Foundation recommends about 800–1000 IU of vitamin D for men and women over the age of 50 years. Vitamin D can be obtained from foods and is manufactured by the skin when exposed to sunlight. Candidates for vitamin D supplements include people who don't eat many foods rich in vitamin D; those who don't expose their faces, arms, and hands to the sun (without sunscreen) for 5–15 minutes a few times each week; and people who live north of an imaginary line roughly between Boston and the Oregon–California border (where the sun is weaker).

- **Vitamin K.** Vitamin K promotes the synthesis of proteins that help keep bones strong. Broccoli and leafy green vegetables are rich in vitamin K.

- **Other nutrients.** Other nutrients that may play an important role in bone health include vitamin C, magnesium, potassium, phosphorus, fluoride, manganese, zinc, copper, and boron.

Several dietary substances may have a *negative* effect on bone health, especially if consumed in excess. These include alcohol, sodium, caffeine, and retinol (a form of vitamin A). Drinking lots of soda, which often replaces milk in the diet, has been shown to increase the risk of bone fractures in teenage girls.

The effect of protein intake on bone mass depends on other nutrients. Protein helps build bone as long as calcium and vitamin D intake are adequate. But if intake of calcium and vitamin D is low, high protein intake can lead to bone loss.

Weight-bearing aerobic exercise helps maintain bone mass throughout life, and strength training improves bone density, muscle mass, strength, and balance. Drinking alcohol only in moderation, refraining from smoking, and managing depression and stress are also important for maintaining strong bones. For people who develop osteoporosis, a variety of medications are available to treat the condition.

---

radical damage after it occurs. Some antioxidants, such as vitamin C, vitamin E, and selenium, are also essential nutrients. Others—such as the carotenoids found in yellow, orange, and deep-green vegetables—are not. Some of the top antioxidant-containing foods and beverages include blackberries, walnuts, strawberries, artichokes, cranberries, brewed coffee, raspberries, pecans, blueberries, cloves, grape juice, baking chocolate, sour cherries, and red wine. Also high in antioxidants are brussels sprouts, kale, cauliflower, and pomegranates.

Phytochemicals Antioxidants fall into the broader category of **phytochemicals,** which are substances found in plant foods that may help prevent chronic disease. In just the past 30 years, researchers have identified and studied hundreds of different compounds found in foods, and many findings are promising. For example, certain substances found in soy foods may help lower cholesterol levels. Sulforaphane, a compound isolated from broccoli and other **cruciferous vegetables,** may render some carcinogenic compounds harmless. Allyl sulfides, a group of chemicals found in garlic and onions, appear to boost the activity of immune cells and lower total cholesterol concentrations.

Berries are rich in antioxidants, vitamins, and dietary fiber.

phytochemical A naturally occurring substance found in plant foods that may help prevent and treat chronic diseases like cancer and heart disease; *phyto* means plant. **TERMS**

Carotenoids found in green vegetables may help preserve eyesight with age. Further research on phytochemicals may extend the role of nutrition to the prevention and treatment of many chronic diseases.

If you want to increase your intake of phytochemicals, it is best to eat a variety of fruits, vegetables, and grains rather than relying on supplements. Like many vitamins and minerals, isolated phytochemicals may be harmful if taken in high doses. In many cases, their health benefits could be the result of many chemical substances working in combination. Eating more fruits and vegetables is a smart alternative to less healthy foods. In contrast, people who rely more on supplements may take them and eat large portions of unhealthy foods.

NUTRITIONAL GUIDELINES: PLANNING YOUR DIET

Scientific and government groups have created a variety of tools to help people design healthy diets: **Dietary Reference Intakes (DRIs)** are standards for nutrient intake designed to prevent nutritional deficiencies and reduce the risk of chronic diseases. The **Dietary Guidelines for Americans** were established to promote health and reduce the risk of major chronic diseases through diet and physical activity. **MyPlate** (formerly MyPyramid) provides a food guidance system to help people apply the Dietary Guidelines for Americans to their own diets.

> Two-thirds of Americans are overweight or obese, yet many are **undernourished in several key nutrients**.

Dietary Reference Intakes (DRIs)

The Food and Nutrition Board of the Institute of Medicine of the National Academies establishes dietary standards, or recommended intake levels, for Americans of all ages. The current set of standards, the Dietary Reference Intakes (DRIs), was introduced in 1997. The DRIs are frequently reviewed and are updated as new nutrition-related information becomes available. The DRIs present different categories of nutrients in an easy-to-read table format. The DRIs have a broad focus, being based on research that looks not just at the prevention of nutrient deficiencies but also at the role of nutrients in promoting health and preventing chronic diseases such as cancer, osteoporosis, and heart disease.

The DRIs include a set of four reference values used as standards for both recommended intakes and maximum safe intakes. The recommended intake of each nutrient is expressed as either a *Recommended Dietary Allowance (RDA)* or an *Adequate Intake (AI)*. An AI is set when there is not enough information available to set an RDA value; regardless of the type of standard used, however, the DRI represents the best available estimate of intake for optimal health. The *Tolerable Upper Intake Level (UL)* is the maximum daily intake that is unlikely to cause health problems in a healthy person.

Because of lack of data, ULs have not been set for all nutrients. The absence of ULs does not mean that people can tolerate chronic intakes of these vitamins and minerals above recommended levels. Like all chemical agents, nutrients can produce adverse effects if intakes are excessive. There is no established benefit from consuming nutrients at levels above the RDA or AI.

Because the DRIs are too cumbersome to use as a basis for food labels, the U.S. Food and Drug Administration (FDA) uses another set of dietary standards, the **Daily Values.** The Daily Values are based on several different sets of guidelines and include standards for fat, cholesterol, carbohydrate, dietary fiber, and selected vitamins and minerals. The Daily Values represent appropriate intake levels for a 2000-calorie diet. The Daily Value percentage on a food label shows how well that food contributes to your recommended daily intake, assuming you follow a 2000-calorie-per-day diet. Food labels are described in detail later in this chapter.

Dietary Guidelines for Americans

To provide general guidance for choosing a healthy diet, the USDA and the U.S. Department of Health and Human Services (HHS) issue the Dietary Guidelines for Americans, revising them every five years. These guidelines are intended for all healthy Americans, including children aged 2 and older.

Following these guidelines promotes health and reduces risk of chronic disease, including heart disease, cancer, diabetes, stroke, osteoporosis, and obesity. Each of the guidelines is supported by an extensive review of scientific and medical evidence.

The 2010 Dietary Guidelines are designed to help Americans make healthy and informed food choices. The main objective of the 2010 report is to encourage improved nutrition and physical activity in the American population, two-thirds of whom are overweight or obese and yet undernourished in several key nutrients. It focuses on the total diet and how to integrate the recommendations into a practical eating pattern that is nutrient-dense and calorie-balanced. And it includes findings on the broad environmental and societal aspects of the American diet—that is, the "food environment."

The 2010 Dietary Guidelines point out the large discrepancy between the recommendations and the actual American diet. Until new guidelines become available (estimated 2015), we will continue to rely on the 2010 guidelines. The most likely change in the 2015 dietary guidelines will be a greater emphasis on limiting added sugars and greater encouragement of physical activity.

General Guidelines   The Dietary Guidelines present two overarching recommendations:

- Maintain calorie balance over time to achieve and sustain a healthy weight.
- Focus on consuming nutrient-dense foods and beverages.

The guidelines highlight several key areas—balancing energy intake to manage weight, reducing certain dietary components, increasing other dietary components, building healthy eating patterns, and making healthy choices in the context of the current food and physical activity environment.

Balancing Energy Intake and Expenditure to Manage Weight   Energy balance—the balance between energy intake and energy expenditure—is the key to weight management. Current high rates of overweight and obesity can be attributed at least in part to people consuming more calories in foods and beverages than they expend in physical activity. In other words, they eat more than they can burn off.

The guidelines recognize that many aspects of American life promote obesity, leading to an "obesogenic food environment." This environment is affected by such factors as an increase in the number of fast-food restaurants in impoverished communities, an increase in meals eaten outside the home, increased portion sizes, sedentary work and home environments, limited availability of safe outdoor walking and recreational spaces, increased dependence on transportation and technological advances that lead to lower energy expenditure on everyday tasks, and reliance on precooked or canned energy-dense foods.

Whereas societal policies can help prevent unhealthy body weights at all stages of the life cyle, managing body weight still remains a personal responsibility.

> The food environment affects both sides of the energy balance equation— it can **promote overconsumption of high-energy foods and/or discourage energy expenditure** in the form of physical activity.

Foods and Food Components to Reduce   In addition to overall energy intake, Americans tend to eat certain foods and food components in excess—in particular, those rich in sodium, solid fats, added sugars, and refined grains. Foods high in these items often replace foods with the needed nutrients in the diet. Key recommendations include the following:

- Reducing daily sodium intake to less than 2300 milligrams (mg) and further reducing intake to 1500 mg if you are 51 or older, are African American, or have hypertension, diabetes, or chronic kidney disease. High sodium intake is associated with high blood pressure.

- Limiting intake of fat and dietary cholesterol. Keep trans fatty acid consumption as low as possible, especially by limiting foods that contain synthetic sources of trans fats, such as partially hydrogenated oils. Consume less than 300 mg per day of dietary cholesterol.

- Reducing the intake of energy from solid fats and added sugars. Most people should consume no more than 5–15% of daily calories from foods in these categories.

- Limiting the consumption of foods that contain refined grains, especially refined grain foods that contain solid fats, added sugars, and sodium.

- Consuming alcohol in moderation—up to one drink per day for women and two drinks per day for men.

Foods and Nutrients to Increase   In general, Americans don't eat a wide enough variety of nutrient-dense foods to obtain all the nutrients they need in the amounts for optimal health. Recommendations include the following:

- Eating more fruits and vegetables, and eating a variety of vegetables, especially dark-green, red, and orange vegetables and beans and peas.

- Consuming at least half of all grains as whole grains, which are a source of iron, B vitamins, and dietary fiber.

- Increasing intake of fat-free or low-fat milk and milk products, such as milk, yogurt, cheese, or fortified soy beverages. They are important sources of calcium, potassium, magnesium, vitamin D, and vitamin A.

- Choosing a variety of protein foods, including seafood, lean meat and poultry, eggs, beans and peas, soy products, and unsalted nuts and seeds. Increase the amount and variety of seafood, and reduce protein foods that are high in solid fats and calories. In addition to protein, these foods provide B vitamins, vitamin E, zinc, and magnesium.

- Using oils to replace solid fats where possible.

- Choosing foods that provide more potassium, dietary fiber, calcium, and vitamin D, which are nutrients of concern in American diets. These foods include vegetables, fruits, whole grains, and milk and milk products.

- Other nutrients are a concern for certain specific population groups, such as folic acid and iron for women who are pregnant or may become pregnant and vitamin B-12 for adults aged 50 or older.

Building Healthy Eating Patterns   There are many different ways to incorporate the individual recommendations of the 2010 Dietary Guidelines into healthy eating patterns that (1) meet nutrient needs; (2) stay within calorie limits; (3) accommodate cultural, ethnic, traditional, and personal preferences; and (4) take into account food cost and availability. In other words, people can eat healthfully in many different ways.

Three eating plans that show how to put the Dietary Guidelines recommendations into action are the USDA Food Patterns, vegetarian adaptations of the USDA Food Patterns, and the DASH Eating Plan.

A general principle in all these diets is that people should eat nutrient-dense foods—foods with little or no solid fats and added sugars—so they get all the needed nutrients without exceeding their daily energy intake requirements. Another principle is that people should get their nutrients from foods rather than from dietary supplements, although supplements or fortification may be helpful for certain populations.

The USDA Food Patterns set recommended amounts of food to eat from each of five food groups and subgroups at different energy levels. They also allow a certain amount of oils, and they limit the amount of energy that should be consumed from solid fats and added sugars (SoFAS). You can use the chart shown in Figure 9.2 to find out the recommended intake of foods in each food group at your energy level. For help determining your energy level, refer to Table 9.4.

The vegetarian adaptations of the USDA Food Patterns include changes in the protein group and, for vegans, in the dairy group. The vegetarian variations, especially the vegan variation, rely on some fortified foods to ensure that the diet provides all required nutrients, such as calcium and vitamin B-12.

The DASH Eating Plan emphasizes fruits, vegetables, fat-free and low-fat milk and milk products, whole grains, fish, poultry, seeds, and nuts. The DASH Eating Plan has been shown to help people lower their blood pressure and cholesterol levels, and it is associated with a lower risk of cardiovascular disease.

Table 9.4	Estimated Daily Calorie Needs		
AGE (YEARS)	SEDENTARY[a]	MODERATELY ACTIVE[b]	ACTIVE[c]
Female			
2–3	1000	1000–1400	1000–1400
4–8	1200–1400	1400–1600	1400–1800
9–13	1400–1600	1600–2000	1800–2200
14–18	1800	2000	2400
19–30	1800–2000	2000–2200	2400
31–50	1800	2000	2200
51+	1600	1800	2000–2200
Male			
2–3	1000–1200	1000–1400	1000–1400
4–8	1400–1600	1400–1600	1600–2000
9–13	1600–2000	1800–2200	2000–2600
14–18	2000–2400	2400–2800	2800–3200
19–30	2400–2600	2600–2800	3000
31–50	2200–2400	2400–2600	2800–3000
51+	2000–2200	2200–2400	2400–2800

[a]A lifestyle that includes only the light physical activity associated with typical day-to-day life

[b]A lifestyle that includes physical activity equivalent to walking about 1.5 to 3 miles per day at 3 to 4 miles per hour (30–60 minutes a day of moderate physical activity), in addition to the light physical activity associated with typical day-to-day life

[c]A lifestyle that includes physical activity equivalent to walking more than 3 miles per day at 3 to 4 miles per hour (60 or more minutes a day of moderate physical activity), in addition to the light physical activity associated with typical day-to-day life

SOURCE: U.S. Department of Agriculture and U.S. Department of Health and Human Services. 2010. *Dietary Guidelines for Americans, 2010,* 7th ed. Washington, DC: U.S. Government Printing Office (http://www.cnpp.usda.gov/publications/dietaryguidelines/2010/policydoc/policydoc.pdf).

The eating pattern associated with many cultures bordering the Mediterranean Sea and referred to as the Mediterranean diet or the Mediterranean-style eating pattern has many features in common with the USDA Food Patterns and the DASH Eating Plan. It emphasizes fruits and vegetables, nuts, olive oil, and grains—often whole grains—and includes only small amounts of meat and full-fat milk and milk products. The Mediterranean diet has been associated with lower rates of heart disease and total mortality.

Helping Americans Make Healthy Choices   A final area covered by the 2010 Dietary Guidelines for Americans is the environment in which people make their food choices. To make healthy choices, individuals need opportunities to obtain healthy foods and engage in physical activity in safe and conducive environments. Significant numbers of Americans—notably members of racial and ethnic minorities, people with disabilities, and people with lower incomes—lack access to affordable, nutritious foods and opportunities for safe physical activity in their neighborhoods.

Daily Amount of Food from Each Group

Food group amounts shown in cups (c) or ounce-equivalents (oz-eq)

Calorie level of pattern	1600	1800	2000	2200	2400	2600	2800	3000
Fruits	1.5 c	1.5 c	2 c	2 c	2 c	2 c	2.5 c	2.5 c
Vegetables	2 c	2.5 c	2.5 c	3 c	3 c	3.5 c	3.5 c	4 c
Dark-green	1.5 c/wk	1.5 c/wk	1.5 c/wk	2 c/wk	2 c/wk	2.5 c/wk	2.5 c/wk	2.5 c/wk
Red and orange	4 c/wk	5.5 c/wk	5.5 c/wk	6 c/wk	6 c/wk	7 c/wk	7 c/wk	7.5 c/wk
Beans and peas (legumes)	1 c/wk	1.5 c/wk	1.5 c/wk	2 c/wk	2 c/wk	2.5 c/wk	2.5 c/wk	3 c/wk
Starchy	4 c/wk	5 c/wk	5 c/wk	6 c/wk	6 c/wk	7 c/wk	7 c/wk	8 c/wk
Other	3.5 c/wk	4 c/wk	4 c/wk	5 c/wk	5 c/wk	5.5 c/wk	5.5 c/wk	7 c/wk
Grains	5 oz-eq	6 oz-eq	6 oz-eq	7 oz-eq	8 oz-eq	9 oz-eq	10 oz-eq	10 oz-eq
Whole grains	3 oz-eq	3 oz-eq	3 oz-eq	3.5 oz-eq	4 oz-eq	4.5 oz-eq	5 oz-eq	5 oz-eq
Enriched grains	2 oz-eq	3 oz-eq	3 oz-eq	3.5 oz-eq	4 oz-eq	4.5 oz-eq	5 oz-eq	5 oz-eq
Protein foods	5 oz-eq	5 oz-eq	5.5 oz-eq	6 oz-eq	6.5 oz-eq	6.5 oz-eq	7 oz-eq	7 oz-eq
Seafood	8 oz/wk	8 oz/wk	8 oz/wk	9 oz/wk	10 oz/wk	10 oz/wk	11 oz/wk	11 oz/wk
Meat poultry, eggs	24 oz/wk	24 oz/wk	26 oz/wk	29 oz/wk	31 oz/wk	31 oz/wk	34 oz/wk	34 oz/wk
Nuts, seeds, soy products	4 oz/wk	4 oz/wk	4 oz/wk	4 oz/wk	5 oz/wk	5 oz/wk	5 oz/wk	5 oz/wk
Dairy	3 c	3 c	3 c	3 c	3 c	3 c	3 c	3 c
Oils	22 g	24 g	27 g	29 g	31 g	34 g	36 g	44 g
Maximum SoFAS limit, calories (% of calories)	121 (8%)	161 (9%)	258 (13%)	266 (12%)	330 (14%)	362 (14%)	395 (14%)	459 (15%)

FIGURE 9.2 **USDA Food Patterns.** To determine an appropriate amount of food from each food group, find the column for your estimated daily energy level. That column shows the recommended daily intake from each group. For a personalized intake plan, visit http://choosemyplate.gov/.

SOURCE: U.S. Department of Agriculture and U.S. Department of Health and Human Services. 2010. *Dietary Guidelines for Americans, 2010,* 7th ed. Washington, DC: U.S. Government Printing Office (http://www.cnpp.usda.gov/publications/dietaryguidelines/2010/policydoc/policydoc.pdf).

The guidelines also recognize the need for *food security* in the United States—defined as the ability to acquire adequate food to meet nutritional needs in a socially acceptable manner. According to the USDA's 2013 economic research report, nearly 15% of the U.S. population is not able to obtain sufficient food to meet basic nutritional needs, and as already noted, many more Americans have diets that provide adequate energy but are deficient in essential nutrients.

The guidelines call on all elements of society, ranging from educators to communities to government policymakers, to implement strategies aimed at improving the food and activity environment in the United States.

USDA's MyPlate

To further help consumers put the Dietary Guidelines for Americans into practice, the USDA also issues the food guidance system known as MyPlate (formerly MyPyramid). MyPlate provides a simple graphic showing how to use the five good groups to build a healthy plate at each meal (Figure 9.3).

FIGURE 9.3 **How to eat for health.** Released in 2011, the USDA's MyPlate is designed as a simple graphic to help Americans apply the Dietary Guidelines for Americans to their own diets.

SOURCE: U.S. Department of Agriculture. 2010. *Choose MyPlate* (http://www.choosemyplate.gov).

Key messages include the following:

- Balancing calories:
  - Enjoy your food, but eat less.
  - Avoid oversized portions.
- Foods to increase:
  - Make half your plate fruits and vegetables.
  - Make at least half your grains whole grains.
  - Switch to fat-free or low-fat (1%) milk.
- Foods to reduce:
  - Compare sodium in foods like soup, bread, and frozen meals, and choose the foods with lower numbers.
  - Drink water instead of sugary drinks.

You can get a personalized version of MyPlate recommendations by visiting ChooseMyPlate.gov. Using the daily food plan feature, you can determine the amount of each food group you need daily based on your calorie allowance. Your plan is personalized based on your age, gender, weight, height, and level of physical activity. Another feature available at ChooseMyPlate.gov is the SuperTracker, which helps consumers create a personalized food and activity plan.

Each food group is described briefly in the following sections. Many Americans have trouble identifying serving sizes, so recommended daily intakes from each group are given in terms of cups and ounces; see the box "Judging Portion Sizes" for additional advice. Another way to track your calories and exercise is through several well-rated smartphone apps, such as MyFitnessPal and SparkPeople.

Whole and Refined Grains A 2000-calorie diet should include 6 ounce-equivalents each day, with half of those servings from whole grains. The key message for consumers is this: *Make at least half of your grains whole grains.* The following items count as a 1 ounce-equivalent:

- 1 slice of bread
- 1 small (2½-inch diameter) muffin
- 1 cup ready-to-eat cereal flakes
- ½ cup cooked cereal, rice, grains, or pasta
- 1 6-inch tortilla

Vegetables A 2000-calorie diet should include 2½ cups of vegetables daily. The key message for the vegetable group is this: *Make half your plate fruits and vegetables.* Each of the following counts as a 1 cup equivalent from the vegetable group:

- 1 cup raw or cooked vegetables
- 2 cups raw leafy salad greens
- 1 cup vegetable juice

Because vegetables vary in the nutrients they provide, it is important to eat a variety of vegetables to obtain maximum nutrition. MyPlate recommends weekly servings from five different subgroups within the vegetables group (see Figure 9.2). Try to eat vegetables from several subgroups each day.

Fruits A 2000-calorie diet should include 2 cups of fruits daily. The key message for the fruit group is this: *Make half your plate fruits and vegetables.* Each of the following counts as a 1 cup equivalent from the fruit group:

- 1 cup fresh, canned, or frozen fruit
- 1 cup fruit juice (100% juice)
- 1 small whole fruit
- ½ cup dried fruit

Choose whole fruits often; they are higher in fiber and often lower in energy than fruit juices. Fruit *juices* typically contain more nutrients and less added sugar than fruit *drinks*.

Dairy Dairy choices should be fat-free or low-fat as much as possible to reduce energy intake. A 2000-calorie diet should include 3 cups of milk or the equivalent daily. Each of the following counts as the equivalent of 1 cup:

- 1 cup milk
- 1 cup yogurt
- ½ cup ricotta cheese
- 1½ ounces natural cheese
- 2 ounces processed cheese

Cottage cheese is lower in calcium than most other cheeses; ½ cup is equivalent to ¼ cup milk.

Protein Foods A 2000-calorie diet should include 5½ ounce-equivalents daily. Each of the following counts as an equivalent to 1 ounce:

- 1 ounce cooked lean meat, poultry, or fish
- ¼ cup cooked dried beans (legumes) or tofu

Studies have shown that most people underestimate the size of their food portions, in many cases by as much as 50%. If you need to retrain your eye, try using measuring cups and spoons and an inexpensive kitchen scale when you eat at home. With a little practice, you'll learn the difference between 3 and 8 ounces of chicken or meat and what a half-cup of rice really looks like. For quick estimates, use the following equivalents:

- 1 teaspoon of margarine = the tip of your thumb

- 1 ounce of cheese = your thumb, four dice stacked together, or an ice cube

- 3 ounces of chicken or meat = a deck of cards

- 1 cup of pasta = a small fist or a tennis ball

- ½ cup of rice or cooked vegetables = an ice cream scoop or one-third of a can of soda

- 2 tablespoons of peanut butter = a ping-pong ball or a large marshmallow

- 1 medium potato = a computer mouse

- 2-ounce muffin or roll = a plum or a large egg

- 2-ounce bagel = a hockey puck or a yo-yo

- 1 medium fruit (apple or orange) = a baseball

- ¼ cup nuts = a golf ball

- Small cookie or cracker = a poker chip

- 1 egg
- 1 tablespoon peanut butter
- ½ ounce nuts or seeds

Choose lean meats and skinless poultry, select a variety of protein foods, and watch serving sizes carefully. Choose at least one serving of plant proteins, such as black beans, lentils, or tofu, every day, and include at least 8 ounces of cooked seafood per week.

Oils Oils are major sources of vitamin E and unsaturated fatty acids, including essential fatty acids, but they are not a food group. A 2000-calorie diet should include 6 teaspoons (27g) of oils per day. A 1 teaspoon serving is the equivalent of the following:

- 1 teaspoon vegetable oil or soft margarine
- 1 tablespoon mayonnaise-type salad dressing

Foods that are mostly oils include nuts, olives, avocados, and some fish. The following portions include about 1 teaspoon of oil: 8 large olives, ⅙ medium avocado, ½ tablespoon peanut butter, and ⅓ ounce roasted nuts.

Solid Fats and Added Sugars (SoFAS) If you consistently choose nutrient-dense foods that are fat-free or low-fat and that contain no added sugars, you can also have a small amount of additional calories in the form of solid fats and added sugars (SoFAS). Figure 9.2 shows the maximum number of SoFAS calories allowed at each calorie level in MyPlate.

Physical Activity The Dietary Guidelines for Americans and MyPlate strongly encourage all Americans to be physically active as much as possible. Daily physical activity improves health, reduces the risk of chronic diseases, and helps people manage body weight. The MyPlate recommendation for adults is 2½ hours of moderate physical activity or 1¼ hours of vigorous physical activity per week, equivalent to the 150 minutes of moderate activity or 75 minutes of vigorous activity recommended in the 2008 Physical Activity Guidelines for Americans.

The Vegetarian Alternative

Vegetarians choose a diet with one basic difference from the diets described previously—they restrict or exclude foods of animal origin (meat, poultry, fish, eggs, and milk). Vegetarian diets tend to be lower in total energy content and calories from total fat, saturated fat, cholesterol, and animal protein while being higher in complex carbohydrates, dietary fiber, potassium, folate, vitamins C and E, carotenoids, and phytochemicals. Individuals who follow a vegetarian diet generally have a lower BMI than nonvegetarians. Many people adopt a vegetarian diet for health reasons, whereas others do so out of concern for the environment, financial reasons, or reasons related to ethics or religion.

Types of Vegetarian Diets There are various vegetarian styles. The wider the variety of the diet eaten, the easier it is to meet nutritional needs. *Vegans* eat only plant foods. *Lacto-vegetarians* eat plant foods and dairy products. *Lacto-ovo-vegetarians* eat plant foods, dairy products, and eggs. Others can be categorized as partial vegetarians, semi-vegetarians, or pesco-vegetarians. The latter—also called pescatarians or pescetarians—have diets that are mainly plant-based but also include fish and other seafoods. Partial vegetarians generally eat plant foods, dairy products, eggs, and usually a small selection of poultry, fish, and other seafood.

A Food Plan for Vegetarians Adapting the USDA Food Patterns and MyPlate for vegetarians requires only a few key modifications. For the meat and beans group, vegetarians can

> **vegetarian** Someone who follows a diet that restricts or eliminates foods of animal origin.

TERMS

WELLNESS ON CAMPUS
Eating Strategies for College Students

All the Time

- Eat a colorful, varied diet. The more colorful your diet is, the more varied and rich in fruits and vegetables it will be. Fruits and vegetables are typically inexpensive, delicious, nutritious, and low in fat.

- Eat breakfast. You'll have more energy in the morning and be less likely to grab an unhealthy snack later on.

- Choose healthy snacks—fruits, vegetables, whole grains, and cereals.

- Drink nonfat milk, water, mineral water, or 100% fruit juice more often than soft drinks or sweetened beverages.

- Pay attention to portion sizes.

- Combine physical activity with healthy eating.

Eating in the Dining Hall

- Choose a meal plan that includes breakfast.

- Decide what you want to eat before you get in line, and stick to your choices.

- Build your meals around whole grains and vegetables. Ask for small servings of meat and high-fat main dishes.

- Choose leaner poultry, fish, or bean dishes without added sugar or high sodium rather than high-fat meats and fried entrees.

- Ask that gravies and sauces be served on the side; limit your intake.

- Choose broth-based or vegetable soups, not cream soups.

- At the salad bar, load up on leafy greens, beans, and fresh vegetables. Avoid mayonnaise-coated salads, bacon, croutons, and high-fat dressings. Put dressing on the side, and dip your fork into it rather than pouring it over the salad.

- Choose fruit for dessert rather than baked goods.

Eating in Fast-Food Restaurants

- Order small single burgers with no cheese instead of double burgers with many toppings.

- Ask for items to be prepared without mayonnaise, tartar sauce, sour cream, or other high-fat sauces. Ketchup, mustard, and fat-free mayonnaise or sour cream are better choices and are available at many fast-food restaurants.

- Choose whole-grain bread for burgers and sandwiches.

- Choose chicken items made from chicken breast, not processed chicken.

- Order vegetable pizzas without extra cheese.

- Try a salad or fruit as a side item. If you can't resist French fries or onion rings, get the smallest size.

Eating on the Run

- Carry items that are small and convenient but nutritious, such as fresh fruits or vegetables, whole-wheat buns or muffins, snack-size cereal boxes, and water.

- Choose whole-grain crackers, pretzels, nuts or seeds, baked chips, low-fat popcorn, or low-fat granola bars from vending machines.

connect ACTIVITY DO IT ONLINE

---

focus on the nonmeat choices of dry beans, nuts, seeds, eggs, and soy foods like tofu. Vegans and other vegetarians who do not consume any dairy products must find other rich sources of calcium. Fruits, vegetables, and whole grains are healthy choices for people following all types of vegetarian diets.

Unlike most animal proteins, most plant proteins do not contain all the necessary amino acids for good health. Thus, a healthy vegetarian diet must emphasize a wide variety of plant foods in order to include all the necessary amino acids. Choosing minimally processed and unrefined foods will maximize nutrient value and provide ample dietary fiber. Daily consumption of a variety of plant foods in amounts that meet total energy needs can provide all needed nutrients, except vitamin B-12 and possibly calcium, iron, zinc, and vitamin D.

Dietary Challenges for Various Population Groups

The Dietary Guidelines for Americans and MyPlate can help nearly anyone create a healthy diet. However, some population groups face special dietary challenges.

College Students Convenient foods are not always the healthiest choices. Students who eat in buffet-style dining halls can easily overeat, and the foods offered are not necessarily high in nutrients or low in fat, sodium, and added sugars. The same is true of meals at fast-food restaurants. See the box "Eating Strategies for College Students" for tips on making healthy eating convenient and affordable.

Older Adults   Nutrient needs do not change much as people age, but because older adults tend to become less active, they don't need as much energy intake to maintain body weight. At the same time, older adults absorb some nutrients less efficiently (e.g., vitamin B-12) because of age-related changes in the digestive tract. For these reasons, older adults should focus on eating nutrient-dense foods. Foods fortified with vitamin B-12 and/or B-12 supplements are recommended for people over age 50, and calcium and vitamin D supplements may be recommended for older adults to reduce bone loss and lower the risk of osteoporosis.

Athletes   Key dietary concerns for athletes are meeting their increased energy requirements and drinking enough fluids during practice and throughout the day to remain fully hydrated. Endurance athletes and athletes in heavy training may also benefit from increasing the amount of carbohydrates in the diet to 60–70% of total daily energy intake; this increase should take the form of complex, rather than simple, carbohydrates. Athletes who need to maintain a low body weight—such as skaters, gymnasts, and wrestlers—must avoid unhealthy eating patterns, which can lead to eating disorders.

People with Special Health Concerns   People with diabetes benefit from a well-balanced diet that is low in simple sugars and high in complex carbohydrates. People with high blood pressure need to control their weight and limit their sodium consumption. If you have a health concern that requires a special diet, discuss your situation with a physician or registered dietitian.

Global Nutrition Transitions

No population seems to be isolated from the effects of a *nutrition transition*, in which the quality and quantity of our diet is changing with globalization, that is, an increased availability of cheap foods, urbanization, and increased sedentary activities. In the United States, as our incomes increase, we eat fewer starches and more meats, vegetable oils, animal fats, and added sugars. The increases in fats and sugars are implicated in cardiovascular disease, obesity, and diabetes. The increases in animal protein and energy-dense foods are advantageous for undernourished people (in 2010 the number of underweight children dropped from 160 million to 102 million) but problematic for overweight people (the number of overweight children rose from 31 million to 44 million).

A PERSONAL PLAN: MAKING INFORMED CHOICES ABOUT FOOD

Understanding the basics of good nutrition should get you started on creating a healthy diet that works for you. But eating for health involves other skills, including how to interpret the labels on food products and dietary supplements, knowing how to handle and prepare food safely, understanding the nutritional content of foods, and the various ways foods can be processed before going to market.

Reading Food Labels

All processed foods regulated by either the FDA or the USDA include standardized nutrition information on their labels. Every food label shows serving sizes and the amounts of fat, saturated fat, trans fat, cholesterol, sodium, total carbohydrate, dietary fiber, sugars, and protein in each serving. To make informed choices about food, learn to read and *understand* food labels (see the box "Using Food Labels").

Dietary Supplements

All government food guidance systems encourage people to meet their nutritional needs with food rather than with vitamin and mineral supplements. Supplements lack the fiber and potentially beneficial phytochemicals that are found only in whole foods. Most Americans can get the vitamins and minerals they need by eating a nutritionally balanced diet of various foods. The use of supplements to reduce heart disease or cancer risk remains controversial, so experts suggest that you avoid taking any nutrient at a level exceeding the Tolerable Upper Intake Level (UL).

Although dietary supplements are sold over the counter, that doesn't necessarily mean they are safe, especially when consumed over a long period of time. Some vitamins and minerals are dangerous when taken in excess. Large doses of particular nutrients can also cause health problems by affecting the absorption of certain vitamins or minerals. For this reason, ask your doctor, your pharmacist, or a dietician before taking any high-dosage supplement.

People Who Benefit from Supplements   In setting the DRIs, the Food and Nutrition Board recommended supplements of particular nutrients for specific groups:

•   Women who are capable of getting pregnant should get 400 µg per day of folic acid (the synthetic form of the vitamin folate) from fortified foods and supplements in addition to folate from a varied diet. This level of folate can reduce the risk of neural tube defects in a developing fetus. Enriched breads, flours, cornmeal, rice, noodles, and other grain products are fortified with folic acid. Folate is found naturally in leafy green vegetables, legumes, oranges, and strawberries.

•   As noted earlier, people over age 50 should eat foods fortified with vitamin B-12, take a B-12 supplement, or combine the two to meet the RDA of 2.4 µg daily. Up to 30% of people over 50 may have trouble absorbing protein-bound B-12 in foods.

CRITICAL CONSUMER
Using Food Labels

The Nutrition Facts panel on a food label is designed to help consumers make food choices based on the nutrients that are most important to good health. In addition to listing nutrient content by weight, the label puts the information in the context of a daily diet of 2000 calories that includes no more than 65 grams of fat (approximately 30% of total calories). For example, if a serving of a particular product has 13 grams of fat, the label will show that the serving represents 20% (13/65) of the daily fat allowance. If your daily diet contains fewer or more than 2000 calories, you need to adjust these calculations accordingly. Doing so will require a good understanding of the information on the food label of a given food.

Food labels contain uniform serving sizes. This means that if you look at different brands of salad dressing, for example, you can compare calories and fat content based on the serving amount. It is important to keep in mind, however, that food label serving sizes may be larger or smaller than MyPlate serving size equivalents. Regulations also require that foods meet strict definitions if their packaging includes the terms *light, low-fat,* or *high-fiber.* Health claims such as "good source of dietary fiber" or "low in fat" on packages are signals that those products can wisely be included in your diet. Overall, the food label is an important tool to help you choose a diet that conforms to MyPlate and the Dietary Guidelines.

Selected Nutrient Claims and What They Mean

Healthy A food that is low in fat, has no more than 360–480 mg of sodium and 60 mg of cholesterol, *and* provides 10% or more of the Daily Value for vitamin A, vitamin C, protein, calcium, iron, or dietary fiber.

Light *or* lite 33% fewer calories or 50% less fat than a similar product.

Reduced *or* fewer At least 25% less of a nutrient than a similar product; can be applied to fat ("reduced fat"), saturated fat, cholesterol, sodium, and calories.

Extra *or* added 10% or more of the Daily Value per serving when compared to what a similar product has.

Good source 10–19% of the Daily Value for a particular nutrient per serving.

High, rich in, *or* excellent source of 20% or more of the Daily Value for a particular nutrient per serving.

Low calorie 40 or fewer calories per serving.

High fiber 5 g or more of fiber per serving.

Good source of fiber 2.5–4.9 g of fiber per serving.

Fat-free Less than 0.5 g of fat per serving.

Low-fat 3 g of fat or less per serving.

Saturated fat-free Less than 0.5 g of saturated fat and 0.5 g of trans fatty acids per serving.

Low saturated fat 1 g or less of saturated fat per serving and no more than 15% of total calories.

Cholesterol-free Less than 2 mg of cholesterol and 2 g or less of saturated fat per serving.

Low cholesterol 20 mg or less of cholesterol and 2 g or less of saturated fat per serving.

Low sodium 140 mg or less of sodium per serving.

Very low sodium 35 mg or less of sodium per serving.

Lean Cooked seafood, meat, or poultry with less than 10 g of fat, 4.5 g or less of saturated fat, and less than 95 mg of cholesterol per serving.

Extra lean Cooked seafood, meat, or poultry with less than 5 g of fat, 2 g of saturated fat, and 95 mg of cholesterol per serving.

NOTE: The FDA has not yet defined nutrient claims relating to carbohydrates, so foods labeled low- or reduced-carbohydrate do not conform to any approved standard.

SOURCE: FDA. 2013. Food Labeling Guide. Appendix C: Health Claims (http://www.fda.gov/FoodLabelingGuide).

1. Serving size: Determine how many servings there are in the food package and compare it to how much you actually eat. You may need to adjust the rest of the nutrient values based on your typical serving size.

2. Calories and calories from fat: Note whether a serving is high in calories and fat. The sample food shown here is low in fat, with only 30 of its 235 calories from fat.

3. Daily Values: Based on a 2000-calorie diet, Daily Value percentages tell you whether the nutrients in a serving of food contribute a lot or a little to your total daily diet.
  5% or less is low
  20% or more is high

4. Limit these nutrients: Look for foods low in fat, saturated fat, trans fat, cholesterol, and sodium.

5. Get enough of these nutrients: Look for foods high in dietary fiber, vitamin A, vitamin C, calcium, and iron.

Nutrition Facts
Serving Size 1 cup (265g)
Servings per Container 2

Amount per Serving

Calories 235   Calories from Fat 30

	% Daily Value*
Total Fat 3g	**5%**
Saturated Fat 1g	**5%**
Trans Fat 0.5g	
Cholesterol 30mg	**10%**
Sodium 775mg	**32%**
Total Carbohydrate 34g	**11%**
Dietary Fiber 9g	**36%**
Sugars 5g	
Protein 18g	

Vitamin A 25%	•	Vitamin C 0%
Calcium 12%	•	Iron 20%

*Percent Daily Values are based on a 2,000 calorie diet. Your daily values may be higher or lower depending on your calorie needs:

		Calories	2,000	2,500
Total Fat	Less than		65g	80
Sat Fat	Less than		20g	25g
Cholesterol	Less than		300mg	300mg
Sodium	Less than		2,400mg	2,400mg
Total Carbohydrate			300g	375g
Dietary Fiber			25g	30g

Calories per gram:
Fat 9 • Carbohydrate 4 • Protein 4

Footnote: This section shows recommended daily intake for two levels of calorie consumption and values for dietary calculations; it's the same on all labels.

- Because of the oxidative stress caused by smoking, smokers should get 35 mg more vitamin C per day than the RDA has set for their age and sex. Supplements aren't usually necessary, however, because this extra vitamin C can easily be found in foods. For example, an 8-ounce glass of orange juice has about 100 mg of vitamin C.

Supplements may be recommended in other cases. Women with heavy menstrual flows, for example, may need extra iron. Older adults, people with dark skin, and people exposed to little sunlight may need extra vitamin D. Other people may benefit from supplementation based on their physical condition, the medicines they take, or their dietary habits.

Before deciding whether to take a vitamin or mineral supplement, consider whether you already eat a fortified breakfast cereal every day. Many breakfast cereals contain almost as many nutrients as a multivitamin pill. If you elect to take a supplement, choose one that contains 50–100% of the Daily Values for vitamins and minerals. Avoid supplements containing large doses of particular nutrients.

Reading Supplement Labels   Dietary supplements include vitamins, minerals, amino acids, herbs, glandular extracts, enzymes, and other compounds. They are available as tablets, capsules, liquids, and powders. Although dietary supplements are often thought to be safe and "natural," they can contain powerful bioactive chemicals that have the potential for harm.

In the United States, dietary supplements are not legally considered drugs and are not regulated the same way drugs are. The FDA does not authorize or test dietary supplements, and supplement manufacturers are not required to demonstrate either safety or effectiveness prior to marketing.

Dietary supplement manufacture is not as closely regulated, and there is no guarantee that a product even contains a given ingredient, let alone in the appropriate amount. In addition, herbs can be contaminated or misidentified at any stage from harvest to packaging.

To provide consumers with more reliable and consistent information about supplements, the FDA requires supplements to have labels similar to those found on foods (see the box "Using Dietary Supplement Labels" for more information). Label statements and claims about supplements are also regulated.

Protecting Yourself against Foodborne Illness

The CDC estimates that about 1000 reported disease outbreaks and approximately 48 million illnesses, 128,000 hospitalizations, and 3000 deaths occur each year in the United States due to foodborne illnesses. Symptoms include diarrhea, vomiting, fever, pain, headache, and weakness. Although the effects of foodborne illnesses are usually not serious, some groups, such as children, pregnant women, individuals with immune deficits and the elderly, are more at risk for severe complications such as rheumatic diseases, seizures, blood poisoning, hemolytic uremic syndrome, and death.

Most cases of foodborne illness are caused by **pathogens**—disease-causing microorganisms. According to the CDC, about 90% of foodborne illnesses and related hospitalizations and deaths in 2010 were due to seven pathogens: *Salmonella* (most often found in eggs, on vegetables, and on poultry); *Norovirus* (most often found in salad ingredients and shellfish); *Campylobacter jejuni* (most often found in meat and poultry); *Toxoplasma* (most often found in meat); *Escherichia coli (E. coli)* O157:H7 (most often found in meat and water); *Listeria monocytogenes* (most often found in lunch meats, sausages, and hot dogs); *Clostridium perfringens* (most often found in meat and gravy). *Salmonella* was the leading cause of hospitalizations and deaths, accounting for 28% of deaths and 35% of hospitalizations.

Another potential threat from food is bovine spongiform encephalopathy (BSE), or "mad cow disease"—a fatal degenerative neurological disease caused by an abnormal protein that forms deposits in the brain. Visit the USDA website for more information (www.usda.gov).

Although foodborne illness outbreaks associated with food-processing plants make headlines, most cases of illness trace back to poor food handling in the home or in restaurants. The Dietary Guidelines for Americans encourage people to follow four basic food safety principles:

- *Clean* hands, food contact surfaces, and vegetables and fruits.
- *Separate* raw, cooked, and ready-to-eat foods while shopping, storing, and preparing foods.
- *Cook* foods to a safe temperature.
- *Chill* (refrigerate) perishable foods promptly.

If you think you may be having a bout of foodborne illness, drink plenty of fluids to prevent dehydration and consult a physician. For more details on handling food safely, see the box "Safe Food Handling."

Although pathogens are usually destroyed during cooking, the U.S. government has taken steps to bring down levels of contamination by improving national surveillance and testing. Raw meat and poultry products are now sold with safe handling and safe cooking instructions, and all packaged, unpasteurized fresh fruit and vegetable juices carry warnings about potential contamination. In 2011 the Food Safety Modernization Act (FSMA) was signed into law to reform the food safety system in the United States and further ensure the safety of the U.S. food supply. The FSMA allows the FDA to focus more on preventing food safety problems than on reacting to problems after they occur.

Careful food handing greatly reduces the risk of foodborne illness.

pathogen   A microorganism that causes disease.   TERMS

CRITICAL CONSUMER
Using Dietary Supplement Labels

Since 1999, specific types of information have been required on the labels of dietary supplements. In addition to basic information about the product, labels include a "Supplement Facts" panel, modeled after the "Nutrition Facts" panel used on food labels (see the label illustrated in this box). Under the Dietary Supplement Health and Education Act (DSHEA) and food labeling laws, supplement labels can make three types of health-related claims:

• *Nutrient content claims,* such as "high in calcium," "excellent source of vitamin C," or "high potency." The claims "high in" and "excellent source of" mean the same as they do on food labels. A "high-potency" single-ingredient supplement must contain 100% of that nutrient's Daily Value; a "high-potency" multi-ingredient product must contain 100% or more of the Daily Value of at least two-thirds of the nutrients present for which Daily Values have been established.

• *Health claims,* if they have been authorized by the FDA or another authoritative scientific body. The association between adequate calcium intake and lower risk of osteoporosis is an example of an approved health claim. Since 2003 the FDA has also allowed so-called *qualified* health claims for situations in which there is emerging but as yet inconclusive evidence for a particular claim. Such claims must include qualifying language such as "scientific evidence suggests but does not prove" the claim.

• *Structure–function claims,* such as "antioxidants maintain cellular integrity" or "this product enhances energy levels." Because these claims are not reviewed by the FDA, they must carry a disclaimer (see the sample label).

Tips for Choosing and Using Dietary Supplements

• Check with your physician before taking a supplement. Many are not meant for children, older adults, women who are pregnant or breastfeeding, people with chronic illnesses or upcoming surgery, or people taking prescription or over-the-counter (OTC) medications. When you visit your doctor, bring a list of all dietary supplements you are taking. Do not take megadoses (more than double the DRI levels) without your doctor's approval.

• Choose brands made by nationally known food and drug manufacturers or house brands from large retail chains. Due to their size and visibility, such sources are likely to have high manufacturing standards.

• Look for the "USP" (United States Pharmacopeia) verification mark on the label, indicating that the product meets minimum safety and purity standards developed under the USP Dietary Supplement Verification Program. The USP mark means that the product (1) contains the listed ingredients, (2) has the declared amount and strength of ingredients, (3) will dissolve effectively, (4) has been screened for harmful contaminants, and (5) has been manufactured using safe, sanitary, and well-controlled procedures. The National Nutritional Foods Association (NNFA) has a self-regulatory testing program for its members; other associations and laboratories, including ConsumerLab.com, also test and rate dietary supplements.

• Follow the label's cautions, directions for use, and dosage.

• If you experience side effects, stop using the product and contact your physician. Report any serious reactions to the FDA's MedWatch monitoring program (800-FDA-1088 or online at http://www.fda.gov/Safety/MedWatch/default.htm).

For More Information about Dietary Supplements

ConsumerLab.com: http://www.consumerlab.com

National Institutes of Health, Office of Dietary Supplements: http://ods.od.nih.gov

U.S. Food and Drug Administration: http://www.fda.gov/food/Dietary Supplements/default.htm

U.S. Department of Agriculture: http://fnic.nal.usda.gov/dietary-supplements

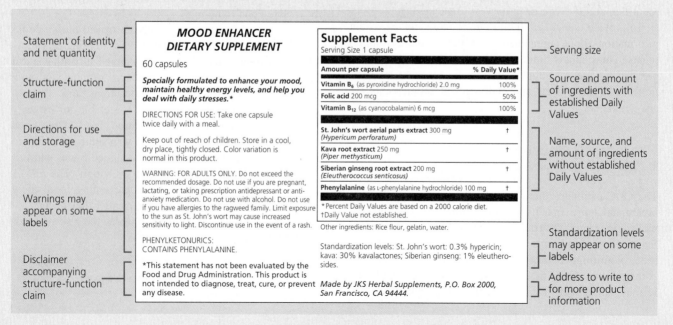

Statement of identity and net quantity

MOOD ENHANCER DIETARY SUPPLEMENT

60 capsules

Structure-function claim

Specially formulated to enhance your mood, maintain healthy energy levels, and help you deal with daily stresses. *

Directions for use and storage

DIRECTIONS FOR USE: Take one capsule twice daily with a meal.

Keep out of reach of children. Store in a cool, dry place, tightly closed. Color variation is normal in this product.

Warnings may appear on some labels

WARNING: FOR ADULTS ONLY. Do not exceed the recommended dosage. Do not use if you are pregnant, lactating, or taking prescription antidepressant or anti-anxiety medication. Do not use with alcohol. Do not use if you have allergies to the ragweed family. Limit exposure to the sun as St. John's wort may cause increased sensitivity to light. Discontinue use in the event of a rash.

PHENYLKETONURICS:
CONTAINS PHENYLALANINE.

Disclaimer accompanying structure-function claim

*This statement has not been evaluated by the Food and Drug Administration. This product is not intended to diagnose, treat, cure, or prevent any disease.

Supplement Facts
Serving Size 1 capsule

Amount per capsule	% Daily Value*
Vitamin B₆ (as pyroxidine hydrochloride) 2.0 mg	100%
Folic acid 200 mcg	50%
Vitamin B₁₂ (as cyanocobalamin) 6 mcg	100%
St. John's wort aerial parts extract 300 mg (*Hypericum perforatum*)	†
Kava root extract 250 mg (*Piper methysticum*)	†
Siberian ginseng root extract 200 mg (*Eleutherococcus senticosus*)	†
Phenylalanine (as ʟ-phenylalanine hydrochloride) 100 mg	†

*Percent Daily Values are based on a 2000 calorie diet.
†Daily Value not established.

Other ingredients: Rice flour, gelatin, water.

Standardization levels: St. John's wort: 0.3% hypericin; kava: 30% kavalactones; Siberian ginseng: 1% eleuthero-sides.

Made by JKS Herbal Supplements, P.O. Box 2000, San Francisco, CA 94444.

Serving size

Source and amount of ingredients with established Daily Values

Name, source, and amount of ingredients without established Daily Values

Standardization levels may appear on some labels

Address to write to for more product information

- Don't buy food in containers that leak, bulge, or are severely dented. Refrigerated foods should be cold, and frozen foods should be solid when you buy them.

- Refrigerate perishable items as soon as possible after purchase. Use or freeze fresh meats within 3–5 days and fresh poultry, fish, and ground meat within 1–2 days.

- Store raw meat, poultry, fish, and shellfish in containers in the refrigerator so that the juices don't drip onto other foods. Keep these items away from other foods, surfaces, utensils, or serving dishes to prevent cross-contamination.

- Thaw frozen food in the refrigerator or in the microwave oven, not on the kitchen counter. Cook foods immediately after thawing.

- Thoroughly wash your hands with warm soapy water for 20 seconds before and after handling food, especially raw meat, fish, shellfish, poultry, or eggs.

- Make sure counters, cutting boards, dishes, utensils, and other equipment are thoroughly cleaned before and after use using hot soapy water. Wash dishcloths frequently.

- If possible, use separate cutting boards for meat, poultry, and seafood and for foods that will be eaten raw. Replace cutting boards once they become worn or develop hard-to-clean grooves.

- Thoroughly rinse and scrub fruits and vegetables with a brush, if possible, or peel off the skin.

- Cook foods thoroughly, especially beef, poultry, fish, pork, wild game, and eggs; cooking kills most microorganisms. Use a food thermometer to ensure that foods are cooked to a safe temperature. Hamburgers should be cooked to at least 160° F. Turn or stir microwaved food to make sure it is heated evenly throughout. When eating out, order hamburger cooked well-done and make sure foods are served piping hot.

- Keep hot foods hot (140°F or above) and cold foods cold (40°F or below). Harmful bacteria can grow rapidly between these two temperatures. Refrigerate foods within two hours of purchase or preparation, and within one hour if the air temperature is above 90°F. Refrigerate foods at or below 40°F and freeze at or below 0°F. Use refrigerated leftovers within 3–4 days.

- Don't eat raw animal products, including raw eggs in homemade hollandaise sauce or eggnog. Use only pasteurized milk and juice, and look for pasteurized eggs, which are now available in some states.

- Cook eggs until they're firm, and fully cook foods containing eggs. Store eggs in the cooler parts of the refrigerator, not in the door, and use them within 3–5 weeks.

- Avoid raw sprouts. Even sprouts grown under clean conditions in the home can be risky because bacteria may be present in the seeds. Cook sprouts before eating them.

- Read the food label and package information, and follow safety instructions such as "Keep Refrigerated" and the "Safe Handling Instructions."

- According to the USDA, "When in doubt, throw it out." Even if a food looks and smells fine, it may not be safe. If you aren't sure that a food has been prepared, served, and stored safely, don't eat it.

Additional precautions are recommended for people at particularly high risk for foodborne illness—pregnant women, young children, older people, and people with weakened immune systems or certain chronic illnesses. If you are a member of one of these groups, don't eat or drink any of the following products: unpasteurized juices; raw sprouts; unpasteurized (raw) milk and products made from unpasteurized milk; raw or undercooked meat, poultry, eggs, fish, and shellfish; and soft cheeses such as feta, Brie, Camembert, or blue-veined cheeses. To protect against *Listeria*, avoid ready-to-eat foods such as hot dogs, luncheon meats, and cold cuts unless they are reheated until they are steaming hot.

Organic Foods

Some people who are concerned about pesticides and other environmental contaminants choose to buy foods that are **organic.** To be certified as organic by the USDA, foods must meet strict production, processing, handling, and labeling criteria. Organic crops must meet limits on pesticide residues. For meat, milk, eggs, and other animal products to be certified organic, animals must be given organic feed and access to the outdoors and may not be given antibiotics or growth hormones. The use of genetic engineering, ionizing radiation, and sewage sludge is prohibited. Products can be labeled "100% organic" if they contain all organic ingredients and "organic" if they contain at least 95% organic ingredients; all such products may carry the USDA organic seal. A product with at least 70% organic ingredients can be labeled "made with organic ingredients" but cannot use the USDA seal.

> **organic** A designation applied to foods grown and produced according to strict guidelines limiting the use of pesticides, nonorganic ingredients, hormones, antibiotics, irradiation, genetic engineering, and other practices. **TERMS**

Some experts recommend that consumers who want to buy organic produce spend their money on those fruits and vegetables that have the highest levels of pesticide residue when grown conventionally (the "dirty dozen"): apples, bell peppers, celery, cherries, imported grapes, nectarines, peaches, pears, potatoes, red raspberries, spinach, and strawberries. Experts also recommend buying organic beef, poultry, eggs, dairy products, and baby food. Fruits and vegetables that carry little pesticide residue whether grown conventionally or organically include asparagus, avocadoes, bananas, broccoli, cauliflower, corn, kiwi, mangoes, onions, papaya, pineapples, and peas. All foods are subject to strict pesticide limits; the debate about the health effects of small amounts of residue is ongoing.

Whether organic foods are better for your health or not, organic farming is better for the environment. Benefits include sustainable farming practices, preservation of biodiversity, healthier soil, protection of water supplies, reduced use of fossil fuels, improved animal welfare, protection of ecosystems, and safer conditions for farmworkers. Buying organic food, buying locally grown foods, and participating in a community garden are ways to support food production that benefits and sustains the environment.

Guidelines for Fish Consumption

A specific area of concern has been mercury contamination in fish. Overall, fish and shellfish are healthy sources of protein, omega-3 fats, and other nutrients. Prudent choices can minimize the risk of any possible negative health effects.

However, according to FDA and Environmental Protection Agency (EPA) guidelines, as well as the Dietary Guidelines for Americans, women who are or may become pregnant and nursing mothers should follow these guidelines to minimize their exposure to mercury:

- Do not eat shark, swordfish, king mackerel, or tilefish.
- Eat 8–12 ounces a week of a variety of fish and shellfish that is lower in mercury, such as shrimp, canned light tuna, salmon, pollock, and catfish. Limit consumption of albacore tuna to 6 ounces per week.
- Check advisories about the safety of recreationally caught fish from local lakes, rivers, and coastal areas; if no information is available, limit consumption to 6 ounces per week.

The same FDA/EPA guidelines apply to children, although they should consume smaller servings.

---

food irradiation The treatment of foods with gamma rays, X-rays, or high-voltage electrons to kill potentially harmful pathogens and increase shelf life.

genetically modified organism (GMO) A plant, animal, or microorganism in which genes have been added, rearranged, or replaced through genetic engineering.

TERMS

Additives in Food

According to the FDA's "Everything Added to Food in the United States (EAFUS)" database, approximately 3000 substances are intentionally added to foods to maintain or improve nutritional quality, maintain freshness, help in processing or preparation, or alter taste or appearance. The most widely used food additives are sugar, salt, and corn syrup; these three plus citric acid, baking soda, vegetable colors, mustard, and pepper account for 98% by weight of all food additives used in the United States.

Additives having potential health concerns include nitrates and nitrites, used in processed meats and associated with the synthesis of cancer-causing agents in the stomach; BHA (Butylated hydroxyanisole) and BHT (butylated hydroxytoluene), used to maintain freshness and possibly associated with an increased risk of some cancers; sulfites, used to keep vegetables from turning brown and associated with severe reactions in sensitive people; and monosodium glutamate (MSG), used as a flavor enhancer and associated with episodes of increased blood pressure and sweating in sensitive people. If you are sensitive to an additive, check food labels when you shop, and ask questions when you eat out.

Food Biotechnology

Modern biotechnology tools, such as genetic engineering and cloning, allow for more precise, productive, and efficient development of crops and livestock. The USDA, FDA, and EPA are the three federal agencies in charge of the regulatory oversight of biotechnology.

Food irradiation is the treatment of foods with gamma rays, X-rays, or high-voltage electrons to kill potentially harmful pathogens, including bacteria, parasites, insects, and fungi that cause foodborne illness. Irradiation also reduces spoilage and extends a product's shelf life.

Even though irradiation has been generally endorsed by agencies such as the World Health Organization (WHO), the CDC, and the American Medical Association (AMA), few irradiated foods are currently on the market due to consumer resistance and skepticism. Studies indicate that when consumers are given information about the process of irradiation and the benefits of irradiated foods, most want to purchase them. All primary irradiated foods (meat, vegetables, and so on) are labeled with the flowerlike Radura symbol and a brief information label; spices and foods that are merely ingredients do not have to be so labeled.

Genetic engineering involves altering the characteristics of a plant, animal, or microorganism by adding, rearranging, or replacing genes in its DNA; the result is a **genetically modified organism (GMO)**. Many GM crops are already grown in the United States. Products made with GMOs include juice, soda, nuts, tuna, frozen pizza, spaghetti sauce, canola oil, chips, salad dressings, and soup.

The potential benefits of GM foods cited by supporters include improved yields overall and in difficult growing conditions, increased disease resistance, improved nutritional content, lower prices, and less pesticide use. Critics of biotechnology argue that unexpected harmful effects may occur. Gene manipulation could elevate levels of naturally occurring toxins or allergens, permanently change the gene pool, reduce biodiversity, and produce pesticide-resistant insects. Experience has shown that GM products are difficult to keep separate from non-GM products. Animal escapes, cross-pollination, and contamination during processing are just a few ways in which GMOs could potentially appear unexpectedly in the food supply or the environment.

Food Allergies and Food Intolerances

For some people, consuming a particular food causes symptoms such as itchiness, swollen lips, or abdominal pain. Adverse reactions like these may be due to a food allergy or a food intolerance, and symptoms may range from annoying to life-threatening.

A true **food allergy** is a reaction of the body's immune system to a food or food ingredient, usually a protein. This immune reaction can occur within minutes of ingesting the food, resulting in symptoms that affect the skin (hives), gastrointestinal tract (cramps or diarrhea), respiratory tract (asthma), or mouth (swelling of the lips or tongue). The most severe response is a systemic reaction called *anaphylaxis,* which involves a potentially life-threatening drop in blood pressure.

Although numerous food allergens have been identified, just eight foods account for more than 90% of the food allergies in the United States: cow's milk, eggs, peanuts, tree nuts (walnuts, cashews, and so on), soy, wheat, fish, and shellfish. Food labels are now required to state the presence of the eight most common allergens in plain language in the ingredient list.

Many people who believe they have food allergies may actually suffer from a much more common source of adverse food reactions—a **food intolerance.** In the case of a food intolerance, the problem usually lies with metabolism rather than with the immune system. Typically the body cannot adequately digest a food or food component, often because of some type of chemical deficiency; in other cases, the body reacts to a particular compound in a food. Lactose intolerance is a fairly common food intolerance. A more serious condition may be intolerance of gluten, a protein component of some grains. The results of a Mayo Clinic study in 2012 concluded that only 1.8 million Americans have a problem that causes the body to attack the small intestine when gluten is ingested and can lead to other debilitating medical problems. Sulfite, a common food additive, can produce severe asthmatic reactions in sensitive individuals.

Food intolerance reactions often produce symptoms similar to those of food allergies, such as diarrhea or cramps, but reactions are typically localized and not life-threatening. Exceptions are gluten and sulfite, which must be avoided by sensitive individuals. Through trial and error, most people with food intolerances can adjust their intake of the trigger food to an appropriate level.

TERMS

food allergy An adverse reaction to a food or food ingredient in which the immune system perceives a particular substance (allergen) as foreign and acts to destroy it.

food intolerance An adverse reaction to a food or food ingredient that doesn't involve the immune system; intolerances are often due to a problem with metabolism.

TIPS FOR TODAY AND THE FUTURE

Opportunities to improve your diet present themselves every day, and small changes add up.

RIGHT NOW YOU CAN:
- Substitute a healthy snack for an unhealthy one.
- Drink a glass of water and put a reusable water bottle in your backpack for tomorrow.
- Plan to make healthy selections when you eat out, such as steamed vegetables instead of french fries, or salmon instead of steak.

IN THE FUTURE YOU CAN:
- Visit the MyPlate website at ChooseMyPlate.gov and use the online tools to create a personalized nutrition plan and begin tracking your eating habits.
- Learn to cook healthier meals. Hundreds of free websites and low-cost cookbooks provide recipes for healthy dishes.

- To function at its best, the human body requires about 45 essential nutrients in certain relative proportions. People get these nutrients from foods; the body cannot synthesize most of them.

- Proteins, made up of amino acids, form muscles and bones and help make up blood, enzymes, hormones, and cell membranes. Foods from animal sources provide complete proteins; plants provide incomplete proteins and must be combined in order to attain the right balance of amino acids. Protein intake should be 10–35% of total daily energy intake.

- Fats, a concentrated source of energy, also help to insulate the body and cushion the organs; 1 tablespoon of vegetable oil per day supplies the essential fats. Dietary fat intake should be 20–35% of total daily energy intake. Unsaturated fats should be favored over trans fats; the evidence for the harmfulness of saturated fat has become questionable.

- Carbohydrates supply energy to the brain and other parts of the nervous system as well as to red blood cells. The body needs about 130 grams of carbohydrates a day, but more is recommended. Carbohydrates should make up 45–65% of total daily energy intake.

- Fiber includes nondigestible carbohydrates provided mainly by plants. Adequate intake of fiber (38 grams per day for men and 25 grams per day for women) can help people manage diabetes and high cholesterol levels and improve intestinal health.

- The 13 vitamins needed in the diet are organic substances that promote specific chemical and cell processes within living tissue. Deficiencies or excesses can cause serious illnesses and even death.

- The approximately 17 minerals needed in the diet are inorganic substances that regulate body functions, aid in the growth and maintenance of body tissues, and help in the release of energy from foods.

- Water is used to digest and absorb food, transport substances around the body, and regulate body temperature.

- Foods contain other substances such as phytochemicals, which may not be essential nutrients but may help reduce chronic disease risk.

- Dietary Reference Intakes (DRIs) are recommended intakes for essential nutrients that meet the needs of healthy people.

- The Dietary Guidelines for Americans are designed to help people make healthy and informed food choices. Following the guidelines promotes health and reduces the risk of chronic disease. The 2010 Dietary Guidelines for Americans present recommendations in several areas: balancing calories to manage weight, reducing certain food components, increasing other food components, building healthy eating patterns, and making healthy choices in the context of the current food and physical activity environment.

- Choosing the right amount of foods from each food group in MyPlate every day ensures that you get enough necessary nutrients without overconsuming calories.

- A vegetarian diet can meet human nutritional needs but must be planned carefully to prevent potential micronutrient deficiencies.

- Almost all foods have labels that show how much fat, cholesterol, protein, fiber, and sodium they contain. Serving sizes are standardized, and health claims are carefully regulated. Dietary supplements also have uniform labels that provide supplement facts.

- Foodborne illnesses from *Salmonella, E. coli, Norovirus,* and other microorganisms are a greater threat to health than food additives and environmental contaminants. Other dietary issues of concern to some people include food irradiation, genetic modification of foods, and food allergies and intolerances.

FOR MORE INFORMATION

BOOKS

Duyff, R. L. 2012. *ADA Complete Food and Nutrition Guide,* 4th ed. Hoboken, NJ: Wiley. *An excellent review of current nutrition information.*

Insel, P., et al. 2014. *Nutrition,* 5th ed. Sudbury, MA: Jones & Bartlett. *An introductory nutrition textbook covering a variety of key topics.*

Teicholz, N. 2014. *The Big Fat Surprise: Why Butter, Meat & Cheese Belong in a Healthy Diet.* New York: Simon & Schuster.

NEWSLETTERS

Environmental Nutrition
    (http://www.environmentalnutrition.com)
Nutrition Action Health Letter from the Center for Science in the Public Interest
    (http://cspinet.org/nah)
Tufts University Health & Nutrition Letter
    (http://www.tuftshealthletter.com)

ORGANIZATIONS, HOTLINES, AND WEBSITES

American Diabetes Association. An organization with the aim of leading the fight against the deadly consequences of diabetes and fighting for those affected by diabetes.

    http://www.diabetes.org

Academy of Nutrition and Dietetics (formerly the American Dietetic Association). Provides a wide variety of nutrition-related educational materials.

    http://www.eatright.org

The *Dietary Guidelines.* The official site for the Dietary Guidelines for Americans, 2010.

    http://www.dietaryguidelines.gov

FDA Center for Food Safety and Applied Nutrition. Offers information about topics such as food labeling, food additives, dietary supplements, and foodborne illness.

    http://www.fda.gov/food

Food Safety Hotlines. Provide information on safe purchase, handling, cooking, and storage of food.

    888-SAFEFOOD (FDA)
    800-535-4555 (USDA)

Fruit and Veggies: More Matters. A nonprofit organization designed to increase consumption of fruits and vegetables to five or more servings a day to improve the health of Americans.

    http://www.fruitsandveggiesmorematters.org

Gateways to Government Nutrition Information. Provides access to government resources relating to food safety and nutrition.

http://www.foodsafety.gov

http://www.nutrition.gov

Harvard School of Public Health: The Nutrition Source. Provides recent key research findings, an overview of the Healthy Eating Plate, and suggestions for building a healthful diet.

http://www.hsph.harvard.edu/nutritionsource

Mayo Clinic: Nutrition Basics. Medical, nutrition, and health information and tools for healthy living.

http://www.mayoclinic.com/health/nutrition-and-healthy-eating/MY00431

MyPlate. Provides personalized dietary plans and interactive food and activity tracking tools.

http://www.ChooseMyPlate.gov

National Academies' Food and Nutrition Board. Provides information about the Dietary Reference Intakes and related guidelines.

http://www.nap.edu/openbook.php?record_id=11537&page=R1

USDA Center for Nutrition Policy and Promotion. Includes information about the Dietary Guidelines and MyPlate.

http://www.cnpp.usda.gov/

USDA Food and Nutrition Information Center. Provides a variety of materials and extensive links relating to the Dietary Guidelines, food labels, MyPlate, and many other topics.

http://www.nal.usda.gov/fnic

SELECTED BIBLIOGRAPHY

American Heart Association. 2012. *Diet and Lifestyle Recommendations* (http://www.heart.org/HEARTORG/GettingHealthy/Diet-and-Lifestyle-Recommendations_UCM_305855_Article.jsp).

American Heart Association. 2012. *Fish and Omega-3 Fatty Acids* (http://www.heart.org/HEARTORG/GettingHealthy/NutritionCenter/HealthyDietGoals/Fish-and-Omega-3-Fatty-Acids_UCM_303248_Article.jsp).

American Heart Association. 2012. *Frequently Asked Questions about "Bad" Fats* (http://www.heart.org/HEARTORG/General/Frequently-Asked-QuestionsAbout-Bad-Fats_UCM_306349_Article.jsp).

Centers for Disease Control and Prevention. 2011. Vital signs: Incidence and trends of infection with pathogens transmitted commonly through food—Foodborne Diseases Active Surveillance Network, 10 U.S. sites, 1996–2010. *Morbidity and Mortality Weekly Report* 60(2): 749–755.

Centers for Disease Control and Prevention. 2012. *CDC and the Food Safety Modernization Act* (http://www.cdc.gov/foodsafety/fsma.html).

Centers for Disease Control and Prevention. 2012. Vital signs: Food categories contributing the most to sodium consumption—United States, 2007–2008. *Morbidity and Mortality Weekly Report* 61(5): 92–98.

Chowdhury, R., et al. 2014. Association of dietary, circulating, and supplement fatty acids with coronary risk: A systematic review and meta-analysis. *Annals of Internal Medicine* 160(6):398–406.

Council for Responsible Nutrition. 2009. *Dietary Supplements: Safe, Regulated and Beneficial* (http://www.crnusa.org/pdfs/CRN_FACT_DSSafeRegulatedBeneficial_09.pdf).

Eckel, R., et al. 2013. AHA/ACC Guideline on lifestyle management to reduce cardiovascular risk: A report of the American College of Cardiology/American Heart Association task force on practice guidelines. *Circulation* 01.cir.0000437740.48606.d1.

El Khoury, D., et al. 2011. Beta glucan: Health benefits in obesity and metabolic syndrome. *Journal of Nutrition and Metabolism* 20, Article ID 851362.

Fink, S. W. 2012. Key articles of dietary interventions that influence cardiovascular mortality. *Pharmacotherapy* 32(4): e54–87.

Finkelstein, E. A., et al. 2012. Obesity and severe obesity forecasts through 2030. *American Journal of Preventive Medicine Online* (http://www.ajpmonline.org/webfiles/images/journals/amepre/AMEPRE_33853-stamped2.pdf).

Food and Nutrition Board, Institute of Medicine. 2011. *Dietary Reference Intakes for Calcium and Vitamin D.* Washington, DC: National Academy Press.

Harvard School of Public Health, Department of Nutrition. 2010. *The Nutrition Source: Knowledge for Healthy Eating* (http://www.hsph.harvard.edu/nutritionsource).

The Hunger Project. 2012. *Know Your World: Facts about Hunger and Poverty* (http://www.thp.org/learn_more/issues/know_your_world_facts_about_hunger_and_poverty).

Jonnalagadda, S. S., et al. 2011. Putting the whole grain puzzle together: Health benefits associated with whole grains—Summary of American Society for Nutrition 2010 Satellite Symposium. *Journal of Nutrition* 14(5): 1011S–1022S.

Kiage, J. N., et al. 2013. Trans fat intake and all-cause mortality in the Reasons for Geographical and Racial Differences in Stroke (REGARDS) cohort. *American Journal of Clinical Nutrition* 97: 1121–1128.

Lasater, G., C. Piernas, and B. M. Popkin. 2011. Beverage patterns and trends among school-age children in the U.S., 1989–2008. *Nutrition Journal* 10:103.

Maki, K. C., et al. 2010. Whole-grain ready-to-eat oat cereal, as part of a dietary program for weight loss, reduces low-density lipoprotein cholesterol in adults with overweight and obesity more than a dietary program including low-fiber control foods. *Journal of the American Dietetic Association* 110(2): 205–214.

National Osteoporosis Foundation. 2014. 54 Million Americans affected by osteoporosis and low bone mass. National Osteoporosis Foundation online news, June 2. (http://nof.org/news/2948).

Ng, M., et al. 2014. Global, regional, and national prevalence of overweight and obesity in children and adults during 1980–2013: A systematic analysis for the Global Burden of Disease Study 2013. The Lancet, DOI: 10.1016/S0140-6736(14)60460-8.

Siri-Tarino, P. W., et al. 2010. Meta-analysis of prospective cohort studies evaluating the association of saturated fat with cardiovascular disease. *American Journal of Clinical Nutrition* 91(3): 535–546.

Trump, D. L., et al. 2010. Vitamin D: Considerations in the continued development as an agent for cancer prevention and therapy. *Cancer Journal* 16(1): 1–9.

Tufts University Health & Nutrition Newsletter, 2014 (June). Does new study mean "Butter is back?"

U.S. Department of Agriculture. 2011. *ChooseMyPlate* (http://www.choosemyplate.gov).

U.S. Department of Agriculture. 2013. Household Food Security in the United States in 2012. Economic Research Report No. (ERR-155) (http://www.ers.usda.gov/publications/err-economic-research-report/err155.aspx).

U.S. Department of Agriculture and Centers for Disease Control and Prevention. 2010. *What We Eat in America* (http://www.ars.usda.gov/Services/docs.htm?docid=15044).

U.S. Department of Agriculture and U.S. Department of Health and Human Services. 2010. *Dietary Guidelines for Americans, 2010,* 7th ed. Washington, DC: U.S. Government Printing Office (http://www.cnpp.usda.gov/publications/dietaryguidelines/2010/policydoc/policydoc.pdf).

U.S. Environmental Protection Agency. 2012. *Fish Consumption Advisories* (http://www.epa.gov/hg/advisories.htm).

U.S. Food and Drug Administration. 2012. *Food Allergies: What You Need to Know* (http://www.fda.gov/food/resourcesforyou/consumers/ucm079311.htm).

BEHAVIOR CHANGE STRATEGY
Improving Your Diet by Choosing Healthy Beverages

This Behavior Change Strategy focuses on choosing healthy beverages to increase intake of nutrients and decrease intake of empty calories from added sugars and fat. This model can be applied to any change you want to make to your diet.

Gather Data and Establish a Baseline

Begin by tracking your beverage consumption in a journal. Write down the types and amounts of beverages you drink, including water. Also note where you were at the time and whether you got the beverage there or brought it with you. At the same time, investigate your options. Find out what other beverages you can easily find during your daily routine. This information will help you put together a successful plan for change.

Analyze Your Data and Set Goals

Evaluate your beverage consumption by dividing your typical daily consumption between healthy and less healthy choices. Use the following guide as a basis, and add other beverages to the lists as needed:

Choose More Often	Servings Daily	Choose Less Often	Servings Daily
Water: plain, mineral, sparkling		Regular soda	
Low-fat or fat-free milk		Whole milk	
Fruit juice (100%)		Fruit beverages made with little fruit juice	
Unsweetened or non-calorie sweetened herbal tea		Sugar-sweetened beverages such as iced tea and sports drinks	
Others		Others	

How many beverages do you consume daily from each category? What would be a healthy and realistic goal for change? For example, if your beverage consumption is currently evenly divided between the "choose more often" and "choose less often" categories (four from each list), you might set a final goal for your behavior change program of increasing your healthy choices by two (to six from the "more often" list and two from the "less often" list).

Develop a Plan for Change

Once you've set your goal, you need to develop strategies that will help you choose healthy beverages more often. Consider the following possibilities:

- Keep healthy beverages on hand. If you live in a dorm, rent a small refrigerator or keep water in a reusable bottle and other healthy choices in the dorm kitchen's refrigerator.

- Plan ahead, and carry a reusable bottle with water or 100% juice in your backpack every day.

- Check food labels on beverages for serving sizes, energy content, and nutrients; compare products to find the healthiest choices, and watch your serving sizes. Use this information to make your "choose more often" list longer and more specific.

- If you eat out frequently, examine all the beverages available at the places you typically eat your meals. You'll probably find that plain water or other healthy choices are available.

You may also need to make changes in your routine to decrease the likelihood that you'll make unhealthy choices. For example, your journal might reveal that you always buy a soda after class when you pass a particular vending machine. If this is the case, try another route that bypasses the machine. Guard against impulse buying by carrying water or a healthy snack with you every day.

To complete your plan, try some of the other behavior change strategies described in Chapter 1: Develop and sign a contract, set up a system of rewards, involve other people in your program, and develop strategies for challenging situations. Once your plan is complete, take action. Keep track of your progress by continuing to monitor and evaluate your beverage consumption.

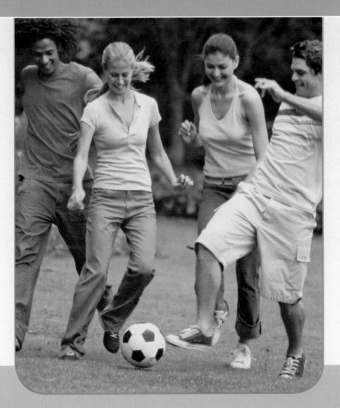

CHAPTER OBJECTIVES

- Define physical fitness, and list the health-related components of fitness
- Explain the wellness benefits of physical activity and exercise
- Describe how to develop each of the health-related components of fitness
- Explain how to choose appropriate exercise equipment, how to eat and drink for exercise, and how to prevent and manage injuries
- Explain and apply different methods for assessing fitness levels
- Put together a personalized exercise program that you enjoy and that will enable you to achieve your fitness goals

CHAPTER **10**

Exercise for Health and Fitness

Your body is a wonderful moving machine made to work best when it is physically active. It readily adapts to practically any level of activity and exercise: The more you ask of your body, the stronger and more fit it becomes. The opposite is also true. Left unchallenged, bones lose their density, joints stiffen, muscles become weak, and the body's energy systems degenerate. To be truly healthy, human beings must be active. If approached correctly, physical activity and exercise can contribute immeasurably to overall wellness, add fun and joy to life, and provide the foundation for a lifetime of fitness.

WHAT IS PHYSICAL FITNESS?

Physical fitness is a set of physical attributes that allow the body to respond or adapt to the demands and stress of physical effort—to perform moderate to vigorous levels of physical activity without becoming overly tired.

Some components of fitness are related to specific activities or sports, whereas others relate to general health. **Health-related fitness** includes cardiorespiratory endurance, muscular strength, muscular endurance, flexibility and body composition. Health-related fitness helps you withstand physical challenges and protects you from diseases.

Cardiorespiratory Endurance

Cardiorespiratory endurance is the ability to perform prolonged, large-muscle, dynamic exercise at moderate to high intensity.

When cardiorespiratory fitness is low, the heart has to work hard during normal daily activities and may not be able to work hard enough to sustain high-intensity physical activity in an emergency. Poor cardiorespiratory fitness is linked

physical fitness   The body's ability to respond or **TERMS** adapt to the demands and stress of physical effort.

health-related fitness   Physical capabilities that contribute to health, including cardiorespiratory endurance, muscular strength, muscular endurance, flexibility, and body composition.

cardiorespiratory endurance   The ability of the body to perform prolonged, large-muscle, dynamic exercise at moderate to high levels of intensity.

with heart disease, diabetes, colon cancer, stroke, depression, anxiety, and premature death from all causes.

Regular **cardiorespiratory endurance training**, however, conditions the heart and metabolism. Endurance training makes the heart stronger and improves the function of the entire cardiorespiratory system. As cardiorespiratory fitness improves, related physical functions also improve. The heart pumps more blood per heartbeat, resting heart rate slows and resting blood pressure decreases, blood volume increases, blood supply to tissues improves, the body can cool itself better, metabolic health improves, which helps the body process fuels and regulate cell function.

A healthy heart can better withstand the strains of daily life, the stress of occasional emergencies, and the wear and tear of time. You can develop cardiorespiratory endurance through activities that involve continuous, rhythmic movements of large muscle groups, such as the legs. Such activities include walking, jogging, cycling, and aerobic dancing.

Muscular Strength

Muscular strength is the amount of force a muscle can produce with a single maximum effort. Strong muscles are important for everyday activities, such as climbing stairs, as well as for emergencies. They help keep the skeleton in proper alignment, preventing back and leg pain and providing the support necessary for good posture. Muscular strength has obvious importance in recreational activities. Strong people can hit a tennis ball harder, kick a soccer ball farther, and ride a bicycle uphill more easily.

Muscle tissue is an important element of overall body composition. Greater muscle mass makes possible a higher rate of metabolism and faster energy use, which help maintain a healthy body weight.

Strength training helps maintain muscle mass, function, and balance in older people, which greatly enhances their quality of life and prevents injuries. Strength training promotes cardiovascular health, reduces the risk of osteoporosis

(bone loss), and prevents premature death from all causes. Muscular strength can be developed by training with weights or by using the weight of the body for resistance during calisthenic exercises such as push-ups and curl-ups.

Muscular Endurance

Muscular endurance is the ability to resist fatigue and sustain a given level of muscle tension—that is, to hold a muscle contraction for a long time or to contract a muscle over and over again.

Muscular endurance is important for good posture and for injury prevention. Muscular endurance helps people cope with the physical demands of everyday life and enhances performance in sports and work. Stressing the muscles with a greater load (weight) than they are accustomed to develops muscle endurance as well as muscular strength. The degree to which strength or endurance develops depends on the type and amount of stress that is applied.

Flexibility

Flexibility is the ability of joints to move through their full range of motion. Flexible, pain-free joints are important for good health and well-being. Inactivity causes the joints to become stiffer with age. Stiffness, in turn, often causes older people to assume unnatural body postures that can stress joints and muscles. Stretching exercises can help ensure a healthy range of motion for all major joints.

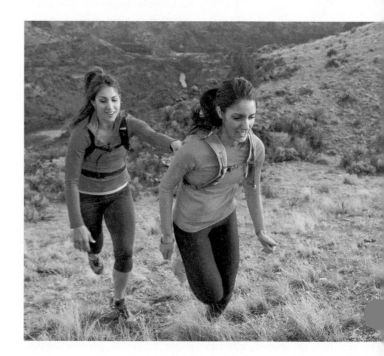

Cardiorespiratory endurance is a critical component of fitness.

Body Composition

Body composition refers to the proportion of fat and **fat-free mass** (muscle, bone, and water) in the body. Healthy body composition involves a high proportion of fat-free mass and an acceptably low level of body fat, adjusted for age and sex. A person with excessive body fat—especially in the abdomen—is more likely to experience health problems, including heart disease, high blood pressure, sexual problems, stroke, joint problems, diabetes, gallbladder disease, cancer, and back pain. The best way to lose fat is through a lifestyle that includes a sensible diet and exercise. The best way to add muscle mass is through resistance training such as weight training.

Skill-Related Components of Fitness

In addition to the five health-related components of physical fitness, the ability to perform a particular sport or activity may depend on **skill-related fitness** components such as speed, power, agility, balance, coordination, and reaction time.

Skill-related fitness tends to be sport-specific and is best developed through practice. Playing a sport can be fun, can help build fitness, and may contribute to other areas of wellness.

> **The best way to lose fat** is through a lifestyle that includes a sensible diet and exercise.

PHYSICAL ACTIVITY AND EXERCISE FOR HEALTH AND FITNESS

Despite the many benefits of an active lifestyle, levels of physical activity remain low for all populations of Americans.

Physical activity is any body movement carried out by the skeletal muscles that requires energy. Different types of physical activity can be arranged on a continuum based on the amount of energy they require. Quick, easy movements such as standing up or walking down a hallway require little energy or effort. More intense, sustained activities such as cycling five miles or running in a race require considerably more.

Exercise refers to a subset of physical activity—planned, structured, repetitive movement of the body intended specifically to improve or maintain physical fitness. To develop fitness, a person must perform enough physical activity to stress the body and cause long-term physiological changes. Moderate-intensity physical activity is essential to health and confers wide-ranging health benefits, but more intense exercise is necessary to improve physical fitness.

In 2011 the American College of Sports Medicine released the newest version of its exercise guidelines for healthy adults. This update followed the 2010 U.S. Surgeon General's report on overweight and obesity in American children and adults, *The Surgeon General's Vision for a Healthy and Fit Nation,* and the landmark 2008 report from the U.S. Department of Health and Human Services, *Physical Activity Guidelines for Americans.* Although each of these reports has a somewhat different focus, they all stress the importance of regular physical activity for health, wellness, and the prevention of chronic diseases and premature death. The 2011 guidelines include the following key recommendations for adults:

• For substantial health benefits, adults should do at least 150 minutes (2.5 hours) a week of moderate-intensity aerobic physical activity, or 75 minutes (1 hour and 15 minutes) a week of vigorous-intensity aerobic physical activity, or an equivalent combination of moderate- and vigorous-intensity aerobic activity. Activity should preferably be spread throughout the week.

• For additional and more extensive health benefits, adults should increase their aerobic physical activity to 300 minutes (5 hours) a week of moderate-intensity activity, or 150 minutes (2.5 hours) a week of vigorous-intensity activity, or an equivalent combination of moderate- and vigorous-intensity activity.

• Adults should also do muscle-strengthening activities that are moderate or high intensity and involve all major muscle groups on two or more days a week.

• Everyone should avoid inactivity.

TERMS

body composition The proportion of fat and fat-free mass (muscle, bone, and water) in the body.

fat-free mass The nonfat components of the human body, consisting of skeletal muscle, bone, and water.

skill-related fitness Physical abilities that contribute to performance in a sport or activity, including speed, power, agility, balance, coordination, and reaction time.

physical activity Any body movement carried out by the skeletal muscles that requires energy.

exercise Planned, structured, repetitive movement of the body intended to improve or maintain physical fitness.

"Too little time" is a common excuse for not being physically active. Learning to manage your time successfully is crucial if you are to maintain a wellness lifestyle. Begin by keeping a record of how you currently spend your time. List each type of activity and the total time you engaged in it on a given day—for example, sleeping, 7 hours; eating, 1.5 hours; studying, 3 hours; and so on. Prioritize your activities according to how important they are to you, from essential to somewhat important to not important at all.

Make changes in your daily schedule by subtracting time from some activities in order to make time for physical activity. Look carefully at your leisure-time activities and your methods of transportation—these are areas where it is easy to build in physical activity. For example, you may choose to reduce the total amount of time you spend playing computer games to make time for an after-dinner bike ride or a walk with a friend. You may decide to watch 10 fewer minutes of television in the morning to change your 5-minute drive to class into a 15-minute walk.

Here are just a few ways to incorporate more physical activity into your daily routine:

- Take the stairs instead of the elevator or escalator.

- Walk to the mailbox, post office, store, bank, or library whenever possible.

- Do at least one chore every day that requires physical activity: Wash the windows or your car, clean your room or house, mow the lawn, or rake the leaves.

- Take study or work breaks to avoid sitting for more than 30 minutes at a time. Get up and walk around the library, your office, or your home or dorm; go up and down a flight of stairs.

- When you take public transportation, get off one stop early and walk to your destination.

- Take the dog for a walk every day.

- If weather or neighborhood safety rule out walking outside, look for alternative locations—an indoor track, an enclosed shopping mall, or even a long hallway.

- Seize every opportunity to get up and walk around. Move more and sit less.

These levels of physical activity promote health and wellness by lowering the risk of high blood pressure, stroke, heart disease, type 2 diabetes, colon cancer, and osteoporosis and by reducing feelings of mild to moderate depression and anxiety.

What's the difference between moderate- and vigorous-intensity physical activity? *2008 Physical Activity Guidelines for Americans* defines moderate-intensity physical activity as activity that causes a noticeable increase in heart rate, such as brisk walking. Vigorous-intensity physical activity is activity that causes rapid breathing and a substantial increase in heart rate, such as jogging. Brisk walking, dancing, swimming, cycling, and yardwork can all help you meet the physical activity recommendations. You can burn the same number of calories by doing a moderate-intensity activity for a longer time or higher-intensity activity for a shorter time.

Ask Yourself

QUESTIONS FOR CRITICAL THINKING AND REFLECTION

Does your current lifestyle include enough physical activity—150 minutes of moderate-intensity activity a week—to support health and wellness? Do you go beyond this level to include enough vigorous activity and exercise to build physical fitness? What changes could you make in your lifestyle to start developing physical fitness?

The daily total of physical activity can be accumulated in multiple bouts of 10 or more minutes—for example, two 10-minute bike rides to and from class and a brisk 10-minute walk to the store. In this lifestyle approach to physical activity, people can choose activities that they find enjoyable and that fit into their daily routine. Everyday tasks at school, work, and home can be structured to contribute to the daily activity total (see the box "Making Time for Physical Activity").

THE BENEFITS OF EXERCISE

As mentioned earlier, the human body is very adaptable. The greater the demands made on it, the more it adjusts to meet the demands—it becomes fit. Over time, immediate, short-term adjustments translate into long-term changes and improvements. (See page T1-4 of the color transparency insert "Touring Lifestyle Behaviors" in Chapter 8.) The goal of regular physical activity is to bring about these kinds of long-term changes and improvements in the body's functioning.

Reduced Risk of Premature Death

Physically active people have a reduced risk of dying prematurely from all causes, with the greatest benefits found in the most active people (Figure 10.1). Physical inactivity increases the risk of premature death and is as important a risk

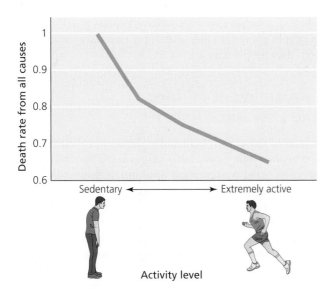

FIGURE 10.1 **Exercise promotes longevity.** The risk of death each year from all causes decreases with increased amounts and intensities of weekly physical activity.

SOURCES: Adapted from a composite of 12 studies involving more than 200,000 men and women. Wen, M. et al. 2013. Physical activity and mortality among middle-aged and older adults in the United States. *Journal of Physical Activity & Health* (published online); Physical Activity Guidelines Advisory Committee. 2008. *Physical Activity Guidelines Advisory Committee Report, 2008.* Washington, DC: U.S. Department of Health and Human Services.

factor as smoking, high blood pressure, obesity, and diabetes. Poor muscle strength also increases the risk of premature death.

A large 15-year study of exercise and mortality found that running even 5 to 10 minutes a day, and at slow speeds (less than 6 miles per hour), benefits adults in the long term.

Improved Cardiorespiratory Functioning

During exercise, the cardiorespiratory system (heart, lungs, and circulatory system) must work harder to meet the body's increased demand for oxygen. Regular cardiorespiratory endurance exercise improves the functioning of the heart and the ability of the cardiorespiratory system to carry oxygen to body tissues. Exercise directly affects the health of your arteries, keeping them from stiffening or clogging with plaque and reducing the risk of cardiovascular disease. Exercise also improves sexual function and general vitality.

More Efficient Metabolism and Improved Cell Health

Endurance exercise improves metabolism—the process that converts food to energy and builds tissue. This process involves oxygen, nutrients, hormones, and enzymes. A physically fit person's body can more efficiently use energy from carbohydrates and fats and better regulate hormones. Exercise may also protect cells from damage from free radicals, which are destructive chemicals produced normally during metabolism, and from inflammation caused by obesity, high blood pressure or cholesterol, nicotine, and overeating. Training activates antioxidants that prevent free radical damage and maintain cell health. Regular physical activity prevents the deterioration of telomeres, which form the protective ends of chromosomes that are vital for cell health and repair.

Improved Body Composition

Exercise can improve body composition in several ways. Endurance exercise significantly increases daily calorie expenditure. It can also slightly raise *metabolic rate,* the rate at which the body burns calories, for several hours after an exercise session. Strength training increases muscle mass, thereby tipping the body composition ratio toward fat-free mass and away from fat. It can also help with losing fat because metabolic rate is directly proportional to fat-free mass: The more muscle mass, the higher the metabolic rate.

Disease Prevention and Management

Regular physical activity lowers your risk of many chronic, disabling diseases.

Cardiovascular Disease A sedentary lifestyle is one of the six major risk factors for cardiovascular disease (CVD), including heart attack and stroke. Sedentary people have CVD death rates significantly higher than those of fit individuals. Physical inactivity increases the risk of CVD by as much as 240%.

The benefits of physical activity begin at moderate levels of exercise and increase as the amount and intensity of activity rises. Exercise positively affects the risk factors for CVD, including cholesterol levels, insulin resistance, and blood pressure. Exercise also directly interferes with the disease process itself, lowering the risk of heart disease and stroke.

CANCER Studies have shown a relationship between increased physical activity and a reduced risk of cancer, but these findings are not conclusive. There is evidence that exercise reduces the risk of colon cancer and promising data that it reduces the risk of cancer of the breast and reproductive organs in women and prostate cancer in men.

Osteoporosis A special benefit of exercise, especially for women, is protection against osteoporosis, a disease that results in loss of bone density and poor bone strength. Weight-bearing exercise, which includes almost everything

> QUICK
> STATS
>
> **69,071**
> **Americans died from diabetes in 2011, making it the 7th leading cause of death that year.**
> —CDC, 2013

except swimming, helps build bone during childhood and the teens and twenties. Strength training and impact exercises such as jumping rope can increase bone density throughout life. With stronger bones and muscles and better balance, fit people are less likely to experience debilitating falls and bone fractures.

Type 2 Diabetes People with diabetes are prone to heart disease, blindness, and severe problems of the nervous and circulatory systems. Exercise prevents the development of type 2 diabetes, the most common form of the disease. Exercise burns excess sugar and makes cells more sensitive to insulin. Exercise also helps keep body fat at healthy levels, which is important because obesity is a key risk factor for type 2 diabetes. For people who have diabetes, physical activity is an important part of treatment.

Improved Psychological and Emotional Wellness

Physically active people enjoy many social, psychological, and emotional benefits, including the following:

• *Reduced anxiety and depression.* Exercise reduces symptoms of anxiety, such as worry and self-doubt, and is associated with a lower risk for panic attacks. Exercise also relieves feelings of sadness and hopelessness and can be as effective as psychotherapy in treating mild to moderate cases of depression.

• *Improved sleep.* Regular physical activity helps people fall asleep more easily; it also improves sleep quality.

• *Reduced stress.* Exercise reduces the body's overall response to all forms of stressors and helps people deal more effectively with stress.

• *Enhanced self-esteem, self-confidence, and self-efficacy.* Exercise can boost self-esteem and self-confidence by providing opportunities for people to succeed and excel. Exercise also improves body image. Sticking with an exercise program increases people's belief in their ability to be active, thereby boosting self-efficacy.

• *Enhanced creativity and intellectual functioning.* Exercise improves alertness and memory in the short term and helps maintain reaction time, short-term memory, and nonverbal reasoning skills over time.

• *Increased opportunities for social interaction.* Exercise provides many chances for people to have positive interactions with other people.

Improved Immune Function

Exercise can have either positive or negative effects on the immune system—the physiological processes that protect us from disease. Moderate endurance exercise boosts immune function, whereas excessive training depresses it. Physically fit people get fewer colds and upper respiratory tract infections than people who are not fit.

Prevention of Injuries and Low-Back Pain

Increased muscle strength and endurance provides protection against injury because it helps people maintain spinal stability, good posture, and appropriate body mechanics when performing everyday activities such as walking, lifting, and carrying. Good muscle endurance in the abdomen, hips, lower back, and legs supports the back in proper alignment and helps prevent low-back pain, which afflicts more than 85% of Americans at some time in their lives.

Improved Wellness for Life

Although people differ in the maximum levels of fitness they can achieve through exercise, the wellness benefits of exercise are available to everyone. Exercising regularly may be the single most important thing you can do now to improve the quality of your life in the future.

DESIGNING YOUR EXERCISE PROGRAM

The best exercise program has two primary characteristics: It promotes your health, and it's fun for you to do. Exercise can provide some of the most pleasurable moments of your day, once you make it a habit. A little thought and planning will help you achieve these goals.

Figure 10.2 shows a physical activity pyramid to guide you in meeting goals for physical activity. If you are sedentary, start at the bottom of the pyramid and gradually increase the moderate-intensity physical activity in your daily life. You don't have to exercise vigorously, but you should experience a moderate increase in your heart and breathing rates. If weight management is a concern for you, begin by achieving the goal of 150 minutes per week and then gradually increase your activity level to 300 minutes per week while reducing caloric intake.

For even greater benefits, move up to the next two levels of the pyramid, which illustrate parts of a formal exercise program. These recommendations are from the ACSM's exercise guidelines, which include cardiorespiratory endurance (aerobic) exercise, strength training, flexibility training, and balance training (for older adults). Such a program will develop all the health-related components of physical fitness. New research shows that high-intensity interval training—repetitions of high-intensity exercise followed by rest—builds fitness rapidly in less time than traditional aerobic training. For a summary of the health and fitness benefits of different levels of physical activity, see Figure 10.3.

Sedentary Activities
Do infrequently
Watching television, surfing the Internet, talking on the telephone

Strength Training
2–3 nonconsecutive days per week (all major muscle groups)
Biceps curls, push-ups, abdominal curls, bench press, calf raises

Flexibility Training
At least 2–3 days per week, ideally 5–7 days per week (all major joints)
Calf stretch, side lunge, step stretch, hurdler stretch

Cardiorespiratory Endurance Exercise
3–5 days per week (20–60 minutes)

Walking, jogging, bicycling, swimming, aerobic dancing, in-line skating, cross-country skiing, dancing, basketball

Moderate-Intensity Physical Activity
150 minutes per week; for weight loss or prevention of weight regain following weight loss, 60–90 minutes per day

Walking to the store or bank, washing windows or your car, climbing stairs, working in your yard, walking your dog, cleaning your room

FIGURE 10.2   Physical activity pyramid.

	Lifestyle physical activity	Moderate exercise program	Vigorous exercise program
Description	Moderate physical activity (150 minutes per week; muscle-strengthening exercises 2 or more days per week)	Cardiorespiratory endurance exercise (20–60 minutes, 3–5 days per week); strength training (2–3 nonconsecutive days per week); and stretching exercises (2 or more days per week)	Cardiorespiratory endurance exercise (20–60 minutes, 3–5 days per week); interval training; strength training (3–4 nonconsecutive days per week); and stretching exercises (5–7 days per week)
Sample activities or program	*One of the following:* • Walking to and from work, 15 minutes each way • Cycling to and from class, 10 minutes each way • Yard work for 30 minutes • Dancing (fast) for 30 minutes • Playing basketball for 20 minutes	• Jogging for 30 minutes, 3 days per week • Weight training, 1 set of 8 exercises, 2 days per week • Stretching exercises, 3 days per week	• Running for 45 minutes, 3 days per week • Intervals: running 400 m at high effort, 4 sets, 2 days per week • Weight training, 3 sets of 10 exercises, 3 days per week • Stretching exercises, 6 days per week
Health and fitness benefits	Better blood cholesterol levels, reduced body fat, better control of blood pressure, improved metabolic health, and enhanced glucose metabolism; improved quality of life; reduced risk of some chronic diseases. Greater amounts of activity can help prevent weight gain and promote weight loss.	All the benefits of lifestyle physical activity, plus improved physical fitness (increased cardiorespiratory endurance, muscular strength and endurance, and flexibility) and even greater improvements in health and quality of life and reductions in chronic disease risk.	All the benefits of lifestyle physical activity and a moderate exercise program, with greater increases in fitness and somewhat greater reductions in chronic disease risk. Participating in a vigorous exercise program may increase risk of injury and overtraining.

FIGURE 10.3   Health and fitness benefits of different amounts of physical activity and exercise.

First Steps

Are you thinking about starting a formal exercise program? A little planning can help make it a success.

Medical Clearance   Previously inactive men over 40 and women over 50 should get a medical examination before beginning an exercise program. Diabetes, asthma, heart disease, and extreme obesity are conditions that may call for a modified program. If you have an increased risk of heart disease because of smoking, high blood pressure, or obesity, get a physical checkup, including an **electrocardiogram (ECG *or* EKG),** before beginning an exercise program.

Basic Principles of Physical Training   To put together an effective exercise program, you should first understand the basic principles of physical training.

SPECIFICITY   To develop a fitness component, you must perform exercises that are specifically designed for that component. This is the principle of **specificity.** Weight training, for example, develops muscular strength but is less effective for developing flexibility or cardiorespiratory endurance. Specificity also applies to the skill-related fitness components and to the different parts of the body. A well-rounded exercise program includes exercises geared to each component of fitness, to different parts of the body, and to specific activities or sports.

PROGRESSIVE OVERLOAD   When the amount of exercise, or overload, is progressively increased, fitness continues to improve. This training principle is called **progressive overload.** Too little exercise has no effect on fitness; too much may cause injury. The appropriate amount depends on your current level of fitness, your genetic capacity to adapt to exercise, your fitness goals, and the fitness components being developed.

The amount of overload needed to maintain or improve a particular level of fitness is determined in four dimensions, represented by the acronym FITT: Frequency Intensity Time and Type.

REST AND RECUPERATION   Fitness gains occur following exercise as the body adapts to the stress of training. Adequate rest is as important to this process as training. Overtraining—an imbalance between training and recovery—leads to injury, illness, and excessive fatigue.

REVERSIBILITY   The body adjusts to lower levels of physical activity the same way it adjusts to higher levels—this is the principle of **reversibility.** When you stop exercising, you can lose up to 50% of fitness improvements within two months. Try to exercise consistently, and don't quit if you miss a few workouts.

INDIVIDUAL DIFFERENCES   There are genetic limits to how much a person can improve fitness, as well as large individual differences between people in their ability to improve fitness, achieve a desirable body composition, and perform and learn sports skills. In studies, some people on a diet and exercise program improve fitness by 50%, whereas others on the same program improve by only 2–3%. It is more difficult for those whose bodies don't respond as well to exercise to make changes in fitness or body fat levels. Elite athletes start out with a genetic advantage over the average person. However, everyone has the capacity to improve fitness and reap the health benefits of exercise.

Selecting Activities   If you have been inactive, begin by gradually increasing the amount of moderate physical activity in your life (the bottom of the activity pyramid shown in Figure 10.2). Once your body adjusts to your new level of activity, you can choose additional activities for your exercise program.

Be sure the activities you choose contribute to your overall wellness and make sense for you. Are you competitive? If so, try racquetball, basketball, or squash. Do you prefer to exercise alone? Then consider cross-country skiing or road running. Have you been sedentary? A walking program may be a good place to start. If you think you may have trouble sticking with an exercise program, find a structured activity that you can do with a friend, a personal trainer, or a group. Be realistic about the constraints presented by some sports, such as accessibility, expense, and time.

Cardiorespiratory Endurance Exercise

Exercises that condition your heart and lungs and improve your metabolism should have a central role in your fitness program.

Frequency   The optimal workout schedule for endurance training is 3–5 days per week. Beginners should start with 3 days and work up to 5 days. Training more than 5 days a week often leads to injury for recreational athletes.

---

electrocardiogram (ECG or EKG)   A recording   TERMS
of the changes in electrical activity of the heart.

specificity   The training principle that the body adapts to the particular type and amount of stress placed on it.

progressive overload   The training principle that placing increasing amounts of stress (in the form of exercise) on the body causes adaptations that improve fitness.

reversibility   The training principle that fitness improvements are lost when demands on the body are lowered.

Ask Yourself

QUESTIONS FOR CRITICAL THINKING AND REFLECTION

Which benefits of exercise are most important to you, and why? For example, is there a history of heart disease or diabetes in your family? Have you thought about how regular exercise could reduce your risks for specific diseases?

One of the best ways to monitor the intensity of cardiorespiratory endurance exercise is to measure your heart rate. It isn't necessary to exercise at your maximum heart rate to improve maximal oxygen consumption. Fitness adaptations occur at lower heart rates with a much lower risk of injury.

According to the American College of Sports Medicine, your target heart rate zone—rates at which you should exercise to experience cardiorespiratory benefits—is between 65% and 90% of your maximum heart rate. To calculate your target heart rate zone, follow these steps:

1. Estimate your maximum heart rate (MHR) by subtracting your age from 220.

2. Multiply your MHR by 65% and 90% to calculate your target heart rate zone. Very unfit people should use 55% of MHR for their training threshold.

For example, a 19-year-old would calculate her target heart rate zone as follows:

MHR = 220 − 19 = 201

65% training intensity = 0.65 × 201 = 131 bpm

90% training intensity = 0.90 × 201 = 181 bpm

To gain fitness benefits, the young woman in our example would have to exercise at an intensity that raises her heart rate to between 131 and 181 bpm.

An alternative method for calculating target heart rate range uses heart rate reserve, the difference between maximum heart rate and resting heart rate. Using this method, target heart rate is equal to resting heart rate plus between 50% (40% for very unfit people) and 85% of heart rate reserve.

Intensity The most misunderstood aspect of conditioning, even among experienced athletes, is training intensity. Intensity is the crucial factor in attaining a significant training effect—that is, in increasing the body's cardiorespiratory capacity. A primary purpose of endurance training is to increase **maximal oxygen consumption ($\dot{V}O_{2max}$)**. $\dot{V}O_{2max}$ represents the cells' maximum ability to use oxygen and is considered the best measure of cardiorespiratory capacity. Intensity of training is the crucial factor in improving $\dot{V}O_{2max}$.

One of the easiest ways to determine exactly how intensely you should work involves measuring your heart rate. It is not necessary or desirable to exercise at your maximum heart rate—the fastest heart rate possible before exhaustion sets in—to improve your cardiorespiratory capacity. Beneficial effects occur at lower heart rates with a much lower risk of injury. Your **target heart rate zone** is the range of rates within which you should exercise to obtain cardiorespiratory benefits. To determine the intensity at which you should exercise, see the box "Determine Your Target Heart Rate."

If you have been sedentary, start by exercising at the lower end of your target heart rate range for at least 4–6 weeks. For people with a very low initial level of fitness, a lower training intensity may be sufficient to achieve improvements in maximal oxygen consumption, especially at the start of an exercise program. Heart-rate monitors make it easy to monitor your heart rate before, during, and after exercise.

Another way scientists describe fitness is in terms of the capacity to increase metabolism (energy usage level) above rest. Scientists use METs to measure the metabolic cost of an exercise. One **MET** represents the body's resting metabolic rate—that is, the energy or calorie requirement of the body at rest. Exercise intensity is expressed in multiples of resting metabolic rate.

Activities that increase metabolism by 6–8 METs are classified as moderate-intensity exercises and are suitable for most people beginning an exercise program.

Time (Duration) A total time of 20–60 minutes per workout is recommended for cardiorespiratory endurance training. Exercise can be done in a single session or several sessions lasting 10 or more minutes. The total duration of exercise depends on its intensity. To improve cardiorespiratory endurance during a moderate-intensity activity such as walking or slow swimming, you should exercise for 45–60 minutes. For high-intensity exercise performed at the top of your target heart rate zone, a duration of 20 minutes is sufficient. Start with less vigorous activities and gradually increase intensity.

Type The best exercises for developing cardiorespiratory endurance stress a large portion of the body's muscle mass for a prolonged period of time. These include walking, jogging, running, swimming, bicycling, and aerobic dance. Many popular sports and recreational activities, such as racquetball, tennis, basketball, and soccer, are also good if the skill level and intensity of the game are sufficient to provide a vigorous workout.

> **maximal oxygen consumption ($\dot{V}O_{2max}$)** The TERMS body's maximum ability to transport and use oxygen.
>
> **target heart rate zone** The range of heart rates that should be reached and maintained during cardiorespiratory endurance exercise to obtain benefits.
>
> **MET** A measure of the metabolic cost of an exercise. One MET represents the body's resting metabolic rate—the energy or calorie requirement of the body at rest; exercise intensity is expressed in multiples of resting metabolic rate.

The Warm-Up and Cool-Down   It is always important to warm up before you exercise and to cool down afterward. Warming up enhances your performance and decreases your chances of injury.

A warm-up session should include low-intensity movements similar to those in the activity that will follow. For example, hit forehands and backhands before a tennis game or jog slowly for 400 meters before progressing to an 8-minute mile. Some people like to include stretching exercises in their warm-up, but experts recommend stretching *after* the active part of your warm-up, when your body temperature is elevated. Studies have found that stretching prior to exercise can temporarily decrease muscle strength and power.

Cooling down after exercise is important to restore the body's circulation to its normal resting condition. When you are at rest, a relatively small percentage of your total blood volume is directed to muscles, but during exercise, as much as 90% of the heart's output is directed to them. During recovery from exercise, continuing to exercising at a low level is important to provide a smooth transition to the resting

state. Cooling down helps regulate the return of blood to your heart. After exercising, avoid taking a hot shower until you have cooled down.

Exercises for Muscular Strength and Endurance

Any program designed to promote health should include exercises that develop muscular strength and endurance.

Types of Strength Training Exercises   Muscular strength and endurance can be developed in many ways, from weight training to calisthenics. Common exercises such as curl-ups, push-ups, pull-ups, and nonweighted squats maintain the muscular strength of most people if they practice them several times a week. To condition and tone your whole body, choose exercises that work the major muscles of the shoulders, chest, back, arms, abdomen, and legs.

To increase muscular strength and endurance, you must do **resistance exercise**—exercises in which your muscles must exert force against a significant amount of resistance. Resistance can be provided by weights, exercise machines, your own body weight, or even objects such as rocks.

Isometric (static) exercises involve applying force without movement, such as when you contract your abdominal muscles. This type of exercise is valuable for toning and strengthening muscles. Isometrics can be practiced anywhere and do not require any equipment. For maximum strength gains, hold an isometric contraction maximally for 6 seconds, and do 5–10 repetitions. Don't hold your breath: Doing so can restrict blood flow to your heart and brain. Within a few weeks, you will notice the effect of this exercise. Isometrics are particularly useful when recovering from an injury.

Isotonic (dynamic) exercises involve applying force with movement, as in weight training exercises such as the bench press. These type of exercises are the most popular for increasing muscle strength and seem to be most valuable for developing strength that can be transferred to other forms of physical activity. They include exercises using barbells, dumbbells, kettlebells, weight machines, and body weight (as in push-ups or curl-ups).

Core Training   The core muscles include those in the abdomen, pelvic floor, sides of the trunk, back, buttocks, hips, and pelvis. They stabilize the spine and help transfer force between the upper and lower body. They stabilize the midsection when you sit, stand, reach, walk, jump, twist, squat, throw, or bend. Strong core muscles make movements more forceful and help prevent back pain.

The best exercises for low-back health are whole-body exercises that force the core muscles to stabilize the spine in many different directions.

TERMS

resistance exercise   Exercise that forces muscles to contract against increased resistance; also called *strength training*.

isometric (static) exercise   The application of force without movement.

isotonic (dynamic) exercise   The application of force with movement.

Weight training exercises are isotonic (dynamic) exercises that involve applying force with movement.

Gender Differences in Muscular Strength   Men are generally stronger than women because their bodies are typically larger overall and a larger proportion of their total body mass is made up of muscle. But when strength is expressed per unit of muscle tissue, men are only 1–2% stronger than women in the upper body and about equal to women in the lower body.

Men also have more testosterone than women. Testosterone promotes the growth of muscle tissue in both males and females, but testosterone levels are about 6–10 times higher in men than in women, so men develop larger muscles. Most women will not develop large muscles from strength training. Resistance exercise helps women reduce their overall body fat levels and reduce fat in the midsection. It also helps them preserve muscle mass as they age. Because men start out with more muscle when they are young and don't lose power as quickly as women, older women often have greater impairment of muscle function than older men.

Choosing Equipment   Many people prefer weight machines to free weights because they are safe, convenient, and easy to use. You set the resistance, sit down at the machine, and start working. Free weights require more care, balance, and coordination to use, but they strengthen your body in ways that are more adaptable to real life.

Choosing Exercises   A complete weight training program works all the major muscle groups: neck, upper back, shoulders, arms, chest, abdomen, lower back, thighs, buttocks, and calves. Different exercises work different muscles, so it usually takes about 8–10 exercises to get a complete workout for general fitness. For example, you can do bench presses to develop the chest, shoulders, and upper arms; pull-ups to work the biceps and upper back; squats to develop the legs and buttocks; toe raises to work the calves; and so on.

Frequency   For general fitness, the American College of Sports Medicine recommends a strength workout frequency of at least two nonconsecutive days per week. This schedule allows your muscles one or more days of rest between workouts to avoid soreness and injury. If you enjoy weight training and would like to train more often, try working different muscle groups on alternate days.

Intensity and Time   The amount of weight (resistance) you lift in weight training exercises is equivalent to intensity in cardiorespiratory endurance training, and the number of repetitions of each exercise is equivalent to time. To improve fitness, you must do enough repetitions of each exercise to temporarily fatigue your muscles. The number of repetitions needed to cause fatigue depends on the amount of resistance: The heavier the weight, the fewer repetitions to reach fatigue. In general, a heavy weight and a low number of repetitions (1–5) build strength, whereas a light weight and a high number of repetitions (10–25) build endurance. For a general fitness program to build both strength and endurance, try

to do 8–12 repetitions of each exercise. For people who are over 50 years of age, 10–15 repetitions of each exercise using a lighter weight is recommended.

To start, choose a weight that you can move easily through 8–12 repetitions. Add weight when you can do more than 12 repetitions of an exercise. If adding weight means you can do only 7 or 8 repetitions before your muscles fatigue, stay with that weight until you can again complete 12 repetitions. If you can do only 4–6 repetitions after adding weight, or if you can't maintain good form, you've added too much and should take some off. As a general guideline, try increases of approximately $\frac{1}{2}$ pound of additional weight for each 10 pounds you are currently lifting.

For developing strength and endurance for general fitness, a single set (a group of repetitions) of each exercise is sufficient, provided you use enough weight to fatigue your muscles. Doing more than one set of each exercise may increase strength development further, and most serious weight trainers do at least three sets of each exercise. If you do more than one set of an exercise, rest long enough between sets (1–5 minutes) to allow your muscles to recover. You should warm up before every weight training session and cool down afterward.

A Caution about Supplements   No nutritional supplement or drug will change a weak person into a strong person. Those changes require regular training that stresses the body and causes physiological adaptations. Supplements or drugs that promise quick, large gains in strength usually don't work and are often dangerous, expensive, or illegal. Over-the-counter supplements are not carefully regulated, and their long-term effects have not been systematically studied.

Flexibility Exercises

Flexibility, or stretching, exercises are important for maintaining the normal range of motion in the major joints of the body. Some exercises, such as running, can decrease flexibility because they require only a partial range of motion. Like a good weight training program, a good stretching program includes exercises for all the major muscle groups and joints of the body: neck, shoulders, back, hips, thighs, hamstrings, and calves. In tandem with core training, flexibility training is important for preventing lower back injuries and maintaining lower back health.

Proper Stretching Technique   Timing determines the best stretching technique: In general, do static stretching after a workout and dynamic or active stretching before a workout. *Static stretching* involves extending to a certain position, then holding it. *Dynamic stretching* is done by actively moving through the joints' ranges of motion. *Ballistic stretching* (known as "bouncing") is dangerous and counterproductive. The safest and most convenient technique for increasing flexibility may be active static stretching with a passive assist. For example, you might do a seated stretch of your calf muscles by contracting the muscles on the top of your shin and by grabbing your feet and pulling them toward you.

Frequency   Do stretching exercises at least 2–3 days per week (but 5–7 days is optimal). If you stretch after cardiorespiratory endurance exercise or strength training, during your cool-down, you may develop more flexibility because your muscles are warmer then and can be stretched farther.

Intensity and Time   Do stretching exercises statically. Stretch to the point of mild discomfort, hold the position for 10–30 seconds, rest for 30–60 seconds, and then repeat, trying to stretch a bit farther. Stretch each muscle group for a total of 60 seconds. Older adults might benefit more from holding a stretch for 30-60 seconds.

Increase your intensity gradually over time. Improved flexibility takes many months to develop. There are large individual differences in joint flexibility. Don't feel you have to compete with others during stretching workouts.

Training in Specific Skills

The final component in your fitness program is learning the skills required for the sports or activities in which you choose to participate. The first step in learning a new skill is getting help. Sports like tennis, golf, and skiing require mastery of basic movements and techniques, so instruction from a qualified teacher or coach can save you hours of frustration and increase your enjoyment. Skill is also important in conditioning activities such as jogging, swimming, and cycling. Even if you learned a sport as a child, additional instruction now can help you refine your technique.

Putting It All Together

Now that you know the basic components of a fitness program, you can put them all together in a program that works for you. See Figure 10.4 for a summary of the FITT principle for the health-related components of fitness.

GETTING STARTED AND STAYING ON TRACK

Once you have a program that fulfills your basic fitness needs and suits your personal tastes, adhering to a few basic principles will help you improve quickly, have fun, and minimize the risk of injury.

Selecting Instructors, Equipment, and Facilities

One of the best places to get help is an exercise class, where an expert instructor can teach you the basics of training and answer your questions. A qualified personal trainer can also get you started on an exercise program or a new form of training. Make sure that your instructor or trainer has proper qualifications, such as a college degree in exercise physiology, kinesiology, or physical education and certification by the American College of Sports Medicine, National Strength and Conditioning Association, International Sports Science Association (ISSA), or another professional organization.

Many websites provide fitness programs, including ongoing support and feedback via e-mail. Many of these sites charge fees, so it is important to review the sites, decide which ones seem most appropriate, and if possible go through a free trial period before subscribing. Also remember to consider the reliability of the information at fitness websites, especially those that also advertise or sell products.

Good equipment will enhance your enjoyment and decrease your risk of injury. Appropriate safety equipment, such as pads and helmets for skateboarding, is particularly important. Before you invest in a new

	Cardiorespiratory Endurance Training	Strength Training	Flexibility Training
Frequency	3–5 days per week	2–3 nonconsecutive days per week	2–3 days per week (minimum); 5–7 days per week (ideal)
Intensity	55/65–90% of maximum heart rate	Sufficient resistance to fatigue muscles	Stretch to the point of tension
Time	20–60 minutes in sessions lasting 10 minutes or more	8–12 repetitions of each exercise, 1 or more sets	2–4 repetitions of each exercise, held for 15–30 seconds
Type	Continuous rhythmic activities using large muscle groups	Resistance exercises for all major muscle groups	Stretching exercises for all major joints

FIGURE 10.4   A summary of the FITT principle for the health-related components of fitness.

Clothing

Modern exercise clothing is attractive, comfortable, and functional. Shorts made of elastic material, such as spandex, hug the body, supplying support. If you prefer, you can wear running shorts and a T-shirt. The main requirement for workout clothes is that they let you move easily but are not so loose that they get caught in the exercise machines or on fences when running outside. Don't wear street clothes when exercising because they can interfere with movement, and sweat, oil, and dirt can ruin them. If you run or cycle on the street, wear bright-colored clothing so motorists can see you.

Breast Support for Women

Breast support is important when running, playing volleyball, or weight training. A good sports bra should support the breasts in all directions, contain little elastic material, absorb moisture freely, and be easily laundered. Seams, hooks, and catches should not irritate the skin.

Footwear

Footwear is perhaps the most important item of equipment for almost any activity. Shoes protect and support your feet and improve your traction. They also help cushion your lower legs against the stress of running or jumping, thereby preventing injuries.

When choosing athletic shoes, first consider the activity you've chosen for your exercise program. Shoes appropriate for different activities have different characteristics. Foot type is another important consideration. If your feet tend to roll inward excessively, you may need additional stability features on the inner side of the shoe to counteract this movement. If your feet tend to roll outward excessively, you may need highly flexible and cushioned shoes that promote foot motion. Most women will get a better fit if they choose shoes that are specially designed for women's feet rather than downsized versions of men's shoes.

Two-thirds of runners experience an injury every year. Most runners strike heel first when using heavily padded running shoes. Barefoot runners strike the ground with their forefoot, which better uses the shock absorbing capacity of the skeleton. Some researchers speculate that using "minimalist" footwear allows people to run more naturally. Other research suggests that traditional running shoes provide a physiological advantage that makes running easier.

Successful Shopping

For successful shoe shopping, keep the following strategies in mind:

- Shop late in the day or, ideally, following a workout. Your foot size increases during the day and after exercise.

- Wear socks like those you plan to wear during exercise.

- Try on both shoes and wear them around for 10 minutes or more. Try walking on an uncarpeted surface. Approximate the movements of your activity: walk, jog, run, jump, and so on.

- Check the fit and style carefully:

  - Is the toe box roomy enough? Your toes will spread out when your foot hits the ground or you push off. There should be at least one thumb's width of space from the longest toe to the end of the toe box.
  - Do the shoes have enough cushioning? Do your feet feel supported when you bounce up and down? Try bouncing on your toes and on your heels.
  - Do your heels fit snugly in the shoe? Do they stay put when you walk, or do they slide up?
  - Are the arches of your feet on top of the shoes' arch supports?
  - Do the shoes feel stable when you twist and turn on the balls of your feet? Try twisting from side to side while standing on one foot.
  - Do you feel any pressure points?

- If you exercise at dawn or dusk, choose shoes with reflective sections for added visibility and safety.

- Replace athletic shoes about every three months or 300–500 miles of jogging or walking.

piece of equipment, investigate it. Try it out at a local gym to make sure that you'll use it regularly. Footwear is an important piece of equipment for almost any activity; see the box "What to Wear" for shopping strategies.

If you are thinking of joining a health club or fitness center, be sure to choose one that has the right programs and equipment available at the times you will use them.

Also make sure the facility is certified. Look for the displayed names American College of Sports Medicine, National Strength and Conditioning Association, American Council on Exercise, or Aerobics and Fitness Association of America. These trade associations have established standards to help protect consumer health, safety, and rights.

Eating and Drinking for Exercise

Most people do not need to change their eating habits when they begin a fitness program. In most cases a well-balanced diet contains all the energy and nutrients needed to sustain an exercise program.

A balanced diet is also the key to improving body composition when you begin to exercise more. One of the promises of a fitness program is a decrease in body fat and an increase in muscle mass. The best way to control body fat is to follow a reduced-calorie diet and to be physically active.

One of the most important principles to follow when exercising is to drink enough water. Sweating during exercise depletes the body's water supply and can lead to dehydration if fluids are not replaced. Serious dehydration can cause reduced blood volume, accelerated heart rate, elevated body temperature, muscle cramps, heat stroke, and other serious problems.

Thirst receptors in the brain make you want to drink fluids, but during heavy or prolonged exercise or exercise in hot weather, thirst alone isn't a good indication of how much fluid you need to drink. As a rule of thumb, drink at least 16 ounces of fluid two hours before exercise and then drink enough during exercise to prevent significant fluid loss in sweat. After exercise, let thirst be your guide to your fluid needs.

Bring a bottle of water when you exercise so you can replace your fluids when they're depleted. For exercise sessions lasting less than 60–90 minutes, cool water is an excellent fluid replacement. For longer workouts, a sports drink that contains water and small amounts of electrolytes (sodium, potassium, and magnesium) and simple carbohydrates (sugar, usually in the form of sucrose or glucose) is recommended.

Managing Your Fitness Program

How can you tell when you're in shape? When do you stop improving and start maintaining? How can you stay motivated? If your program is going to become an integral part of

your life, and if the principles behind it are going to serve you well in the future, these questions are key.

Start Slowly, Get in Shape Gradually   An exercise program can be divided into three phases:

- *Beginning phase.* The body adjusts to the new type and level of activity.
- *Progress phase.* Fitness increases.
- *Maintenance phase.* The targeted level of fitness is sustained over the long term.

When beginning a program, start slowly to give your body time to adapt to the stress of exercise. Choose activities carefully according to your fitness status.

Exercising Consistently   Steady fitness improvement comes when you overload your body consistently over time. The best way to ensure consistency is to record the details of your workouts in a journal: how far you ran, how much weight you lifted, and so on. This record will help you evaluate your progress and plan workout sessions intelligently. Don't increase your exercise volume by more than 5–10% per week. Table 10.1 shows how the amount of overload is increased gradually over time.

Assessing Your Fitness   When are you in shape? It depends. One person may be out of shape running a mile in

Table 10.1	Sample Progression for an Endurance Program		
STAGE/WEEK	FREQUENCY (days/ week)	INTENSITY* (beats/minute)	TIME (duration in minutes)
Initial stage			
1	3	120–130	15–20
2	3	120–130	20–25
3	4	130–145	20–25
4	4	130–145	25–30
Improvement stage			
5–7	3–4	145–160	25–30
8–10	3–4	145–160	30–35
11–13	3–4	150–165	30–35
14–16	4–5	150–165	30–35
17–20	4–5	160–180	35–40
21–24	4–5	160–180	35–40
Maintenance stage			
25+	3–5	160–180	20–60

*The target heart rates shown here are based on calculations for a healthy 20-year-old with a resting heart rate of 60 beats per minute. The program progresses from an initial target heart rate of 50% to a maintenance range of 70–85% of heart rate reserve.

SOURCE: Adapted from American College of Sports Medicine. 2013. *ACSM's Guidelines for Exercise Testing and Prescription*, 9th ed. Philadelphia: Wolters Kluwer/Lippincott Williams & Wilkins Health. Reprinted with permission from the publisher.

5 minutes, but another may be in shape running a mile in 12 minutes. Your ultimate level of fitness depends on your goals, your program, and your natural ability. The important thing is to set goals that make sense for you.

Preventing and Managing Athletic Injuries

It is important that you learn how to deal with injuries so they don't derail your fitness program or escalate into chronic problems (see Table 10.2). Some injuries require medical attention. See a physician right away if you suffer a head or eye injury, a possible ligament injury, a broken bone, or an internal disorder such as chest pain, fainting, or intolerance to heat. Also seek medical attention for apparently minor injuries that do not get better within a reasonable amount of time.

For minor cuts and scrapes, stop the bleeding and clean the wound with soap and water. Treat soft tissue injuries (muscles and joints) with the R-I-C-E principle: rest, ice, compress, and elevate the injured area.

After 36–48 hours, if the swelling has disappeared, apply heat to relieve pain, relax muscles, and reduce stiffness.

Immerse the affected area in warm water or apply warm compresses, a hot water bottle, or a heating pad.

To prevent injuries, follow a few basic guidelines:

- Stay in condition: Haphazard exercise programs invite injury.
- Warm up thoroughly before exercising.
- Use proper body mechanics when lifting objects or executing sports skills.
- Don't exercise when you're ill or overtrained (experiencing extreme fatigue due to overexercising).
- Use the proper equipment.
- Don't return to your normal exercise program until athletic injuries have healed.

You can minimize the risk of injury by following safety guidelines, respecting signals from your body that something may be wrong, and treating injuries promptly. Use special caution in heat or humidity (over 80°F and/or 60% humidity): Exercise slowly, rest frequently in the shade, wear clothing that breathes, and drink plenty of fluids. Slow

Table 10.2	Care of Common Exercise Injuries and Discomforts	
INJURY	**SYMPTOMS**	**TREATMENT**
Blister	Accumulation of fluid in one spot under the skin	Don't pop or drain it unless it interferes too much with your daily activities. If it does pop, clean the area with antiseptic and cover with a bandage. Do not remove the skin covering the blister.
Bruise (contusion)	Pain, swelling, and discoloration	R-I-C-E: rest, ice, compression, elevation.
Fracture and/or dislocation	Pain, swelling, tenderness, loss of function, and deformity	Seek medical attention, immobilize the affected area, and apply cold.
Joint sprain	Pain, tenderness, swelling, discoloration, and loss of function	R-I-C-E. Apply heat when swelling has disappeared. Stretch and strengthen affected area.
Muscle cramp	Painful, spasmodic muscle contractions	Gently stretch for 15–30 seconds at a time and/or massage the cramped area. Drink fluids and increase dietary salt intake if exercising in hot weather.
Muscle soreness or stiffness	Pain and tenderness in the affected muscle	Stretch the affected muscle gently; exercise at a low intensity; apply heat. Nonsteroidal anti-inflammatory drugs, such as ibuprofen, help some people.
Muscle strain	Pain, tenderness, swelling, and loss of strength in the affected muscle	R-I-C-E. Apply heat when swelling has disappeared. Stretch and strengthen the affected area.
Plantar fasciitis	Pain and tenderness in the connective tissue on the bottom of your feet	Apply ice, take nonsteroidal anti-inflammatory drugs, and stretch. Wear night splints when sleeping.
Shin splint	Pain and tenderness on the front of the lower leg; sometimes also pain in the calf muscle	Rest. Apply ice to the affected area several times a day and before exercise; wrap with tape for support. Stretch and strengthen muscles in the lower legs. Purchase good-quality footwear and run on soft surfaces.
Side stitch	Pain on the side of the abdomen	Stretch the arm on the affected side as high as possible; if that doesn't help, try bending forward while tightening the abdominal muscles.
Tendinitis	Pain, swelling, and tenderness of the affected area	R-I-C-E. Apply heat when swelling has disappeared. Stretch and strengthen the affected area.

SOURCE: Fahey, T. D., P. M. Insel, and W. T. Roth. 2015. *Fit and Well: Core Concepts and Labs in Physical Fitness and Wellness*, 11th ed. New York: McGraw-Hill. Copyright © 2015 The McGraw-Hill Companies, Inc.

- **Set realistic goals.** Unrealistically high goals will discourage you.

- **Sign a contract and keep a fitness journal.** A journal can help keep your program on track, identify problems, and give you a continuing sense of accomplishment.

- **Start slowly and increase your intensity and duration gradually.** Overzealous exercising can result in discouraging discomfort and injuries. Your program is meant to last a lifetime. The important first step is to break your established pattern of inactivity.

- **Make your program fun.** Participate in a variety of different activities that you enjoy. Vary the routes you take when walking, running, or biking.

- **Exercise with a friend.** The social side of exercise is important to many people.

- **Focus on the positive.** Concentrate on the improvements you get from your program, and how good you feel during and after exercise.

- **Revisit and revise.** If your program turns out to be unrealistic, revise it. Expect to make many adjustments in your program along the way.

- **Expect fluctuation.** On some days your progress will be excellent, but on others you'll barely be able to drag yourself through your scheduled activities.

- **Expect lapses.** Don't let lapses discourage you or make you feel guilty. Instead make a renewed commitment to your exercise program.

- **Plan ahead for difficult situations.** Think about what circumstances might make it tough to keep up with your fitness routine, and develop strategies for sticking with your program. For example, devise a plan for your program during vacation, travel, bad weather, and so on.

- **Reward yourself.** Give yourself frequent rewards for sticking with your program.

- **Renew your attitude.** If you notice you're slacking off, try to list the negative thoughts and behaviors that are causing you to lose interest. Devise a strategy to reduce negative thoughts and behaviors. Make changes in your program plan and reward system to help renew your enthusiasm and commitment.

- **Review your goals.** Visualize what it will be like to reach them, and keep these pictures in your mind as an incentive to stick to your program.

connect
ACTIVITY
DO IT ONLINE

down or stop if you begin to feel uncomfortable. During hot weather, exercise in the early morning or evening when temperatures are lowest.

Staying with Your Program   Once you have attained your desired level of fitness, you can maintain it by exercising regularly at a consistent intensity, 3–5 days a week. In general, if you exercise at the same intensity over a long period, your fitness will level out and can be maintained easily.

Adapt your program to changes in environment or schedule. Don't use wet weather or a new job as an excuse to give up your fitness program. If you walk in the summer, dress appropriately and walk in the winter as well. If you can't go out because of darkness or an unsafe neighborhood, walk in a local shopping mall or on campus or join a gym and walk on a treadmill.

What if you run out of steam? Although good health is an important *reason* to exercise, it's a poor *motivator*.

Find specific suggestions for staying with your program in the box "Maintaining Your Exercise Program" and in the Behavior Change Strategy box at the end of the chapter.

Cross-training can add variety to your workouts. Cross trainers learn to handle their bodyweight by practicing gymnastics, pull-ups, dips, rope climbing, push-ups, handstands, pirouettes, flips, and splits. They also do aerobics, but the emphasis is on speed and intensity. Cross-training programs, such as CrossFit, attempt to develop well-rounded fitness by including exercises that build cardiovascular and respiratory endurance, stamina, strength, flexibility, power, speed, coordination, agility, balance, and accuracy.

cross-training   Participating in two or more activities to develop a variety of fitness components.   **TERMS**

Connect to Your Choices

Have you ever thought about how you came to have the physical activity patterns you have? Many factors can influence our physical activity and exercise choices, some not as obvious as others. Was your family physically active when you were growing up? Do you have access to a fitness center or facilities and equipment for working out? Do you hang out with people who make physical activity part of their daily lives—or with couch potatoes?

What are the external factors that influence your choices about exercise? What are your inner motivations and core values, and how do they affect your choices? Based on what you learned in this chapter, will you make some different choices in the future? If so, what will they be?

Go online to Connect to complete this activity: www.mcgraw-hillconnect.com

TIPS FOR TODAY AND THE FUTURE

Physical activity and exercise offer benefits in nearly every area of wellness. Even a low to moderate level of activity provides valuable health benefits.

RIGHT NOW YOU CAN:

- Go outside and take a brisk 15-minute walk.
- Look at your calendar for the rest of the week and write in some physical activity—such as walking, running, or playing Frisbee—on as many days as you can. Schedule the activity for a specific time and stick to it.
- Call a friend and invite him or her to start planning a regular exercise program with you.

IN THE FUTURE YOU CAN:

- Schedule a session with a qualified personal trainer who can evaluate your current fitness level and help you set personalized fitness goals.
- Create seasonal workout programs for the summer, spring, fall, and winter. Develop programs that are varied but consistent with your overall fitness goals.

SUMMARY

- The five components of physical fitness most important to health are cardiorespiratory endurance, muscular strength, muscular endurance, flexibility, and body composition.

- Exercise improves the functioning of the heart and the ability of the cardiorespiratory system to carry oxygen to the body's tissues. It also increases metabolic efficiency and improves body composition.

- Exercise lowers the risk of cardiovascular disease by improving blood fat levels, reducing high blood pressure, and interfering with the disease process that causes coronary artery blockage.

- Exercise reduces the risk of cancer, osteoporosis, and diabetes. It improves immune function and psychological health and helps prevent injuries and low-back pain.

- Most people should accumulate at least 150 minutes per week of moderate-intensity or 75 minutes of vigorous-intensity physical activity. Longer-duration or more vigorous activity produces additional health and fitness benefits.

- Cardiorespiratory endurance exercises stress a large portion of the body's muscle mass. Endurance exercise should be performed 3–5 days per week for a total of 20–60 minutes per day. Intensity can be evaluated by measuring the heart rate.

- Warming up before exercising and cooling down afterward improve your performance and decrease your chances of injury.

- Exercises that develop muscular strength and endurance involve exerting force against a significant resistance. A strength training program for general fitness typically involves one or more sets of 8–12 repetitions of 8–10 exercises performed on at least 2 nonconsecutive days per week.

- A good stretching program includes exercises for all the major muscle groups and joints of the body. Do a series of active, static stretches at least 2–3 days per week. Hold each stretch for 10–30 seconds and do 2–4 repetitions. Stretch when muscles are warm.

- Instructors, equipment, and facilities should be chosen carefully to enhance enjoyment and prevent injuries.

- A well-balanced diet contains all the energy and nutrients needed to sustain a fitness program. When exercising, remember to drink enough fluids.

- Rest, ice, compression, and elevation (R-I-C-E) are treatments for minor muscle and joint injuries.

FOR MORE INFORMATION

BOOKS

Swain, D. P. 2013. *ACSM's Resource Manual for Guidelines for Exercise Testing and Prescription,* 7th ed. Philadelphia: Lippincott Williams & Wilkins.

Andrews, J. R., and D. Yaeger. 2013. *Any Given Monday: Sports Injuries and How to Prevent Them for Athletes, Parents, and Coaches—Based on My Life in Sports Medicine.* New York:

Scribner. *A primer on sports injuries for athletes, parents, and coaches.*

Fahey, T. 2013. *Basic Weight Training for Men and Women,* 8th ed. New York: McGraw-Hill. *Weight training and plyometric exercises for fitness, weight control, and improved sports performance.*

Fahey, T., P. Insel, and W. Roth. 2015. *Fit and Well: Core Concepts and Labs in Physical Fitness and Wellness,* 11th ed. New York: McGraw-Hill. *A comprehensive guide to developing a complete fitness program.*

Hawkins, J. D. and S. Hawkins. 2013. *Walking for Fun and Fitness.* Independence, KY: Cengage Learning. *Discusses walking as a fitness method and a way to avoid diseases such as diabetes.*

John, D. 2013. *Intervention: Course Correction for the Athlete and Trainer.* Santa Cruz, CA: On Target Publications. *A superb guidebook to building whole body fitness using a combination of traditional and functional training exercises.*

Nieman, D. C. 2011. *Exercise Testing and Prescription: A Health-Related Approach,* 7th ed. New York: McGraw-Hill. *A comprehensive discussion of the effect of exercise and exercise testing and prescription.*

ORGANIZATIONS, HOTLINES, AND WEBSITES

American Alliance for Health, Physical Education, Recreation, and Dance (AAHPERD). A professional organization dedicated to promoting quality health and physical education programs.

http://www.aahperd.org

American College of Sports Medicine (ACSM). The principal professional organization for sports medicine and exercise science. Provides brochures, publications, and audio- and videotapes.

http://www.acsm.org

American Council on Exercise (ACE). Promotes exercise and fitness; the website features fact sheets on many consumer topics, including choosing shoes, cross-training, and steroids.

http://www.acefitness.org

American Heart Association: Start! Walking for a Healthier Lifestyle. Provides practical advice for people of all fitness levels plus an online fitness diary.

http://www.startwalkingnow.org/about_start.jsp

CDC Physical Activity Information. Provides information about the benefits of physical activity and suggestions for incorporating moderate physical activity into daily life.

http://www.cdc.gov/physicalactivity/

Disabled Sports USA. Provides sports and recreation services to people with physical or mobility disorders.

http://www.dsusa.org

MedlinePlus: Exercise and Physical Fitness. Provides links to news and reliable information about fitness and exercise from government agencies and professional associations.

http://www.nlm.nih.gov/medlineplus/exerciseandphysicalfitness
  .html

President's Council on Physical Fitness and Sports (PCPFS). Provides information about PCPFS programs and publications, including fitness guides and fact sheets.

http://www.fitness.gov

http://www.presidentschallenge.org

Robert Wood Johnson Foundation. Promotes the health and health care of Americans through research and distribution of information on healthy lifestyles; publishes an annual report on the status of the national obesity problem.

http://www.rwjf.org

Shape Up America! A nonprofit organization that provides information and resources for exercise, nutrition, and weight loss.

http://www.shapeup.org

The following link provides information about a wide variety of activities and fitness issues; evaluate commercial sites carefully.

CrossFit. A cross-training method involving a variety of exercises and unaccustomed physical challenges. The program includes franchised health clubs and training facilities. The website provides extensive information on cross-training, nutrition, exercise techniques, and sports psychology.

http://www.crossfit.com

SELECTED BIBLIOGRAPHY

American College of Sports Medicine. 2013. *ACSM's Guidelines for Exercise Testing and Prescription,* 9th ed. Philadelphia: Wolters Kluwer/ Lippincott Williams & Wilkins Health. American Heart Association. 2013. Heart Disease and Stroke Statistics—2013 Update. *Circulation* 127(1): e6–e245.

Bostrom, P., et al. 2012. A PGC1-alpha-dependent myokine that drives brown-fat-like development of white fat and thermogenesis. *Nature* 481: 463–468.

Burd, N. A., et al. 2012. Muscle time under tension during resistance exercise stimulates differential muscle protein sub-fractional synthetic responses in men. *Journal of Physiology* 590: 351–362.

Centers for Disease Control and Prevention. 2013. Adult participation in aerobic and muscle-strengthening physical activities—United States, 2011. *Morbidity and Mortality Weekly Report* 62(17): 326–330.

Curlik, D. M. and T. J. Shors. 2013. Training your brain: Do mental and physical (MAP) training enhance cognition through the process of neurogenesis in the hippocampus? *Neuropharmacology* 64(1): 506–514.

Denis, G. V. and M. S. Obin. 2013. Metabolically healthy obesity: Origins and implications. *Molecular Aspects of Medicine* 34(1): 59–70.

Deusinger, S. S. 2012. Exercise intervention for management of obesity. *Pediatric Blood Cancer* 58(1): 135–139.

Egan, B., and J. R. Zierath. 2013. Exercise metabolism and the molecular regulation of skeletal muscle adaptation. *Cell Metabolism* 17(2): 162–184.

Fahey, T. D., P. M. Insel, and W. T. Roth. 2015. *Fit & Well: Core Concepts and Labs in Physical Fitness and Wellness,* 11th ed. New York: McGraw-Hill.

Garber, C. E., et al. 2011. Quantity and quality of exercise for developing and maintaining cardiorespiratory, musculoskeletal, and neuromotor fitness in apparently healthy adults: Guidance for prescribing exercise. *Medicine & Science in Sports & Exercise* 43(7):1334–1359.

Gibala, M. J., et al. 2012. Physiological adaptations to low-volume, high-intensity interval training in health and disease. *Journal of Physiology* 590(5): 1077–1084.

Hamer, M., and G. O'Donovan. 2010. Cardiorespiratory fitness and metabolic risk factors in obesity. *Current Opinion in Lipidology* 21(1): 1–7.

Lee, D., et al. 2014. Leisure-Time running reduces all-cause and cardiovascular mortality risk. *Journal of the American College of Cardiology* 64(5):472–481.

McGill, S. M., et al. 2012. Kettlebell swing, snatch, and bottoms-up carry: Back and hip muscle activation, motion, and low back loads. *Journal of Strength & Conditioning Research* 26: 16–27.

McGill, S. M., et al. 2013. Low back loads while walking and carrying: Comparing the load carried in one hand or in both hands. *Ergonomics* 56(2): 293–302.

Schnohr, P., et al. 2013. Longevity in male and female joggers: The Copenhagen City Heart Study. *American Journal of Epidemiology* 177(7): 683–689.

Swain, D. P. 2013. *ACSM's Resource Manual for Guidelines for Exercise Testing and Prescription,* 7th ed. Philadelphia: Lippincott Williams and Wilkins.

U.S. Department of Health and Human Services. 2008. *2008 Physical Activity Guidelines for Americans.* Hyattsville, MD: HHS. ODPHP Publication U0036.

U.S. Department of Health and Human Services. 2010. *The Surgeon General's Vision for a Healthy and Fit Nation.* Rockville, MD: HHS, Office of the Surgeon General.

Vissers, D., et al. 2013. The effect of exercise on visceral adipose tissue in overweight adults: A systematic review and meta-analysis. *PLOS ONE* 8(2): e56415.

Planning a Personal Exercise Program

Although most people recognize the importance of incorporating exercise into their lives, many find it difficult to do. No single strategy will work for everyone, but the general steps outlined here should help you create an exercise program that fits your goals, preferences, and lifestyle. A carefully designed contract and program plan can help you convert your vague wishes into a detailed plan of action. And the strategies for program compliance outlined here and in Chapter 1 can help you enjoy and stick with your program for the rest of your life.

Step 1: Set Goals

Setting specific goals to accomplish by exercising is an important first step in a successful fitness program because it establishes the direction you want to take. Your goals might be specifically related to health, such as lowering your blood pressure and risk of heart disease, or they might relate to other aspects of your life, such as improving your tennis game or the fit of your clothes. If you can decide why you're starting to exercise, it can help you keep going.

Step 2: Select Activities

As discussed in the chapter, the success of your fitness program depends on the consistency of your involvement. Select activities that encourage your commitment: The right program will be its own incentive to continue, but poor activity choices provide obstacles and can turn exercise into a chore.

When choosing activities for your fitness program, consider the following:

- Is this activity fun? Will it hold my interest over time?

- Will this activity help me reach the goals I have set?

- Will my current fitness and skill level enable me to participate fully in this activity?

- Can I easily fit this activity into my daily schedule? Are there any special requirements (facilities, partners, equipment, etc.) that I must plan for?

- Can I afford any special costs required for equipment or facilities?

- If I have special exercise needs due to a particular health problem, does this activity conform to those exercise needs? Will it enhance my ability to cope with my specific health problem?

Using these guidelines listed, select a number of sports and activities.

Step 3: Make a Commitment

By completing a contract, you make a firm commitment and will be more likely to follow through until you meet your goals.

Step 4: Begin and Maintain Your Program

Start slowly to allow your body time to adjust. Be realistic and patient—meeting your goals will take time. The following guidelines may help you start and stick with your program:

- Set aside regular periods for exercise. Choose times that fit in best with your schedule, and stick to them. Allow an adequate amount of time for warm-up, cool-down, and a shower.

- Take advantage of any opportunity for exercise that presents itself (for example, walk to class or take stairs instead of an elevator).

- Do what you can to avoid boredom. Do stretching exercises or jumping jacks to music, or watch the evening news while riding your stationary bicycle.

- Exercise with a group that shares your goals and general level of competence.

- Vary the program. Change your activities periodically. Alter your route or distance if biking or jogging. Change racquetball partners, or find a new volleyball court.

- Establish mini-goals or a point system, and work rewards into your program. Until you reach your main goals, a series of small rewards will help you stick with your program. Rewards should be things you enjoy that are easily obtainable.

Step 5: Record and Assess Your Progress

Keeping a record that notes the daily results of your program will help remind you of your ongoing commitment to your program and give you a sense of accomplishment. Create daily and weekly program logs that you can use to track your progress. Record the activity frequency, intensity, time, and type. Keep your log handy, and fill it in immediately after each exercise session. Post it in a visible place to remind you of your activity schedule and to provide incentive for improvement.

SOURCE: Adapted from Kusinitz, I., and M. Fine. 1995. *Your Guide to Getting Fit,* 3rd ed. Mountain View, CA: Mayfield.

CHAPTER OBJECTIVES

- Discuss different methods for assessing body weight and body composition

- Explain factors that may contribute to a weight problem, including genetic, physiological, lifestyle, and psychosocial factors

- Explain the health risks associated with overweight and obesity

- Describe lifestyle factors that contribute to weight gain and loss, including the roles of diet, exercise, and emotions

- Identify and describe the symptoms of eating disorders and the health risks associated with them

- Design a personal plan for successfully managing body weight

CHAPTER **11**

Weight Management

Achieving and maintaining a healthy body weight is a public health priority and a serious challenge for many Americans. According to standards developed by the National Institutes of Health (NIH), 68.8% of American adults are overweight, including 35.7% who are obese (Table 11.1). Of adult men, an estimated 35.5% are obese, and of adult women, an estimated 35.8% are obese. One study predicted that if current rates continue, 42% of Americans will be obese by the year 2050. As millions struggle to lose weight, others fall into dangerous eating patterns such as binge eating or self-starvation.

Although not completely understood, managing body weight is not a mysterious process. It's basically a matter of balancing the calories you take in with calories you expend in daily activities—in other words, eating a moderate diet and being physically active. To manage your weight

successfully, you must coordinate many aspects of your life—including nutrition, physical activity, and stress control—over the long term.

BASIC CONCEPTS OF WEIGHT MANAGEMENT

Energy Balance

The key to achieving and maintaining a healthy body weight and keeping a healthy ratio of fat to fat-free mass across the lifespan is **energy balance** (Figure 11.1). You take in energy (calories) from the food you eat. Your body uses energy (calories) to maintain vital body functions (resting metabolism), to digest food, and to fuel physical activity. When *energy in* equals *energy out*, you maintain your current weight. To change your weight and body composition, you must tip the energy balance equation in a particular direction. If you take in more calories daily than your body burns (a *positive* energy balance), the excess calories will be stored as fat and you will gain weight over time. If you eat fewer calories than you burn each day (a *negative* energy

> **energy balance** A condition that occurs when energy intake equals energy expenditure; the key to achieving and maintaining a healthy body weight.
>
> TERMS

Table 11.1	Weight of Americans Aged 20 and Older, 2009–2010	
GROUP	PERCENT OVERWEIGHT*	PERCENT OBESE
Both sexes	68.8	35.7
All races, male	74.1	35.5
All races, female	64.5	35.8
White, male	74.0	36.2
White, female	59.5	32.2
African American, male	69.9	38.8
African American, female	82.1	58.5
Latino, male	81.7	37.0
Latino, female	75.7	41.4

*Includes obesity.

SOURCE: Flegal, K. M., et al. 2012. Prevalence of obesity and trends in the distribution of body mass index among U.S. adults, 1999–2010. *Journal of the American Medical Association* 307(5) (published online January 17).

ENERGY IN
Food calories

ENERGY OUT
Physical activity 20–30%
Food digestion ±10%
Resting metabolism 65–70%

FIGURE 11.1   **The energy balance equation.**

balance), you will lose some of the stored fat and probably lose weight.

If we look at the energy balance equation today as expressed for the general American population, the equation is tipped heavily toward the energy-in side. Our environment is rich in large portion sizes; high-fat, high-calorie foods; and palatable, easily available, and inexpensive foods. Unfortunately the energy-out side of the equation has not compensated for increased energy intake. Instead we've decreased work-related physical activity, decreased activity associated with daily living, and increased time spent in sedentary pastimes like TV watching and computer use. The good news, however, is that you control both parts of the energy balance equation.

Determining Healthy Body Weight

For a variety of reasons, many individuals struggle with body dissatisfaction and are concerned about their weight. But how do you decide if you are at a healthy weight? How thin is too thin and at what point does being overweight present a health risk?

overweight   Body weight above the recommended range for good health.

obesity   Severe overweight, characterized by an excessive accumulation of body fat; may also be defined in terms of some measure of total body weight.

essential fat   Fat incorporated in various tissues of the body; critical for normal body functioning.

TERMS

QUICK STATS

In 1970, **15%** of adult Americans were obese. In 2012, more than **35.7%** were obese.

—National Center for Health Statistics

Overweight is defined as total body weight above the recommended range for good health, as determined by large-scale population surveys. **Obesity** is defined as a more serious degree of overweight that carries multiple health risks. Both terms are used to identify weight ranges that are associated with increased likelihood of certain diseases and health problems.

Several methods can be used to measure and evaluate body weight and percent body fat. These assessments can help you establish reasonable goals and set a starting point for current and future decisions about weight loss and weight gain. Three methods used to determine how your current weight might be affecting your health are body composition, body mass index (BMI), and body fat distribution.

Body Composition and Its Importance

The human body can be divided into fat-free mass and body fat. Fat-free mass is composed of all the body's nonfat tissues: bone, water, muscle, connective tissue, organ tissues, and teeth. A certain amount of body fat is necessary for the body to function. Fat is incorporated into the nerves, brain, heart, lungs, liver, mammary glands, and other body organs and tissues. It is the main source of stored energy in the body. It also cushions body organs and helps regulate body temperature. This **essential fat** makes up about 3–5% of total body weight in men and about 8–12% in women. The percentage is higher in women due to fat deposits in the breasts, uterus, and other sex-specific sites.

Most of the fat in the body is stored in fat cells, or **adipose tissue,** located under the skin (**subcutaneous fat**) and around major organs (**visceral fat** or *intra-abdominal fat*). People have a genetically determined number of fat cells, but these cells can increase or decrease in size depending on how much fat is being stored, which in turn depends on several factors, including age, sex, metabolism, diet, and activity level. The primary source of excess body fat is excess calories consumed in the diet—that is, calories consumed in excess of calories expended in metabolism, physical activity, and exercise.

When looking at body composition, one important consideration is the proportion of the body's total weight that is fat—the **percent body fat.** For example, two women may both be 5 feet, 5 inches tall and weigh 130 pounds. But one woman may have only 15% of her body weight as fat, whereas the other woman could have 34% body fat. Although neither woman is overweight by most standards, the second woman is considered overfat.

Methods for determining percent body fat provide only an estimate of the amount of body fat (or adipose tissue) and the amount of lean body mass (or lean tissue) you have. A healthy body fat range for men is considered to be about 12–20%, and for women, about 20–30%. Men with more than 25% body fat are considered obese, as are women with more than 33% body fat.

Skinfold Measurement

Skinfold measurement is a simple and practical way to assess body composition based on the amount of subcutaneous fat. A technician measures the thickness of skinfolds at several different sites on the body with a device, called calipers, that painlessly "pinches" the folds of skin and its underlying fat at various locations of the body. The measurements are used in formulas that calculate body fat percentages. When performed by a skilled technician, this method can estimate body fat within a 3% to 4% margin of error, which means that if your skinfold measurement shows that you have 20% body fat, this value could be accurate between 17% and 23% body fat.

Bioelectrical Impedance Analysis (BIA)

In this method, a very low level of electrical current is sent through a person's body, transmitting current from one point to another. The electrical conduction through the body favors the path of the fat-free tissues over the fat tissues, so the amount of resistance to the current is related to the amount of fat-free tissue in the body. Percent body fat is calculated from the measurements of resistance to the current. One disadvantage to this method is that, for the most accurate results, the person being tested must have followed the suggested guidelines for food and fluid intake, as well as restrictions on exercise prior to the test. BIA can estimate your body fat with an error of about 3% to 4%.

Hydrostatic Weighing

In hydrostatic (underwater) weighing, a person is first weighed on a traditional scale. Then the person is submerged and weighed under water. Muscle has a higher density than water, and fat has a lower

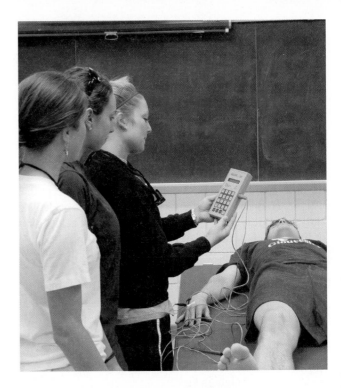

These students are using bioelectrical impedance analysis to estimate percent body fat.

density than water, so people with more fat tend to "float" and weigh less under water, whereas lean people tend to "sink" and weigh more under water. The amount of water displaced is used to calculate percent body fat. Under the best circumstances, underwater weighing can estimate body fat within a 2% to 3% margin of error.

The Bod Pod

This specialized body composition analysis device called the Bod Pod uses air displacement instead of water. A person sits in a chamber for about 5 minutes, and computerized pressure sensors determine the amount of air displaced by the person's body to determine percentage of body fat.

Scanning Procedures

High-tech scanning procedures are very accurate means of assessing body composition, but they require expensive equipment. These procedures include computed tomography (CT), magnetic resonance imaging (MRI), dual-energy X-ray absorptiometry (DEXA), and dual-photon absorptiometry. Other procedures include near

---

adipose tissue   Connective tissue in which fat is stored.   TERMS

subcutaneous fat   Fat located under the skin.

visceral fat   Fat located around major organs; also called *intra-abdominal fat.*

percent body fat   The percentage of total body weight that is composed of fat.

infrared reactance (Futrex 1100) and total body electrical conductivity (TOBEC). Considered to be very accurate, these techniques are generally offered only at medical or research facilities.

Determining Body Mass Index

Body mass index (BMI) is a measure of body weight that is useful for estimating a person's weight status and for classifying the health risks of body weight if more sophisticated methods aren't available. BMI is based on the concept that weight should be proportional to height. Easy to calculate and rate, BMI is a fairly accurate measure of the health risks of body weight for most average (nonathletic) people. BMI is correlated with body fat, but it does not directly measure body fat.

BMI is calculated by dividing your body weight (expressed in kilograms or pounds) by the square of your height (expressed in meters or inches). You can look up your BMI in the chart in Figure 11.2, or you can use the following formula to calculate it more precisely:

$$BMI = \frac{\text{weight in kg}}{(\text{height in meters})^2}$$

or

$$\frac{\text{weight in pounds}}{(\text{height in inches})^2} \times 703 \text{ (conversion factor)}$$

Body weight status is categorized as underweight, healthy weight, overweight, or obese in comparison with what is considered healthy for a given height. Under standards issued by the National Institutes of Health and adopted by the Dietary Guidelines for Americans, a BMI between 18.5 and 24.9 is considered healthy, a BMI of 25 or above is classified as overweight, and a BMI of 30 or above is classified as obese. A person with a BMI below 18.5 is classified as underweight, although low BMI values may be healthy in some cases if they are not the result of smoking, an eating disorder, or an underlying disease.

BMI is a valuable tool for assessing weight, but it is not such a good tool for determining body composition. Like height–weight tables, it does not distinguish between fat weight and fat-free weight. It can also be inaccurate for some groups, including short people (under 5 feet tall), muscular athletes, and older adults with little muscle mass due to inactivity or an underlying disease. People in these groups should use one of the methods described in the next section for estimating percent body fat to assess whether their weight and body composition are healthy.

> **body mass index (BMI)** A measure of relative body weight that takes height into account and is highly correlated with more direct measures of body fat; calculated by dividing total body weight (in kilograms) by the square of height (in meters). **TERMS**

	<18.5 Underweight		18.5–24.9 Normal						25–29.9 Overweight					30–34.9 Obesity (Class I)					35–39.9 Obesity (Class II)					≥40 Extreme obesity
BMI	17	18	19	20	21	22	23	24	25	26	27	28	29	30	31	32	33	34	35	36	37	38	39	40
Height												Body Weight (pounds)												
4' 10"	81	86	91	96	101	105	110	115	120	124	129	134	139	144	148	153	158	163	168	172	177	182	187	192
4' 11"	84	89	94	99	104	109	114	119	124	129	134	139	144	149	154	159	163	168	173	178	183	188	193	198
5'	87	92	97	102	108	113	118	123	128	133	138	143	149	154	159	164	169	174	179	184	190	195	200	205
5' 1"	90	95	101	106	111	117	122	127	132	138	143	148	154	159	164	169	175	180	185	191	196	201	207	212
5' 2"	93	98	104	109	115	120	126	131	137	142	148	153	159	164	170	175	181	186	191	197	202	208	213	219
5' 3"	96	102	107	113	119	124	130	136	141	147	153	158	164	169	175	181	186	192	198	203	209	215	220	226
5' 4"	99	105	111	117	122	128	134	140	146	152	157	163	169	175	181	187	192	198	204	210	216	222	227	233
5' 5"	102	108	114	120	126	132	138	144	150	156	162	168	174	180	186	192	198	204	210	216	222	229	235	241
5' 6"	105	112	118	124	130	136	143	149	155	161	167	174	180	186	192	198	205	211	217	223	229	236	242	248
5' 7"	109	115	121	128	134	141	147	153	160	166	173	179	185	192	198	204	211	217	224	230	236	243	249	256
5' 8"	112	118	125	132	138	145	151	158	165	171	178	184	191	197	204	211	217	224	230	237	244	250	257	263
5' 9"	115	122	129	136	142	149	156	163	169	176	183	190	197	203	210	217	224	230	237	244	251	258	264	271
5' 10"	119	126	133	139	146	153	160	167	174	181	188	195	202	209	216	223	230	237	244	251	258	265	272	279
5' 11"	122	129	136	143	151	158	165	172	179	187	194	201	208	215	222	230	237	244	251	258	265	273	280	287
6'	125	133	140	148	155	162	170	177	184	192	199	207	214	221	229	236	243	251	258	266	273	280	288	295
6' 1"	129	137	144	152	159	167	174	182	190	197	205	212	220	228	235	243	250	258	265	273	281	288	296	303
6' 2"	132	140	148	156	164	171	179	187	195	203	210	218	226	234	242	249	257	265	273	281	288	296	304	312
6' 3"	136	144	152	160	168	176	184	192	200	208	216	224	232	240	248	256	264	272	280	288	296	304	312	320
6' 4"	140	148	156	164	173	181	189	197	206	214	222	230	238	247	255	263	271	280	288	296	304	312	321	329

FIGURE 11.2 **Body mass index (BMI).** To determine your BMI, find your height in the left column. Move across the appropriate row until you find the weight closest to your own. The number at the top of the column is the BMI at that height and weight.

SOURCES: Ratings from National Heart, Lung, and Blood Institute. 1998. *Clinical Guidelines on the Identification, Evaluation, and Treatment of Overweight and Obesity in Adults: The Evidence Report.* Bethesda, MD: National Institutes of Health; U.S. Departments of Agriculture and Health and Human Services. 2005. *Dietary Guidelines for Americans,* 6th ed. Washington, DC: Government Printing Office.

Determining Body Fat Distribution

To complete the assessment and evaluation of your current body weight, it is important to also consider how fat is distributed throughout your body. The location of fat on your body is an important indicator of health, as it is known to affect your risk for various diseases.

Two of the simplest methods for measuring body fat distribution are waist circumference measurement and waist-to-hip ratio calculation. In the first method, waist circumference is measured using a tape measure placed around your abdomen at the top of your hip bone. A waist circumference of ≥40 inches (102 cm) for men or ≥35 in (88 cm) for women is associated with an increased risk for chronic disease for most adults. In the second method a mathematic formula (waist circumference divided by hip circumference) is used to find your waist-to-hip ratio. A waist-to-hip ratio above 0.94 for young men and above 0.82 for young women is associated with an increased risk of heart disease and diabetes. The reason for the increased risk associated with abdominal obesity appears to be that visceral fat is more easily mobilized and sent into the bloodstream, increasing disease-related blood fat levels.

Visceral fat contains many biologically active substances such as inflammatory chemicals and growth factors, which can adhere to the lining of blood vessels, cause insulin resistance, and have a negative influence on cardiovascular health. Subcutaneous fat tends to be soft and flabby (whereas visceral fat is hard) and is not metabolically active the way visceral fat is.

Men and postmenopausal women tend to store fat in the upper regions of their bodies, particularly in the abdominal area, as visceral fat. People with this pattern of fat distribution, called *android obesity*, are said to be apple-shaped. Premenopausal women usually store fat in the hips, buttocks, and thighs, as subcutaneous fat. People with this pattern, called *gynoid obesity*, are said to be pear-shaped.

FACTORS CONTRIBUTING TO EXCESS BODY FAT

Body weight and body composition may be determined by multiple factors that vary with each individual. These factors can be grouped into genetic, physiological, lifestyle, and psychosocial factors.

Genetic Factors

Estimates of the genetic contribution to obesity vary widely, from about 25% to 40% of an individual's body fat. Scientists have so far identified more than 600 genes associated with obesity. Genes influence body size and shape, body fat distribution, and metabolic rate. Genetic factors also affect the ease with which weight is gained as a result of overeating and where on the body extra weight is added.

If both parents are obese, their children have an 80% risk of being obese; children with only one obese parent face a 50% risk of becoming obese. In studies that compared adoptees and their biological parents, the weights of the adoptees were found to be more like those of the biological parents than those of the adoptive parents, again indicating a strong genetic link.

Hereditary influences, however, must be balanced against the contribution of environmental factors. Not all children of obese parents become obese, and normal-weight parents may have overweight children. Environmental factors like diet and exercise are probably responsible for such differences. Thus the *tendency* to develop obesity may be inherited, but the expression of this tendency is affected by environmental influences.

The set-point theory suggests that our bodies are designed to maintain a normal and generally stable weight within a narrow range, or at a "set point," despite the variability in energy intake and expenditure. This theory is based on the idea that the rate at which our body burns calories adjusts according to the amount of food that we eat, but it does not imply that we cannot maintain weight loss.

It is true that some people have a harder time losing weight and maintaining weight loss than others. However, with increased exercise and attention to diet, even those with a genetic tendency toward obesity can maintain a healthy body weight. And regardless of genetic factors, lifestyle choices remain the cornerstone of successful weight management.

Physiological Factors

Metabolism is a key physiological factor in the regulation of body fat and body weight. Hormones and fat cell types also play a role.

Metabolism   Metabolism is the sum of all the vital processes by which food energy and nutrients are made available to and used by the body. The largest component of metabolism, **resting metabolic rate (RMR),** is the energy required to maintain vital body functions, including respiration, heart rate, body temperature, and blood pressure, while the body is at rest. As shown in Figure 11.1, RMR accounts for about 65–70% of daily energy expenditure. The energy required to digest food accounts for as much as 10% of daily energy expenditure. The remaining 20–30% is expended during physical activity.

Both genetics and behavior affect metabolic rate. Men, who have a higher proportion of muscle mass than women, have a higher RMR because muscle tissue is more metabolically

> **resting metabolic rate (RMR)**   The energy required to maintain vital body functions, including respiration, heart rate, body temperature, and blood pressure, while the body is at rest.
>
> TERMS

active than fat. A higher RMR means that a person burns more calories while at rest and can therefore take in more calories without gaining weight.

Weight loss or gain also affects metabolic rate. When a person loses weight, both RMR and the energy required to perform physical tasks decrease. The reverse occurs when weight is gained. One of the reasons why exercise is so important during a weight loss program is that exercise, especially resistance training, helps maintain muscle mass and metabolic rate.

Hormones   Hormones clearly play a role in the accumulation of body fat, especially for females. Hormonal changes at puberty, during pregnancy, and at menopause contribute to the amount and location of fat accumulation. One hormone thought to be linked to obesity is *leptin*. Secreted by the body's fat cells, leptin is carried to the brain, where it appears to let the brain know how big or small the body's fat stores are. With this information, the brain can regulate appetite and metabolic rate accordingly. However, as most of us will admit, hunger is often *not* the primary reason we overeat. Cases of obesity based solely or primarily on hormone abnormalities do exist, but they are rare.

Fat Cells   The amount of fat (adipose tissue) the body can store is a function of the number and size of fat (adipose) cells.

Some people are born with an above-average number of fat cells and thus have the potential for storing more energy as body fat. Overeating at critical times, such as in childhood, can cause the body to create more fat cells. If a person loses weight, fat cell content is depleted, but it is unclear whether the number of fat cells can be decreased.

Lifestyle Factors

Although genetic and physiological factors may increase the risk for excess body fat, they are not sufficient to explain the increasingly high rate of obesity seen in the United States. The gene pool has not changed dramatically in the past 60 years, but the rate of obesity among Americans has more than doubled. Clearly other factors are at work—particularly lifestyle factors such as increased eating and decreased physical activity.

Eating   Americans have access to plenty of calorie-dense foods, and many have eating habits that contribute to weight gain. Most overweight adults admit to eating more than they should of high-fat, high-sugar, high-calorie foods. Americans eat out more frequently now than in the past and rely more heavily on fast food and packaged convenience foods. Restaurant and convenience food portion sizes tend to be large, and the foods themselves are likely to be high in fat, sugar, and calories and low in nutrients. In addition, many people underestimate the actual number of calories they eat.

The popularity of sugar-free soft drinks does not appear to be helping people lose weight, though it is not yet clear why this may be the case. Compared to people who don't drink soda, people who drink more than one soda per day, either regular or diet, are more likely to be obese, develop metabolic syndrome, and have high blood pressure.

Physical Activity   Activity levels among Americans are declining, beginning in childhood and continuing throughout life. Incidence of overweight is consistently linked to excessive screen time—whether time spent watching TV, playing video games, or using computers. Fewer than 5% of American adults participate in daily physical activity for at least 30 minutes.

An "Obesogenic" Environment   The 2010 Dietary Guidelines for Americans focused attention on the "obesogenic" environment in which most Americans live. This environment promotes overconsumption of calories while at the same time discourages physical activity. Food and activity choices are influenced by the communities in which individuals live, their socioeconomic status, religion and culture, and geographic location. People living in areas with limited access to healthy foods and opportunities for physical activity do not have the same options for choosing a healthy lifestyle as do people living in more enriched environments.

Psychosocial Factors

Many people have learned to use food as a means of coping with stress and negative emotions. When food and eating become the primary means of regulating emotions, binge eating or other disturbed eating patterns can develop.

Obesity is strongly associated with socioeconomic status. The prevalence of obesity in women and children tends to go down as income level goes up, though it stays the same in men. These differences may reflect the greater sensitivity and concern for a slim physical appearance among upper-income women, as well as greater access to information about nutrition, to low-fat and low-calorie foods, and to opportunities for physical activity. It may also reflect the greater acceptance of obesity among certain ethnic groups, as well as different cultural values related to food choices.

In some families and cultures, food is used as a symbol of love and caring. In such cases, it may be difficult to change established eating patterns because they are linked to cultural and family values.

EXCESS BODY FAT AND WELLNESS

The amount and distribution of fat in the body can have profound effects on health. Obesity doubles mortality rates and can reduce life expectancy by 10–20 years. In fact, if the current trends in overweight and obesity (and their related health problems) continue, some experts predict that the average American's life expectancy will soon decline by 5 years.

Obese people have an increased risk of death from all causes compared with people of normal weight. Obesity is associated with a number of chronic conditions such as diabetes, cardiovascular disease, many kinds of cancer, impaired immune function, gallbladder and kidney diseases, skin problems, impotence, sleep and breathing disorders, back pain, arthritis, and other bone and joint disorders. Obesity is also associated with complications of pregnancy, menstrual irregularities, urine leakage (stress incontinence), increased surgical risk, and psychological disorders and problems (such as depression, low self-esteem, and body dissatisfaction). Researchers who conducted a 16-year study that looked at over 9,000 adults aged 51 to 77 years concluded that over 7% of deaths after age 51 were due to issues directly related to being overweight. In addition, studies show decrease in the quality of life (measured by such things as self-image, bullying, bodily pain, quality of food intake, physical activity, and screen time) in overweight and obese children and adolescents compared to those of normal weight. It is also important to realize that small weight losses—5% to 10% of total body weight—can lead to significant health improvements.

There is debate over the health risks for people who are overweight but not obese (BMI of 25 to 29), particularly for people who are overweight and physically active. These risks depend in part on an individual's overall health and other risk factors, such as high blood pressure, unhealthy cholesterol levels, body fat distribution, tobacco use, and level of physical activity.

Diabetes

About 26 million Americans have one of the two major types of **diabetes mellitus,** a disease that disrupts normal metabolism. About 5–10% of people with diabetes have a form known as type 1 diabetes, a disease that usually begins in childhood or adolescence and is not related to obesity. The remaining 90–95% of people with diabetes have type 2 diabetes, a disease that is strongly associated with excess body fat. The prevalence of type 2 diabetes has been rising dramatically in parallel with the increase in prevalence of obesity. In 2011 almost 2 million new cases of diabetes were diagnosed in adults over the age of 20, and an estimated 7.0 million people are believed to have undiagnosed diabetes.

Diabetes involves the production of the hormone insulin by the pancreas. In normal metabolism, the pancreas secretes insulin, which stimulates cells to take up blood sugar (glucose) to produce energy. In diabetes, this process is disrupted, causing a buildup of glucose in the bloodstream. In type 1 diabetes, the body's immune system, triggered by a viral infection or some other environmental factor, destroys the insulin-producing cells in the pancreas. Little or no insulin is produced, so daily doses of insulin are required. In type 2 diabetes, the pancreas doesn't produce enough insulin, or body cells are resistant to insulin (called *insulin resistance*), or both. This condition can develop slowly, and about 25% of type 2 diabetics are unaware of their condition. About one-third of people with type 2 diabetes must take insulin; others may take medications that increase insulin production or stimulate the cells to take up glucose.

A third type of diabetes, called *gestational diabetes*, occurs in about 7% of women during pregnancy. The condition usually disappears after pregnancy, but about half of women who experience it eventually develop type 2 diabetes. *Prediabetes* is a condition in which blood sugar levels are higher than normal but not high enough for a diagnosis of full-blown diabetes. About 79 million Americans have prediabetes, and most will develop type 2 diabetes unless they adopt preventive lifestyle measures. The warning signs of diabetes include frequent urination, extreme hunger or thirst, unexplained weight loss, extreme fatigue, blurred vision, frequent infections, tingling or numbness in the hands or feet, and generalized itching with no rash.

Complications of diabetes include kidney failure; nerve damage; circulation problems and amputations; retinal damage and blindness; and increased rates of heart attack, stroke, and hypertension. Diabetes is currently the seventh leading cause of death in the United States.

The major risk factors for diabetes are age, obesity, physical inactivity, a family history of diabetes, and lifestyle. Ethnicity also plays a role, with Native Americans, Alaska Natives, African Americans, and Hispanics having higher rates than Asian Americans and white Americans. Excess body fat reduces cell sensitivity to insulin, and insulin resistance is almost always a precursor of type 2 diabetes. Nearly 90% of people with type 2 diabetes are overweight when diagnosed, including 55% who are obese.

It is estimated that 90% of cases of type 2 diabetes could be prevented if people adopted healthy lifestyle behaviors, including regular physical activity, a moderate diet to control body fat, and modest weight loss. Even a small amount of weight loss can be beneficial. For people with prediabetes, lifestyle measures are more effective than medication for delaying or preventing the development of diabetes. Exercise (endurance and/or strength training) makes cells more sensitive to insulin and helps stabilize blood glucose levels; it also helps keep body fat at healthy levels. Regular exercise and a healthy diet are often sufficient to control type 2 diabetes. There is no cure for diabetes, but it can be successfully managed by keeping blood sugar levels within safe limits through diet, exercise, and, if necessary, medication.

Heart Disease and Other Chronic Conditions

Obesity is one of the six major controllable risk factors for heart disease. Excess body fat is strongly associated with hypertension, unhealthy cholesterol and triglyceride levels, and impaired heart function. Many overweight and obese people—especially those who are sedentary and eat a poor diet—also suffer from a group of symptoms called *metabolic*

diabetes mellitus   A disease that disrupts normal metabolism, interfering with cells' ability to take in glucose for energy production.

TERMS

According to popular belief, college students typically gain 15 pounds in their first year at school—the infamous "freshman 15." Is this the fate of all college students, or is it a myth that adds stress for body-conscious young adults?

Research indicates that the truth lies somewhere between these two scenarios. Although many people do gain weight in the first year at college, the amount of weight gain varies. A study that looked at a group of male and female students during their first three years of college found significant three-year gains for weight, BMI, percent body fat, and fat mass, with weight gain highest during freshman and junior years. Studies also find that weight gain tends to be less than 5 pounds. Other studies concluded that freshmen gain between 2.5 and 3.5 pounds, on average, during their first year. This is only half a pound more than is gained by individuals of the same age who are not attending college. Reasons for the weight gain include newfound food independence, changes in eating habits, stress, and social comparison and the influence of roommates and friends.

Although 5 pounds may not seem like a lot of weight, it still can pose a health risk or contribute to lower self-esteem. Changes in body composition—specifically, increased body fat—can become a troublesome pattern for students. Even if they don't have a spike in weight during their first year, college-educated individuals tend to experience a moderate but steady weight gain during and after college.

More importantly, whether the weight gain is 5 pounds, 15 pounds, or even more, freshman weight gain is avoidable!

Try following these tips and guidelines for avoiding freshman weight gain:

- Eat when you are hungry and not for emotional reasons; stop when you are satisfied.

- Watch portion sizes, and avoid second and third servings.

- Follow a daily schedule for your meals and snack times.

- Try not to go longer than 3–4 hours without eating. Don't skip meals—especially breakfast.

- Plan ahead so that you have healthy snacks in your room or home.

- Avoid late-night eating.

- Be more physically active.

SOURCES: Zagorsky, J. L., and P. K. Smith. 2011. The freshman 15: Critical time for obesity intervention or media myth? *Social Science Quarterly*, 92(5): 1389–1407; Smith-Jackson, T., and J. J. Reed. 2012. Freshman women and the "Freshman 15": Perspectives on prevalence and causes of college weight gain. *Journal of American College Health*, 60(1): 14–20; Wansink, B., et al. 2013. College cafeteria snack food purchases become less healthy with each passing week of the semester. *Public Health Nutrition* 16(7): 1291–1295; Gropper, S.S., et al. 2012. Weight and body composition changes during the first three years of college. *Journal of Obesity*, 25 September; Gillen, M. M., and E. S. Lefkowitz. 2011. The "freshman 15": Trends and predictors in a sample of multiethnic men and women. *Eating Behaviors* 12(4): 261–266.

syndrome. Symptoms include insulin resistance, high blood pressure, high blood glucose, unhealthy cholesterol levels, chronic inflammation, and abdominal fat. Metabolic syndrome increases the risk of heart disease.

ADOPTING A HEALTHY LIFESTYLE FOR SUCCESSFUL WEIGHT MANAGEMENT

A good time to develop a lifestyle for successful weight management is during early adulthood, when healthy behavior patterns have a better chance of taking a firm hold.

Diet and Eating Habits

In contrast to *dieting*, which involves some form of food restriction, the term *diet* refers to your daily food choices. Everyone has a diet, but not everyone is dieting. You need to develop a way of eating that you enjoy and that enables you to maintain a healthy body composition. Use MyPlate or the DASH Eating Plan as the basis for a healthy diet. For weight management, pay special attention to total calories, portion sizes, energy density, fat and carbohydrate intake, and eating habits.

Total Calories MyPlate suggests approximate daily energy needs based on gender, age, and activity level. However, energy balance may be a more important consideration for weight management than total calories consumed. To maintain your current weight you have to burn the same number of calories that you take in. To lose weight, you must decrease your calorie intake and/or increase the number of calories you burn; to gain weight, the reverse is true.

The best approach for weight loss is combining an increase in physical activity with moderate calorie restriction. Don't go on a crash diet. To maintain weight loss, you may need to maintain some degree of the calorie restriction you used to lose the weight. Therefore, you need to adopt a level of food intake that provides all the essential nutrients that you can live with over the long term. For many people, maintaining weight loss is more difficult than losing the weight in the first place.

Portion Sizes Overconsumption of total calories is closely tied to portion sizes. Many Americans are unaware that the portions of packaged foods and of foods served at restaurants have increased in size, and most of us significantly underestimate the amount of food we eat. Studies have found that the larger the meal, the more calories people tend to eat. Portion size is associated with body weight, so limiting portion sizes is critical for maintaining a healthy body weight.

Energy (Calorie) Density   Experts also recommend that you pay attention to *energy density*—the number of calories per ounce or gram of weight in a food. Ice cream, potato chips, croissants, crackers, and cakes and cookies are examples of foods high in energy density. Studies suggest that it isn't consumption of a certain amount of fat or calories in food that reduces hunger and leads to feelings of fullness and satisfaction; rather, it is consumption of a certain weight of food. Foods that are low in energy density have more volume and bulk—that is, they are relatively heavy but have few calories. Examples include air-popped popcorn, fat-free yogurt with fruit, and fresh fruits and vegetables.

As you decrease foods high in energy density, increase foods high in nutrient density—foods that are low in calories and high in nutrients. Strategies for lowering the energy density of your diet while at the same time increasing its nutrient density include the following:

- Eat fruit with breakfast and for dessert.
- Add extra vegetables to sandwiches, casseroles, stir-fry dishes, pizza, pasta dishes, and fajitas.
- Start meals with a bowl of broth-based soup; include a green salad or fruit salad.
- Snack on fresh fruits and vegetables rather than crackers, chips, or other energy-dense snack foods.
- Limit serving sizes of energy-dense foods such as butter, mayonnaise, cheese, chocolate, fatty meats, and croissants.
- Limit snack foods that are fried, are high in added sugars (including reduced-fat products), or contain trans fats.

Eating Habits   Equally important to weight management is the habit of eating regular meals daily, including breakfast and snacks. Eating every 3 to 4 hours can help to fuel healthy metabolism, maintain muscle mass, and prevent between-meal hunger that often leads to unhealthy snacking. Balance your meals with whole grains, lean protein, fiber-rich fruits and vegetables, low-fat dairy, and small amounts of healthy fats. For breakfast choose a high-fiber cereal that is low in added sugar with fat-free milk on most days; save pancakes and waffles for special occasions unless they are whole-grain.

A good goal is to eat in moderation; no foods need to be entirely off-limits, though some should be eaten judiciously.

Physical Activity and Exercise

Physical activity and exercise burn calories and keep the metabolism geared to using food for energy instead of storing it as fat. Exercise has a positive effect on metabolism.

Regular physical activity improves cardiovascular and respiratory health, enhances mood, results in a higher quality of sleep, increases self-esteem, and gives us a sense of accomplishment. All of these changes enhance our ability to engage in long-term healthful lifestyle behaviors.

Thinking and Emotions

The way you think about yourself and your world influences, and is influenced by, how you feel and how you act. Often people with low self-esteem mentally compare the actual self to an internally held picture of an "ideal self," an image based on perfectionistic goals and beliefs about how they and others should be. The more these two pictures differ, the larger the impact on self-esteem and the more likely the presence of negative emotions.

Besides the internal picture we carry of ourselves, all of us carry on an internal dialogue about events happening to us and around us. This *self-talk* can be self-deprecating or positively motivating, depending on our beliefs and attitudes. Having realistic beliefs and goals and practicing positive self-talk and problem solving support a healthy lifestyle.

Coping Strategies

Appropriate coping strategies help you deal with the stresses of life. They are also an important lifestyle factor in weight management. Those who overeat might use food to alleviate loneliness or to serve as a pickup for fatigue, as an antidote to boredom, or as a distraction from problems.

Those who recognize that they are misusing food in such ways can consciously attempt to find new coping strategies and begin to use food appropriately—to fuel life's activities, to foster growth, and to bring pleasure, but *not* as a way to manage stress.

APPROACHES TO OVERCOMING A WEIGHT PROBLEM

Americans spend approximately $62 billion on weight loss efforts every year, including diet plans, diet products, and health club memberships. If you are overweight, you may already be creating a plan to lose weight and keep it off. You have many options.

Ask Yourself   **?**

QUESTIONS FOR CRITICAL THINKING AND REFLECTION

Have you ever used food as an escape when you were stressed out or distraught? Were you aware of what you were doing at the time? How can you avoid using food as a coping mechanism in the future?

Doing It Yourself

If you need to lose weight, focus on adopting the healthy lifestyle described throughout this book. The right weight for you will naturally evolve, and you won't have to diet. Combine modest cuts in energy intake with exercise, and avoid very low-calorie diets. (In general, a low-calorie diet should provide 1200–1500 calories per day.) Producing a negative energy balance of 250–1000 calories per day can result in the recommended weight loss of 0.5–2.0 pounds per week.

Most low-calorie diets cause a rapid loss of body water at first. When this phase passes, weight loss declines. As a result, dieters are often misled into believing that their efforts are not working. They then give up, not realizing that smaller, mostly fat, losses later in the diet are actually better than the initial larger, mostly fluid losses. Reasonable weight loss is 8–10% of body weight over six months.

Many diets can cause weight loss if the diet is maintained; however, the real difficulty is finding a safe and healthy pattern of food choices and physical activity that results in long-term maintenance of a healthy body weight and reduced risk of chronic disease (see the box "Is Any Diet Best for Weight Loss?"). A registered dietitian or nutritionist can recommend an appropriate plan for you when you want to lose weight on your own.

Dietary Supplements and Diet Aids

Dietary supplements marketed for weight loss are subject to fewer regulations than over-the-counter (OTC) medications. According to the Federal Trade Commission (FTC), more than half of advertisements for weight loss products make representations that are likely to be false. And although the FTC will order companies to stop making baseless and bogus product claims when monitors become aware of them, consumers are urged to critically evaluate any product that sounds too good to be true.

Formula Drinks and Food Bars Canned diet drinks, powders used to make shakes, and diet food bars and snacks are designed to achieve weight loss by substituting for some or all of a person's daily food intake. However, most people find it difficult to use these products for long periods, and muscle loss and other serious health problems may result if they are used as the sole source of nutrition for an extended period. Use of such products sometimes results in rapid short-term weight loss, but the weight is typically regained because users don't learn to change their eating and lifestyle behaviors.

Herbal Supplements Most herbal weight loss products work by increasing urination (causing water loss); by stimulating the central nervous system (causing the body's activities to speed up or increasing metabolism); or by affecting levels of brain chemicals (causing appetite suppression). Herbs are marketed as dietary supplements, so there is little information about effectiveness, proper dosage, drug interactions, or side effects. In addition, labels may not accurately reflect the ingredients and dosages present, and safe manufacturing practices are not guaranteed. Weight loss occurs only while the product is being taken.

The FDA has banned the sale of ephedra (*ma huang* in Chinese medicine), stating that it presented a significant and unreasonable risk to human health. Ephedrine, the active ingredient in ephedra, is structurally similar to amphetamine and was widely used in weight loss supplements. It may suppress appetite, but adverse effects have included elevated blood pressure, panic attacks, seizures, insomnia, and increased risk of heart attack or stroke, particularly when combined with another stimulant such as caffeine.

> **QUICK STATS**
>
> A 16-ounce whole-milk latte has **265 calories;** beverages have a huge impact on calorie intake.
>
> —CDC, 2011

Other Supplements Fiber is another common ingredient in OTC diet aids, promoted for appetite control. Many diet aids contain only 3 or fewer grams of fiber, which does not contribute much toward the recommended daily intake of 25–38 grams. Other popular dietary supplements include chitosan, chromium picolinate, conjugated linoleic acid, glucomannan, carnitine, green tea extract, pyruvate, calcium, B vitamins, and a number of products labeled "fat absorbers," "fat blockers," and "starch blockers." Research has not found these products to be effective, and many have potentially adverse side effects.

Weight Loss Programs

Weight loss programs come in a variety of types, including noncommercial support organizations, commercial programs, websites, and clinical programs. According to the NIH, safe and effective weight loss programs should include

- Healthy eating plans that reduce calories but do not exclude specific foods or food groups.

- Tips on ways to increase moderate-intensity physical activity.

- Tips on healthy habits that also keep your cultural needs in mind, such as lower-fat versions of your favorite foods.

- Slow and steady weight loss. Depending on your starting weight, experts recommend losing weight at a rate of ½ to 2 pounds per week.

- A recommendation for medical evaluation and care if you have health problems, are taking medication, or are planning to follow a special formula diet that requires monitoring by a doctor.

- A plan to keep the weight off after you have lost it.

Many popular weight loss plans promote specific food choices and macronutrient combinations. Research findings have been mixed, but two points are clear: Total calorie intake matters, and the best diet is probably the one you can stick with.

Low-Carbohydrate Diets

Some low-carb diets advocate fewer than 10% of total calories from carbohydrates, compared to the 45–65% recommended by the Food and Nutrition Board. Some suggest daily carbohydrate intake below the 130 grams needed to provide essential carbohydrates in the diet. Low-carb diets that advocate switching to "healthy carbs" are better for you than the more extreme versions.

Low-Fat Diets

Many experts advocate diets that are relatively low in fat, high in carbohydrates, and moderate in protein. If you try a low-fat, high-carb diet, you still need to pay attention to the quality of the carbohydrates you consume, focusing on whole grains, and to your total calorie intake. A low-fat diet is not a license to consume excess calories, even in low-fat foods.

High-Protein Diets

High-protein diets advocate high protein intake, moderate fat intake, and low carbohydrate intakes. These diets can be low in fiber, whole grains, vegetables, and fruits and so may lack some essential nutrients. Diets high in protein and fat have been linked to an increased risk of heart disease, high blood pressure, and cancer. Studies find that following a diet with a normal protein-to-carbohydrate ratio (1 gram of protein to 2 grams of carbohydrate) promoted more improvements in body fat, waist circumference, and waist-to-hip ratio than following either a low-protein diet (1 gram of protein to 4 grams of carbohydrate) or a high-protein diet (1 gram of protein to 1 gram of carbohydrate) and is probably superior in reducing long-term chronic disease risk.

How Do Different Diets Measure Up?

A study comparing weight loss among adults assigned to one of four reduced-calorie diets differing in percentages of protein, carbohydrate, and fat found that weight loss at two years was similar for all four diets (about 9 pounds). Weight loss was strongly associated with attendance at group sessions. Other studies have also found little difference in weight loss among popular reduced-calorie diets; most resulted in modest weight loss and reduced heart disease risk factors. The more closely people adhered to each diet, the more weight they lost.

Adding exercise helps people lose weight and improve disease risk factors. A study found that when overweight and obese people added exercise and weight loss to the DASH Eating Plan, they experienced greater reductions in blood pressure and greater improvements in insulin sensitivity and lipid levels than those who follow the DASH diet alone or regular diet plans.

Energy Balance Counts: The National Weight Control Registry

Future research may determine that certain macronutrient patterns are somewhat more helpful for disease reduction in people with particular risk profiles. In terms of weight loss, however, such differences among diets are likely overshadowed by the importance of total calorie intake and physical activity. Important lessons about energy balance can be drawn from the National Weight Control Registry—an ongoing study of people who have lost significant amounts of weight and kept it off. The average participant in the registry has lost 71 pounds and kept the weight off for more than five years. Nearly all participants use a combination of diet and exercise to manage their weight. Greater weight regain in this group of individuals comes as a result of decreases in physical activity, having less dietary restraints, less individual monitoring of body weight, and increases in percentage of energy intake from fat. This study illustrates that to lose weight and keep it off, you must decrease daily calorie intake and/or increase daily physical activity—and continue to do so over your lifetime.

SOURCES: Campbell, D. D., and K. A. Meckling. 2012. Effect of the protein: Carbohydrate ratio in hypoenergetic diets on metabolic syndrome risk factors in exercising overweight and obese women. *British Journal of Nutrition,* 16 January: 1–14; Thomas, J.G. 2014. Weight-loss maintenance for 10 years in the National Weight Control Registry. *American Journal of Preventive Medicine* 46(1): 17–23; Papadaki, A., et al. 2013. Impact of weight loss and maintenance with ad libitum diets varying in protein and glycemic index content on metabolic syndrome. *Nutrition.* 23 December (e-pub first).

Noncommercial Weight Loss Programs Noncommercial programs such as TOPS (Take Off Pounds Sensibly) and Overeaters Anonymous (OA) mainly provide group support. They do not advocate any particular diet but do recommend seeking professional advice for creating an individualized plan. These types of programs are generally free. Your physician or a registered dietitian can also provide information and support for weight loss.

Commercial Weight Loss Programs Commercial weight loss programs typically provide group support, nutrition education, physical activity recommendations, and behavior modification advice. Some also make available packaged foods to assist in following dietary advice.

In addition to the features of a safe and effective program outlined earlier, commercial weight loss programs should provide information about all fees and costs,

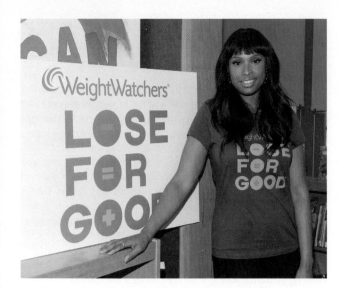

Weight Watchers is one of the best-known commercial weight loss programs. Singer and actor Jennifer Hudson lost 80 pounds and became a spokesperson for the program.

including those of supplements and prepackaged foods, as well as data on risks and expected outcomes of participating in the program. They should also have a registered dietitian on staff along with qualified counselors and health professionals.

A strong commitment and a plan for maintenance are especially important because only about 10–15% of program participants maintain their weight loss—the rest gain back all or more than they had lost. One study found that important predictors of weight loss and maintenance of weight loss in commercial programs include daily self-monitoring; an increased intake of vegetables, fruit, and low-fat dairy products; decreased intake of sweets; regular exercise; and adequate water consumption. A strong predictor of weight gain was frequent television viewing.

Online Weight Loss Programs Most weight loss websites combine self-help with group support through chat rooms, bulletin boards, and e-newsletters. Many sites offer online self-assessment for diet and physical activity habits as well as a meal plan; some provide access to a staff professional for individualized help. Many are free, but some charge a weekly or monthly fee. Research suggests that this type of program provides an alternative to in-person diet counseling and can lead to weight loss for some people.

Clinical Weight Loss Programs Medically supervised clinical programs are usually located in a hospital or other medical setting. Designed to help those who are severely obese, these programs typically involve a closely monitored, very low-calorie diet. The cost of a clinical program is usually high, but insurance may cover part of the fee for those with obesity-related health problems.

Prescription Drugs

The medications most often prescribed for weight loss are appetite suppressants that reduce feelings of hunger or increase feelings of fullness. Appetite suppressants usually work by increasing levels of catecholamine or serotonin—two brain chemicals that affect mood and appetite.

All prescription weight loss drugs have potential side effects. Reported side effects include sleeplessness, nervousness, and euphoria, as well as increases in blood pressure and heart rate, headaches, constipation or diarrhea, dry mouth, and insomnia.

Only one prescription medication is approved for long-term use (up to two years). This medication, Xenical (orlistat), is a lipid inhibitor that works by blocking fat absorption in the intestines. Orlistat prevents about 30% of the fat in food from being digested. Similar to the fat substitute olestra, orlistat reduces the absorption of fat-soluble vitamins and antioxidants. Therefore, taking a vitamin supplement is highly recommended for people taking orlistat. Side effects include diarrhea, cramping, and other gastrointestinal problems if users do not follow a low-fat diet. Alli is an FDA-approved, lower-dose version of orlistat that is sold over the counter.

Prescription medications work best in conjunction with behavior modification. Studies have generally found that appetite suppressants produce modest weight loss—about 5–22 pounds above the loss expected with nondrug obesity treatments. Unfortunately weight loss tends to level off or reverse after 4–6 months on a medication, and many people regain the weight they've lost when they stop taking the medication.

Prescription drugs are recommended only in certain cases: for people who have been unable to lose weight with nondrug options and who have a BMI over 30 (or over 27 if two or more additional risk factors such as diabetes and high blood pressure are present).

Surgery

According to the National Health and Nutrition Examination Survey (NHANES), it is estimated that 6.3% of adult Americans age 20 years and older have a BMI greater than 40, qualifying them as extremely or "morbidly" obese. The number of severely obese people has nearly doubled in the

Ask Yourself

QUESTIONS FOR CRITICAL THINKING AND REFLECTION

Why do you think people continue to buy into fad diets and weight loss gimmicks, even though they are constantly reminded that the key to weight management is lifestyle change? Have you ever tried a fad diet or weight loss supplement? If so, what were your reasons for trying it? What were the results?

last two decades. Extreme obesity is a serious medical condition that is often complicated by other health problems such as diabetes, heart disease, arthritis, and sleep disorders. Surgical intervention may be necessary as a treatment of last resort. According to the NIH, weight loss (bariatric) surgery is recommended for patients with a BMI greater than 40, or greater than 35 with obesity-related illnesses.

Bariatric surgery modifies the gastrointestinal tract by changing either the size of the stomach or how the intestine drains, thereby reducing food intake. The keys to success with surgical weight loss procedures are adequate follow-up and continued motivation so that eating patterns and lifestyle behaviors are permanently changed.

PROBLEMS ASSOCIATED WITH VERY LOW LEVELS OF BODY FAT

Health experts have generally viewed very low levels of body fat—less than 8–12% for women and 3–5% for men—as a threat to wellness. Extreme leanness has been linked with reproductive, circulatory, and immune system disorders. Extremely lean people may experience muscle wasting and fatigue. They are also more likely to suffer from dangerous eating disorders.

In physically active women and girls, particularly those involved in sports where weight and appearance are important (ballet, gymnastics, skating, and distance running, for example), a condition called the **female athlete triad** may develop. The triad consists of three interrelated disorders: abnormal eating patterns (and excessive exercising), followed by **amenorrhea** (absence of menstruation), followed by decreased bone density (premature osteoporosis). Prolonged amenorrhea can cause bone density to erode to a point that a woman in her twenties will have the bone density of a woman in her sixties. Left untreated, the triad can lead to decreased physical performance, increased incidence of bone fractures, disturbances of heart rhythm and metabolism, and even death.

BODY IMAGE

The collective picture of the body as seen through the mind's eye, **body image** consists of perceptions, images, thoughts, attitudes, and emotions. A negative body image is characterized by dissatisfaction with the body in general or some part of the body in particular. People may be dissatisfied with their bodies for a variety of reasons, including sociocultural forces and factors that are specific to life stages.

Losing weight or getting cosmetic surgery does not necessarily improve body image. However, improvements in body image may occur in the absence of changes in weight

or appearance. Many experts now believe that body image issues must be dealt with as part of treating obesity and eating disorders. Developing a positive body image is an important aspect of psychological wellness and an important component of successful weight management.

Severe Body Image Problems

Poor body image can cause significant psychological distress. A person can become preoccupied with a perceived defect in appearance, thereby damaging self-esteem and interfering with relationships. Adolescents and adults who have a negative body image are more likely to diet restrictively, eat compulsively, or develop some other form of disordered eating.

When dissatisfaction becomes extreme, the condition is called *body dysmorphic disorder* (*BDD*). Although many people are dissatisfied with some part of their body or their appearance, these concerns usually do not constantly occupy their thoughts. Individuals with BDD are constantly preoccupied and upset about body imperfections, such as thinking their nose is too big or that their hair is never right. They cannot seem to stop checking or obsessing about their appearance, often focusing on slight flaws that are not obvious to others. Low self-esteem is common. Individuals with BDD may spend hours every day thinking about their flaws and looking at themselves in mirrors; they may desire and seek repeated cosmetic surgeries. BDD affects about 2% of Americans, males and females in equal numbers. It usually begins before age 18 but can begin in adulthood.

This condition is related to obsessive-compulsive disorder and can lead to depression, social phobia, and suicide if left untreated. An individual with BDD needs to get professional evaluation and treatment. Medication and therapy can help people with BDD.

In some cases, body image may bear little resemblance to fact. A person suffering from the eating disorder anorexia nervosa typically has a severely distorted body image—she believes herself to be fat even when she has become

female athlete triad A condition consisting of three interrelated disorders: abnormal eating patterns (and excessive exercising) followed by lack of menstrual periods (amenorrhea) and decreased bone density (premature osteoporosis).   **TERMS**

amenorrhea The absence of menstruation.

body image The mental representation a person holds about his or her body at any given time, consisting of perceptions, images, thoughts, attitudes, and emotions about the body.

Ask Yourself

QUESTIONS FOR CRITICAL THINKING AND REFLECTION

Describe your own body image in the fewest words possible. What satisfies you most and least about your body? Do you think your self-image is in line with the way others see you?

emaciated. Distorted body image is also a hallmark of *muscle dysmorphia*, a disorder experienced by some bodybuilders and other active people who see themselves as small and out of shape despite being very muscular. Those who suffer from muscle dysmorphia may let obsessive exercise interfere with their work and relationships. They may also use steroids and other potentially dangerous muscle-building drugs.

EATING DISORDERS

Problems with body weight and weight control are not limited to excessive body fat. A growing number of people, especially adolescent girls and young women, experience **eating disorders**—psychological disorders characterized by severe disturbances in body image, eating patterns, and eating-related behaviors. The major eating disorders are anorexia nervosa, bulimia nervosa, and binge-eating disorder. In the United States, up to 24 million people of all ages and genders suffer from an eating disorder (anorexia, bulimia, and binge-eating disorder). Many more people have abnormal eating habits and attitudes about food that disrupt their lives, even though these habits do not meet the criteria for a major eating disorder.

Anorexia Nervosa

A person with **anorexia nervosa** does not eat enough food to maintain a reasonable body weight. An estimated 0.5–3.7% of women suffer from anorexia nervosa in their lifetime. Although it can occur earlier or later, anorexia typically develops during puberty and the late teenage years, with an average age of onset of about 19 years.

Characteristics of Anorexia Nervosa People with anorexia have an intense fear of gaining weight or becoming fat. Their body image is so distorted that even when emaciated they

Exercise is a healthy practice, but people with eating disorders sometimes exercise compulsively, building their lives around their workouts. Compulsive exercise can lead to injuries, low body fat, and other health problems.

think they are fat. People with anorexia may engage in compulsive behaviors or rituals that help keep them from eating, though some may also binge and **purge.** They often use vigorous and prolonged exercise to reduce body weight as well. Although they may express a great interest in food, even taking over the cooking responsibilities for the rest of the family, their own diet becomes more and more restricted. People with anorexia nervosa often hide or hoard food without eating it.

People with anorexia are typically introverted, emotionally reserved, and socially insecure. They are often model children who rarely complain and are anxious to please others and win their approval. Although school performance is typically above average, they are often critical of themselves and not satisfied with their accomplishments. For people with anorexia nervosa, their entire sense of self-esteem may be tied up in their evaluation of their body shape and weight.

Health Risks of Anorexia Nervosa Because of extreme weight loss, females with anorexia often stop menstruating, become intolerant of cold, and develop low blood

eating disorder TERMS A serious disturbance in eating patterns or eating-related behavior, characterized by a negative body image and concerns about body weight or body fat.

anorexia nervosa An eating disorder characterized by a refusal to maintain body weight at a minimally healthy level and an intense fear of gaining weight or becoming fat; self-starvation.

purging The use of vomiting, laxatives, excessive exercise, restrictive dieting, enemas, diuretics, or diet pills to compensate for food that has been eaten and that the person fears will produce weight gain.

pressure and heart rate. They develop dry skin that is often covered by fine body hair like that of a newborn. Their hands and feet may swell and take on a blue tinge.

Anorexia nervosa has been linked to a variety of medical complications, including disorders of the cardiovascular, gastrointestinal, endocrine, and skeletal systems. When body fat is virtually gone and muscles are severely wasted, the body turns to its own organs in a desperate search for protein. Death can occur from heart failure caused by electrolyte imbalances. About 1 in 10 women with anorexia dies of starvation, cardiac arrest, or other medical complications—the highest death rate for any psychiatric disorder. Depression is also a serious risk: About half the fatalities related to anorexia are suicides.

Bulimia Nervosa

A person suffering from **bulimia nervosa** engages in recurrent episodes of binge eating followed by purging. Bulimia is often difficult to recognize because sufferers conceal their eating habits and usually maintain a normal weight, although they may experience weight fluctuations of 10–15 pounds. Although bulimia usually begins in adolescence or young adulthood, it has begun to emerge at increasingly younger (11–12 years) and older (40–60 years) ages; the average age of onset is about 20 years.

Characteristics of Bulimia Nervosa During a binge, a bulimic person may rapidly consume thousands of calories. This is followed by an attempt to get rid of the food by purging, usually by vomiting or using laxatives or diuretics. During a binge, bulimics feel as though they have lost control and cannot stop or limit how much they eat. Some binge and purge only occasionally; others do so many times every day.

People with bulimia may appear to eat normally, but they are rarely comfortable around food. Binges usually occur in secret and can become nightmarish—uncontrollably raiding the kitchen for food, going from one grocery store to another to buy food, or stealing food. During the binge, food acts as an anesthetic, blocking out feelings. Afterward, bulimics feel physically drained and emotionally spent. They usually feel deeply ashamed and disgusted with both themselves and their behavior and terrified that they will gain weight from the binge.

Major life changes such as leaving for college, getting married, having a baby, or losing a job can trigger a binge-purge cycle. At such times, stress is high and the person may have no good outlet for emotional conflict or tension. As with anorexia nervosa, bulimia sufferers are often insecure and depend on others for approval and self-esteem. They may hide difficult emotions such as anger and disappointment from themselves and others. Binge eating and purging become a way of dealing with feelings.

Health Risks of Bulimia Nervosa The binge-purge cycle of bulimia places a tremendous strain on the body and can have serious health effects. Contact with vomited stomach acids erodes tooth enamel. Bulimic people often develop tooth decay because they binge on foods that are high in simple sugars. Repeated vomiting or the use of laxatives, in combination with deficient calorie intake, can damage the liver and kidneys and cause cardiac arrhythmia. Chronic hoarseness and esophageal tearing with bleeding may also result from vomiting. More rarely, binge eating can lead to rupture of the stomach. Although many bulimic women maintain normal weight, even a small weight loss to lower-than-normal weight can cause menstrual problems. And although less often associated with suicide or premature death than anorexia, bulimia is associated with increased depression, excessive preoccupation with food and body image, and sometimes disturbances in cognitive functioning.

Binge-Eating Disorder

Binge-eating disorder (BED) affects 3% to 5% of American women and 2% of men. It is characterized by uncontrollable eating, usually followed by feelings of guilt and shame about weight gain. Common eating patterns are eating more rapidly than normal, eating until uncomfortably full, eating when not hungry, and preferring to eat alone. Binge eaters may eat large amounts of food throughout the day, with no planned mealtimes. Many people with binge-eating disorder mistakenly see rigid dieting as the only solution to their problem. However, rigid dieting usually causes feelings of deprivation and a return to overeating.

Compulsive overeaters rarely eat because of hunger. Instead food is used as a means of coping with stress, conflict, and other difficult emotions or to provide solace and entertainment. People who do not have the resources to deal effectively with stress may be more vulnerable to binge-eating disorder. Inappropriate overeating often begins during childhood. In some families, eating may be used as an activity to fill otherwise empty time. Parents may reward children with food for good behavior or withhold food as a means of punishment, thereby creating distorted feelings about the experience of eating.

TERMS

bulimia nervosa An eating disorder characterized by recurrent episodes of binge eating and purging—overeating and then using compensatory behaviors such as vomiting, laxatives, and excessive exercise to prevent weight gain.

binge-eating disorder (BED) An eating disorder characterized by episodes of binge eating and a lack of control over eating behavior in general.

Binge eaters are almost always obese, so they face all the health risks associated with obesity. In addition, binge eaters may have higher rates of depression and anxiety.

Borderline Disordered Eating

People with borderline disordered eating have some symptoms of eating disorders but do not meet the full diagnostic criteria for anorexia, bulimia, or binge-eating disorder. Behaviors such as excessive dieting, occasional bingeing or purging, or the inability to control eating turn food into the enemy and create havoc in the lives of millions of Americans.

How do you know if you have disordered eating habits? When thoughts about food and weight dominate your life, you have a problem. If you're convinced that your worth as a person hinges on how you look and how much you weigh, it's time to get help. Other danger signs include frequent feelings of guilt after a meal or snack, any use of vomiting or laxatives after meals, or overexercising or severely restricting your food intake to compensate for what you've already eaten.

If you suspect you have an eating problem, don't go it alone or delay getting help because disordered eating habits can develop into a full-blown eating disorder. Check with your student health or counseling center—nearly all colleges have counselors and medical personnel who can help you or refer you to a specialist if needed.

Treating Eating Disorders

Anorexia nervosa treatment first involves averting a medical crisis by restoring adequate body weight; then the psychological aspects of the disorder can be addressed. The treatment

of bulimia nervosa or binge-eating disorder involves first stabilizing the eating patterns, then identifying and changing the patterns of thinking that led to disordered eating, and then improving coping skills. Concurrent problems, such as depression, anxiety, and other mental disorders may be present and must also be addressed.

Treatment of eating disorders usually involves a combination of psychotherapy and medical management. The therapy may be done individually or in a group; sessions involving the entire family may be recommended. A support or self-help group can be a useful adjunct to such treatment.

WHAT IS THE RIGHT WEIGHT FOR YOU?

To answer the question of what you should weigh, let your lifestyle be your guide. Don't focus on a particular weight as your goal. Instead focus on living a lifestyle that includes eating moderate amounts of healthful foods, getting plenty of exercise, thinking positively, and learning to cope with stress. Then let the pounds fall where they may. For most people, the result will be close to recommended weight ranges. For some, their weight will be somewhat higher than societal standards—but right for them. By letting a healthy lifestyle determine your weight, you can avoid developing unhealthy patterns of eating and a negative body image. Knowing when you've reached the limits of healthy change—and learning to accept those limits—is crucial for overall wellness.

A balanced, realistic attitude toward weight management is part of overall wellness. Many healthy people do not fit society's image of ideal body size and shape.

connect™

Connect to Your Choices

Have you ever thought about how you came to have the body weight and body composition you have? Many factors can influence our weight management choices, some not as obvious as others. Do you choose high-calorie, high-fat snacks because those types of foods are easy to prepare? Do you take a ride or drive short distances when you could walk? Does your TV or computer lure you into hours of sedentary entertainment?

What are the external factors that influence your choices about weight management? What are your inner motivations and core values, and how do they affect your choices? Based on what you learned in this chapter, will you make some different choices in the future? If so, what will they be?

Go online to Connect to complete this activity: www.mcgraw-hillconnect.com

TIPS FOR TODAY AND THE FUTURE

Many approaches work, but the simplest formula for weight management is moderate food intake coupled with regular exercise.

RIGHT NOW YOU CAN:

- Assess your weight management needs. Do you need to gain weight, lose weight, or stay at your current weight?
- List five things you can do to add more physical activity (not just exercise) to your daily routine.
- Identify the foods you regularly eat that may be sabotaging your ability to manage your weight.

IN THE FUTURE YOU CAN:

- Make an honest assessment of your current body image. Is it accurate and fair, or is it unduly negative and unhealthy? If your body image presents a problem, consider getting professional advice on how to view yourself realistically.
- Keep track of your energy needs to determine whether your energy balance equation is correct. Use this information as part of your long-term weight management efforts.

SUMMARY

- Body composition is the relative amounts of fat-free mass and fat in the body. *Overweight* and *obesity* refer to body weight or the percentage of body fat that exceeds what is associated with good health.

- The key to weight management is maintaining a balance of calories in (food) and calories out (resting metabolism, food digestion, and physical activity).

- Standards for assessing body weight and body composition include body mass index (BMI) and percent body fat.

- Too much or too little body fat is linked to health problems; the distribution of body fat can also be a significant risk factor for many kinds of health problems.

- An inaccurate or negative body image is common and can lead to psychological distress.

- Genetic factors help determine a person's weight, but the influence of heredity can be overcome with attention to lifestyle factors.

- Physiological factors involved in the regulation of body weight and body fat include metabolic rate, hormonal influences, and the size and number of fat cells.

- Nutritional guidelines for weight management include consuming a moderate number of calories; limiting portion sizes, energy density, and the intake of fat, simple sugars, refined carbohydrates, and protein to recommended levels; and developing an eating schedule and rules for food choices.

- Activity guidelines for weight management emphasize daily physical activity and regular sessions of cardiorespiratory endurance exercise and strength training.

- Weight management requires developing positive self-talk and self-esteem, realistic weight and body composition goals, and a repertoire of appropriate techniques for handling stress and other emotional and physical challenges.

- People can be successful at long-term weight loss on their own by combining diet and exercise.

- OTC diet aids and supplements, and formal weight loss programs should be assessed for safety and efficacy.

- Professional help is needed in cases of severe obesity; medical treatments include prescription drugs, surgery, and psychological therapy.

- Dissatisfaction with weight and shape are common to all eating disorders. Anorexia nervosa is characterized by self-starvation, distorted body image, and an intense fear of gaining weight. Bulimia nervosa is characterized by recurrent episodes of uncontrolled binge eating and frequent purging. Binge-eating disorder involves binge eating without regular use of compensatory purging.

FOR MORE INFORMATION

BOOKS

American Heart Association. 2011. *American Heart Association No-Fad Diet, 2nd Edition: A Personal Plan for Healthy Weight Loss*. New York: Clarkson Potter. *Provides guidelines for successful weight management.*

American Psychiatric Association. 2013. *Diagnostic and Statistical Manual of Mental Disorders (DSM-5),* 5th ed. Washington, DC: American Psychiatric Publishing.

Costin, C., and G. S. Grabb. 2011. *8 Keys to Recovery from an Eating Disorder: Effective Strategies from Therapeutic Practice and Personal Experience*. New York: Norton. *A motivating description of the recovery process, written by two therapists who interweave their personal narratives with clinical strategies.*

Dillon, E. 2009. *Issues That Concern You: Obesity*. New York: Greenhaven Press. *A collection of perspectives on the causes of obesity, its management, and its impact on individuals and society.*

Mayo Clinic. 2012. *Mayo Clinic's Essential Diabetes Book*, 2nd ed. Rochester, MN: Mayo Clinic. *A user-friendly guide to diabetes.*

Samuelson, D. A., and A. D. Salzburg. 2011. *The Weight Loss Surgery Workbook: Deciding on Bariatric Surgery, Preparing for the Procedure, and Changing Habits for Post-Surgery Success.* Oakland, CA: New Harbinger Publications. *A step-by-step workbook that guides patients through the process of weight loss surgery; written by a psychologist and a physician.*

ORGANIZATIONS, HOTLINES, AND WEBSITES

American Diabetes Association. Provides information, a free newsletter, and referrals to local support groups; the website includes an online diabetes risk assessment.

    http://www.diabetes.org

Calorie Control Council. This site includes a variety of interactive calculators, including an Exercise Calculator that estimates the calories burned from various forms of physical activity.

http://www.caloriecontrol.org

Centers for Disease Control and Prevention: Obesity. The home page for accessing all the CDC's information about overweight and obesity, their health risks, statistics, and diet and exercise.

http://www.cdc.gov/obesity/index.html

FDA Center for Food Safety and Applied Nutrition: Dietary Supplements. Provides background facts and information on the current regulatory status of dietary supplements, including compounds marketed for weight loss.

http://www.fda.gov/Food/DietarySupplements/default.htm

National Heart, Lung, and Blood Institute (NHLBI): Aim for a Healthy Weight. Provides information and tips on diet and physical activity, as well as a BMI calculator.

http://www.nhlbi.nih.gov/health/public/heart/obesity/lose_wt

National Institute of Diabetes and Digestive and Kidney Diseases (NIDDK): Weight-Control Information Network. Provides information and referrals for problems related to obesity, weight control, and nutritional disorders.

http://win.niddk.nih.gov

RESOURCES FOR PEOPLE CONCERNED ABOUT EATING DISORDERS

Eating Disorder Referral and Information Center
http://www.edreferral.com

Eating Disorders Coalition for Research, Policy and Action
http://www.something-fishy.org

MedlinePlus: Eating Disorders
http://www.nlm.nih.gov/medlineplus/eatingdisorders.html

National Association of Anorexia Nervosa and Associated Disorders
630-577-1330 (help line)
http://www.anad.org

National Eating Disorders Association
800-931-2237
http://www.nationaleatingdisorders.org

National Institute of Mental Health: Eating Disorders
http://www.nimh.nih.gov/health/topics/eating-disorders/index.shtml

SELECTED BIBLIOGRAPHY

American Academy of Child and Adolescent Psychiatry. 2011. *Obesity in Children and Teens* (http://www.aacap.org/cs/root/facts_for_families/obesity_in_children_and_teens).

American Diabetes Association. 2011. *Diabetes Statistics* (http://www.diabetes.org/diabetes-basics/diabetes-statistics/).

Buttitta, M., et al. 2014. Quality of life in overweight and obese children and adolescents: A literature review. *Quality of Life Research*, (19 November 2013.e-pub).

Campbell, I., et al. 2011. Eating disorders, gene–environment interactions, and epigenetics. *Neuroscience & Biobehavioral Reviews* 35(3): 784–793.

Canfi, A., et al. 2011. Effect of changes in the intake of weight of specific food groups on successful body weight loss during a multi-dietary strategy intervention trial. *Journal of the American College of Nutrition* 30(6): 491–501.

Centers for Disease Control and Prevention. 2011. *National Diabetes Fact Sheet: General Information and National Estimates on Diabetes and Prediabetes in the United States, 2011*. Atlanta: U.S. Department of Health and Human Services, CDC.

Centers for Disease Control and Prevention. 2011. *Rethink Your Drink. Healthy Weight: It's Not a Diet, It's a Lifestyle* (http://www.cdc.gov/healthyweight/healthy_eating/drinks.html).

Centers for Disease Control and Prevention. 2012. *Genomics and Health: Genes and Obesity* (http://www.cdc.gov/genomics/resources/diseases/obesity/obesedit.htm).

Champagne, C. M., et al. 2011. Dietary intakes associated with successful weight loss and maintenance during the Weight Loss Maintenance trial. *Journal of the American Dietetic Association* 111(12): 1826–1835.

Dingemans, A. E., et al. 2012. Body dysmorphic disorder in patients with an eating disorder: Prevalence and characteristics. *International Journal of Eating Disorders* 45(4): 562–569.

Drewnowski, A., and P. Eichelsdoerfer. 2010. Can low-income Americans afford a healthy diet? *Nutrition Today* 44(6): 246–249.

Federal Trade Commission. 2011. *Facts for Consumers: Dietary Supplements* (http://www.ftc.gov/bcp/edu/pubs/consumer/health/hea11.shtm).

Federal Trade Commission. 2011. *Facts for Consumers: Weighing the Evidence in Diet Ads* (http://www.ftc.gov/bcp/edu/pubs/consumer/health/hea03.shtm).

Flegal, K., et al. 2012. Prevalence of obesity and trends in the distribution of body mass index among U.S. adults, 1999–2010. *Journal of the American Medical Association* 307(5), published online January 17.

Guedes, E.P., et al. 2013. Body composition and depressive/anxiety symptoms in overweight and obese individuals with metabolic syndrome. *Diabetology & Metabolic Syndrome* 5(1): 82.

Holland, L. A., et al. 2014. Defining features of unhealthy exercise associated with disordered eating and eating disorder diagnoses. *Psychology of Sport and Exercise* 15(1): 116–123.

Hutchesson, M. J., et al. 2013. Changes to dietary intake during a 12-week commercial web-based weight loss program: A randomized controlled trial. *European Journal of Clinical Nutrition*, 16 October (online first).

Kleiman, S., et sl. 2012. Drinking to our health: Can beverage companies cut calories while maintaining profits? *Obesity Reviews* 12(3): 258–274.

Kushner, R. F., et al. 2013. Obesity consults—comprehensive obesity management in 2013: Understanding the shifting paradigm. *Obesity* 21(Suppl 2): S1–S15.

Lasikiewicz, N., et al. 2014. Psychological benefits of weight loss following behavioural and/or dietary weight loss interventions. A systematic research review. *Appetite* 72:123–137.

Mayo Clinic. 2011. *Gastric Bypass Surgery* (http://www.mayoclinic.com/health/g.astric-bypass/MY00825/DSECTION=results).

Micali, N., et al. 2013. Frequency and patterns of eating disorder symptoms in early adolescence. *Journal of Adolescent Health,* 13 December.

Nakamura, K., et al. 2013. Adipokines: A link between obesity and cardiovascular disease. *Journal of Cardiology*, 16 December.

Noser, A., and V. Zeigler-Hill. 2013. Investing in the ideal: Does objectified body consciousness mediate the association between appearance contingent self-worth and appearance self-esteem in women? *Body Image*, 24 December.

Ogden, C. L., and M. D. Carroll. 2011. *Prevalence of Overweight, Obesity, and Extreme Obesity among Adults: United States, Trends 1960–1962 through 2007–2008* (http://www.cdc.gov/nchs/data/hestat/obesity_adult_07_08/obesity_adult_07_08.htm).

Ogden, C. L., et al. 2012. Prevalence of obesity in the United States, 2009–2010. NCHS Data Brief, No. 82 (http://www.cdc.gov/nchs/data/data_briefs/db82.pdf).

Pedersen, E., et al. 2013. High protein weight loss diets in obese subjects with type 2 diabetes mellitus. *Nutrition, Metabolism & Cardiovascular Diseases*, 2 December.

Postrach, E., et al. 2013. Determinants of successful weight loss after using a commercial web-based weight reduction program for six months: Cohort study. *Journal of Medical Internet Research* 15(10).

Pritchard, S. J., et al. 2013. A randomized trial of the impact of energy density and texture of a meal on food and energy intake, satiation, satiety, appetite and palatability responses in healthy adults. *Clinical Nutrition,* 25 October.

Sax, H. C. 2011. Selecting the "best" weight loss procedure: More may be better. *Archives of Surgery* 146(2): 155.

Schmidt, M. E., et al. 2012. Systematic review of effective strategies for reducing screen time among young children. *Obesity*, 5 January (http://www.nature.com/oby/journal/vaop/ncurrent/full/oby2011348a.html, e-pub ahead of print).

Slevec, J. H., and M. Tiggemann. 2011. Predictors of body dissatisfaction and disordered eating in middle-aged women. *Clinical Psychology Review* 31(4): 515–524.

Tiggemann, M., and A. McCourt. 2013. Body appreciation in adult women: Relationships with age and body satisfaction. *Body Image* 10(4): 624–627.

Tong, J., et al. 2013. A two-stage epidemiologic study on prevalence of eating disorders in female university students in Wuhan, China. *Social Psychiatry and Psychiatric Epidemiology,* 7 June.

Urquhart, C. S., and T. V. Mihalynuk. 2011. Disordered eating in women: Implications for the obesity pandemic. *Canadian Journal of Dietetic Practice and Research* 72(1): e115–125.

U.S. Department of Agriculture and U.S. Department of Health and Human Services. 2011. *Dietary Guidelines for Americans, 2010,* 7th ed. Washington, DC: U.S. Government Printing Office (http://www.health.gov/dietaryguidelines/dga2010/DietaryGuidelines2010.pdf, p. 24, accessed January 15, 2014).

U.S. Department of Health and Human Services. 2012. *Healthy People 2020: Nutrition and Weight Status* (http://healthypeople.gov/2020/topicsobjectives2020/overview.aspx?topicid=29).

Webb J. B., et al. 2013. Do you see what I see?: An exploration of inter-ethnic ideal body size comparisons among college women. *Body Image* 10(3): 369–379.

Whitham, C., et al. 2013. Weight maintenance over 12 months after weight loss resulting from participation in a 12-week randomized controlled trial comparing all meal provision to self-directed diet in overweight adults. *Journal of Human Nutrition and Dietetics,* 18 November.

Williams, R. A., et al. 2013. Assessment of satiety depends on the energy density and portion size of the test meal. *Obesity*, 8 August.

Yanovski, S. Z., and J. A. Yanovski. 2014. Long-term drug treatment for obesity: A systematic and clinical review. *Journal of the American Medical Association* 311(1): 74–86.

Zheng, H., et al. 2013. Obesity and mortality risk: New findings from body mass index trajectories. *American Journal of Epidemiology* 178(11): 1591–1599.

BEHAVIOR CHANGE STRATEGY
Creating a Personal Weight Management Plan

The behavior management plan described in Chapter 1 provides an excellent framework for a weight management program. Following are some suggestions about specific ways you can adapt that general plan to control your weight.

Motivation and Commitment

Make sure you are motivated and committed before you begin. Failure at weight loss is a frustrating experience that can make it more difficult to lose weight in the future. Think about why you want to lose weight. Make a list of your reasons for wanting to lose weight, and post it in a prominent place.

Setting Goals

Choose a reasonable weight you think you would like to reach over the long term, and be willing to renegotiate it as you get further along. Break down your long-term weight and behavioral goals into a series of short-term action-oriented goals.

Creating a Negative Energy Balance

When your weight is constant, you are burning approximately the same number of calories as you are taking in. To tip the energy balance toward weight loss, you must consume fewer calories, or burn more calories through physical activity, or both. To generate a negative energy balance, it's usually best to begin by increasing activity level rather than decreasing your calorie consumption.

Physical Activity

Consider how you can increase your energy output simply by increasing routine physical activity, such as walking or taking the stairs. If you are not already involved in a regular exercise routine aimed at increasing endurance and building or maintaining muscle mass, seek help from someone who is competent to help you plan and start an appropriate exercise routine. If you are already doing regular physical exercise, evaluate your program according to the guidelines in Chapter 10.

Diet and Eating Habits

If you can't generate a large enough negative energy balance solely by increasing physical activity, you may want to supplement exercise with modest cuts in your calorie intake. Your goal is to make small changes in your diet that you can maintain for a lifetime. Focus on cutting your intake of trans fats and added sugars and on eating a variety of nutritious foods in moderation. Don't skip meals, fast, or go on a very low-calorie diet or a diet that is unbalanced.

Self-Monitoring

Keep a record of your weight and behavior change progress. Try keeping a record of everything you eat. Write down what you plan to eat, in what quantity, *before* you eat. You'll find that just having to record something that is not OK to eat is likely to stop you from eating it. Also, keep track of your daily activities and your formal exercise program so you can monitor increases in physical activity.

Putting Your Plan into Action

- Examine the environmental cues that trigger poor eating and exercise habits, and devise strategies for dealing with them. Anticipate problem situations, and plan ways to handle them more effectively.

- Create new environmental cues that will support your new healthy behaviors. Move fruits and vegetables to the front of the refrigerator.

- Get others to help. Talk to friends and family members about what they can do to support your efforts. Find a buddy to join you in your exercise program.

- Give yourself lots of praise and rewards. Focus attention on your accomplishments and achievements and congratulate yourself. Plan special nonfood treats for yourself, such as a walk or a movie. Reward yourself often and for anything that counts toward success.

- If you slip, don't waste time on self-criticism. Think positively instead of getting into a cycle of guilt and self-blame.

- Don't get discouraged. Be aware that, although weight loss is bound to slow down after the first loss of body fluid, the weight loss at this slower rate is more permanent than earlier, more dramatic, losses.

- Remember that weight management is a lifelong project. You need to adopt reasonable goals and strategies that you can maintain over the long term.

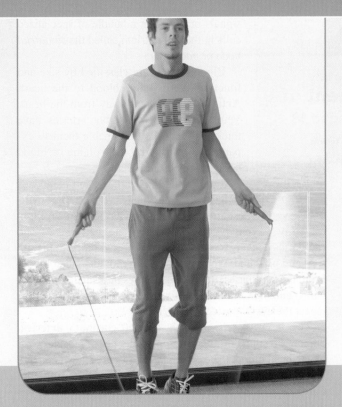

CHAPTER **12**

Cardiovascular Disease and Cancer

Cardiovascular disease (CVD) affects more than 81 million Americans and is the leading cause of death in the United States, claiming one life every 34 seconds—more than 2,500 Americans every day. Heart attacks and strokes are the number one and number four causes of death, respectively, making them the most common life-threatening manifestations of CVD. Cancer is the second leading cause of human death in the United States and is responsible for nearly one in four deaths, claiming over 580,000 lives annually—more than 1600 each day.

Although genes, age, and environmental factors play roles in the development of these diseases, CVD and cancer are primarily lifestyle diseases, linked to many lifestyle factors. The following sections provide information that can help you maintain a healthy heart for life and reduce your risks of developing cancer.

THE CARDIOVASCULAR SYSTEM

The **cardiovascular system (CVS)** consists of the heart and blood vessels, which includes both arteries and veins. Together they move blood throughout the body (see page T2-2 of the color transparency insert "Touring the Cardiorespiratory System"). When the lungs are included, the system is known as the *cardiorespiratory* or *cardiopulmonary system*.

The heart is a four-chambered, fist-sized muscle located just beneath the sternum (breastbone). It pumps deoxygenated (oxygen-poor) blood to the lungs and delivers oxygenated (oxygen-rich) blood to the rest of the body. Blood actually travels through two separate circulatory systems. The right side of the heart pumps blood to the lungs in what is called **pulmonary circulation,** and the left side pumps blood through the rest of the body in the **systemic circulation.**

---

cardiovascular disease (CVD)　The collective term for various diseases of the heart and blood vessels.

cardiovascular system (CVS)　The system that circulates blood through the body; consists of the heart and blood vessels.

pulmonary circulation　The part of the circulatory system controlled by the right side of the heart: the circulation of blood between the heart and the lungs.

systemic circulation　The part of the circulatory system controlled by the left side of the heart: the circulation of blood between the heart and the rest of the body.

TERMS

The path of blood flow through the heart and cardiorespiratory system is illustrated on page T2-3 of the color transparency insert "Touring the Cardiorespiratory System."

Oxygen-poor blood travels through large vessels, the **venae cavae,** into the heart's right upper chamber, the right **atrium.** After the right atrium fills, it contracts and pumps blood into the heart's right lower chamber, the right **ventricle.** When the right ventricle is full, it contracts and pumps blood through the pulmonary artery into the lungs. In the lungs, blood picks up oxygen and discards carbon dioxide, which is expelled during exhalation. The newly oxygenated blood flows from the lungs through the pulmonary veins into the heart's left atrium. After the left atrium fills, it contracts and pumps blood into the left ventricle. When the left ventricle is full, it pumps blood through the **aorta**—the body's largest artery—for distribution to the rest of the body's blood vessels. The period of the heart's contraction is called **systole**; the period of relaxation is called **diastole**.

The heartbeat—the sequence of contractions of the heart's four chambers—is controlled by nerve impulses. These signals originate in a bundle of specialized cells in the right atrium called the *sinoatrial node* or *pacemaker.*

Blood vessels are classified by size and function. **Veins** carry blood to the heart. **Arteries** carry blood away from the heart. Veins have thin walls, but arteries have thick elastic walls that enable them to expand and relax with the volume of blood being pumped through them.

After leaving the heart, the aorta branches into smaller and smaller vessels. The smallest arteries branch still further into **capillaries**—tiny vessels with walls only one cell thick. The capillaries deliver oxygen- and nutrient-rich blood to the tissues and pick up oxygen-poor, carbon dioxide–laden blood. From the capillaries, this blood empties into small veins (*venules*) and then into larger veins that return it to the heart to repeat the cycle.

Two large vessels, the right and left **coronary arteries,** branch off the aorta and supply the heart muscle with oxygenated blood. (The coronary arteries are shown on page T2-3 of the color transparency insert "Touring the Cardiorespiratory System.") Blockage of a coronary artery is the leading cause of heart attacks.

RISK FACTORS FOR CARDIOVASCULAR DISEASE

Researchers have identified a variety of factors associated with an increased risk of developing CVD. They are grouped into two categories: major risk factors and contributing risk factors.

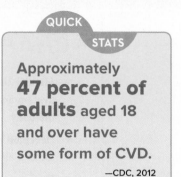

Monitoring blood pressure is a key strategy for the prevention of CVD. Blood pressure can be measured during a health care visit, at home with a home blood pressure monitor, or at a drugstore.

TERMS

vena cava   Either of two large veins (superior vena cava and inferior vena cava) through which blood is returned to the right atrium of the heart (plural, *venae cavae*).

atrium   Either of the two upper chambers of the heart in which blood collects before passing to the ventricles (plural, *atria).*

ventricle   Either of the two lower chambers of the heart that pump blood to the lungs and other parts of the body.

aorta   The largest artery in the body that receives blood from the left ventricle and distributes it to the body.

systole   The contraction phase of the heart.

diastole   The relaxation phase of the heart.

vein   A vessel that carries blood to the heart.

artery   A vessel that carries blood away from the heart.

capillary   A small blood vessel that exchanges oxygen and nutrients between the blood and the tissues.

coronary artery   One of the system of arteries branching from the aorta that provides blood to the heart muscle.

Some risk factors are linked to controllable aspects of lifestyle and can therefore be changed, referred to as modifiable risk factors. Others are beyond our control.

Modifiable Risk Factors

The American Heart Association (AHA) has identified five major risk factors for CVD that can be changed: tobacco use, high blood pressure, poor diet, physical inactivity, and diabetes. Most Americans, including young adults, have at least one major risk factor for CVD.

Tobacco Use Nearly one in five deaths is attributable to smoking. People who smoke a pack of cigarettes a day have twice the risk of heart attack as nonsmokers; smoking two or more packs a day triples the risk. When smokers have heart attacks, they are two to three times more likely than nonsmokers to die from them. Cigarette smoking also doubles the risk of stroke.

Smoking harms the cardiovascular system in the following ways. It damages the lining of arteries. It reduces the level of high-density lipoproteins (HDL), or "good" cholesterol and raises the levels of triglycerides and low-density lipoproteins (LDL), or "bad" cholesterol. Nicotine increases blood pressure and heart rate. The carbon monoxide in cigarette smoke displaces oxygen in the blood, reducing the amount of oxygen available to the body. Smoking causes **platelets** to stick together in the bloodstream, leading to clotting, and it speeds the development of fatty deposits in the arteries.

You don't have to smoke to be affected. The risk of developing heart disease increases up to 30% among those exposed to environmental tobacco smoke (ETS), also known as second-hand smoke, at home or at work. Researchers estimate that nearly 46,000 nonsmokers die from heart disease each year as a result of exposure to ETS.

High Blood Pressure High blood pressure, or **hypertension,** is a risk factor for many forms of cardiovascular disease, including heart attacks and strokes.

Blood pressure, the force exerted by the blood on the vessel walls, is created by the pumping action of the heart. High blood pressure occurs when too much force is exerted against

the walls of the arteries. Many factors affect blood pressure, such as exercise or excitement. Short periods of high blood pressure are normal, but chronic high blood pressure is a health risk.

Health care professionals measure blood pressure with a stethoscope and an instrument called a *sphygmomanometer.* Blood pressure is expressed as two numbers—for example, 120 over 80—and measured in millimeters of mercury (mm Hg). The first number is the *systolic* blood pressure; the second is the *diastolic* blood pressure. A normal blood pressure reading for a healthy adult is below 120 systolic and below 80 diastolic. CVD risk increases when blood pressure rises above that level. High blood pressure in adults is defined as equal to or greater than 140 over 90 mm Hg (Table 12.1).

In about 90% of people with high blood pressure, the underlying cause is unknown. This type of high blood pressure is called *primary* (or *essential*) *hypertension,* and is probably due to a combination of genetic and environmental factors, including obesity, stress, excessive alcohol intake, inactivity, and a high-fat, high-salt diet. In the remaining 10% of people, the condition is caused by an identifiable underlying illness, and is referred to as *secondary*

> **TERMS**
>
> **platelets** Cells in the blood that are necessary for the formation of blood clots.
>
> **hypertension** Sustained abnormally high blood pressure.

Table 12.1	Blood Pressure Classification for Healthy Adults		
CATEGORY[a]	SYSTOLIC (mm Hg)		DIASTOLIC (mm Hg)
Normal[b]	below 120	and	below 80
Prehypertension	120–139	or	80–89
Hypertension[c]			
Stage 1	140–159	or	90–99
Stage 2	160 and above	or	100 and above

[a]When systolic and diastolic pressure fall into different categories, the higher category should be used to classify blood pressure status.
[b]The risk of death from heart attack and stroke begins to rise when blood pressure is above 115/75.
[c]Based on the average of two or more readings taken at different physician visits. In people older than 50, systolic blood pressure greater than 140 is a much more significant CVD risk factor than diastolic blood pressure.

SOURCE: National Heart, Lung, and Blood Institute. 2011. *The Seventh Report of the Joint National Committee on Prevention, Detection, Evaluation, and Treatment of High Blood Pressure.* Bethesda, MD: National Heart, Lung, and Blood Institute. National Institutes of Health (NIH Publication No. 03-5233). These guidelines are under development according to the NIH National Heart, Lung, and Blood Institute (www.nhlbi.nih.gov/guidelines/current.htm, accessed June 2, 2014).

Ask Yourself

QUESTIONS FOR CRITICAL THINKING AND REFLECTION

How often do you think about the health of your heart? Are there certain situations that make you aware of your heart rate, or make you wonder how strong your heart is?

hypertension. Although hypertension often cannot be cured, it can be managed with lifestyle changes and medications.

CAUSES   High blood pressure results from an increased output of blood by the heart or from increased resistance to blood flow in the arteries. The latter condition can be caused by constriction of smooth muscle surrounding the arteries or by **atherosclerosis,** a disease process that causes arteries to become clogged and narrowed. Atherosclerosis also scars and hardens arteries, making them less elastic and further increasing blood pressure. When a person has high blood pressure, the heart must work harder than normal to force blood through the narrowed and stiffened arteries, straining both the heart and the arteries.

High blood pressure is often called a "silent killer" because it usually has no symptoms. A person may have high blood pressure for years without realizing it. But during that time, it slowly damages vital organs and increases the risk of heart attack, congestive heart failure, stroke, kidney failure, and blindness.

Recent research has shed new light on the importance of lowering blood pressure to improve cardiovascular health. The risk of death from heart attack or stroke begin to rise when blood pressure is above 115 over 75 mm Hg, well below the traditional 140 over 90 mm Hg cutoff for a diagnosis of hypertension. People with blood pressure in this lower range, referred to as "prehypertension," are at increased risk of heart attack and stroke as well as at significant risk of developing full-blown hypertension.

PREVALENCE   Hypertension is common. About 31% of adults have hypertension, and 30% have prehypertension (defined as systolic pressure of 120–139 and/or diastolic pressure of 80–89 mm Hg). The incidence of high blood pressure increases with age, but it does occur among children and young adults. Women can sometimes develop hypertension during pregnancy (the blood pressure will usually return to normal following pregnancy). The rate of hypertension is highest in African Americans (43–46%). Among African Americans, compared with other groups, the disorder is often more severe, more resistant to treatment, and more likely to be fatal at an early age.

TREATMENT   Hypertension cannot be cured, but it can be controlled. Because hypertension has no early warning signs, it's crucial to have your blood pressure tested at least once every two years (and more often if you have other CVD risk factors). In fact, experts now advise that anyone with hypertension or prehypertension monitor their own blood pressure several times each week.

Lifestyle changes are recommended for everyone with prehypertension and hypertension. These changes include weight reduction, regular exercise, a healthy diet, and moderation of alcohol use. The DASH diet is recommended specifically for people with high blood pressure.

Sodium restriction is also helpful for most people with hypertension. The 2010 Dietary Guidelines for Americans recommend restricting sodium consumption to less than 2300 mg per day and to less than 1500 mg per day for people with hypertension, African Americans, and middle-aged and older adults.

For people whose blood pressure is not adequately controlled with lifestyle changes, medication can be prescribed.

High Cholesterol   *Cholesterol* is a fatty, waxlike substance that circulates through the bloodstream. It is an important component of cell membranes, sex hormones, vitamin D, the fluid that coats the lungs, and the protective sheaths around nerves. Adequate cholesterol is essential for the proper functioning of the body. Excess cholesterol, however, can clog arteries and increase the risk of CVD. There are two primary sources of cholesterol: the liver, which manufactures it, and dietary sources.

GOOD VERSUS BAD CHOLESTEROL   Cholesterol is carried in the blood in protein-and-lipid packages called **lipoproteins. Low-density lipoproteins (LDLs)** (26 nm) shuttle cholesterol from the liver to the organs and tissues that require it. LDL is known as "bad" cholesterol because if there is more than the body can use, the excess is deposited in the blood vessels. If coronary arteries are blocked, the result may be a heart attack; if an artery carrying blood to the brain is blocked, a stroke may occur. **High-density lipoproteins (HDLs),** or "good" cholesterol, are the smallest of the lipoproteins (6–12.5 nm). They shuttle unused cholesterol back to the liver for recycling. By removing cholesterol from blood vessels, HDL helps protect against atherosclerosis.

BLOOD CHOLESTEROL GUIDELINES   The risk for cardiovascular disease increases with higher blood cholesterol levels, especially LDL. The National Cholesterol Education Program (NCEP) recommends lipoprotein testing at least once every five years for all adults, beginning at age 20. The recommended test measures total cholesterol, LDL cholesterol, HDL cholesterol, and triglycerides (another blood fat). In general, high LDL, total cholesterol, and triglyceride levels, combined with low HDL levels, are associated with a higher risk for CVD. You can reduce this risk by

---

TERMS

atherosclerosis   A form of CVD in which the inner layers of artery walls are made thick and irregular by plaque deposits; arteries become narrow and blood supply can be reduced.

lipoproteins   Protein and lipid substances in the blood that carry fats and cholesterol; classified according to size, density, and chemical composition.

low-density lipoprotein (LDL)   A lipoprotein containing a moderate amount of protein and a large amount of cholesterol, which tends to become deposited on artery walls and increase the risk of heart disease; also known as "bad" cholesterol.

high-density lipoprotein (HDL)   A lipoprotein containing relatively little cholesterol that helps transport cholesterol out of the arteries and thus protects against heart diseases; also known as "good" cholesterol.

lowering LDL, total cholesterol, and triglycerides. Raising HDL is important because a high HDL level seems to offer protection from CVD even in cases where total cholesterol is high. This appears to be especially true for women.

In 2013 the American College of Cardiology (ACC) and the AHA released updated guidelines on the treatment of high blood cholesterol. These new guidelines suggest assessing a person's risk of developing cardiovascular disease over the next 10 years, and treating this level. The ACC and AHA identified four groups of people who would benefit from treatment of high blood cholesterol levels (see Table 12.2).

The updated cholesterol guidelines have been controversial because they have eliminated the previous guidelines for targeting specific levels of LDL and HDL based on people's individual risk. Rather than target specific LDL and HDL levels, the new guidelines suggest statin therapy administered at different intensity doses. *Statins* are cholesterol-lowering medications. *High-intensity* therapy is defined as a statin dosage that reduces the LDL level by greater than or equal to 50%, whereas *moderate-intensity* therapy reduces LDL level by 30–50%. These medications dramatically reduce the risk

> Exercise is thought to be **the closest thing we have to a magic bullet** against heart disease.

of CVD in individuals with high cholesterol levels, and may even decrease CVD risk in those without high cholesterol levels.

BENEFITS OF CONTROLLING CHOLESTEROL People can cut their heart attack risk by about 2% for every 1% that they reduce their total blood cholesterol levels. Previous studies have shown that people who treat their high total cholesterol can reduce their risk of heart attack by 40%. Your primary goal should be to reduce your LDL to healthy levels.

Physical Inactivity An estimated 40–60 million Americans are so sedentary that they are at high risk for developing CVD. Exercise is thought to be the closest thing we have to a "magic bullet" to fight against heart disease. It lowers CVD risk by helping to decrease blood pressure and resting heart rate, increase HDL levels, maintain desirable weight, improve the condition of blood vessels, and prevent or control diabetes. One study found that women who accumulated at least three hours of brisk walking each week cut their risk of heart attack and stroke by more than 50%.

Obesity Death from CVD is two to three times more likely in obese people (body mass index, or BMI ≥ 30) than it is in lean people (BMI 18.5–24.9), and for every 5-unit increase in BMI, a person's risk of death from coronary heart disease increases by 30%.

Excess body fat is strongly associated with hypertension, high cholesterol levels, insulin resistance, diabetes, physical inactivity, and increasing age. With excess weight, there is also more blood to pump and the heart has to work harder. This causes chronically elevated pressures within the heart chambers that can lead to ventricular **hypertrophy** (enlargement). Eventually the heart muscle can start to fail, known as congestive heart failure.

Diabetes As described in Chapter 11, *diabetes mellitus* is a disorder characterized by elevated blood glucose levels due to an insufficient supply or inadequate action of insulin. Diabetes doubles the risk of CVD for men and triples the risk for women. The most common cause of death in adults with diabetes is CVD.

People with diabetes have higher rates of other CVD risk factors, including hypertension, obesity, and unhealthy blood lipid levels (typically, high triglyceride levels and low HDL levels). The elevated blood glucose and insulin levels that occur in diabetes can damage the endothelial cells that line the arteries, making them more vulnerable to atherosclerosis.

Table 12.2

Groups Who Benefit from Treatment of High Cholesterol

1. **People with known cardiovascular disease**, including previous heart attacks, chest pain due to partially clogged arteries, history of invasive treatment for clogged arteries, previous stroke, or previous clogged arteries in the limbs. These patients cannot have a history of heart failure or kidney failure.
2. **People with high LDL levels, above 190 mg/dL.**
3. **People ages 40–75 with a history of diabetes**, and an LDL level 70–189 mg/dL. These patients cannot have a known history of cardiovascular disease.
4. **People ages 40–75 without diabetes or known cardiovascular disease** but with a high risk of developing it over the next 10 years and an LDL level over 70 mg/dL.*

*10-year cardiovascular risk is calculated using a new tool available on the AHA website:

http://my.americanheart.org/professional/StatementsGuidelines /PreventionGuidelines/Prevention-Guidelines_UCM_457698 _SubHomePage.jsp

SOURCE: Stone, N. J., et al. 2013. ACC/AHA Guideline on the treatment of blood cholesterol to reduce atherosclerotic cardiovascular risk in adults. A report of the American College of Cardiology/American Heart Association Task Force on Practice Guidelines. *Journal of the American College of Cardiology.*

hypertrophy Abnormal enlargement of an organ. TERMS

Diabetics also often have platelet and blood coagulation abnormalities that increase the risk of heart attack and stroke. People with prediabetes (when the blood sugar levels are elevated, but not high enough to diagnose diabetes) also face a significantly increased risk of CVD.

In people with prediabetes, a healthy diet and exercise are more effective than medication at preventing diabetes. For people with diabetes, a healthy diet, exercise, and careful control of glucose levels are recommended to reduce the chances of developing complications. Even people whose diabetes is under control face a high risk of CVD, so control of other risk factors is critical.

Contributing Risk Factors That Can Be Changed

Other CVD risk factors that can be changed include triglyceride levels and psychological and social factors.

High Triglyceride Levels   Like cholesterol, **triglycerides** are blood fats that are obtained from food and manufactured by the body. High triglyceride levels are a reliable predictor of heart disease, especially if associated with other risk factors, such as low HDL levels, obesity, and diabetes. Factors contributing to elevated triglyceride levels include excess body fat, physical inactivity, cigarette smoking, type 2 diabetes, excessive alcohol intake, very high-carbohydrate diets, and certain diseases and medications.

A full lipid profile should include testing and evaluation of triglyceride levels (see Table 12.2). For people with borderline high triglyceride levels, increased physical activity, reduced intake of added sugars, and weight reduction can help bring levels down into the healthy range. For people with high triglyceride levels, drug therapy may be recommended if initial strategies are ineffective. Moderating alcohol intake and avoiding use of tobacco products are also important.

Insulin Resistance and Metabolic Syndrome   As people gain weight and become less active, their muscles, fat, and liver become less sensitive to the effect of insulin—a condition known as *insulin resistance* (or prediabetes). As the body becomes increasingly insulin resistant, the pancreas must secrete more and more insulin (hyperinsulinemia) to keep glucose levels within a normal range. Eventually even high levels of insulin may become insufficient, and blood glucose levels start to rise (hyperglycemia), resulting in type 2 diabetes.

Those who have insulin resistance tend to have several other related risk factors. This cluster of abnormalities is called *metabolic syndrome* or *insulin resistance syndrome* (Table 12.3).

Table 12.3	Defining Characteristics of Metabolic Syndrome*	
Abdominal obesity (waist circumference)		
Men	>40 in (>102 cm)	
Women	>35 in (>88 cm)	
Triglycerides	≥150 mg/dl	
HDL cholesterol		
Men	< 40 mg/dl or drug-treated	
Women	< 50 mg/dl or drug-treated	
Blood pressure	≥ 130/≥ 85 mmHg or drug-treated	
Fasting glucose	≥ 100 mg/dl or drug-treated	

*A person is diagnosed with metabolic syndrome if she or he has three or more of the risk factors listed here.

SOURCE: Adapted with permission of the American Heart Association from Table 2. Grundy, S. M., et al. 2005. Diagnosis and management of the metabolic syndrome: An American Heart Association/National Heart, Lung, and Blood Institute scientific statement. *Circulation* 112: 2735.

Metabolic syndrome significantly increases the risk of CVD—more so in women than in men. It is estimated that about 34% of the adult U.S. population has metabolic syndrome.

To reduce your risk of developing metabolic syndrome, choose a healthy diet and get plenty of aerobic exercise. Reducing calorie intake to prevent weight gain or losing weight if needed also reduces insulin resistance. Eating more protein, vegetables, and fiber while limiting fat, added sugars, and starches may be beneficial.

Psychological and Social Factors   Many of the psychological and social factors that influence other areas of wellness are also important risk factors for CVD.

STRESS   Excessive stress can strain the heart and blood vessels over time and contribute to CVD (see Figure 12.1). If you are healthy, you can tolerate the cardiovascular responses that take place during stress. But if you already have CVD, stress can lead to adverse outcomes such as abnormal heart rhythms (arrhythmias) and heart attacks.

CHRONIC HOSTILITY AND ANGER   Certain traits in the hard-driving "Type A" personality—hostility, cynicism, and anger—are associated with increased risk of heart disease.

SUPPRESSING PSYCHOLOGICAL DISTRESS   Consistently suppressing anger and other negative emotions may also be hazardous to a healthy heart. People who hide psychological distress appear to have higher rates of heart disease than people who experience similar distress but share it with others.

DEPRESSION   Depression appears to increase the risk of CVD in healthy people, and it definitely increases the risk of adverse cardiac events in those who already have heart disease.

---

triglyceride   A type of blood fat that can be a predictor of heart disease.

TERMS

FIGURE 12.1 **The effects of stress and emotions on the cardiovascular system.**

SOURCE: Adapted from Rozanski, A, et al. 1999. Impact of psychological factors on the pathogenesis of cardiovascular disease and implications for therapy. *Circulation* 99: 2192–2217.

The relationship between depression and CHD is complex and not fully understood. Depressed people may be more likely to smoke or be sedentary. They may not consistently take prescribed medications, and they may not cope well with having an illness or undergoing a medical procedure. Depression also causes physiological changes; for example, it elevates basal levels of stress hormones, which induce a variety of stress-related responses.

ANXIETY Chronic anxiety and anxiety disorders (such as phobias and panic disorder) are associated with up to a three-fold increased risk of coronary heart disease, heart attack, and sudden cardiac death. People with anxiety are more likely to have a subsequent adverse cardiac event after having a heart attack.

SOCIAL ISOLATION Social isolation and low social support (living alone, or having few friends or family members) are associated with an increased incidence of CHD and poorer outcomes after the first diagnosis of CHD. A strong social support network is a major antidote to stress. Friends and family members can also promote and support a healthy lifestyle.

LOW SOCIOECONOMIC STATUS Low socioeconomic status and low educational attainment are also associated with an increased risk of CVD. These associations are complex and likely due to a variety of factors, including lifestyle, diet, and access to health care, among others.

Alcohol and Drugs Although moderate drinking may have health benefits for some people, drinking alcohol in excess raises blood pressure and can increase the risk of stroke and heart failure. Stimulant drugs, particularly cocaine and methamphetamines—and associated stimulants, such as designer drugs including ecstasy (MDMA)—can also cause serious cardiac problems, including heart attack, stroke, and sudden cardiac death. Injection drug use can cause heart infections and stroke.

Major Risk Factors That Can't Be Changed

A number of major risk factors for CVD cannot be changed. These include family history of CVD (heredity), aging, male gender, and ethnicity.

Heredity Multiple genes contribute to the development of CVD and its associated risk factors, such as high cholesterol, hypertension, diabetes, and obesity. Having a favorable set of genes decreases your risk of developing CVD; having an unfavorable set of genes increases your risk. Risk, however, may be modified by lifestyle factors.

Aging About 70% of all heart attack victims are age 65 or older, and about 75% who suffer fatal heart attacks are over 65. For people over 55, the incidence of stroke more than doubles in each successive decade. However, even people in their thirties and forties, especially men, can have heart attacks.

Gender Although CVD is the leading killer of both men and women in the United States, men face a greater risk of heart attack than women, especially earlier in life. Until age 55, men also have a greater risk of hypertension. The incidence of stroke is also higher for males than females, until age 65. By age 75, however, this gender gap nearly disappears.

Ethnicity Rates of heart disease vary among ethnic groups in the United States, with African Americans having much higher rates of hypertension, heart disease, and stroke than other groups (see the box "Gender, Ethnicity, and CVD"). Puerto Rican Americans, Cuban Americans, and Mexican Americans are also more likely to suffer from high blood pressure and angina (a warning sign of blocked coronary arteries) than non-Hispanic white Americans. Asian Americans historically have had far lower rates of CVD than white Americans.

DIVERSITY MATTERS
Gender, Ethnicity, and CVD

CVD is the leading cause of death for all Americans, but significant differences exist between men and women and between white Americans and African Americans in the incidence, diagnosis, and treatment of this deadly disease.

CVD in Women

CVD has been thought of as a "man's disease," but it actually kills more women than men. Polls indicate that women vastly underestimate their risk of dying of a heart attack and overestimate their risk of dying of breast cancer. In reality, nearly one in three women dies of CVD, whereas one in 34 dies of breast cancer. And although CVD typically does not develop in women younger than age 50, recent research suggests that the number of CVD deaths in women age 35–45 may be increasing.

The hormone estrogen, produced naturally by a woman's ovaries until menopause, improves blood lipid concentrations and reduces other CVD risk factors. For several decades, many physicians encouraged menopausal women to take hormone replacement therapy (HRT), which includes estrogen, to relieve menopause symptoms and presumably to reduce their risk of CVD. However, some studies found that HRT may actually *increase* a woman's risk for heart disease.

Women presenting with CVD are less likely than men to report chest pain, and are also likely to report other symptoms, which may obscure their diagnosis. These additional symptoms include fatigue, weakness, shortness of breath, nausea, vomiting, and pain in the abdomen, neck, jaw, and back. Women are also more likely to have pain at rest, during sleep, or with mental stress.

Women should be aware of their CVD risk factors and consult with a physician to assess their risk and determine the best way to prevent CVD.

CVD in African Americans

African Americans are at substantially higher risk of death from CVD than other groups. The rate of hypertension among African Americans is among the highest of any ethnic group in the world. African Americans tend to develop hypertension at an earlier age than Caucasian Americans, and their average blood pressures are much higher. African Americans have a higher risk of stroke, have strokes at younger ages and, if they survive, have more significant stroke-related disabilities. Some experts recommend that blacks be treated with antihypertensive drugs when blood pressure reaches 130/80 rather than the typical 140/90 cutoff for hypertension.

A number of genetic and biological factors may contribute to CVD in African Americans. They may be more sensitive to dietary sodium, leading to greater blood pressure elevation in response to a given amount of sodium. African Americans may also experience less dilation of blood vessels in response to stress, an attribute that also raises blood pressure.

Heredity also plays a large role in the tendency to develop diabetes, another important CVD risk factor that is more common in blacks than whites. However, Latinos are even more likely to develop diabetes and insulin resistance, and at a younger age, than African Americans. There is variation within the Latino population, however; a higher prevalence of diabetes occurs among Mexican Americans and Puerto Ricans and a relatively lower prevalence among Cuban Americans.

Low income, which usually means reduced access to health care, is another factor that likely contributes to the high incidence of CVD among ethnic minority groups.

Discrimination may also play a role in CVD. Physicians and hospitals may treat the medical problems of ethnic minorities differently than those of Caucasians. Discrimination, low income, and other forms of deprivation may also increase stress, which is linked with hypertension and CVD. Lack of access to care, such as insurance coverage and availability of high-tech cardiac equipment in hospitals that serve minorities, may also play a role.

All Americans, regardless of ethnicity, are advised to have their blood pressure checked regularly, exercise on a regular basis, eat a healthy diet, manage stress, and avoid tobacco products. Tailoring your lifestyle to your particular ethnic risk may also be helpful in some cases. Discuss your particular risk profile with your physician to help identify the lifestyle changes most appropriate for you.

Inflammation   Inflammation plays a key role in the development of CVD. When an artery is injured by hypertension, smoking, cholesterol, or other factors, the body's response is to produce inflammation. A substance called *C-reactive protein (CRP)* is released into the bloodstream during the inflammatory response, and high levels of CRP indicate a substantially elevated risk of heart attack and stroke. It has also been proposed that CRP may harm the coronary arteries. Gum disease involves another type of inflammation that may moderately influence the progress of coronary heart disease.

Possible Risk Factors Currently Being Studied

In recent years other possible risk factors for cardiovascular disease have been identified. Elevated levels of homocysteine, an amino acid circulating in the blood, are associated with an increased risk of CVD. Homocysteine appears to damage the lining of blood vessels, resulting in inflammation and the development of fatty deposits in artery walls. These changes can lead to the formation of clots and blockages in arteries, which in turn can cause heart attacks and strokes.

Several infectious agents have been identified as possible culprits in the development of CVD. *Chlamydia pneumoniae,* a common cause of flulike respiratory infections, has been found in sections of clogged, damaged arteries but not in sections of healthy arteries. This effect may be secondary to the inflammation that many of these infectious agents produce in the body.

Other factors currently under investigation include a particular type of LDL called lipoprotein(a), blood levels of iron, and blood levels of uric acid.

MAJOR FORMS OF CARDIOVASCULAR DISEASE

According to the CDC, heart diseases killed approximately 596,000 Americans in 2011. Figure 12.2 shows the death rates among various ethnic groups due to heart disease in 2008, the most recent year for which data are available.

The main forms of CVD are atherosclerosis, coronary artery disease and heart attack, stroke, peripheral arterial disease (PAD), congestive heart failure, congenital heart disease, rheumatic heart disease, and heart valve problems. Many forms are interrelated and have elements in common; we treat them separately here for the sake of clarity. Hypertension, which is both a major risk factor and a form of CVD, was described earlier in the chapter.

Atherosclerosis

Atherosclerosis is a form of arteriosclerosis, or thickening and hardening of the arteries. In atherosclerosis, arteries become narrowed by deposits of fat, cholesterol, and other

substances (see page T2-4 of the color transparency insert "Touring the Cardiorespiratory System"). The process begins when the endothelial cells (cells that line the arteries) become damaged, most likely through a combination of factors such as smoking, high blood pressure, high insulin or glucose levels, and deposits of oxidized LDL particles. The body's response to this damage results in inflammation and changes in the artery lining that create a magnet for LDL, platelets, and other cells. These cells build up and cause a bulge in the wall of the artery. As these deposits, called **plaques,** accumulate in artery walls, the arteries lose their elasticity and their ability to expand and contract, restricting blood flow. Once narrowed by a plaque, an artery is vulnerable to blockage by blood clots.

If the heart, brain, or other organs are deprived of blood and the oxygen it carries, the effects of atherosclerosis can be deadly. Coronary arteries, which supply the heart with blood, are particularly susceptible to plaque buildup, a condition called **coronary heart disease (CHD)** or *coronary artery disease (CAD).* The blockage of a coronary artery causes a heart attack, and blockage of a cerebral artery (leading to the brain) causes a stroke. Blockage of an artery in a limb causes *peripheral arterial disease,* a condition that causes pain and may require amputation of the affected limb.

The main risk factors for atherosclerosis are tobacco use or abuse, physical inactivity, high blood cholesterol levels, high blood pressure, and diabetes. Atherosclerosis often begins in childhood: Autopsy studies of young trauma victims have revealed atherosclerosis of the coronary arteries in adolescents.

Coronary Artery Disease and Heart Attack

The most common form of heart disease is coronary artery disease caused by atherosclerosis. When one of the coronary arteries becomes blocked, the result is a **heart attack,** or *myocardial infarction (MI).* Although a heart attack may come without warning, it usually results from a chronic disease process.

Heart attack symptoms may include chest pain or pressure; arm, neck, or jaw pain; difficulty breathing; excessive sweating; nausea and vomiting; and loss of consciousness. Most people having a heart attack suffer chest pain, but about one-third of heart attack victims do not. Women, ethnic minorities, older adults, and people with diabetes are the most likely groups to experience heart attacks without chest pain.

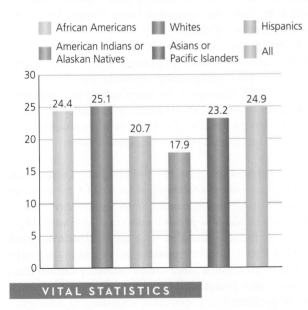

VITAL STATISTICS

FIGURE 12.2 **Percentage of deaths due to heart disease, by ethnic group.**

SOURCE: Heron, M. 2012. Deaths: Leading causes for 2008. *National Vital Statistics Reports* 60(6).

Legend:
- African Americans
- American Indians or Alaskan Natives
- Whites
- Asians or Pacific Islanders
- Hispanics
- All

Values: 24.4, 25.1, 20.7, 17.9, 23.2, 24.9

plaque   A deposit of fatty (and other) substances on the inner wall of an artery.   TERMS

coronary heart disease (CHD)   Heart disease caused by atherosclerosis in the arteries that supply blood to the heart muscle; also called *coronary artery disease (CAD).*

heart attack   Damage to, or death of, heart muscle, resulting from a failure of the coronary arteries to deliver enough blood to the heart; also known as *myocardial infarction (MI).*

Angina   Arteries narrowed by disease may still be open enough to deliver sufficient amounts of oxygenated blood to the heart. At times, however—during stress or exertion, for example—the heart needs more oxygen than can flow through narrowed arteries. When the need for oxygen exceeds the supply, chest pain, called **angina pectoris,** may occur. Angina pain is usually felt as an extreme tightness in the chest and heavy pressure behind the breastbone or in the shoulder, neck, arm, hand, or back.

Angina may be controlled in a number of ways (with drugs and surgical or nonsurgical procedures), but its course is unpredictable. Over a period ranging from hours to years, the narrowing may go on to full blockage and a heart attack.

Arrhythmias and Sudden Cardiac Death   The pumping of the heart is controlled by electrical impulses from the sinus node that maintain a regular heartbeat of 60–100 beats per minute. If this electrical conduction system is disrupted, the heart may beat too quickly, too slowly, or in an irregular fashion—a condition known as an **arrhythmia.** Arrhythmias can cause symptoms ranging from imperceptible to severe and even fatal.

Sudden cardiac death, also called *cardiac arrest,* is most often caused by an arrhythmia called *ventricular fibrillation,* a kind of quivering of the ventricle that makes it ineffective in pumping blood. If ventricular fibrillation continues for more than a few minutes, it is generally fatal. Cardiac defibrillation, in which an electrical shock is delivered to the heart, can be effective in jolting the heart into a more efficient rhythm. Training in the use of AEDs is available from organizations such as the American Red Cross and the American Heart Association.

Helping a Heart Attack Victim   Most deaths from heart attacks occur within two hours of the first onset of symptoms. Unfortunately, however, many heart attack victims wait more than two hours before getting help. If you

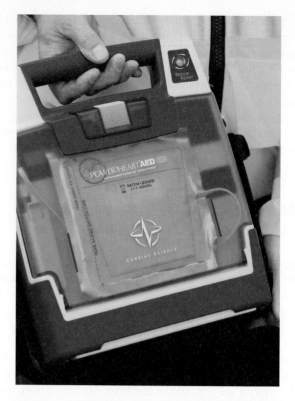

Automated external defibrillators can save the lives of individuals experiencing sudden cardiac arrest. AEDs are becoming more common in public places.

or someone you are with has any of the warning signs of heart attack listed in the box "What to Do in Case of a Heart Attack, Stroke, or Cardiac Arrest," take immediate action. Call for help—even if the person denies there is something wrong. Many experts also suggest that the heart attack victim *chew* and swallow one adult aspirin tablet (325 mg) as soon as possible after symptoms begin. Aspirin has an immediate anticlotting effect.

If the victim loses consciousness, a qualified person should immediately check for a pulse and start administering emergency **cardiopulmonary resuscitation (CPR)** if no pulse is found. Damage to the heart muscle increases with time. If the person receives emergency care quickly enough, a clot-dissolving agent or emergency invasive procedure can be used to break up the clot in the coronary artery.

Detecting and Treating Heart Disease   Currently the most common initial screening tool for CAD is the stress, or exercise, test. During an exercise stress test, a patient runs or walks on a treadmill or pedals a stationary cycle while being monitored for abnormalities with an **electrocardiogram (ECG or EKG).** Certain characteristic changes in the heart's electrical activity while under stress can reveal particular heart problems, such as restricted blood flow. Exercise testing can also be performed in conjunction with imaging techniques that provide pictures of the heart, which can help pinpoint abnormal areas of the heart. Imaging techniques include echocardiography, **magnetic resonance imaging (MRI),** and positron emission tomography (PET), among others.

angina pectoris   Pain in the chest, and often in the left arm and shoulder, caused by the heart muscle not receiving enough oxygenated blood. The pain is usually brought on by exercise or stress.

arrhythmia   A change in the heartbeat's normal, regular pattern.

sudden cardiac death   A nontraumatic, unexpected death from sudden cardiac arrest, most often due to arrhythmia; in most instances, victims have underlying heart disease.

cardiopulmonary resuscitation (CPR)   A technique involving mouth-to-mouth breathing and/or chest compressions to keep oxygen flowing to the brain.

electrocardiogram (ECG or EKG)   A test to detect cardiac abnormalities by evaluating the electrical activity in the heart.

magnetic resonance imaging (MRI)   A computerized imaging technique that uses a strong magnetic field to create detailed pictures of body structures.

TERMS

What to Do in Case of a Heart Attack, Stroke, or Cardiac Arrest

Warning Signs of Heart Attack

Some heart attacks are obvious, sudden, and intense—think of the "movie heart attack," where no one doubts what's happening. However, most heart attacks instead start slowly, with only mild pain or discomfort. Often people affected aren't sure what's wrong and wait too long before getting help. Here are signs that can mean a heart attack is happening:

- **Chest discomfort:** Heart attacks often involve discomfort in the chest that lasts more than a few minutes, or that goes away and comes back. It can feel like uncomfortable pressure, squeezing, fullness, or pain.

- **Discomfort in other areas of the upper body:** Symptoms can include pain or discomfort in one or both arms, the back, neck, jaw, or stomach.

- **Shortness of breath:** May occur with or without chest discomfort.

- **Other signs:** These may include breaking out in a cold sweat, nausea, vomiting, or lightheadedness.

Not all of the signs described above occur in every heart attack. As with men, women most commonly experience chest pain or discomfort, but are somewhat more likely than men to experience some of the other more vague symptoms, particularly shortness of breath, nausea/vomiting, and back or jaw pain.

If you or someone you're with has chest discomfort, especially with one or more of the other signs, don't wait longer than a few minutes (no more than five) before calling for help.

Calling 911 is almost always the fastest way to get lifesaving treatment. Emergency medical services staff can begin treatment when they arrive—up to an hour sooner than if someone gets to the hospital by car. The staff are also trained to revive someone whose heart has stopped. Patients with chest pain who arrive by ambulance usually receive faster treatment at the hospital, too. Today medications and treatments are available that weren't available in the past, but they must be given relatively quickly after the heart attack to be effective.

If you can't access emergency medical services (EMS), have someone drive you to the hospital right away. If you're the one having symptoms, don't drive yourself unless you have absolutely no other option.

Warning Signs of Stroke

- Sudden numbness or weakness of the face, arm, or leg, especially on one side of the body

- Sudden confusion or trouble speaking or understanding.

- Sudden trouble seeing in one or both eyes.

- Sudden trouble walking, dizziness, or loss of balance or coordination.

- Sudden severe headache with no known cause.

If you or someone with you has one or more of these signs, don't delay! Immediately call 911 or the emergency medical services (EMS) number so an ambulance (ideally with advanced life support) can be sent for you. Also, check the time so you'll know when the first symptoms appeared. It's very important to take immediate action. If given within three hours of the start of symptoms, a clot-busting drug called tissue plasminogen activator (tPA) can reduce long-term disability for the most common type of stroke. tPA is the only FDA-approved medication for the treatment of stroke within three hours of symptom onset.

Signs of Cardiac Arrest

Cardiac arrest strikes immediately and without warning. Here are the signs:

- Sudden loss of responsiveness.

- No response to tapping on the shoulders.

- No normal breathing. The victim does not take a normal breath when you tilt the head up and check for at least five seconds.

If these signs of cardiac arrest are present, tell someone to call 911 and to get an automated external defibrillator (AED) if one is available before you begin CPR. Use the AED as soon as it arrives.

SOURCE: Adapted from American Heart Association. 2014. *Warning Signs of Heart Attack, Stroke, & Cardiac Arrest* (http://www.heart.org /HEARTORG/Conditions/911-Warnings-Signs -of-a-Heart-Attack_UCM_305346_Sub HomePage.jsp). Copyright © 2007 American Heart Association. Reprinted with permission.

connect
ACTIVITY
DO IT ONLINE

If symptoms or noninvasive tests suggest coronary artery disease, the next step is usually a coronary **angiogram**, a test that can identify arterial narrowing or blockages. If a problem is found, it is commonly treated with **balloon angioplasty**, a procedure that opens the blocked artery.

Other treatments, ranging from medication to major surgery, are also available. Along with a low-fat diet, regular exercise, and smoking cessation, one frequent recommendation

TERMS

angiogram A picture of the arterial system taken after injecting a dye that is opaque to X-rays.

balloon angioplasty A technique in which a catheter with a deflated balloon on the tip is inserted into an artery; the balloon is then inflated at the point of obstruction in the artery, pressing the plaque against the artery wall to improve blood supply.

for people at intermediate to high risk for CVD is to take a low-dose (81 mg) aspirin tablet every day. Aspirin helps prevent platelets in the blood from sticking to arterial plaques and forming clots, and it also reduces inflammation. Prescription drugs can help control heart rate, dilate arteries, lower blood pressure, and reduce the strain on the heart—improving both the quality and length of life in heart patients. In patients with coronary artery disease, cholesterol-lowering statins are effective in preventing heart attacks; statins also have beneficial anti-inflammatory effects.

TERMS

stroke Impeded blood supply to some part of the brain resulting in the destruction of brain cells; also called a *cerebrovascular accident (CVA).*

ischemic stroke Impeded blood supply to the brain caused by a clot obstructing a blood vessel.

thrombus A blood clot in a blood vessel that usually remains at the point of its formation.

embolus A blood clot that breaks off from its place of origin in a blood vessel and travels through the bloodstream.

hemorrhagic stroke Impeded blood supply to the brain caused by the rupture of a blood vessel.

Stroke

A **stroke,** also called a *cerebrovascular accident (CVA),* occurs when the blood supply to the brain is cut off and brain tissue subsequently dies.

Types of Strokes

There are two major types of strokes (Figure 12.3).

ISCHEMIC STROKE An **ischemic stroke** is caused by a blockage in a blood vessel. There are two types of ischemic strokes. A *thrombotic stroke* is caused by a **thrombus,** which is a blood clot that forms in a cerebral or carotid artery that has been narrowed or damaged by atherosclerosis. An *embolic stroke* is caused by an **embolus,** which is a wandering blood clot that is carried in the bloodstream and may become wedged in a cerebral artery. Ischemic strokes account for 87% of all strokes.

HEMORRHAGIC STROKE A **hemorrhagic stroke** occurs when a blood vessel in the brain bursts, spilling blood into the surrounding tissue. Cells normally nourished by the vessel are deprived of blood and cannot function. In addition, accumulated blood from the burst vessel may put pressure on surrounding brain tissue, causing damage and even death. There are two types of hemorrhagic strokes. In an *intracerebral hemorrhage*, a blood vessel ruptures within the brain. About 10%

HEMORRHAGIC STROKE
- 13% of strokes.
- Caused by ruptured blood vessels followed by blood leaking into tissue.
- Usually more serious than ischemic stroke.

Subarachnoid hemorrhage
- A bleed into the space between the brain and the skull.
- Develops most often from an *aneurysm*, a weakened, ballooned area in the wall of an artery.

Intracerebral hemorrhage
- A bleed from a blood vessel inside the brain.
- Often caused by high blood pressure and the damage it does to arteries.

ISCHEMIC STROKE
- 87% of strokes.
- Caused by blockages in brain blood vessels; potentially treatable with clot-busting drugs.
- Brain tissue dies when blood flow is blocked.

Embolic stroke
- Caused by *emboli*, blood clots that travel from elsewhere in the body to the brain blood vessels.
- 25% of embolic strokes are related to atrial fibrillation.

Thrombotic stroke
- Caused by *thrombi*, blood clots that form where an artery has been narrowed by atherosclerosis.
- Most often develops when part of a thrombus breaks away and causes a blockage in a downstream artery.

FIGURE 12.3 Types of stroke.

SOURCE: Adopted from *Harvard Health Letter,* April 2000. Harvard University. Artwork by Harriet Greenfield, reprinted with permission.

of strokes are caused by intracerebral hemorrhages. In a *subarachnoid hemorrhage,* a blood vessel on the brain's surface ruptures and bleeds into the space between the brain and the skull. About 3% of strokes are of this type.

Hemorrhages can be caused by head injuries or the bursting of a malformed blood vessel, or **aneurysm,** which is a blood-filled pocket that bulges out from a weak spot in the artery wall. Aneurysms in the brain may remain stable and never break. But when they do, the result is a hemorrhagic stroke. Aneurysms may be caused or worsened by hypertension.

The Effects of a Stroke

The interruption of the blood supply to any area of the brain prevents the nerve cells there from functioning—in some cases causing death. Stroke survivors usually have some lasting disability. A stroke may cause paralysis, walking disability, speech impairment, memory loss, or changes in behavior. The severity of the stroke and how long the effects last depend on which brain cells have been injured, how widespread the damage is, how effectively the body can restore the blood supply, and how rapidly other areas of the brain can take over the functions of the damaged areas.

Detecting and Treating Stroke

Effective treatment requires the prompt recognition of symptoms and correct diagnosis of the type of stroke.

Many people have strokes without knowing it. These "silent strokes" do not cause any noticeable symptoms while they are occurring. Although they may be mild, silent strokes leave their victims at a higher risk for subsequent and more serious strokes. They also contribute to loss of mental and cognitive skills.

Some stroke victims have a **transient ischemic attack (TIA),** or "ministroke," days, weeks, or months before they have a full-blown stroke. A TIA produces temporary stroke-like symptoms, such as weakness or numbness in an arm or a leg, speech difficulty, or dizziness. These symptoms are brief, often lasting just a few minutes, and do not cause permanent damage. TIAs should be taken as warning signs of a stroke, however, and anyone with a suspected TIA should get immediate medical attention.

A person with stroke symptoms should be rushed to the hospital. A **computed tomography (CT)** scan, which uses a computer to construct an image of the brain from X-rays, can assess brain damage and determine the type of stroke. Newer techniques using MRI and ultrasound are becoming increasingly available and should improve the speed and accuracy of stroke diagnosis.

If tests reveal that a stroke is caused by a blood clot—and if help is sought within a few hours of the onset of symptoms—the person can be treated with the same kind of clot-dissolving drugs that are used to treat coronary artery blockages. If the clot is dissolved quickly enough, brain damage is minimized and symptoms may disappear.

If tests reveal that a stroke was caused by a cerebral hemorrhage, drugs may be prescribed to lower the blood pressure, which will usually be high. Careful diagnosis is crucial, because administering clot-dissolving drugs to a person suffering a hemorrhagic stroke could cause more bleeding and potentially more brain damage.

If detection and treatment of stroke come too late, rehabilitation and prevention of further events is the only treatment. Although damaged or destroyed brain tissue does not normally regenerate, nerve cells in the brain can make new pathways, and some functions can be taken over by other parts of the brain. Some spontaneous recovery starts immediately after a stroke and continues for a few months.

Some people recover completely in a matter of days or weeks, but most stroke victims who survive must adapt to some disability.

Peripheral Arterial Disease

Peripheral arterial disease (PAD) refers to atherosclerosis in the leg or arm arteries, which can eventually limit or completely obstruct blood flow. The same process that occurs in the heart arteries can occur in any artery of the body.

The risk of PAD is significantly increased in people with diabetes and people who use tobacco products. The likelihood of needing an amputation is increased in those who continue to use tobacco products, and PAD in people with diabetes tends to be extensive and severe.

Symptoms of PAD include claudication and rest pain. *Claudication* is aching or fatigue in the affected leg with exertion, particularly walking, which resolves with rest. Claudication occurs when leg muscles do not get adequate blood and oxygen supply. *Rest pain* occurs when the limb artery is unable to supply adequate blood and oxygen even when the body is not physically active. This occurs when the artery is significantly narrowed or completely blocked. PAD is the leading cause of amputation in people over age 50.

> The same disease process that occurs in the heart arteries can occur in any artery of the body.

Congestive Heart Failure

When the heart has been damaged by high blood pressure or other disease conditions and cannot maintain its regular pumping rate and

---

aneurysm   A sac formed by a distention or dilation TERMS of the artery wall.

transient ischemic attack (TIA)   A small stroke; usually a temporary interruption of blood supply to the brain, causing numbness or difficulty with speech.

computed tomography (CT)   The use of computerized X-ray images to create a cross-sectional depiction (scan) of tissue density.

peripheral arterial disease (PAD)   Atherosclerosis in the arteries in the legs (or less commonly, the arms) that can impede blood flow and lead to pain, infection, and loss of the affected limb.

force, fluid begins to back up. When extra fluid seeps through capillary walls, edema (swelling) results, usually in the legs and ankles, but sometimes in other parts of the body as well. Fluid can collect in the lungs and interfere with breathing, particularly when a person is lying down. This condition is called **pulmonary edema,** and the entire process is known as **congestive heart failure.**

Treatment includes reducing the workload on the heart, modifying salt intake, and using drugs that help the body eliminate excess fluid.

The risk of heart failure increases with age, and being overweight is a significant independent risk factor.

Other Forms of Heart Disease

Other, less common, disorders and diseases also affect the heart.

Congenital Heart Defects   About 40,000 children born each year in the United States have a defect or malformation of the heart or major blood vessels. These conditions are collectively referred to as **congenital heart defects,** and they cause about 3600 deaths a year. The most common congenital defects are holes in the wall that divides the chambers of the heart. Such defects cause the heart to produce a distinctive sound, making diagnosis relatively simple. Another common defect is *coarctation of the aorta—* a narrowing, or constriction, of the aorta. Most of the common congenital defects can now be accurately diagnosed and treated with medication or surgery.

Hypertrophic cardiomyopathy (HCM) occurs in approximately 1 out of every 600 people in the United States and is the most common cause of sudden death among athletes younger than age 35. It causes the heart muscle to become hypertrophic (enlarged). People with hypertrophic

cardiomyopathy are at high risk for sudden death, mainly due to serious arrhythmias. Hypertrophic cardiomyopathy may be identified by a **murmur** and diagnosed using echocardiography. Possible treatments include medication and a pacemaker or an internal defibrillator.

Rheumatic Heart Disease   **Rheumatic fever,** a consequence of certain types of untreated streptococcal throat infections, is a leading cause of heart failure worldwide. Rheumatic fever can permanently damage the heart muscle and heart valves, a condition called *rheumatic heart disease (RHD).* Symptoms of strep throat include the sudden onset of a sore throat, painful swallowing, fever, swollen glands, headache, nausea, and vomiting. If left untreated, up to 3% of strep infections progress into rheumatic fever.

Heart Valve Disorders   Age, previous heart attacks, congenital defects, and certain types of infections can cause abnormalities in the valves between the chambers of the heart.

The most common heart valve disorder is **mitral valve prolapse (MVP),** which occurs in about 3% of the population. MVP is characterized by a billowing of the mitral valve, which separates the left ventricle and left atrium, during ventricular contraction. Most people with MVP have no symptoms and do not need treatment.

PROTECTING YOURSELF AGAINST CARDIOVASCULAR DISEASE

CVD can begin very early in life. Reducing CVD risk factors when you are young can pay off with many extra years of life and health.

Eat Heart-Healthy

For most Americans, eating a heart-healthy diet involves decreasing fat and cholesterol intake, eating a high-fiber diet, reducing sodium intake and increasing potassium intake, avoiding excessive alcohol consumption, and eating foods rich in omega-3 fatty acids. In addition to these familiar guidelines, a few specifics pertain to heart health:

• *Plant stanols and sterols:* Plant stanols and sterols, found in some types of trans-fat–free margarines and other products, reduce the absorption of cholesterol in the body and help lower LDL levels.

TERMS

pulmonary edema   The accumulation of fluid in the lungs.

congestive heart failure (CHF)   A condition resulting from the heart's inability to pump enough blood to keep up with the body's metabolic needs; blood backs up in the veins leading to the heart, causing an accumulation of fluid in various parts of the body.

congenital heart defect   A defect or malformation of the heart or its major blood vessels, present at birth.

hypertrophic cardiomyopathy (HCM)   An inherited condition in which there is an enlargement of the heart muscle, especially the muscle between the two ventricles.

murmur   An abnormal heart sound indicating turbulent blood flow through a valve or hole in the heart.

rheumatic fever   A disease, mainly of children, characterized by fever, inflammation, and pain in the joints. It often damages the heart valves and muscle, a condition called rheumatic heart disease.

mitral valve prolapse (MVP)   A condition in which the mitral valve billows out during ventricular contraction, allowing leakage of blood from the left ventricle into the left atrium.

- *Folic acid, vitamin B-6, and vitamin B-12:* These vitamins lower homocysteine levels, and folic acid has also been found to reduce the risk of hypertension.

- *Calcium:* Diets rich in calcium may help prevent hypertension and possibly stroke by reducing insulin resistance and platelet aggregation.

- *Vitamin D:* There appears to be a close association between vitamin D deficiency and cardiovascular disease. However, studies have failed to show benefits to replacement of low vitamin D levels with supplemental dietary vitamin D.

- *Soy protein:* Replacing some animal proteins with soy protein (such as tofu) may help lower LDL cholesterol.

- *Healthy carbohydrates:* Healthy carbohydrates are important for people with insulin resistance, prediabetes, or diabetes.

- *Total calories:* Reduced calorie intake helps control body weight—an extremely important risk factor for CVD.

A diet plan that reflects many of the recommendations described here is the DASH diet. The DASH study found that a diet low in fat and high in fruits, vegetables, and low-fat dairy products reduces blood pressure. It is one of the eating patterns recommended in the 2010 Dietary Guidelines for Americans.

Exercise Regularly

You can significantly reduce your risk of CVD with a moderate amount of physical activity. In addition to aerobic exercise for building and maintaining cardiovascular health, strength training helps reduce body fat and improves lipid levels and glucose metabolism. The more exercise you get, the less likely you are to develop or die from CVD.

Avoid Tobacco Products

The number-one risk factor for CVD that you can control is smoking. If you smoke, quit. If you don't smoke, don't start. If you live or work with people who smoke, take steps to prevent or stop the exposure.

Know and Manage Your Blood Pressure and Cholesterol Levels

If you have no CVD risk factors, have your blood pressure measured by a trained professional at least once every two years. Yearly tests are recommended if you have risk factors. If your blood pressure is high, follow your physician's advice on how to lower it. All people aged 20 and over should have their cholesterol checked at least once every five years.

Develop Effective Ways to Handle Stress and Anger

To reduce the psychological and social risk factors for CVD, develop effective strategies for handling the stress in your life. Shore up your social support network, and try some of the techniques described in Chapter 2 for managing stress.

WHAT IS CANCER?

Cancer is the abnormal, uncontrolled multiplication of cells, which can ultimately cause death if left untreated.

Tumors

Most cancers take the form of tumors, although not all tumors are cancerous. A **tumor** (or *neoplasm*) is a mass of tissue that serves no physiological purpose.

Benign (noncancerous) **tumors** are made up of cells similar to the surrounding normal cells and are enclosed in a membrane that prevents them from penetrating neighboring tissues. They are dangerous only if their physical presence interferes with body functions. A benign brain tumor, for example, can cause death if it blocks the blood supply to the brain.

The term **malignant tumor** is synonymous with cancer. A malignant tumor can invade surrounding structures, including blood vessels, the **lymphatic system,** and nerves. It can also spread to distant sites via the blood and lymphatic circulation, producing invasive tumors in almost any part of the

cancer   The abnormal, uncontrolled multiplication **TERMS** of cells.

tumor   A mass of tissue that serves no physiological purpose; also called a *neoplasm*.

benign tumor   A tumor that is not cancerous.

malignant tumor   A tumor that is capable of spreading and thus is cancerous.

lymphatic system   A system of vessels that returns proteins, lipids, and other substances from fluid in the tissues to the circulatory system.

body. A few cancers, like leukemia (cancer of the blood), do not produce a mass but still have the fundamental property of rapid, uncontrolled cell proliferation. For this reason, such diseases are malignant and are considered to be a form of cancer.

Cancer begins when a change (or mutation) in a cell occurs that allows the cell to grow and divide when it should not. Normally (in adults) cells multiply at a rate just sufficient to replace dying cells. In contrast, a malignant cell divides into new cells without regard for normal control mechanisms and gradually produces a mass of abnormal cells, or a tumor. A pea-sized mass is made up of about a billion cells, so a single tumor cell must go through many divisions, often taking years, before the tumor grows to a noticeable size.

Eventually a tumor becomes large enough to cause symptoms or to be directly detected. In the breast, for example, a tumor may be felt as a lump or diagnosed as cancer by an X-ray or **biopsy.** In less accessible locations, like the lung, a tumor may be noticed only after it has grown considerably and may then be detected only by an indirect symptom, such as a persistent cough or unexplained bleeding. In the case of leukemia, changes in the blood are eventually noticed as increasing fatigue, infection, or abnormal bleeding.

Metastasis

Metastasis is the spread of cancer cells from one part of the body to another. Metastasis occurs because cancer cells do not stick to each other as strongly as normal cells do and therefore may move away from the site of the *primary tumor* (the cancer's original location). After cancer cells break away, they can pass through the lining of lymph or blood vessels to invade nearby tissue. They can also travel to different parts of the body where they establish new cancer cells. This traveling and seeding process is called *metastasizing,* and the new tumors are called *secondary tumors* or *metastases.* The ability of cancer cells to metastasize makes early cancer detection critical. To cure cancer, every cancerous cell must be removed or destroyed. Once cancer cells enter either the lymphatic system or the bloodstream, it is extremely difficult to stop their spread to other organs of the body.

Remission

A significant number of cancer cases go into **remission,** which in some cases lasts for years. In remission, signs and symptoms of cancer disappear, and the disease is considered

to be under control. Remission typically results from treatment, but rarely some cancer patients enter remission spontaneously.

THE CAUSES OF CANCER

Although scientists do not know everything about what causes cancer, they have identified genetic, environmental, and lifestyle factors that increase the risk of developing cancer.

The Role of DNA

Heredity and genetics are important factors in a person's risk of cancer. Certain genes may predispose some people to cancer, and specific genetic mutations have been associated with cancer.

Some mutations are inherited, and others are caused by environmental agents including radiation, certain viruses, and chemical substances in the air pollution. An example of an inherited mutation is BRCA1 (breast cancer gene 1). Women who inherit an altered copy of this gene face a significantly increased risk of breast and ovarian cancer. Testing and identification of hereditary cancer risks can be helpful for some people, especially if it leads to increased attention to controllable risk factors and better medical screening.

Tobacco Use

Smoking is responsible for at least 80% of lung cancers and 30% of all cancer deaths. Overall, tobacco use is responsible for nearly one in five American deaths—approximately 443,000 premature deaths each year. The U.S. Surgeon General has reported that tobacco use is a direct cause of several types of cancer besides lung and bronchial cancer including larynx, mouth, pharynx, esophagus, stomach, pancreas, kidneys, bladder, and cervix.

Dietary Factors

How important is diet in cancer prevention? The relationship between food and cancer risk is complex and controversial. The foods you eat contain many biologically active compounds, and your food choices may either increase your cancer risk by exposing you to potentially dangerous compounds or reduce your risk by eating potentially protective ones.

The following dietary factors may affect cancer risk:

• *Dietary fat and meat:* Diets high in fat and meat may contribute to certain cancers, including colon, stomach, and prostate cancer. Certain types of fats may be riskier than others. Omega-6 polyunsaturated fats are associated with a higher risk of certain cancers; omega-3 fats are not.

---

biopsy   The removal of a small piece of body tissue to allow for microscopic examination; a needle biopsy uses a needle to remove a small sample of tissue, but some biopsies require surgery.

metastasis   The spread of cancer cells from one part of the body to another.

remission   A period during the course of cancer in which there are no symptoms or other evidence of disease.

TERMS

- **Alcohol:** Alcohol is associated with an increased incidence of several cancers. Women who have two to five drinks daily have about 1.5 times the cancer risk of women who drink no alcohol. Alcohol and tobacco interact as risk factors for oral cancer.

- **Fried foods:** High levels of the chemical acrylamide (a probable human carcinogen) are found in starch-based foods that have been fried or baked at high temperatures, especially french fries and certain types of snack chips and crackers.

- **Fiber:** Further study is needed to clarify the relationship between fiber intake and cancer risk, but experts still recommend a high-fiber diet for its overall positive effect on health.

- **Fruits and vegetables:** Researchers have identified many mechanisms by which food components may act against cancer. Some may prevent carcinogens from forming in the first place or block them from reaching or acting on target cells. Others boost enzymes that detoxify carcinogens and render them harmless. Some essential nutrients help reduce the harmful effects of carcinogens; for example, vitamin C, vitamin E, selenium, and the **carotenoids** (vitamin A precursors) may help block cancer by acting as antioxidants.

Many other anti-cancer agents in the diet fall under the broader heading of **phytochemicals,** which are substances in plants that help protect against chronic diseases. One of the first to be identified was sulforaphane, a potent anti-carcinogen found in broccoli and other cruciferous vegetables, such as cauliflower, Brussels sprouts, and cabbage. Most fruits and vegetables contain beneficial phytochemicals, and researchers are just beginning to identify them.

Inactivity and Obesity

The American Cancer Society (ACS) recommends maintaining a healthy weight throughout life by balancing caloric intake with physical activity, and by achieving and maintaining a healthy weight if you are currently overweight or obese. Being overweight or obese is linked with increased risk mortality from several kinds of cancer, including breast and colon cancer.

Carcinogens in the Environment

Some carcinogens occur naturally in the environment, like viruses and the sun's UV rays. Others are manufactured or synthetic substances that show up occasionally in the general environment but more often in the work environments of specific industries.

Microbes It is estimated that 15–20% of the world's cancers are caused by microbes, including viruses, bacteria, and parasites, although the percentage is much lower in industrialized countries like the United States. Certain types of human papillomavirus are known to cause oropharyngeal cancer, cervical cancer, and other cancers, and the *Helicobacter pylori* bacterium has been linked to stomach cancer. Hepatitis viruses B and C together cause as many as 80% of the world's liver cancers.

Ingested Chemicals Some of the compounds added to foods are potentially dangerous, including the nitrates and nitrites found in processed meat. Although nitrates and nitrites are not themselves carcinogenic, they can combine with substances in the stomach and be converted to nitrosamines, which are highly potent carcinogens. Foods cured with nitrites, as well as those cured by salt or smoke, have been linked to esophageal and stomach cancer, and they should be eaten only in modest amounts.

Environmental and Industrial Pollution Pollutants in the air have long been suspected of contributing to the incidence of lung cancer.

Although fewer than 2% of cancer deaths are caused by general environmental pollution, such as substances in our air and water, exposure to carcinogenic materials in the workplace is a more serious problem. Occupational exposure to specific carcinogens may account for about 4% of cancer deaths. With increasing industry and government regulation, we can anticipate that the industrial sources of cancer risk will continue to diminish, at least in the United States.

Radiation All sources of radiation are potentially carcinogenic, including medical X-rays, radioactive substances (radioisotopes), and **ultraviolet (UV) radiation** from the sun. Successful efforts have been made to reduce the amount of radiation needed for mammograms, dental X-rays, and medical X-rays. Sunlight is also a potential carcinogen, and care should be taken to avoid excessive exposure.

DETECTING, DIAGNOSING, AND TREATING CANCER

Early cancer detection often depends on our willingness to be aware of changes in our own body and to make sure we keep up with recommended screening tests. Although

---

Ask Yourself

QUESTIONS FOR CRITICAL THINKING AND REFLECTION

What do you think your risks for cancer are? Do you have a family history of cancer, or have you been exposed to carcinogens? How about your diet and exercise habits? What can you do to reduce your risks?

---

phytochemical A naturally occurring substance found in plant foods that may help prevent chronic diseases such as cancer and heart disease; *phyto* means "plant." **TERMS**

ultraviolet (UV) radiation Light rays of a specific wavelength emitted by the sun; most UV rays are blocked by the ozone layer in the upper atmosphere.

treatment success varies with individual cancers, cure rates have increased—sometimes dramatically—in this century, especially for cancers that are diagnosed at their early stages.

Detecting Cancer

Self-monitoring is the first line of defense against cancer. By being aware of the risk factors in your own life, your immediate family's cancer history, and your own history, you may bring a problem to the attention of a physician long before it would have been detected at a routine physical. In addition to self-monitoring, the ACS recommends routine cancer checkups, as well as specific screening tests for certain cancers (Table 12.4).

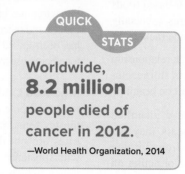

QUICK STATS

Worldwide, **8.2 million** people died of cancer in 2012.

—World Health Organization, 2014

Diagnosing and Treating Cancer

Methods for determining the exact location, type, and extent of a cancer continue to improve.

A biopsy may be performed to confirm the type of tumor. Several diagnostic imaging techniques have replaced exploratory surgery for some patients. They include MRIs, CT scanning, and ultrasonography.

Chemotherapy, or the use of medications to kill cancer cells, works by interfering with DNA synthesis and replication in rapidly dividing cells. Normal cells, which usually grow slowly, are not significantly destroyed by these drugs. However, some normal tissues such as intestinal, hair, and blood-forming cells are always growing, and damage to these tissues produces the unpleasant side effects of chemotherapy, including nausea, vomiting, diarrhea, and hair loss.

---

chemotherapy The treatment of cancer with chemicals that selectively destroy cancerous cells.

carcinoma Cancer that originates in epithelial tissue (skin, glands, and lining of internal organs).

sarcoma Cancer arising from bone, cartilage, or striated muscle.

lymphoma A tumor originating from lymphatic tissue.

leukemia Cancer of the blood or the blood-forming cells.

oncologist A specialist in the diagnosis and treatment of cancer.

hematologist A specialist in the diagnosis and treatment of blood disorders, including cancers such as leukemia and lymphoma.

five-year survival rate The percentage of patients diagnosed with a certain disease who will be alive five years after the date of diagnosis; used to estimate the prognosis of a particular disease.

TERMS

Radiation therapy uses a beam of X-rays or gamma rays directed at the tumor to kill tumor cells. With sophisticated techniques, the harmful rays are directed precisely at the cancerous cells, in order to minimize damage to surrounding normal cells. Occasionally, when an organ is small enough, such as the prostate gland, radioactive seeds are surgically placed inside the cancerous organ to destroy the tumor. Radiation therapy is usually less toxic for the patient than either surgery or chemotherapy, and can be performed on an outpatient basis. For most cancers, surgery is a definitive treatment.

TYPES AND INCIDENCE OF CANCER

Figure 12.4 shows the most common types of cancer and the incidence of each type. Cancers are classified according to the types of cells that give rise to them:

• **Carcinomas** arise from *epithelia*—tissues that cover external body surfaces, line internal tubes and cavities, and form the secreting portion of glands. This type of cancer is the most common. Major sites include the skin, breast, uterus, prostate, lungs, and gastrointestinal tract.

• **Sarcomas** arise from connective and fibrous tissues such as muscle, bone, cartilage, and the membranes covering muscles and fat.

• **Lymphomas** are cancers of the lymph nodes, part of the body's infection-fighting system.

• **Leukemias** are cancers of the blood-forming cells, which reside chiefly in the bone marrow.

Cancers vary greatly in how easily they can be detected and how well they respond to treatment. For example, certain types of skin cancer are easily detected, grow slowly, and are easy to remove; virtually all of these cancers are cured. Cancer of the pancreas, on the other hand, is difficult to detect or treat, and few patients survive the disease. In general, it is difficult for an **oncologist** or **hematologist** to predict how a specific cancer will behave because every one arises from a unique set of changes in a single cell.

Most of the 1.6 million people in the United States who are diagnosed with cancer each year will be cured, or live many years past their initial cancer diagnosis. In fact, the American Cancer Society (ACS) estimates that the **five-year relative survival rate** for all cancers diagnosed between 2002 and 2008 is 68%. These statistics exclude more than 1 million cases of the curable types of skin cancer.

Death rates from cancer are not declining as fast as those from heart disease, in large part because of the differing effects that quitting smoking has on disease risk. Heart-related damage of smoking reverses more quickly and more significantly than the cancer-related damage from smoking. Smoking-related gene mutations cannot be reversed,

Table 12.4

Screening Guidelines for the Early Detection of Cancer in Average-Risk Asymptomatic People

CANCER SITE	POPULATION	TEST OR PROCEDURE	FREQUENCY
Breast	Women, age 20+	Breast self-examination	Optional. Beginning in their early 20s, women should be told about the benefits and limitations of breast self-examination (BSE). The importance of prompt reporting of any new breast symptoms to a health professional should be emphasized. Women who choose to do BSE should receive instruction and have their technique reviewed on the occasion of a periodic health examination. It is acceptable for women to choose not to do BSE or to do BSE irregularly.
		Clinical breast examination	For women in their 20s and 30s, and higher-risk men starting at age 35, it is recommended that clinical breast examination (CBE) be part of a periodic health examination, preferably at least every three years. Asymptomatic women aged 40 and over should continue to receive a clinical breast examination as part of a periodic health examination, preferably annually.
		Mammography	For all women and those men at higher risk, begin annual mammography at age 40.[a]
Colorectal[b]	Men and women, age 50+	*Tests that find polyps and cancer:*	
		Flexible sigmoidoscopy,[c] or	Every five years, starting at age 50
		Colonoscopy, or	Every 10 years, starting at age 50
		Double-contrast barium enema (DCBE),[c] or	Every five years, starting at age 50
		CT colonography (virtual colonoscopy)[c]	Every five years, starting at age 50
		Tests that mainly find cancer:	Annual, starting at age 50
		Fecal occult blood test (FOBT) with at least 50% test sensitivity for cancer, or fecal immuno-chemical test (FIT) with at least 50% test sensitivity for cancer[c] or	Annual, starting at age 50. Testing at home with adherence to the manufacturer's recommendation for collection techniques and a number of samples is recommended. FOBT with a single stool sample collected on the clinician's fingertip during a digital rectal examination in the health care setting is not recommended. Guaiac-based toilet bowl FOBT tests also are not recommended. In comparison with guaiac-based tests for the detection of occult blood, immunochemical tests are more patient-friendly, and are likely to be equal or better in sensitivity and specificity. There is no justification for repeating FOBT in response to an initial positive finding.
Prostate	Men, age 50+	Prostate-specific antigen test (PSA) with or without digital rectal examination (DRE)	Men who have at least a 10-year life expectancy should have an opportunity to make an informed decision with their health care provider about screening for prostate cancer after receiving information about the uncertainties, risks, and potential benefits associated with prostate cancer screening. Prostate cancer screening should not occur without an informed decision-making process.
Cervix	Women, age 21–29 30–65 >65	Pap test Pap test + HPV DNA test	Cervical cancer screening should begin at 21 years of age. Screening should be done every 3 years. [d] Every 5 years[d] An alternative is screening with a Pap test alone every 3 years[d] A woman should stop screening unless she had a serious cervical pre-cancer or cancer in the last 20 years. Women who have had a total hysterectomy may choose to stop cervical cancer screening.
Endometrial	Women, at menopause		At the time of menopause, women at average risk should be informed about risks and symptoms of endometrial cancer and strongly encouraged to report any unexpected bleeding or spotting to their physicians.
Cancer-related checkup	Men and women, age 20+		During a periodic health examination, the cancer-related checkup should include examination for cancers of the thyroid, testicles, ovaries, lymph nodes, oral cavity, and skin, as well as health counseling about tobacco, sun exposure, diet and nutrition, risk factors, sexual practices, and environmental and occupational exposures.

[a]Beginning at age 40, annual clinical breast examination should be performed prior to mammography.

[b]Individuals with a personal or family history of colorectal cancer or adenomas, inflammatory bowel disease, or high-risk genetic syndromes should continue to follow the most recent recommendations for individuals at increased or high risk.

[c]Colonoscopy should be done if test results are positive.

[d]Doctors may suggest a woman be screened more often if she has certain risk factors, such as a history of diethylstilbestrol (DES) exposure, HIV infection, or a weak immune system.

SOURCE: American Cancer Society. 2013. *Cancer Facts and Figures, 2013.* Atlanta: American Cancer Society, Inc. Reprinted by the permission of the American Cancer Society, Inc., from www.cancer.org. All rights reserved.

New cases	Deaths	Male	Female	New cases	Deaths
30,220 (4%)	5,730 (2%)	Oral cavity and pharynx	Brain and other nervous system	10,560 (1%)	6,230 (2%)
43,890 (5%)	6,470 (2%)	Melanoma of the skin	Thyroid	47,790 (6%)	1,060 (.4%)
116,000 (14%)	86,930 (28%)	Lung and bronchus	Melanoma of the skin	32,210 (4%)	3,240 (1%)
14,660 (2%)	12,450 (4%)	Esophagus	Lung and bronchus	108,210 (13%)	72,330 (26%)
24,600 (3%)	15,870 (5%)	Liver and intrahepatic bile duct	Breast	232,670 (29%)	40,000 (15%)
23,530 (3%)	20,170 (7%)	Pancreas	Liver and intrahepatic bile duct	8,590 (1%)	7,130 (3%)
39,140 (5%)	8,900 (3%)	Kidney and renal pelvis	Kidney and renal pelvis	24,780 (3%)	4,960 (2%)
71,830 (8%)	26,270 (9%)	Colon and rectum	Pancreas	22,890 (3%)	19,420 (7%)
56,390 (7%)	11,170 (4%)	Urinary bladder	Colon and rectum	65,000 (8%)	24,040 (9%)
233,000 (27%)	29,480 (10%)	Prostate	Ovary	21,980 (3%)	14,270 (5%)
30,100 (4%)	14,040 (5%)	Leukemia	Uterine corpus	52,630 (7%)	8,590 (3%)
38,270 (5%)	10,470 (3%)	Non-Hodgkin lymphoma	Leukemia	22,280 (3%)	10,050 (4%)
855,220 (100%)	310,010 (100%)	All sites	Non-Hodgkin lymphoma	32,530 (4%)	8,520 (3%)
			All sites	810,320 (100%)	275,710 (100%)

VITAL STATISTICS

FIGURE 12.4 **Estimated number of new cancer cases and deaths by sex, US, 2014.** Estimated new cases are based on 1995–2010 incidence rates reported by the North American Association of Central Cancer Registries, representing 89% of the US population. Estimated deaths are based on 1995–2010 US mortality data, National Center for Health Statistics, Centers for Disease Control and Prevention.

SOURCE: American Cancer Society. 2014. *Cancer Facts and Figures, 2014*. Atlanta: American Cancer Society.

Ask Yourself

QUESTIONS FOR CRITICAL THINKING AND REFLECTION

Most people think of cancer as a death sentence, but is that necessarily true? Have you or has anyone you know had an experience with cancer? If so, what was the outcome? Have you ever considered whether you might be at increased risk for some types of cancer? Have you taken any steps to reduce your risk?

although other mechanisms can sometimes control cellular changes. If heart disease death rates continue to decline faster than cancer death rates, cancer may overtake heart disease as the leading cause of death among Americans of all ages.

Still, many more people could be saved from cancer. The overwhelming majority of skin cancers could be prevented by protecting the skin from excessive sun exposure, and the majority of lung cancer could be prevented by avoiding exposure to tobacco smoke. Thousands of cases of colon, breast, and uterine cancer could be prevented by

improving the diet and controlling body weight. Regular screenings and self-examinations have the potential to save an additional 100,000 lives per year.

COMMON CANCERS

In this section we look at some of the most common cancers and their causes, prevention, and treatment.

Lung Cancer

Lung cancer accounts for about 14% of all new cancer diagnoses and is the most common cause of cancer death in the United States: It is responsible for about 160,000 deaths each year. Since 1987 lung cancer has surpassed breast cancer as the leading cause of cancer death in women.

Risk Factors The chief risk factor for lung cancer is tobacco smoke, which currently accounts for 30% of all cancer deaths and 90% of lung cancer deaths. When smoking is combined with exposure to other carcinogens, such as asbestos particles or certain pollutants, the risk of cancer can be multiplied by a factor of 10 or more. Exposure to environmental tobacco smoke (ETS) increases the risk of lung cancer.

> QUICK STATS
>
> **13.7 million**
> Americans with a history of cancer were alive in January 1, 2012.
> —American Cancer Society, 2013

Detection and Treatment Lung cancer is difficult to detect at an early stage and hard to cure even when detected early. Symptoms of lung cancer do not usually appear until the disease has advanced to the invasive stage. Signs and symptoms such as a persistent cough, chest pain, or recurring bronchitis may be the first indication of a tumor's presence. A diagnosis can usually be made by chest X-ray or by studying the cells in sputum.

If caught early, localized cancers can be treated with surgery alone. The majority of patients are diagnosed with advanced disease, however, and radiation and chemotherapy are often used in addition to surgery. The five-year survival rate for all stages combined is only 16%. Phototherapy, gene therapy, and immunotherapy (vaccines) are being studied in the hope of improving these statistics.

Colon and Rectal Cancer

Another common cancer in the United States is colon and rectal cancer (also called *colorectal cancer*). Although there are effective screening methods for colorectal cancer, it is the third most common type of cancer.

Risk Factors Age is a key risk factor for colon and rectal cancer, with more than 91% of cases diagnosed in people aged 50 and older. Heredity also plays a role. Many cancers arise from preexisting **polyps,** which are small growths on the wall of the colon that may gradually develop into malignancies. The tendency to form colon polyps appears to be determined by specific genes, so many colon cancers may be due to inherited gene mutations.

Excessive alcohol use and smoking may increase the risk of colorectal cancer. Regular physical activity appears to reduce a person's risk, whereas obesity increases risk. A diet rich in red and processed meats increases risk, whereas eating fruits, vegetables, and whole grains is associated with lower risk. However, research findings on whether dietary fiber prevents colon cancer have been mixed. Studies have suggested a protective role for folic acid, magnesium, vitamin D, and calcium; in contrast, high intake of refined carbohydrates, simple sugars, and smoked meats and fish may increase risk.

Regular use of nonsteroidal anti-inflammatory drugs such as aspirin and ibuprofen may decrease the risk of colon cancer and other cancers of the digestive tract. However, these agents are not currently recommended for colorectal cancer prevention, although there are several ongoing studies to determine if the protective benefit of these drugs is greater than the risk of other negative health effects.

Detection and Treatment If identified early, precancerous polyps and early-stage cancers can be removed before they become malignant or spread. Because polyps may bleed as they progress, common warning signs of colon cancer are bleeding from the rectum and a change in bowel habits.

Regular screening tests are recommended beginning at age 50 (earlier for people with a family history of the disease or who are otherwise at high risk). A yearly stool blood test can detect small amounts of blood in the stool long before obvious bleeding would be noticed. More involved screening tests are recommended at 5- or 10-year intervals.

Surgery is the primary treatment for colon and rectal cancer. Radiation and chemotherapy may be used before surgery to shrink a tumor or after surgery to destroy any remaining cancerous cells. The five-year survival rate is 90% for colon and rectal cancers detected early and 64% overall.

Breast Cancer

Breast cancer is the most common cancer in women. In men, breast cancer occurs only rarely. In the United States, about one woman in eight will develop breast cancer during her lifetime. About 232,000 American women are diagnosed with breast cancer each year. About 40,000 women die from breast cancer each year.

Fewer than 2% of breast cancer cases occur in women under age 35, but incidence rates increase quickly with age. About 50% of cases are diagnosed in women age 45–65.

Risk Factors Genetics play a very important role in breast cancer. A woman who has two close relatives with breast cancer is more than four times more likely to develop the disease than a woman who has no close relatives with it. However, even though genetic factors are important, inherited mutations in breast cancer susceptibility genes account for only approximately 5–10% of all breast cancer cases.

Other risk factors include early onset of menstruation, late onset of menopause, having no children or having a first child after age 30, current use of hormone replacement therapy, obesity, and alcohol use. Estrogen may be a unifying element for many of these risk factors. Estrogen circulates in a woman's body in high concentrations between puberty and menopause. Fat cells also produce estrogen, and estrogen levels are higher in obese women. Alcohol can interfere with estrogen metabolism in the liver and increase estrogen levels in the blood. Estrogen promotes the growth of cells in responsive sites, including the breast and the uterus, so any factor that increases estrogen exposure may raise breast cancer risk.

polyp A small, usually harmless mass of tissue that projects from the inner surface of the colon or rectum. **TERMS**

A dramatic drop in rates of breast cancer from 2001 to 2004 was attributed in part to reduced use of hormone replacement therapy by women over 50 beginning in July 2002. Millions of women stopped taking the hormones after research from the Women's Health Initiative linked hormone replacement therapy with an increased risk of breast cancer and heart disease.

Eating a low-fat, vegetable-rich diet, exercising regularly, limiting alcohol intake, and maintaining a healthy body weight can minimize the chance of developing breast cancer, even for women at risk from family history or other factors. Despite some popular myths, studies have shown that breast cancer incidence is not increased by underwire bras, antiperspirants, breast implants, or abortions.

Early Detection   A cure is most likely if breast cancer is detected early, so regular screening is a good investment, even for younger women. The ACS advises a three-part personal program for the early detection of breast cancer:

- *Mammography:* The ACS recommends a **mammogram** (low-dose breast X-ray) every year for women over 40. Some groups have argued that between ages 40 and 50 the rates of false positive mammograms are higher and thus women should not begin receiving mammograms until age 50. However, most organizations in the United States still recommend beginning screening with mammograms at age 40.

Studies show that magnetic resonance imaging (MRI) may be better than mammography at detecting breast abnormalities in some women. The ACS recommends both an annual mammogram and an annual MRI for women who are at high risk for breast cancer. **Ultrasonography** is often used as a follow-up test if a mammogram reveals an abnormality in breast tissue.

- *Clinical breast exam:* Women between ages 20 and 39 should have a clinical breast exam every three years, and women aged 40 and older should have one every year before their scheduled mammogram.

- *Breast self-exams:* Breast self-exam (BSE) allows a woman to become familiar with her breasts, so she can alert her health care provider to any changes. Women who choose to do breast self-exams should begin at age 20 (see the box "How to Perform a Breast Self-Exam").

Breast pain or tenderness is usually associated with benign conditions such as menstruation rather than breast cancer. The first physical signs of breast cancer are more likely to be a lump, swelling, or thickening; skin irritation or dimpling; or nipple pain, scaliness, or retraction. Although most breast lumps are benign, any breast lump should be brought to the attention of a health care provider.

Treatment   If a lump is detected, it may be scanned by ultrasonography and biopsied to see if it is cancerous. In most cases, the lump is found to be a cyst or other harmless growth, and no further treatment is needed. If the lump contains cancer cells, a variety of surgeries may be indicated, ranging from a lumpectomy (removal of the lump and surrounding tissue) to a mastectomy (removal of the breast).

Analyzing the tumor specimen with special stains can help predict the risk of breast cancer recurrence and help identify women who will benefit most from additional therapy; women can then make more informed treatment decisions. Treatment with the **monoclonal antibodies,** such as trastuzumab, is an option for about 15–20% of patients diagnosed with breast cancer.

If the tumor is discovered before it has spread to the adjacent lymph nodes or outside the breast, the patient has about a 98% chance of surviving more than five years. The relative survival rate for all stages is 90% at five years.

Strategies for Prevention   A number of drugs have been proposed for the prevention of breast cancer, especially in high-risk patients. A family of drugs called *selective estrogen receptor modulators* (*SERMs*) acts like estrogen in some tissues of the body but blocks estrogen's effects in others. One SERM, tamoxifen, has long been used in breast cancer treatment because it blocks the action of estrogen in breast tissue. In 1998 the FDA approved the use of tamoxifen to reduce the risk of breast cancer in healthy women who are at high risk for the disease. However, the drug has serious potential side effects, including increased risk of blood clots and uterine cancer. Another SERM, raloxifene, was approved in 2007 for the reduction of invasive breast cancer risk in postmenopausal women at high risk for breast cancer. Compared to tamoxifen, raloxifene has been shown to pose a slightly lower risk of blood clots and uterine cancer, but the risk is still higher than that of a placebo. Raloxifene has also been shown to improve bone mineral density.

Prostate Cancer

The prostate gland is located at the base of the bladder in men and completely surrounds the male's urethra; if enlarged, it can block the flow of urine. Prostate cancer is the most common cancer in men and the second leading cause of cancer death in men. Nearly 239,000 new cases are diagnosed each year, and more than 30,000 American men die from the disease each year.

Risk Factors   Age is the strongest predictor of risk, with approximately 60% of cases of prostate cancer diagnosed in men over age 65. Inherited genetic predisposition may be responsible for 5–10% of cases, and men with a family

---

mammogram   A low-dose X-ray of the breasts used to check for early signs of breast cancer.

ultrasonography   An imaging method in which sound waves are bounced off body structures to create an image on a TV monitor; also called *ultrasound*.

monoclonal antibody   An antibody designed to bind to a specific cancer-related target.

TERMS

It is acceptable for women to choose not to do BSE or to do BSE once in a while. Women who choose not to do BSE should still be aware of the normal look and feel of their breasts and report any changes to their doctor right away.

The best time for a woman to examine her breasts is when the breasts are not tender or swollen. Women who examine their breasts should have their technique reviewed during their periodic health exams by their health care professional.

Women with breast implants can do BSE. It may be helpful to have the surgeon help identify the edges of the implant so that you know what you are feeling. There is some thought that the implants push out the breast tissue and may actually make it easier to examine. Women who are pregnant or breast-feeding can also choose to examine their breasts regularly.

How to Examine Your Breasts

• Lie down and place your right arm behind your head. The exam is done while lying down, not standing up. This is because when lying down the breast tissue spreads evenly over the chest wall and is as thin as possible, making it much easier to feel all the breast tissue.

• Use the finger pads of the three middle fingers on your left hand to feel for lumps in the right breast. Use overlapping dime-sized circular motions of the finger pads to feel the breast tissue.

• Use three different levels of pressure to feel all the breast tissue. Light pressure is needed to feel the tissue closest to the skin; medium pressure to feel a little deeper; and firm pressure to feel the tissue closest to the chest and ribs. It is normal to feel a firm ridge in the lower curve of each breast but you should tell your doctor if you feel anything else out of the ordinary. If you're not sure how hard to press, talk with your doctor or nurse. Use each pressure level to feel the breast tissue before moving on to the next spot.

• Move around the breast in an up and down pattern starting at an imaginary line drawn straight down your side from the underarm and moving across the breast to the middle of the chest bone (sternum or breastbone). Be sure to check the entire breast area going down until you feel only ribs and up to the neck or collar bone (clavicle).

• There is some evidence to suggest that the up-and-down pattern (sometimes called the vertical pattern) is the most effective pattern for covering the entire breast, without missing any breast tissue.

• Repeat the exam on your left breast, putting your left arm behind your head and using the finger pads of your right hand to do the exam.

• While standing in front of a mirror with your hands pressing firmly down on your hips, look at your breasts for any changes of size, shape, contour, or dimpling, or redness or scaliness of the nipple or breast skin. (The pressing down on the hips position contracts the chest wall muscles and enhances any breast changes.)

• Examine each underarm while sitting up or standing and with your arm only slightly raised so you can easily feel in this area. Raising your arm straight up tightens the tissue in this area and makes it harder to examine.

This procedure for doing breast self-exam is different from previous recommendations. These changes represent an extensive review of the medical literature and input from an expert advisory group. There is evidence that this position (lying down), the area felt, pattern of coverage of the breast, and use of different amounts of pressure increase a woman's ability to find abnormal areas.

history of the disease should be particularly vigilant about screening. African American men and Jamaican men of African descent have the highest rates of prostate cancer of any groups in the world. Both genetic and lifestyle factors may be involved.

Diets high in calories, dairy products, and animal fats and low in plant foods have also been implicated as possible culprits, as have obesity, inactivity, and a history of sexually transmitted diseases. Type 2 diabetes and insulin resistance are also associated with prostate cancer. Soy foods, tomatoes, and cruciferous vegetables are being investigated for their possible protective effects.

Detection Warning signs of prostate cancer can include changes in urinary frequency, weak or interrupted urine flow, painful urination, and blood in the urine.

Techniques for early detection include a digital rectal examination and the **prostate-specific antigen (PSA) test.** Currently there is insufficient data in support of or against routine screening with the PSA test. The ACS recommends that men be provided information about the benefits and limitations of the tests and that both the exam and the PSA test be offered annually, beginning at age 50, for men who are at average risk of prostate cancer, do not have any major medical problems, and have a life expectancy of at least 10 years. Men at high risk, including African Americans and those with a family history of the disease, should consider beginning screening at age 45. Men with multiple family members who have been diagnosed with the disease should begin screening at age 40.

PSA testing has been a subject of controversy among experts for several years because of its tendency to yield misleading results, leading to further testing, including biopsies, that can potentially cause harm. In older men, most prostate cancers are not deadly, making treatment pointless and potentially harmful.

Treatment   Treatments vary based on the stage of the cancer and the age of the patient. A small, slow-growing tumor in an older man may be treated with watchful waiting and no initial therapy because he is more likely to die from another cause before his cancer becomes life-threatening. More aggressive treatment would be indicated for younger men or those with more advanced cancers. Treatment may involve *radical prostatectomy* (surgical removal of the prostate). Although radical surgery has an excellent cure rate, it is major surgery and often results in **incontinence** and/or erectile dysfunction. Minimally invasive surgery, which utilizes a laparoscopic or robotic approach, can sometimes be performed with fewer complications and quicker recovery.

A less invasive alternative involves surgical implantation of radioactive seeds. Radiation from the seeds destroys the tumor and much of the normal prostate tissue but leaves surrounding tissue relatively untouched. Alternative or additional treatments include external radiation, hormonal therapy, cryotherapy, and chemotherapy. Several new treatments for advanced prostate cancer have recently been approved by the U.S. Food and Drug Administration (FDA). A cancer vaccine, known as sipuleucel-T, was approved for some men with hormone-refractory advanced prostate cancer. Drugs recently approved for the treatment of metastatic prostate cancer that is resistant to hormonal therapy and chemotherapy include abiraterone and enzalutamide. Survival rates for all stages of this cancer have improved steadily since 1940; the five-year survival rate is now nearly 100%.

Cancers of the Female Reproductive Tract

Several types of cancer can affect the female reproductive tract, and a few of these cancers are relatively common.

Cervical Cancer   Cancer of the cervix occurs in women in their twenties and thirties. Virtually all cases of cervical cancer stem from infection by the human papillomavirus (HPV), a group of about 100 related viruses that also cause common warts and genital warts. When certain types of HPV are introduced into the cervix, usually by an infected sex partner, the virus infects cervical cells, causing them to divide and grow. If unchecked, this growth can develop into cervical cancer. Cervical cancer is associated with multiple sex partners and is extremely rare in women who have not had heterosexual intercourse. Smoking, immunosuppression, and prolonged use of oral contraceptives also have been associated with increased risk.

Screening for the changes in cervical cells that precede cancer is done chiefly by means of the **Pap test.** During a pelvic exam, loose cells are scraped from the cervix and examined under a microscope to see whether they are normal. If cells are abnormal but not yet cancerous, the patient has a condition commonly referred to as *cervical dysplasia.* Sometimes such abnormal cells spontaneously return to normal, but in about one-third of cases the cellular changes progress toward malignancy. If this happens, the abnormal cells must be removed, either surgically or with a cryoscopic (ultra-cold) probe or localized laser treatment. Without timely surgery, the malignant cells invade the cervical wall and spread to the uterus and adjacent lymph nodes. At this stage, chemotherapy and radiation may be used to kill the cancer cells, but chances for a complete cure are reduced.

Because the Pap test is highly effective, all women between ages 21 and 65 should be tested. The recommended schedule for testing depends on risk factors, the type of Pap test performed, and whether the Pap test is combined with HPV testing. Two HPV vaccines have been approved by the FDA for the prevention of cervical cancer. Women who receive one of the vaccines should continue to receive routine Pap tests because the vaccines do not protect against all types of the virus.

Uterine, or Endometrial, Cancer   Cancer of the lining of the uterus (the *endometrium*) most often occurs after the age of 55. The risk factors are similar to those for breast cancer, including prolonged exposure to estrogen, early onset of menstruation, late menopause, never having been pregnant, and obesity. Type 2 diabetes is also associated with increased risk. The use of oral contraceptives and hormone therapy that contain estrogen plus progestin do not appear to increase risk.

---

prostate-specific antigen (PSA) test   A screening test for prostate cancer that measures blood levels of prostate-specific antigen (PSA).

incontinence   The inability to control the flow of urine.

Pap test   A scraping of cells from the cervix for examination under a microscope to detect cancer.

TERMS

Endometrial cancer often presents with abnormal vaginal bleeding in a postmenopausal woman. It is treated surgically, commonly by *hysterectomy,* or removal of the uterus. Radiation treatment, hormones, and chemotherapy may be used in addition to surgery. When the tumor is detected at an early stage, about 95% of patients are alive and disease-free five years later. When the disease has spread beyond the uterus, the five-year survival rate is less than 67%.

Ovarian Cancer   Although ovarian cancer is rare compared with cervical or uterine cancer, it causes more deaths than the other two combined. About 22,000 patients were diagnosed with ovarian cancer in 2013 and an estimated 14,000 deaths resulted from this cancer. Early symptoms may include increased abdominal size and bloating, urinary urgency, and pelvic pain. It cannot be detected by Pap tests or any other simple screening method and is often diagnosed late in its development, when surgery and other therapies are unlikely to be successful.

The risk factors are similar to those for breast and endometrial cancer: increasing age (most ovarian cancer occurs after age 60), never having been pregnant, a family history of breast or ovarian cancer, obesity, and specific genetic mutations including *BRCA1* and *BRCA2.* A high number of ovulations appear to increase the chance that a cancer-causing genetic mutation will occur, so anything that lowers the number of lifetime ovulation cycles—pregnancy, breastfeeding, or use of oral contraceptives—reduces a woman's risk of ovarian cancer.

Women with symptoms or who are at high risk because of family history should have thorough pelvic exams at regular intervals. Ovarian cancer is treated by surgical removal of both ovaries, the fallopian tubes, and the uterus. Radiation and chemotherapy are sometimes used in addition to surgery. When the tumor is localized to the ovary, the five-year survival rate is 92%. However, it is diagnosed this early only 15% of the time. For all stages, the five-year survival rate is only 44%.

Skin Cancer

Skin cancer is the most common type of cancer, but it is often not included in cancer incidence and mortality statistics because many types of skin cancer are easily curable. Of the approximate 3.5 million cases of skin cancer diagnosed each year, about 76,000 are of the most serious type, **melanoma.**

Risk Factors   Almost all cases of skin cancer can be traced to excessive exposure to ultraviolet (UV) radiation from the sun, including longer-wavelength ultraviolet A (UVA) and shorter-wavelength ultraviolet B (UVB) radiation. UVB radiation causes sunburns and can damage the eyes and the immune system. UVA is less likely to cause an immediate sunburn, but it damages connective tissue and leads to premature aging of the skin, giving it a wrinkled, leathery appearance. Both UVA and UVB radiation have been linked to the development of skin cancer, and the National Toxicology Program has declared both solar and artificial sources of UV radiation, including sunlamps and tanning beds, to be known human carcinogens. Tanning, either under direct sunlight or in a tanning bed, is a known cause of skin cancer. (Tanning lamps and tanning salon beds emit mostly UVA radiation.)

Both severe, acute sun reactions (sunburns) and chronic low-level sun reactions (suntans) can lead to skin cancer. People with fair skin have less natural protection against skin damage from the sun and a higher risk of developing skin cancer, whereas people with naturally dark skin have a considerable degree of protection. Caucasians are about 10 times more likely than African Americans to develop melanoma, but African Americans and Latinos are still at risk.

Severe sunburns in childhood have been linked to a significantly increased risk of skin cancer in later life, so children in particular should be protected. According to the Skin Cancer Foundation, the risk of skin cancer doubles in people who have had five or more sunburns in their lifetime. Because of damage to the ozone layer of the atmosphere, there is a chance that we may all be exposed to increasing amounts of UV radiation in the future. Other risk factors for skin cancer include having many moles (particularly large ones), spending time at high altitudes, and a family history of the disease.

Types of Skin Cancer   There are three main types of skin cancer, named for the types of skin cells from which they develop. **Basal cell carcinoma** (usually benign) and **squamous cell carcinoma** (malignant) together account for about 95% of the skin cancers diagnosed each year. They are usually found in chronically sun-exposed areas, such as the face, neck, hands, and arms. They usually appear as pale, waxlike, pearly nodules or red, scaly, sharply outlined patches. These cancers are often painless, although they may bleed, crust, and form an open sore on the skin.

Melanoma is by far the most dangerous skin cancer because it spreads so rapidly. It can occur anywhere on the body, but the most common sites are the back, chest, abdomen, and lower legs. A melanoma usually appears at the site of a preexisting mole. The mole may begin to enlarge, become mottled or varied in color (colors can include blue, pink, and white), or develop an irregular surface or irregular borders. Tissue invaded by melanoma may also itch, burn, or bleed easily.

Prevention   One of the major steps you can take to protect yourself against all forms of skin cancer is to avoid lifelong overexposure to sunlight. Blistering, peeling sunburns from unprotected sun exposure are particularly dangerous, but suntans—whether from sunlight or from tanning lamps—also increase your risk of developing skin cancer later in life.

---

melanoma   A malignant tumor of the skin that arises from pigmented cells, usually a mole.   **TERMS**

basal cell carcinoma   Benign skin cancer of the base of the outermost layer of the skin.

squamous cell carcinoma   Malignant cancer of the surface of the outermost layer of the skin.

Sunscreens and Sun-Protective Clothing

If you consistently use sun-protective clothing, sunscreen, and common sense, you can lead an active outdoor life *and* protect your skin against most sun-induced damage.

Clothing

• Wear long-sleeved shirts and long pants. Consider clothing made from special sun-protective fabrics; these garments have an ultraviolet protection factor (UPF) rating, similar to the SPF for sunscreens.

• Wear a hat. A good choice is a broad-brimmed hat or a legionnaire-style cap that covers the ears and neck. Wear sunscreen on your face even if you are wearing a hat.

• Wear sunglasses. Exposure to UV rays can damage the eyes and cause cataracts.

Sunscreen

• Use a sunscreen and lip balm with a sun protection factor (SPF) of 15 or higher. An SPF rating refers to the amount of time you can stay out in the sun before you burn, compared with not using sunscreen. For example, a product with an SPF of 15 would allow you to remain in the sun without burning 15 times longer, on average, than if you didn't apply sunscreen.

• Shake sunscreen before applying. Apply it 30 minutes before exposure to allow it time to bond to the skin. Reapply sunscreen frequently and generously to all sun-exposed areas. Reapply sunscreen 15–30 minutes after sun exposure begins and then every two hours after that and/or following activities, such as swimming, that could remove sunscreen.

Time of Day and Location

• Avoid sun exposure between 10 a.m. and 4 p.m., when the sun's rays are most intense.

• Consult the day's UV index, which predicts UV levels on a 0–11+ scale, to get a sense of the amount of sun protection you'll need. UV index ratings are available in local newspapers, from the weather bureau, or from certain websites.

Tanning Salons

• Avoid tanning salons. Tanning beds and lamps emit mostly UVA radiation, increasing your risk of premature skin aging (such as wrinkles) and skin cancer.

• If you really want a tan, consider using a sunless tanning product. Lotions, creams, and sprays containing the color additive dihydroxyacetone (DHA) are approved by the FDA for tanning.

People of every age, especially babies and children, need to be protected from the sun with **sunscreens** and protective clothing. For a closer look at sunlight and skin cancer, see the box "Sunscreens and Sun-Protective Clothing."

Detection and Treatment   Make it a habit to examine your skin regularly. Most of the spots, freckles, moles, and blemishes on your body are normal; you were born with some of them, and others appear and disappear throughout your life. But if you notice an unusual growth, discoloration, sore that does not heal, or mole that undergoes a sudden or progressive change, see your physician or dermatologist immediately.

Figure 12.5 illustrates the characteristics that may signal a melanoma—asymmetry, border irregularity, color change, a diameter greater than ¼ inch and evolution of the size, shape, or color of the mole. If someone in your family has had multiple skin cancers or melanomas, consult a dermatologist for a complete skin examination and discussion of your particular risk.

In 2011 the FDA approved two new therapies for metastatic melanoma. Ipilimumab is a monoclonal antibody that activates the body's anti-cancer immune response and vemurafenib targets a specific gene mutation in melanoma. For melanoma, the five-year survival rate is 98% if the tumor is

A—Asymmetry: Is one half unlike the other?

B—Border irregularity: Does it have an uneven, scalloped edge rather than a clearly defined border?

C—Color variation: Is the color uniform, or does it vary from one area to another, from tan to brown to black, or from white to red to blue?

¼ in. D—Diameter larger than ¼ inch: At its widest point, is the growth as large as, or larger than, a pencil eraser?

Ordinary Mole

E—Evolving: A mole or skin lesion that looks different from the rest or has any change in size, shape, color, elevation, or another trait, or any new symptom such as bleeding, itching, or crusting.

Changing in size, shape and color

FIGURE 12.5   The ABCDE test for melanoma. To see a variety of photos of melanoma and benign moles, visit the National Cancer Institute's Visuals Online site (http://visualsonline.cancer.gov).

---

sunscreen   A substance used to protect the skin from UV rays; usually applied as a lotion, cream, or spray.   TERMS

The best time to perform a testicular self-exam is after a warm shower or bath, when the scrotum is relaxed.

First, stand in front of a mirror and look for any swelling of the scrotum. Then examine each testicle with both hands. Place the index and middle fingers under the testicle and the thumbs on top. Roll the testicle gently between the fingers and thumbs. Don't worry if one testicle seems slightly larger than the other; that's common. Also, expect to feel the epididymis, which is the soft, sperm-carrying tube at the rear of the testicle.

Perform a self-exam each month. If you find a lump, swelling, or nodule, see a physician right away. The abnormality may not be cancer, but only a physician can make a diagnosis.

Other possible signs of testicular cancer include a change in the way a testicle feels, a sudden collection of fluid in the scrotum, a dull ache in the lower abdomen or groin, a feeling of heaviness in the scrotum, or pain in a testicle or the scrotum.

SOURCES: Testicular Cancer Resource Center. 2012. *How to Do a Testicular Self Examination* (http://tcrc.acor.org/tcexam.html); National Cancer Institute. 2013. *General Information about Testicular Cancer* (http://www.cancer.gov/cancertopics/pdq/treatment/testicular/Patient).

---

localized but only 62% if the cancer has spread to adjacent lymph nodes. Improvements in survival are anticipated with the use of these new targeted treatments.

Head and Neck Cancers

Head and neck cancers—cancers of the oral cavity, pharynx, larynx, and nasal cavity—can be traced principally to cigarette, cigar, or pipe smoking, the use of spit tobacco, and the excessive consumption of alcohol. These risk factors work together to multiply a person's risk of oral cancer. The incidence of head and neck cancer is twice as great in men as in women, and the disease is most frequent in men over 40.

Chemotherapy, radiation, and surgery are the primary methods of treatment for head and neck cancers. Patients often endure intense mouth and throat inflammation and some require disfiguring surgeries, but many can be cured. Among those who survive, a significant number will develop another primary cancer of the head and neck. The five-year survival rate is about 61%.

Testicular Cancer

Testicular cancer is relatively rare, accounting for only 1% of cancer in men (about 8000 cases per year), but it is the most common cancer in men aged 20–35. It is much more common among white Americans and among men whose fathers had testicular cancer than among Latinos, Asian Americans, or African Americans. Men with undescended testicles are at increased risk for testicular cancer, and for this reason that condition should be corrected in early childhood. Self-examination may help in the early detection of testicular cancer (see the box "Testicle Self-Examination"). Tumors are treated by surgical removal of the testicle and, if the tumor has spread, by chemotherapy; radiation treatment is used only rarely. The five-year survival rate for testicular cancer is 95%.

Ask Yourself

QUESTIONS FOR CRITICAL THINKING AND REFLECTION

Has anyone you know had cancer? If so, what type of cancer was it? What were its symptoms? Based on the information presented so far in this chapter, did the person have any of the known risk factors for the disease?

connect™

Connect to Your Choices

Have you ever thought about where you get your behaviors and habits related to CVD and cancer? Many factors can influence our behaviors and habits, some not as obvious as others. When you were growing up, did your family avoid risk-increasing behaviors like smoking and being physically inactive? Currently do you live on a campus or in a community where smoking is discouraged and physical activity is encouraged? Do the people in your social circle value tanned skin? Does your health clinic offer programs to help tobacco users quit or to promote and facilitate physical activity?

What are the external factors that influence your choices about cancer–related behaviors and choices? What are your inner motivations and core values, and how do they affect your choices? Based on what you learned in this chapter, will you make some different choices in the future? If so, what will they be?

Go online to Connect to complete this activity: www.mcgraw-hillconnect.com

Other Cancers

Several other cancers affect a significant number of people each year. Some have identifiable risk factors, particularly smoking and obesity, that are controllable. Causes of others are still under investigation.

SUMMARY

- The cardiovascular system circulates blood throughout the body. The heart pumps blood to the lungs via the pulmonary artery and to the body via the aorta.

- Atherosclerosis is a progressive hardening and narrowing of arteries that can lead to restricted blood flow and even complete blockage.

- The six major risk factors for CVD that can be changed or controlled are tobacco use/misuse, high blood pressure, unhealthy cholesterol levels, inactivity, overweight or obese body habitus, and diabetes.

- Hypertension occurs when blood pressure exceeds normal levels most of the time. It weakens the heart, scars and hardens arteries, and can damage the eyes and kidneys.

- Physical inactivity, obesity, and diabetes are interrelated and are associated with high blood pressure and unhealthy cholesterol levels.

- Contributing risk factors that can be changed include high triglyceride levels and psychological and social factors.

- Risk factors for CVD that can't be changed include being over 65, being male, being African American, and having a family history of CVD.

- Heart attacks are usually the result of a long-term disease process. Warning signs of a heart attack include chest discomfort, shortness of breath, nausea, and sweating.

- A stroke occurs when the blood supply to the brain is cut off by a blood clot or hemorrhage. A transient ischemic attack (TIA) may be a warning sign of an impending stroke.

- Congestive heart failure occurs when the heart's pumping action becomes less efficient and fluid collects in the lungs or in other parts of the body.

- CVD risk can also be reduced by exercising regularly, avoiding tobacco and environmental tobacco smoke, knowing and managing your blood pressure and cholesterol levels, and developing effective ways of handling stress and anger.

- Cancer is the abnormal, uncontrolled multiplication of cells; it can cause death if untreated.

- One in two men and one in three women will develop cancer.

- Mutational damage to a cell's DNA can lead to rapid and uncontrolled growth of cells; mutagens include radiation, viral infection, and chemical substances in food and air.

- Other possible causes of cancer include inactivity and obesity, certain types of infections and chemicals, and radiation.

- Self-monitoring and regular screening tests are essential to early cancer detection. Methods of cancer diagnosis include MRI scanning, CT scanning, and ultrasound.

- Treatment methods usually consist of some combination of surgery, chemotherapy, and radiation. Research continues to show promise in these and other areas.

- Lung cancer kills more people than any other type of cancer. Tobacco smoke is the primary cause.

- Colon and rectal cancer are linked to age, heredity, obesity, and a diet rich in red meat and low in fruits and vegetables. Most colon cancers arise from preexisting polyps.

- Breast cancer affects about one in eight women in the United States. Although there is a genetic component to breast cancer, diet and hormones are also risk factors.

- Prostate cancer is chiefly a disease of aging; diet and lifestyle probably are factors in its occurrence. Early detection is possible through rectal examinations and PSA blood tests.

- Cancers of the female reproductive tract include cervical, uterine, and ovarian cancer. The Pap test is an effective screening test for cervical cancer.

- Abnormal cellular changes in the epidermis, often a result of exposure to the sun, cause skin cancer, as does chronic exposure to certain chemicals. Skin cancers include basal cell carcinoma, squamous cell carcinoma, and melanoma.

- Head and neck cancers are caused primarily by smoking, excess alcohol consumption, and use of smokeless tobacco.

- Testicular cancer can be detected early through self-examination.

Touring the Cardiorespiratory System

> ## The Cardiorespiratory System

> ## The Heart and Lungs

> ## Atherosclerosis: The Process of Cardiovascular Disease

> ## Diabetes: A Disorder of Metabolism

GOALS OF THE TOUR

1. **The Cardiorespiratory System.** Identify the parts of the cardiorespiratory system and the pattern of blood flow through the body.

2. **The Heart and Lungs.** Identify the chambers of the heart and describe the flow of blood through the right side of the heart to the lungs (pulmonary circulation) and through the left side of the heart to the body (systemic circulation).

3. **Atherosclerosis.** Explain the process of cardiovascular disease and compare and contrast the outcomes affecting the heart and the brain.

4. **Diabetes.** Describe how the body uses digested food for energy and growth and how this process is disrupted when a person has diabetes.

The Cardiorespiratory System

1 Identify the parts of the cardiorespiratory system and the pattern of blood flow through the body.

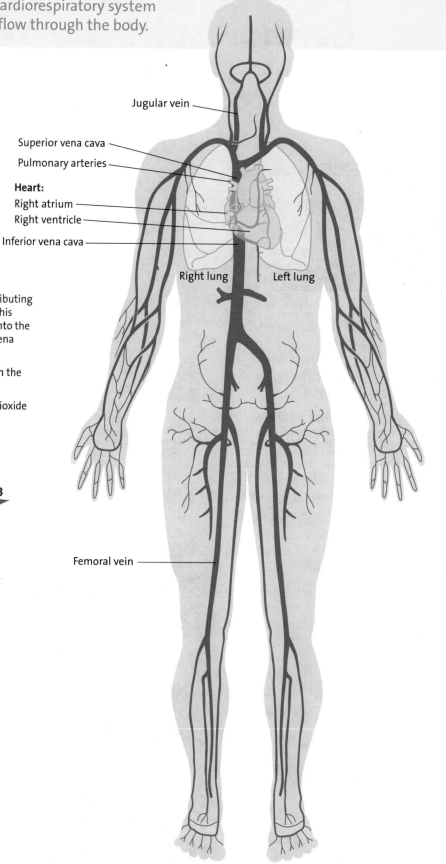

Jugular vein

Superior vena cava

Pulmonary arteries

Heart:

Right atrium

Right ventricle

Inferior vena cava

Right lung   Left lung

Femoral vein

Return of deoxygenated blood to the heart

1. Blood travels through the body, distributing oxygen and picking up carbon dioxide. This waste-laden, oxygen-poor blood flows into the right side of the heart via the superior vena cava and the inferior vena cava.

2. From there, blood is pumped through the pulmonary arteries into the lungs.

3. In the lungs, blood discards carbon dioxide and picks up oxygen.

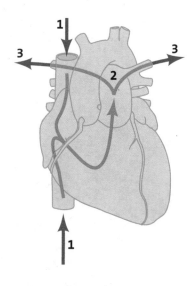

The Heart and Lungs

Identify the chambers of the heart and describe the flow of blood through the right side of the heart to the lungs (pulmonary circulation) and through the left side of the heart to the body (systemic circulation).

2

Blood is supplied to the heart muscle by the right and left coronary arteries, which branch off the aorta.

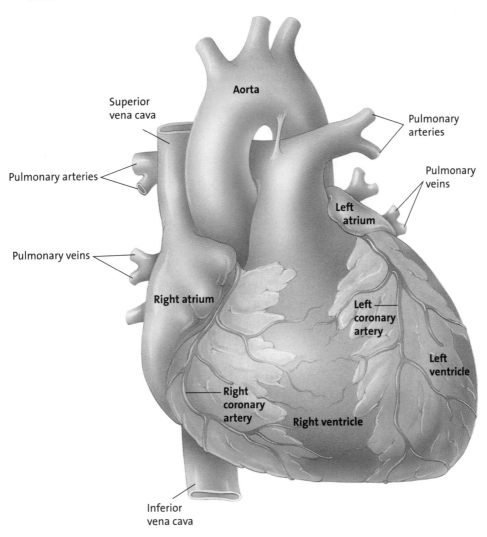

Aorta

Superior vena cava

Pulmonary arteries

Pulmonary arteries

Pulmonary veins

Pulmonary veins

Left atrium

Right atrium

Left coronary artery

Left ventricle

Right coronary artery

Right ventricle

Inferior vena cava

Atherosclerosis: The Process of Cardiovascular Disease

3 Explain the process of cardiovascular disease and compare and contrast the outcomes affecting the heart and the brain.

1. A healthy artery allows blood to flow through freely.

2. Plaque buildup begins when endothelial cells lining the arteries are damaged by smoking, high blood pressure, oxidized LDL cholesterol, and other causes. Excess cholesterol particles collect beneath these cells.

Coronary arteries

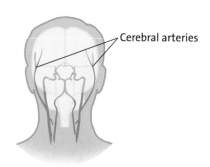

Cerebral arteries

Diabetes: A Disorder of Metabolism

Describe how the body uses digested food for energy and growth and how this process is disrupted when a person has diabetes.

Normal metabolism

1. When a meal is consumed, food is broken down into nutrients that the body can use to produce energy and build and nourish cells. Carbohydrates are broken down into glucose, which is the body's primary source of energy.

2. When glucose enters the bloodstream, the pancreas secretes the hormone insulin, which allows glucose to enter body cells.

Glucose

Bloodstream

Insulin

Liver

Pancreas

Body cells

Stomach

Kidney

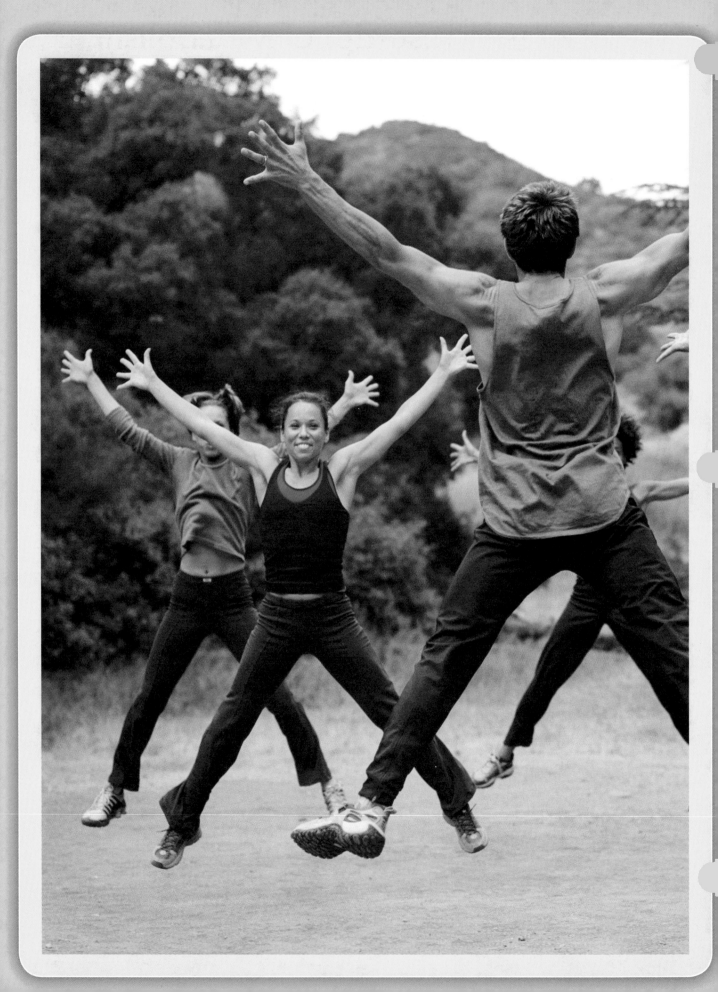

BOOKS

Chatham, J. 2012. *The DASH Diet Health Plan: Low-Sodium, Low-Fat Recipes to Promote Weight Loss, Lower Blood Pressure, and Prevent Diabetes.* Berkeley, CA: Rockridge Press. *A compilation of the findings of the medical and scientific community, alongside dozens of DASH diet recipes, to make it easy to put the DASH diet into action.*

Johnson, G. 2013. *The Cancer Chronicles.* New York: Random House. *Assessment of theories and recent advances in the war on cancer, prompted by the author's wife's personal battle with the disease, revealing deep truths about life itself.*

Mostyn, B. 2012. *Pocket Guide to Low Sodium Foods,* 3rd ed. Olympia, WA: InData Publishing. *Lists thousands of low-sodium products that can be purchased in supermarkets, as well as low-sodium choices available in many restaurants.*

Mukherjee, S. 2010. *The Emperor of All Maladies.* New York: Scribner. *An attempt to write the biography of cancer, this encyclopedic history of scientific progress includes stories of cancer patients and of heroic researchers, but its main character is the disease itself as it has been diagnosed, treated, and thought about over the last 4000 years.*

Sikka, M. 2014. *A Breast Cancer Alphabet.* New York: Crown Publishers.

ORGANIZATIONS, HOTLINES, AND WEBSITES

American Academy of Dermatology. Provides information about skin cancer prevention.

http://www.aad.org

American Cancer Society. Provides a wide range of free materials on the prevention and treatment of cancer.

http://www.cancer.org

American Heart Association. Provides information about hundreds of topics relating to cardiovascular disease; the AHA's website links to several sites focusing on specific heart-related topics.

http://www.heart.org (general information)

American Institute for Cancer Research. Provides information about lifestyle and cancer prevention, especially nutrition.

http://www.aicr.org

Cancer Guide: Steve Dunn's Cancer Information Page. Links to many good cancer resources on the Internet and advice about how to make best use of the information.

http://www.cancerguide.org

Clinical Trials. Information about clinical trials for new cancer treatments can be accessed at the following sites:

http://www.cancer.gov/clinicaltrials

http://www.centerwatch.com

Dietary Approaches to Stop Hypertension (DASH). Provides information about the design, diets, and results of the DASH study, including tips on how to follow the DASH diet at home.

http://www.nhlbi.nih.gov/health/public/heart/hbp/dash

EPA/Sunwise. Information about the UV index and the effects of sun exposure, with links to sites with daily UV index ratings for cities in the United States and other countries.

http://www.epa.gov/sunwise/uvindex.html

Harvard School of Public Health: Disease Risk Index. Includes interactive risk assessments as well as tips for preventing common cancers.

http://www.diseaseriskindex.harvard.edu/update

MedlinePlus: Blood, Heart, and Circulation Topics. Provides links to reliable sources of information on many topics relating to cardiovascular health.

http://www.nlm.nih.gov/medlineplus/bloodheartandcirculation.html

MedlinePlus Cancer Information. Provides news and links to reliable information on a variety of cancers and cancer treatment.

http://www.nlm.nih.gov/medlineplus/cancers.html

National Cancer Institute. Provides information about treatment options, screening, and clinical trials.

http://www.cancer.gov

National Cholesterol Education Program (NCEP): Cholesterol Counts for Everyone. Provides information about cholesterol for people with heart disease and people who want to avoid it.

http://www.nhlbi.nih.gov/about/ncep/

National Comprehensive Cancer Network (NCCN). Presents treatment guidelines for physicians and patients related to the treatment of various cancers; these guidelines were developed by a group of leading cancer centers.

http://www.nccn.org

National Heart, Lung, and Blood Institute. Provides information about and interactive applications for a variety of topics relating to cardiovascular health and disease, including cholesterol, smoking, obesity, hypertension, and the DASH diet.

http:// http://www.nhlbi.nih.gov/

National Stroke Association. Provides information and referrals for stroke victims and their families as well as a stroke risk assessment.

http://www.stroke.org/site/PageNavigator/HOME

National Toxicology Program. The federal program that creates regular reports listing the substances that are known or reasonably assumed to cause cancer in humans.

http://ntp-server.niehs.nih.gov

Oncolink/The University of Pennsylvania Cancer Center Resources. Contains information about different types of cancer and answers to frequently asked questions.

http://www.oncolink.org

The Human Heart: An On-Line Exploration. An online museum exhibit containing information about the structure and function of the heart, how to monitor your heart's health, and how to maintain a healthy heart.

http://www.fi.edu/learn/heart/

SELECTED BIBLIOGRAPHY

Adly, G., and R. Plakogiannis. 2013. Reinitiating aspirin therapy for primary prevention of cardiovascular events in a patient post–aspirin-induced upper gastrointestinal bleed: A case report and review of literature. *Annals of Pharmacotherapy,* published online February 5.

American Cancer Society. 2014. *Cancer Facts and Figures 2014.* Atlanta: American Cancer Society.

American Cancer Society. 2012. *Cancer Treatment and Survivorship Facts & Figures 2012–2013.* Atlanta: American Cancer Society.

American Cancer Society. 2012. *Colorectal Cancer Facts & Figures 2012.* Atlanta: American Cancer Society.

American Cancer Society. 2013. *Breast Cancer Facts and Figures 2013–2014.* Atlanta, GA: American Cancer Society.

American Heart Association. 2013. *Heart Disease and Stroke Statistics, 2013 Update.* Dallas: American Heart Association.

Broomall, E. M., et al. 2010. Epidemiology, clinical manifestations, and recent advances in vaccination against human papillomavirus. *Postgraduate Medicine* 122(2): 121–129.

Centers for Disease Control and Prevention. 2011. National and state vaccination coverage among adolescents aged 13 through 17 years—United States, 2010. *Morbidity and Mortality Weekly Reports* 60(33): 1117–1123.

Centers for Disease Control and Prevention. 2011. Vital signs: Prevalence, treatment, and control of high levels of low-density lipoprotein cholesterol—United States, 1999–2002 and 2005–2008. *Morbidity and Mortality Weekly Report* 60(4):109–14 (http://www.cdc.gov/mmwr/preview/mmwrhtml/mm6004a5.htm?s_cid=mm6004a5_w).

Centers for Disease Control and Prevention. 2011. Vital signs: Current cigarette smoking among adults aged ≥18 years—United States, 2005–2010. *Morbidity and Mortality Weekly Report* 60(35): 1207–1212.

Després, Jean-Pierre. 2012. Body fat distribution and risk of cardiovascular disease: An update. *Circulation* 126: 1301–1313.

Go, A. S., et al. 2014. AHA statistical update: Heart disease and stroke statistics—2014 update: A report from the American Heart Association.*Circulation* 129: e28–e292.

Gommans, J., et al. 2009. Preventing strokes: The assessment and management of people with transient ischemic attack. *New Zealand Medical Journal* 122(1293): 50–60.

Mendis, S., et al., eds. 2011. *Global Atlas on Cardiovascular Disease Prevention and Control.* Geneva, Switzerland: World Health Organization (in collaboration with the World Heart Federation and World Stroke Organization).

Mirmiran, P., et al. 2009. Fruit and vegetable consumption and risk factors for cardiovascular disease. *Metabolism* 58(4): 460–468.

Müller, D., et al. 2006. How sudden is sudden cardiac death? *Circulation* 114(11): 1146–1150.

National Cancer Institute, National Institutes of Health. 2011. *Radon and Cancer* (http://www.cancer.gov/cancertopics/factsheet/Risk/radon).

National Center for Health Statistics. 2012. Deaths: Final data for 2010. *National Vital Statistics Reports* 60(6).

National Center for Health Statistics. 2013. Deaths: Final data for 2010. *National Vital Statistics Reports* 61(4): 1–118. Hyattsville, MD: NCHS.

National Human Genome Research Institute. 2014. *A Brief Guide to Genomics Fact Sheet* (http://www.genome.gov/18016863).

Robert, C., et al. 2011. Ipilimumab plus dacarbazine for previously untreated metastatic melanoma. *New England Journal of Medicine* 364: 2517–2526.

Samet, J., et al. 2009. Lung cancer in never smokers: Clinical epidemiology and environmental risk factors. *Clinical Cancer Research* 15(18): 5626–5645.

Schiller, J. S., et al. 2012. Summary health statistics for U.S. adults: National Health Interview Survey, 2010. National Center for Health Statistics. *Vital Health Stat* 10(252).

Stone, N. J., et al. 2013. ACC/AHA guideline on the treatment of blood cholesterol to reduce atherosclerotic cardiovascular risk in adults: A report of the American College of Cardiology/American Heart Association Task Force on Practice Guidelines. *Journal of the American College of Cardiology,* 12 November (published online).

U.S. Preventive Services Task Force. 2008. Screening for prostate cancer: U.S. Preventive Services Task Force recommendation statement. *Annals of Internal Medicine* 149(3): 185–191.

Willershausen, I. et al. 2013. Association between chronic periodontal and apical inflammation and acute myocardial infarction. *Odontology,* 21 April.

Modifying Your Diet for Heart Health and Cancer Prevention

Gradually modifying you diet to include less saturated and trans fat and more fruits and vegetables can help you avoid both CVD and cancer in the future. Begin by assessing your current diet. Keep a record of everything you eat for a week. At the end of the week you can evaluate your diet and start taking steps to modify it.

Reducing the Saturated and Trans Fat in Your Diet

The American Heart Association recommends that no more than 1% of the calories in your diet come from trans fats. Similarly, the report of the 2010 Dietary Guidelines Advisory Committee recommends that Americans avoid trans fat and saturated fat from industrial sources completely and consume only small amounts (less than 0.5% of calories) from natural sources. Hydrogenated fats, products made with them, and deep-fried fast food are high in trans fats. Although food manufacturers are phasing out trans fats, it's important to read labels to see how much trans fat a product contains. If a product contains less than 0.5% trans fat, the manufacturer is allowed to list trans fat content as 0%.

To see how your diet measures up, keep track of everything you eat for three days in your health journal. Information about the calorie and fat content of foods is available on many food labels, in books, and on the Internet.

At the end of the monitoring period, write in the calories and grams of trans fat for the foods you've eaten. Determine the percentage of daily calories as fat that you consumed for each day: Multiply grams of trans fats by 9 (fat has 9 calories per gram) and then divide by total calories. For example, if you consumed 30 grams of trans fats and 2100 calories on a particular day, then your trans fat consumption as a percentage of total calories would be calculated as $30 \times 9 = 270$ calories of fat $\div$ 2100 total calories = 0.13, or 13%.

To plan healthy changes, take a close look at your food record. Do you choose many foods high in fat? Do you limit your portion sizes to those recommended by MyPlate? Try making healthy substitutions. Instead of a grilled cheese sandwich, try turkey, or substitute a plain baked potato for french fries. If you frequently eat in fast-food restaurants, try finding an appealing alternative— and recruit some friends to join you. When you choose foods that are rich in fat, *watch your portion sizes carefully,* and try to balance your choices throughout the day.

Most Americans need to double the amount of fruits and vegetables they eat every day. Begin by monitoring your diet for one or two weeks to assess your current intake; then look for ways to incorporate these foods into your diet in easy and tasty ways. Here are some tips to get you started.

Breakfast

- Drink pure fruit juice every morning.
- Add raisins, berries, or sliced fruit to cereal, pancakes, or waffles. Top bagels with tomato slices.
- Try a fruit smoothie made from fresh or frozen fruit and orange juice or low-fat yogurt.

Lunch

- Choose vegetable soup or salad with your meal.
- Replace potato chips or french fries with cut-up vegetables.
- Add vegetables such as roasted peppers, cucumber slices, shredded carrots, avocado, or salsa to sandwiches.

Dinner

- Choose a vegetarian main course, such as stir-fry or vegetable stew. Have at least two servings of vegetables with every dinner.
- Substitute vegetables for meat in casseroles and pasta and chili recipes.
- At the salad bar, pile your plate with healthful vegetables and use low-fat or nonfat dressing.

Snacks and On the Go

- Keep ready-to-eat-fruits and vegetables on hand (apples, plums, pears, and carrots).
- Keep small packages of dried fruit in the car (try dried apples, apricots, peaches, pears, and raisins).

The All-Stars

Different fruits and vegetables contribute different vitamins, phytochemicals, and other nutrients, so be sure to get a variety. The following types of produce are particularly rich in nutrients and phytochemicals:

- Cruciferous vegetables (broccoli, cauliflower, cabbage, bok choy, brussels sprouts, kohlrabi, turnips, etc.).
- Citrus fruits.
- Berries.
- Dark green leafy vegetables.
- Deep yellow, orange, and red fruits and vegetables.

CHAPTER OBJECTIVES

- Identify the body's physical and chemical barriers to infection, and explain how the immune system responds to an invading microorganism

- Describe the step-by-step process by which infectious diseases are transmitted

- Identify the major types of pathogens and describe the common diseases they cause

- Explain how HIV infection affects the body and how it is transmitted, diagnosed, and treated

- Discuss the symptoms, risks, and treatments for the other major STIs

- Discuss steps you can take to prevent infections, including STIs, and strengthen your immune system

CHAPTER **13**

Immunity and Infection

ountless microscopic organisms live around, on, and in us. Although most microbes are beneficial, many of them can cause **infections** and infectious diseases including sexually transmitted infections. For the most part, the vigilance of our immune system keeps them at bay and our bodies healthy. The immune system protects us not just from **pathogens** but also from cancer.

This chapter introduces you to the mechanisms of immunity and infection, as well as strategies for keeping yourself well in a world of disease-causing microorganisms.

THE BODY'S DEFENSE SYSTEM

Our bodies have very effective ways of protecting themselves against invasion by foreign organisms. The immune system is the body's collective set of defenses that includes surface barriers as well as the specialized cells, tissues, and organs that carry out the immune reponse. The first line of defense is a formidable array of physical and chemical barriers. When these barriers are breached, cellular processes of the immune system come into play. Together these defenses provide an effective response to nearly all the invasions our bodies experience.

Physical and Chemical Barriers

The skin, the body's largest organ, prevents many microorganisms from entering the body. Although many bacterial and fungal organisms live on the surface of the skin, few can penetrate it except through a cut or break.

Wherever there is an opening in the body, or an area without skin, other barriers exist. All body cavities and passages that are exposed to the external environment are lined with mucous membranes, which secrete mucus and contain cells designed to prevent the passage of unwanted organisms and particles. These areas include the mouth, nostrils, eyelids, bronchioles, vagina, and other organs of the respiratory, digestive, and urogenital tracts. The surface of both skin and mucous membranes is made of epithelial tissue, which consists of one or more layers of closely packed cells with almost

---

infection Invasion of the body by a microorganism. **TERMS**

pathogen A microorganism that causes disease.

no space between cells. The fluids that cover epithelial tissue, such as tears, saliva, and vaginal secretions, are rich in enzymes and other proteins that break down and destroy many microorganisms.

The respiratory tract is lined not only with mucous membranes but also with cells having hairlike protrusions called *cilia.* The cilia sweep foreign matter up and out of the respiratory tract. Particles that are not caught by this mechanism may be expelled from the system by a cough.

The Immune System: Cells, Tissues, and Organs

Beyond surface barriers, the **immune system** operates through a remarkable information network involving billions of cellular defenders that rush to protect the body when a threat arises. The immune system can be thought of as two systems. The innate immune system consists of cells that can recognize pathogenic microorganisms and are the first responders to those pathogens. The adaptive immune system consists of cells that can recognize pathogenic microorganisms and have the remarkable ability to improve and accelerate their responses after exposure to those pathogens. It is also very specific, operating through mechanisms that work like a lock and key. The complete elimination of a pathogen involves the coordinated activities of both systems.

The immune system works through the action of different types of white blood cells, which are continuously produced in the bone marrow.

Cells of the Innate Immune System
The cells of the innate immune system recognize pathogens as "foreign" and kill them, but they cannot develop a memory of these pathogens. Thus they respond the same way no matter how many times a pathogen invades. *Neutrophils,* one type of white blood cell, travel in the bloodstream to areas of invasion, attacking and ingesting pathogens. *Eosinophils,* white blood cells that occur in mucosal tissues such as those in the gastrointestinal tract and the mammary glands, provide innate immunity to certain microbes. *Macrophages,* or "big eaters," act as scavengers, devouring pathogens and worn-out cells. *Natural killer cells* directly destroy virus-infected cells and cells that have turned cancerous. *Dendritic cells,* which reside in tissues, engulf pathogens and activate lymphocytes.

Cells of the Adaptive Immune System
The cells of the adaptive immune system are white blood cells called **lymphocytes.** The two main types of lymphocytes are T cells and B cells, which differ in function. Whereas cells of the innate immune system can recognize a cell as foreign, lymphocytes are capable of exquisite specificity and of immunological memory.

> The immune system has a remarkable ability: It can **distinguish foreign cells from the body's own cells.**

Antigens and Antibodies All of your body cells display markers on their surface that identify them as "self" to lymphocytes. Invading microbes also display markers, and these markers identify them as foreign, or "nonself," to lymphocytes. Nonself markers that trigger an immune response are known as **antigens.**

Antibodies are specialized proteins that circulate in your bloodstream and are present in most body fluids. Produced by white blood cells, they have complementary markers on their surface that work with antigens like a lock and key, allowing them to recognize and neutralize specific microbes. When an antibody encounters an antigen with a complementary pattern, it locks onto it and neutralizes it or tags it for attack by immune system cells.

T Cells and B Cells When a B cell lymphocyte or T cell lymphocyte encounters the antigen for which it is specific, it proliferates, producing many more lymphocytes that are specific to the same antigen. These daughter cells then differentiate into cells with specific immune functions and attack the invading organisms. **B cells** become plasma cells that secrete antibodies. **T cells** differentiate into helper T cells, killer T cells, or suppressor T cells (also called regulatory T cells.) Some B and T cells become memory B and T cells, which can mount a rapid and powerful response should they encounter the same invader months or even years in the future.

The Inflammatory Response When injured or infected, the body reacts by producing an inflammatory response. Macrophages engulf the invading microbe and produce substances that convey danger to other cells of the immune system. The resulting inflammatory response

---

TERMS

immune system   The body's collective system of defenses that includes surface barriers as well as the specialized cells, tissues, and organs that carry out the immune reponse.

lymphocyte   A type of white blood cell that carries out important functions in the immune system.

antigen   A marker on the surface of a foreign substance that immune system cells recognize as nonself; a foreign antigen's presence in the body triggers the immune response.

antibody   A specialized protein, produced by white blood cells, that can recognize and neutralize specific microbes.

B cell   A type of lymphocyte with specific immune system functions; B cells mature in the bone marrow and produce antibodies.

T cell   A type of lymphocyte with specific immune system functions; T cells arise in bone marrow and mature in the thymus.

triggered by **histamine** causes blood vessels to dilate and fluid to flow out of capillaries into the injured tissue. This activity produces increased heat, swelling, and redness in the affected area. White blood cells are drawn to the area and attack the invaders, in many cases destroying them. This entire reaction is the immune response, as described in the next section. At the site of infection there may be *pus*—a collection of dead white blood cells and debris resulting from the encounter.

The Immune Response   The immune response can be thought of as happening in four phases (Figure 13.1).

- *Phase 1: Recognition.* Dendritic cells are drawn to the site of the injury and consume the foreign cells. They then migrate to nearby lymphoid tissue, where they activate T cells by displaying the foreign cells' antigen on their surfaces. Natural killer cells and other early responders destroy infected cells.

- *Phase 2: Proliferation.* Helper T cells specific to the antigen multiply rapidly and stimulate the proliferation of killer T cells and B cells. Cytokines, which are chemical messengers secreted by lymphocytes and other cells of the immune system, help regulate and coordinate the immune response.

- *Phase 3: Elimination.* Elimination of pathogens occurs one of two ways, depending on whether the pathogens reproduce outside or inside of cells: In *antibody-mediated*

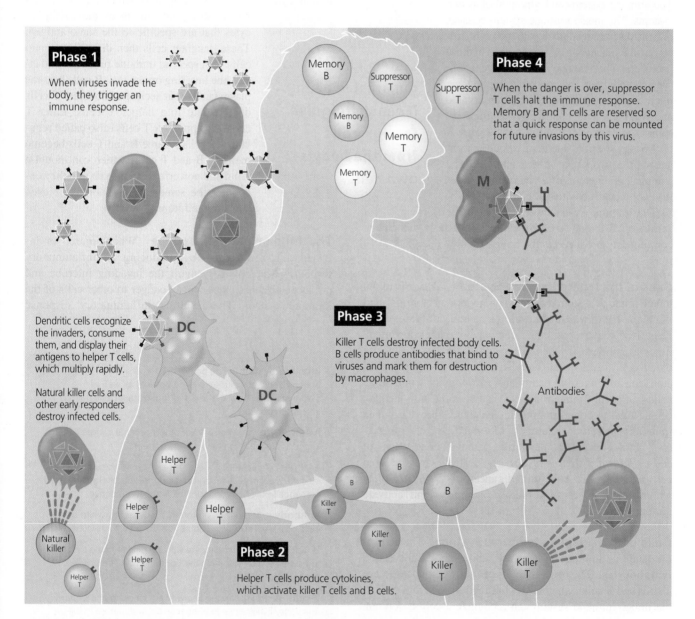

FIGURE 13.1   The immune response.   Once invaded by a pathogen, the body mounts a complex series of reactions to destroy the invader. Pictured here are the phases of the immune response as the body responds to a virus.

immune response, B cells are activated to become antibody-producing factories that release antibodies into the blood stream. These antibodies bind to their target extracellular pathogens (pathogens *outside* the cells), marking them for destruction by macrophages and other cells of the immune system. Antibodies are not, however, effective against pathogens that reproduce inside cells. These pathogens are eliminated by various cell types, including killer T cells, in an action known as *cell-mediated immune response*. In this response, the killer T cells actually kill the infected cells, thereby eliminating the pathogen that is *within* the infected cells.

- *Phase 4: Slowdown.* Regulatory molecules and suppressor T cells inhibit lymphocyte proliferation and induce lymphocyte death, causing a slowdown of activity. This process restores "resting" levels of B and T cells. Some memory T and B cells remain in the body, where they can initiate a rapid response if the same pathogen reappears in the future.

Immunity   After an infection, survival often confers **immunity;** that is, an infected person will not be susceptible to the same pathogen again. This insusceptibility is because some of the lymphocytes created during phase 2 of the immune response are reserved as memory T and B cells. As part of the acquired immune response, they continue to circulate in the blood and lymphatic system for years or even for the rest of the person's life. If the same antigen enters the body again, the memory T and B cells recognize and destroy it before it can cause illness. This subsequent response takes only a few days to initiate and prevents illness. The ability of memory lymphocytes to remember previous infections is known as **acquired immunity**.

The Lymphatic System   The lymphatic system consists of a network of vessels that carry a clear fluid called lymph. It also includes organs and structures, including the spleen and the lymph nodes, that function as part of the immune system. The lymphatic vessels pick up excess fluid from body tissues; the fluid passes through the lymph nodes, where macrophages and dendritic cells congregate. They help clear the fluid of debris and pathogens. Lymph nodes are also the sites where T cells and B cells are activated. When these nodes are actively involved in fighting an infection, they fill with cells. Physicians use the location of swollen lymph nodes as a clue to an infection's location and cause.

Immunization

The ability of the immune system to remember previously encountered organisms and retain its strength against them is the basis for **immunization**. When a person is immunized,

the immune system is primed with an antigen similar to the pathogenic organism but not as dangerous. The body responds by producing antibodies, which prevent serious infection if the person is exposed to the disease organism itself. The preparations used to manipulate the immune system are known as **vaccines.**

Active immunity, a condition in which the vaccinated person produces his or her own antibodies to the microorganism, can be acquired by vaccination or naturally when a person is infected and mounts an immune response to the pathogen. This contrasts with *passive immunity,* which is conferred by injecting gamma globulin (antibodies) produced by other human beings or animals who have recovered from a given disease.

Immunization has become a source of public debate among people who question whether vaccinations actually do more harm than good. In the past century vaccines have helped to increase the average American lifespan by approximately 30 years—and have done so with an excellent safety record. Nevertheless, misinformation about vaccines has spread raising concerns about their efficacy and safety.

Vaccines are approved by the Advisory Committee on Immunization Practices—the advisors for the Centers for Disease Control and Prevention (CDC)—and the Committee on Infectious Diseases—the advisors for the American Academy of Pediatrics (AAP).

To further ensure their safety, vaccines are tested in larger numbers of people for longer periods of time than drugs are before being licensed. For example, the human papillomavirus (HPV) vaccine was tested in 30,000 women, the conjugate pneumococcal vaccine was tested in 40,000 children, and each of the current rotavirus vaccines were tested in 70,000 children before being licensed. No other medication receives this degree of scrutiny.

Additionally, safety mechanisms such as the Vaccine Adverse Event Reporting System (VAERS) and the Vaccine Safety Datalink Project monitor adverse events reported after licensure. Side effects from immunization are usually

> **QUICK STATS**
>
> **27** common diseases can be prevented by vaccines.
>
> —CDC, 2012

immunity   Resistance to infection.   **TERMS**

acquired immunity   The body's ability to mobilize the cellular memory of a pathogen's attack to prevent subsequent illness; acquired through the normal immune response and through vaccination.

immunization   The process of conferring a person with immunity to a pathogen by administering a vaccine.

vaccines   A preparation of killed or weakened microorganisms, inactivated toxins, or components of microorganisms that is administered to stimulate an immune response; a vaccine protects against future infection by the pathogen.

Ask Yourself

?

QUESTIONS FOR CRITICAL THINKING
AND REFLECTION

What are your views on government-required child
vaccinations? What has shaped your views on this issue?

mild, such as soreness at the injection site. Any risk from a vaccine must be balanced against the risk posed by the diseases it prevents. For example, the global death rate from diphtheria is 5–10%, compared to less than 1% in countries that offer vaccinations.

Allergy: The Body's Defense System Gone Haywire

Allergies result from a hypersensitive and overactive immune system. The immune system reacts to a harmless substance such as pollen or animal dander as if it were a harmful pathogen. For the most part, allergy symptoms— stuffy nose, sneezing, wheezing, skin rashes, and so on—are the result of the immune response.

Substances that provoke allergies are known as **allergens**. Common allergens include pollen, animal dander, dust mites and cockroaches, mold and mildew, insect stings, and some foods.

The Allergic Response   Most allergic reactions are due to an immune response that leads to the release of large amounts of histamine and other compounds that cause allergic symptoms. Histamine has many effects, including increasing the inflammatory response and stimulating mucus production. In the nose, histamine may cause congestion and sneezing; in the eyes, itchiness and tearing; in the skin, redness, swelling, and itching; in the intestines, bloating and cramping; and in the lungs, coughing, wheezing, and shortness of breath. In some people, an allergen can trigger an **asthma** attack. Symptoms often occur immediately, within minutes of exposure.

---

allergy   A disorder caused by the body's exaggerated response to foreign chemicals and proteins; also called *hypersensitivity*.

TERMS

allergen   A substance that triggers an allergic reaction.

asthma   A disease in which chronic inflammation and periodic constriction of the airways cause wheezing, shortness of breath, and coughing.

anaphylaxis   A severe systemic hypersensitive reaction to an allergen characterized by difficulty breathing, low blood pressure, heart arrhythmia, seizure, and sometimes death.

incubation   The period when bacteria or viruses are actively multiplying inside the body's cells; usually a period without symptoms of illness.

The most serious, but rare, kind of allergic reaction is **anaphylaxis,** which results from a release of histamine throughout the body. Anaphylactic reactions can be life threatening because symptoms may include swelling of the throat, extremely low blood pressure, fainting, heart arrhythmia, and seizures. Anaphylaxis is a medical emergency, and treatment requires immediate injection of epinephrine.

Dealing with Allergies   If you suspect you might have an allergy, visit your physician or an allergy specialist. You may be able to avoid or minimize exposure to allergens by changing your environment or behavior. For example, removing carpets from the bedroom and using special bedding can reduce dust mite contact.

There are also medications available for allergy sufferers. Many over-the-counter antihistamines are effective at controlling symptoms, and prescription corticosteroids delivered by aerosol markedly reduce allergy symptoms. A third approaach is immunotherapy, in which a person is desensitized to a particular allergen through the administration of gradually increasing doses of the allergen over a period of months or years.

THE SPREAD OF DISEASE

The immune system is operating at the cellular level at all times, maintaining its vigilance when you're well and fighting invaders when you're sick.

Symptoms and Contagion

The symptoms you experience during an illness are related to the phase of infection and the actions of your immune system. During the first phase of infection, **incubation,** when viruses or bacteria are actively multiplying before the immune system has gathered momentum, you may not have any symptoms of the illness, but you may be contagious. During the second and third phases you may "feel a cold coming on." Symptoms first appear during the *prodromal period,* which follows incubation. If you have acquired immunity, the infection may be eradicated during the incubation period or the prodromal period. In this case it does not develop into a full-blown illness.

Many symptoms of an illness are actually due to the body's immune response rather than to the actions or products of the invading organism. For example, fever is caused by the release of certain cytokines during the immune response that cause the body's thermostat to be reset to a higher level. The resulting elevated temperature helps the body fight against pathogens by enhancing immune responses.

You may be contagious before you experience any symptoms, which means that you can transmit an illness without knowing you're infected or catch an illness from someone who doesn't appear to be sick. On the other hand, your symptoms may continue after the pathogens have been mostly destroyed, when you are no longer infectious.

The Chain of Infection

Infectious diseases are transmitted from one person to another through a series of steps—a chain of infection.

The cycle begins with a *pathogen*, which has a natural environment—called a **reservoir**—in which it typically lives. This reservoir can be a person, an animal, or an environmental space like soil or water. A person who is the reservoir for a pathogen may be ill or may be an asymptomatic carrier who, although having no symptoms, can spread infection. To transmit infection, the pathogen must leave the reservoir through some *portal of exit*. In the case of a human reservoir, portals of exit include saliva, the mucous membranes, blood, feces, and nose and throat discharges. Next, there has to be a means of transmission: Transmission can occur directly or indirectly. In *direct transmission,* the pathogen is passed from one person to another without an intermediary.

In *indirect transmission,* animals or insects such as rats, ticks, and mosquitoes serve as **vectors,** carrying the pathogen from one host to another. Pathogens can also be transmitted via contaminated soil, food, or water or from inanimate objects, such as eating utensils, doorknobs, and handkerchiefs.

To infect a new host, a pathogen must have a *portal of entry* into the body. Pathogens can enter through direct contact with or penetration of the skin or mucous membranes, inhalation, or ingestion. Pathogens that enter the skin or mucous membranes can cause a local infection of the tissue, or they may penetrate into the bloodstream or lymphatic system, thereby causing a **systemic infection**.

Once in the *new host,* a variety of factors determine whether the pathogen will be able to establish itself and cause infection. If conditions are right, the pathogen will multiply and produce disease in the new host, who then becomes a reservoir from which a new chain of infection can be started.

Interrupting the chain of infection at any point can prevent disease. Strategies for breaking the chain include both public health measures and individual action. For example, a pathogen's reservoir can be isolated or destroyed, as when a sick individual is placed under quarantine or when insects or animals carrying pathogens are killed. Public sanitation practices, such as sewage treatment and the chlorination of drinking water, can also kill pathogens. Transmission can be disrupted through strategies like hand washing and the use of face masks. Immunization and the treatment of infected hosts can stop the pathogen from multiplying, producing a serious disease, and being passed on to a new host.

Epidemics and Pandemics

The rapid spread of a disease or health condition is called an **epidemic.** Although the word is usually used in reference to infectious diseases, it is also used for health conditions that are not caused by an infectious organism. For example, it is often said that obesity and diabetes have reached epidemic proportions in the United States.

In an epidemic, the occurrence of the disease is greater than what is expected normally. Thus, the common cold, which occurs with great frequency, is never classified as an epidemic. Conversely, the term *epidemic* is used to refer to outbreaks of diseases that are not widespread. For example, when 10 infants died in California in 2010 from whooping cough, the incident was referred to as an epidemic.

A **pandemic** is an epidemic that has spread across a large area, such as an entire nation, a continent, or even the world. In contrast to the term *epidemic,* the term *pandemic* refers exclusively to infectious disease. Human history has been punctuated by numerous pandemics of various diseases, including bubonic plague, smallpox, and influenza. One of the most severe influenza pandemics occurred in 1918–1919, following World War I, when 20–40% of the world's population became ill and as many as 40 million people died.

Not all widespread infectious diseases are pandemics. An infectious disease is said to be endemic when it habitually exists in a

> In an epidemic, the occurrence of the disease is greater than normally expected. Because the common cold occurs frequently, it is **never classified as an epidemic.**

reservoir A natural environment in which a pathogen typically lives.

vector An insect, rodent, or other organism that carries and transmits a pathogen from one host to another.

systemic infection An infection spread by the blood or lymphatic system to large portions of the body.

epidemic A rapidly spreading disease or health-related condition.

pandemic A widespread epidemic.

TERMS

certain region. Endemic diseases generally occur at low frequency in particular populations or regions. For example, malaria is endemic to low-altitude areas of northern and eastern South Africa.

H1N1 Influenza   In 2009 an outbreak of influenza caused by a virus never before identified as a cause of human illness sparked fears of a worldwide influenza pandemic. Most people had no immunity to this new strain, initially called swine flu and subsequently labeled H1N1 influenza A virus. This strain resulted from a combination of genes from four different viruses: two from swine flu viruses, one from an avian (bird) flu virus, and one from a human flu virus. The addition of the gene from a human virus meant that humans could be infected with it, and, because it was new, they would have no prior immunity. In June 2009, the World Health Organization (WHO) declared that a pandemic was under way. By February 2010, the WHO reported up to 86 million cases and up to nearly 18,000 deaths. By May of that year, flu activity had tapered off and declined to normal levels, but the WHO continues to track trends globally, and the CDC continues to recommend H1N1 vaccination for persons aged 6 months to 24 years and people aged 25–64 years who are at high risk.

H5N1 Influenza   Since 1998 scientists have been monitoring the progress of another influenza A virus known as H5N1, or avian (bird) influenza. This strain infects chickens, ducks, and geese as well as wild birds; it doesn't pass easily to humans or among humans, but when it does, it is deadly. According to the World Health Organization, as of February 2014, 650 people worldwide had been infected with H5N1, and 386 of them had died.

PATHOGENS AND DISEASE

The pathogens that cause infectious diseases include bacteria, viruses, fungi, protozoa, parasitic worms, and prions (Figure 13.2). Infections can occur almost anywhere in or on the body. Examples of common infections are *bronchitis,* infection of the airways *meningitis,* infection of the tissue surrounding the brain and spinal cord; and *conjunctivitis,* infection of the layer of cells surrounding the eyes.

---

bacterium   A microscopic single-celled organism that may be helpful or harmful to humans; plural, *bacteria.*

pneumonia   Inflammation of the lungs, typically caused by infection or exposure to chemical toxins or irritants.

meningitis   Infection of the meninges (membranes covering the brain and spinal cord).

TERMS

Bacteria

The most abundant living things on earth are **bacteria,** which are single-celled organisms that usually reproduce by splitting in two to create a pair of identical cells. Bacteria are often classified by their shape: bacilli (rod-shaped), cocci (spherical), spirochete (spiral-shaped), or vibrios (comma-shaped).

Many species of bacteria are beneficial, but some are pathogenic, causing disease in their hosts. About 100 species of bacteria can cause disease in humans. We harbor both helpful and harmful bacteria on our skin and in our gastrointestinal and reproductive tracts. The human colon contains helpful bacteria that produce certain vitamins and help digest nutrients. Helpful bacteria also keep harmful bacteria in check by competing for food and resources and secreting substances toxic to pathogenic bacteria.

Pneumonia   Inflammation of the lungs, called **pneumonia**, may be caused by infection with bacteria, viruses, or fungi, or by contact with chemical toxins or irritants. Pneumonia can be serious if the alveoli (air sacs) become clogged with fluid, thus preventing oxygen from reaching the bloodstream. Pneumonia often follows another illness, such as a cold or the flu, but the symptoms are typically more severe—fever, chills, shortness of breath, increased mucus production, and cough. Pneumonia is one of the 10 leading causes of death for Americans; people most at risk for severe infection include those under age 2 and over age 75 and those with chronic health problems such as heart disease, asthma, or HIV. Worldwide, pneumonia is the leading cause of death for children under 5 years of age.

The most common cause of bacterial pneumonia is *Streptococcus pneumoniae,* or pneumococcus. A vaccine is available for pneumoccocal pneumonia and is recommended for all adults aged 65 and older and others at risk. Mycoplasma is a very small bacterium; *M. pneumoniae* causes a mild form of pneumonia often called "walking pneumonia." Outbreaks of infection with mycoplasmas are relatively common among young adults, especially in crowded settings such as dormitories. Bacterial pneumonia can be treated with antibiotics.

Meningitis   Inflammation of the *meninges,* the protective membranes covering the brain and spinal cord, is called **meningitis**. Most cases of meningitis are viral; they are usually mild and go away on their own. Bacterial meningitis, however, can be life-threatening and requires immediate treatment with antibiotics. Symptoms of meningitis include fever, a severe headache, stiff neck, sensitivity to light, and confusion. Immediate treatment is needed because death can occur within hours.

The disease is fatal in about 10% of cases, and about 10–20% of people who recover have permanent disabilities, including brain damage, seizures, and hearing loss. Today *Neisseria meningitidis* (meningococcus) and *Streptococcus pneuumoniae* (pneumococcus) are the leading causes of

Type of Organism	Selected Pathogens	Associated Diseases
Bacteria Microscopic single-celled organisms	*Bordetella pertussis* *Borrelia burgdorferi* *Chlamydia* *Clostridium tetani* *Helicobacter pylori* *Legionella pneumophila* *Mycobacterium tuberculosis* Mycoplasma *Neisseria* Rickettsia Staphylococcus Streptococcus	Pertussis (whooping cough) Lyme disease Pneumonia (*C. pneumoniae*), chlamydia (*C. trachomatis*) Tetanus Peptic ulcers Legionnaire's disease Tuberculosis Pneumonia, ear infections, sore throat, urethritis Gonorrhea (*N. gonorroeae*), meningitis (*N. meningitidis*) Rocky Mountain spotted fever, typhus Boils and other skin infections, toxic shock syndrome Strep throat, skin infections, pneumonia, rheumatic fever and rheumatic heart disease, necrotizing fasciitis
Viruses Infectious agents consisting of a protein shell enclosing DNA or RNA	Coronavirus, rhinovirus Epstein-Barr virus Hepatitis viruses Herpes simplex 1 and 2 Human immunodeficiency virus Human papillomaviruses Influenza viruses A and B Paramyxovirus Rhabdovirus Togavirus Varicella-zoster	Severe acute respiratory syndrome (SARS), common cold Infectious mononucleosis Hepatitis (inflammation of the liver) Cold sores, genital herpes HIV/AIDS Warts, cervical cancer Flu Measles, mumps Rabies Rubella Chicken pox, shingles
Fungi Single- or multicelled organisms (e.g., yeasts, molds)	*Candida albicans* *Cryptococcus neoformans* Dermatophyte fungi *Histoplasma capsulatum* *Coccidioides immitis*	Yeast infections, thrush Pneumonia, meningitis Athlete's foot, jock itch, ringworm, nail infections Histoplasmosis Coccidioidomycosis
Protozoa Single-celled organisms	*Entamoeba histolytica* *Giardia lamblia* *Plasmodia* *Trichomonas vaginalis* *Trypanosoma brucei*	Amoebic dysentery Giardiasis Malaria Trichomoniasis African sleeping sickness
Parasitic worms Worms that feed and live on or in a host	*Ancylostoma duodenale* *Ascaris lumbricoides* Beef, pork, or fish tapeworms *Enterobius vermicularis* *Necator americanus* Schistosoma	Ancylostomiasis (hookworm infection) Ascariasis (roundworm infection) Tapeworm infection Pinworm infection Hookworm infection Cercarial dermatitis (swimmer's itch), schistosomiasis
Prions Proteinaceous infectious particles	PrP^{Sc}	Creutzfeldt-Jakob disease (CJD)

FIGURE 13.2 **Pathogens and associated infectious diseases.**

bacterial meningitis, particularly in adolescents and young adults (see the box "Meningococcal Meningitis and College Students).

Strep Throat and Other Streptococcal Infections

The **streptococcus** bacterium can cause streptococcal pharyngitis, or strep throat, which is characterized by a red, sore throat with white patches on the tonsils, swollen lymph nodes, fever, and headache. Typically it is spread from an infected individual through close contact via respiratory droplets that are released when the infected person sneezes or coughs. If left untreated, strep throat can develop into the more serious rheumatic fever.

A particularly virulent type of streptococcus can invade the bloodstream, spread to other parts of the body, and produce dangerous systemic illness. It can also cause a serious but rare infection of the deeper layers of the skin, a condition called necrotizing fasciitis or "flesh-eating strep."

> **streptococcus** Any of a genus (*Streptococcus*) of spherical bacteria; streptococcal species can cause skin infections, strep throat, rheumatic fever, pneumonia, scarlet fever, and other diseases. **TERMS**

Meningococcal Meningitis and College Students

When meningitis is caused by the bacterium *Neisseria meningitidis,* it is called meningococcal meningitis. Although rates of this disease have been declining since the 1990s, it still causes deaths. The disease is spread by the exchange of respiratory and throat secretions (as in coughing and sneezing) and through person-to-person contact (as in kissing); it can readily spread among people living in close quarters.

In the United States nearly 30% of meningitis cases occur in adolescents and young adults, and there is an increased risk in college students. Lifestyle factors, such as crowded living situations, irregular sleep patterns, sharing of personal items, bar patronage, and smoking (active or passive) all increase the risk for meningococcal meningitis.

A vaccine is available that protects against four of the five most common strains of meningitis. Because rates of the disease rise beginning in early adolescence and peak between ages 15 and 20, the CDC and the American College Health Association recommend vaccination for all unvaccinated first-year college students living in dormitories, and some schools require it. In 2012 Texas became the first state to require all college students, even those living off campus, to be vaccinated against meningitis.

A person diagnosed with meningococcal meningitis is treated with antibiotics, and often those who have direct contact with the patient, such as housemates, roommates, and romantic partners, are also given antibiotics. Besides being vaccinated, you can protect yourself against meningococcal meningitis by getting enough sleep, not smoking and not being around tobacco smoke, and avoiding people who are sick.

SOURCES: Centers for Disease Control and Prevention. 2012. *Meningitis* (http://www.cdc.gov/meningitis/index.html); American College Health Association. 2009. *Meningitis on Campus* (http://www.acha.org/projects_programs/meningitis/disease_info.cfm).

Toxic Shock Syndrome and Other Staphylococcal Infections

The spherical-shaped **staphylococcus** bacterium can cause infections ranging from minor skin infections such as boils to very serious conditions such as blood infections and pneumonia.

Staphylococcus aureus is responsible for many cases of toxic shock syndrome (TSS). The bacteria produce a toxin that results in tissue damage, widespread coagulation of blood in the blood vessels, and ultimately organ failure.

A very serious antibiotic-resistant infection is caused by a staphylococcus bacterium known as methicillin-resistant *Staphylococcus aureus* (MRSA). Many cases of MRSA infection occur in hospitalized patients, and these infections tend to be severe. MRSA is also common in the community (outside hospital settings), where it usually infects the skin, causing painful lesions that resemble infected spider bites. The spread of MRSA infection is associated with places where people are in close contact with one another, such as locker rooms and playing fields; athletes are particularly at risk and should keep any cuts or abrasions covered.

QUICK STATS

One-third of the world's population is infected with tuberculosis.

—CDC, 2012

Tuberculosis

Caused by the bacterium *Mycobacterium tuberculosis,* **tuberculosis (TB)** is a chronic bacterial infection that usually affects the lungs, though it can affect other organs as well. TB is spread via the respiratory route. Symptoms include coughing, fatigue, night sweats, weight loss, and fever. Between 10 and 15 million Americans have been infected with *M. tuberculosis* and continue to carry it. Only about 10% of people with latent TB infections actually develop an active case of the disease; the immune system usually prevents the disease from becoming active. In the United States, active TB is most common among people infected with HIV, recent immigrants from countries where TB is endemic, and those who live in inner cities.

Many strains of tuberculosis respond to antibiotics, but only over a course of treatment lasting 6–12 months. Failure to complete treatment can lead to relapse and the development of strains of antibiotic-resistant bacteria. Multidrug-resistant TB (MDR TB) is resistant to at least two of the best anti-TB drugs. Extensively drug-resistant TB (XDR TB) is resistant to those drugs as well as some second-line drugs. XDR TB is relatively rare, but patients with this form of TB have fewer and less effective treatment options. TB is a leading cause of death in people with HIV infection.

Tickborne Infections

Lyme disease is spread by the bite of a tick that is infected with the spiral-shaped bacterium *Borrelia burgdorferi.* The deer tick is responsible for transmitting Lyme disease bacteria to humans in the northeastern and north-central United States; on the Pacific Coast, the culprit is the western black-legged tick.

staphylococcus Any of a genus (*Staphylococcus*) of spherical, clustered bacteria commonly found on the skin or in the nasal passages; staphylococcal species may enter the body and cause conditions such as boils, pneumonia, toxic shock syndrome, and severe skin infections.

TERMS

tuberculosis (TB) A chronic bacterial infection that usually affects the lungs.

Symptoms of Lyme disease vary but typically occur in three stages. In the first stage, about 80% of victims develop a bull's-eye-shaped red rash expanding from the area of the bite, usually about two weeks after the bite occurs. The second stage occurs weeks to months later in 10–20% of untreated patients; symptoms may involve the nervous and cardiovascular systems and can include impaired coordination, partial facial paralysis, and heart rhythm abnormalities. These symptoms usually disappear on their own within a few weeks. The third stage, which occurs in about half of untreated people, can develop months or years after the tick bite and usually consists of chronic or recurring arthritis. Lyme disease is preventable by avoiding contact with ticks or by removing a tick before it has had the chance to transmit the infection.

Rocky Mountain spotted fever is also transmitted via tick bites. It is characterized by sudden onset of fever, headache, and muscle pain, followed by development of a spotted rash.

Other Bacterial Infections   The following are a few of the many other infections caused by bacteria:

- *Ulcers:* Up to 90% of ulcers are caused by infection with the bacterium *Helicobacter pylori*. If tests show the presence of *H. pylori*, antibiotics often cure the infection and the ulcers.

- *Tetanus:* Also known as lockjaw, tetanus is caused by the bacterium *Clostridium tetani,* which thrives in deep puncture wounds and produces a deadly toxin. Worldwide more than 200,000 people die from tetanus each year.

- *C. diff:* Another type of *Clostridium* bacteria, called *Clostridium difficile* (*C. diff*), has joined MRSA as a major emerging threat in American health care settings, particularly hospitals. It causes inflammation of the colon, resulting in diarrhea, fever, and nausea. The CDC recommends that doctors, nurses, and other health care providers wash their hands frequently to reduce the spread of the bacterium.

- *Pertussis:* Also known as whooping cough, pertussis is a highly contagious respiratory illness caused by the bacterium *Bordetella pertussis.* Those at high risk include infants and children who are too young to be fully vaccinated. Adolescents and adults become susceptible when immunity from vaccination wanes, so a booster shot is recommended at 11–12 years or during adolescence and thereafter every 10 years.

- *Urinary tract infections (UTIs):* Infection of the bladder and urethra is most common among sexually active women, but UTIs can occur in anyone. The bacterium *Escherichia coli* (E. coli) is the most common infectious agent, responsible for about 80% of all UTIs.

Antibiotic Treatments   **Antibiotics** are both naturally occurring and synthetic substances that can kill bacteria. Most antibiotics work in a similar fashion: They interfere with the reproduction of bacteria. Antibiotics are among the most widely prescribed and most effective drugs. Overuse of antibiotics has led to an increase in bacterial resistance to their effects. When exposed to antibiotics, resistant bacteria can grow and flourish while the antibiotic-sensitive bacteria die off. Antibiotic-resistant strains of many common bacteria have developed, including strains of gonorrhea, salmonella, and tuberculosis. Antibiotic resistance is a major factor contributing to the rise in problematic infectious diseases.

Resistance is promoted when people fail to take the full course of an antibiotic or when they inappropriately take antibiotics for viral infections. Another possible source of resistance is the use of antibiotics in agriculture, which is estimated to account for 50–80% of the 25,000 tons of antibiotics used annually in the United States.

You can help prevent the development of antibiotic-resistant strains of bacteria by using antibiotics properly. Don't ask your doctor for an antibiotic every time you get sick. Antibiotics are helpful for bacterial infections but are ineffective against viruses. Use antibiotics as directed, and finish the full course of medication even if you begin to feel better. Never take an antibiotic without a prescription. If you take an antibiotic for a viral infection, your illness will not improve.

> **Antibiotics are not effective against viral illnesses.**
> Talk to your doctor before taking antibiotics.

Viruses

A **virus** is a microscopic organism consisting of genetic material covered by a protein coat. Viruses lack the enzymes essential to energy production and protein synthesis in normal animal cells, and they can replicate only inside the cells of another organism. Once a virus is inside the host cell, it sheds its protein covering and exploits the host's cellular machinery to produce more viruses like itself. Most contagious diseases are caused by viruses.

The Common Cold   A cold may be caused by any of more than 200 different viruses that attack the lining of the nasal passages. Cold viruses are almost always transmitted by hand-to-hand contact. To lessen your risk of contracting a cold, wash your hands frequently; if you touch someone else, avoid touching your face until after you've washed your

---

antibiotics   Synthetic or naturally occurring substances used as drugs to kill bacteria.

virus   A very small infectious agent composed of nucleic acid (DNA or RNA) surrounded by a protein coat; lacks an independent metabolism and reproduces only within a host cell.

TERMS

lds. If you catch a cold, over-the-counter cold remedies may relieve your symptoms, but they do not eliminate the virus. The jury is still out on whether other remedies, including zinc gluconate lozenges, Echinacea, and vitamin C, relieve symptoms or shorten the duration of a cold. Antibiotics will not help a cold, unless a bacterial infection is also present, such as a sinus infection.

Influenza   Commonly called the flu, **influenza** is an infection of the respiratory tract caused by the influenza virus. Compared to the common cold, influenza is a more serious illness, usually including a fever and extreme fatigue. Most people who get the flu recover within 1–2 weeks, but some develop potentially life-threatening complications, such as pneumonia. The highest rates of infection occur in children. Influenza is highly contagious and is spread via respiratory droplets.

The most effective way of preventing the flu is through annual vaccination. The CDC recommends vaccination for all people aged 6 months and older.

Chicken Pox, Cold Sores, and Other Herpesvirus Infections   The **herpesviruses** are a large group of viruses. Once infected, the host is never free of the virus. The virus lies latent within certain cells and becomes active periodically, producing symptoms. The family of herpesviruses includes the varicella-zoster virus, which causes chicken pox and shingles; herpes simplex virus (HSV) types 1 and 2, which cause cold sores and the STI herpes; and epstein-barr virus (EBV), which causes infectious mononucleosis.

Two herpesviruses that can cause severe infections in people who have a suppressed immune system are cytomegalovirus (CMV), which infects the lungs, brain, colon, and eyes, and human herpesvirus 8 (HHV-8), which has been linked to Kaposi's sarcoma, a cancer of the connective tissue.

Viral Hepatitis   Viral **hepatitis** is a term used to describe several different infections that cause inflammation of the liver. Hepatitis is usually caused by one of the three most common hepatitis viruses. Hepatitis A virus (HAV) causes the mildest form of the disease and is usually transmitted by food or water contaminated by sewage or an infected person. Hepatitis B virus (HBV) is usually transmitted sexually. Hepatitis C virus (HCV) can also be transmitted sexually, but it is much more commonly passed through direct contact with infected blood via injection drug use or—prior to the development of screening tests—blood transfusions. HBV and, to a lesser extent, HCV can also be passed from a pregnant woman to her child.

Symptoms of acute hepatitis infection can include fatigue, **jaundice,** abdominal pain, loss of appetite, nausea, and diarrhea. Most people recover from hepatitis A within a month or so. However, 5–10% of people infected with HBV and 85–90% of people infected with HCV become chronic carriers of the virus, capable of infecting others for the rest of their lives. Some chronic carriers remain asymptomatic, while others slowly develop chronic liver disease, cirrhosis, or liver cancer.

There are effective vaccines for hepatitis A and B. The extent of HCV infection has been only recently recognized, and most infected people are unaware of their condition. To ensure proper treatment and prevention, testing for HCV may be recommended for people at risk, including people who have injected drugs (even once), who received a blood transfusion or a donated organ prior to July 1992, who have engaged in high-risk sexual behavior, or who have had body piercing, tattoos, or acupuncture involving unsterile equipment.

Human Papillomavirus (HPV)   The more than 100 different types of HPV cause a variety of warts (noncancerous skin tumors), including common warts on the hands, plantar warts on the soles of the feet, and genital warts around the genitalia. Depending on their location, warts may be removed using over-the-counter preparations or professional methods such as laser surgery or cryosurgery. Because HPV infection is chronic, warts can reappear despite treatment. HPV causes the majority of cases of cervical cancer. Two HPV vaccines are available and recommended for girls age 9–12, but may also be taken up to age 26. Experts now advise that boys receive HPV vaccine to protect them against genital warts and prevent certain cancers later in life.

Treating Viral Illnesses   Antiviral drugs typically work by interfering with some part of the viral life cycle; for example, they may prevent a virus from entering body cells or from successfully reproducing within cells. Antivirals are currently available to fight infections caused by HIV, influenza, herpes simplex, varicella-zoster, HBV, and HVC. Most other viral diseases must simply run their course.

Fungi

A **fungus** is an organism that reproduces by spores and feeds on organic matter. Only about 50 of the many thousands of species of fungi cause disease in humans, and these diseases are usually

---

TERMS

influenza   Infection of the respiratory tract by the influenza virus, which is highly infectious and prone to variation; the form changes so rapidly that every year new strains arise; commonly known as the flu.

herpesvirus   A large family of viruses responsible for cold sores, mononucleosis, chicken pox, shingles, and the STI herpes; causes latent infections.

hepatitis   Inflammation of the liver, which can be caused by infection, drugs, or toxins.

jaundice   Increased bile pigment levels in the blood, characterized by yellowing of the skin and the whites of the eyes.

fungus   A single-celled or multicelled organism that reproduces by spores and feeds on organic matter; examples include molds, mushrooms, and yeasts. Fungal diseases include yeast infections, athlete's foot, and ringworm.

restricted to the skin, mucous membranes, and lungs. Some fungal diseases are extremely difficult to treat because spores are an especially resistant dormant stage of the organism.

Candida albicans is a common fungus found naturally in the vagina of most women. When excessive growth occurs, the result is itching and discomfort, commonly known as a yeast infection.

Other common fungal conditions, including athlete's foot, jock itch, and ringworm, affect the skin. These three conditions are usually mild and easy to cure. Fungi can also cause systemic diseases that are severe, life-threatening, and extremely difficult to treat. Fungal infections can be especially deadly in people with impaired immune systems.

Protozoa

Protozoa are single-celled organisms that can cause a range of diseases in humans. Millions of people in developing countries suffer from protozoal infections.

Malaria, caused by a parasitic protozoan of the genus *Plasmodium,* is a major killer worldwide; each year there are 350–500 million new cases of malaria globally and more than 1 million deaths, mostly among infants and children. Drug-resistant strains of malaria have emerged, requiring new medicines.

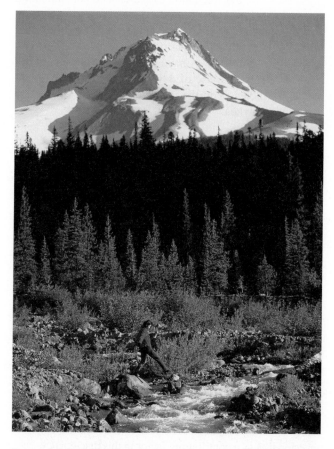

Even seemingly pristine mountain streams can be contaminated with the protozoan *Giardia lamblia,* as many unwary hikers and campers have discovered. Symptoms of giardiasis include abdominal pain, bloating, and diarrhea.

Giardiasis is caused by *Giardia lamblia,* a single-celled parasite that lives in the intestines of humans and animals. Giardiasis is characterized by nausea, diarrhea, bloating, and abdominal cramps, and it is among the most common waterborne diseases in the United States. People may become infected with *Giardia* if they consume contaminated food or water.

Parasitic Worms

The **parasitic worms** are the largest organisms that can enter the body to cause infection. They include tapeworms, hookworms, pinworms, and flukes. They cause a variety of relatively mild infections, primarily, of the intestines. Worm infections generally originate from contaminated food or drink and can be prevented by careful attention to hygiene.

Emerging Infectious Diseases

Emerging infectious diseases are infections whose incidence in humans has increased or threatens to increase in the near future. They include both known diseases that have experienced a resurgence, such as tuberculosis and cholera, and diseases that were previously unknown or confined to specific areas, such as the Ebola and West Nile viruses.

Selected Infections of Concern Although the chances of the average American contracting an exotic infection are very low, emerging infections are a concern to public health officials and represent a challenge to all nations in the future.

WEST NILE VIRUS A mini-outbreak of encephalitis in New York in 1999 led to identification of this virus, which had previously been restricted to Africa, the Middle East, and parts of Europe. Since 1999, the virus has spread across the United States and caused more than 27,605 cases of human illness and 1086 deaths. West Nile virus is carried by birds and then passed to humans when mosquitoes bite first an infected bird and then a person. Most people who are bitten have few or no symptoms, but the virus can cause permanent brain damage or death in some.

> **protozoan** A microscopic single-celled organism that often produces recurrent, cyclical attacks of disease; plural, *protozoa.*
>
> **malaria** A severe, recurrent, mosquito-borne infection caused by the parasitic protozoan *Plasmodium.*
>
> **giardiasis** An intestinal disease caused by the parasitic protozoan *Giardia lamblia.*
>
> **parasitic worm** A pathogen that causes intestinal and other infections; includes tapeworms, hookworms, pinworms, and flukes.
>
> TERMS

SEVERE ACUTE RESPIRATORY SYNDROME (SARS) In February 2003 SARS appeared in southern China and quickly spread to more than 15 countries; it is a form of pneumonia that is fatal in 5–15% of cases. SARS is caused by a type of coronavirus found in wildlife that may have crossed the species barrier. By 2004 SARS had been responsible for more than 8000 illnesses and 800 deaths, but there have been no new cases reported since 2004.

ROTAVIRUS The leading viral cause of gastroenteritis, an intestinal inflammation that results in vomiting and diarrhea, rotavirus infects almost every child at one time or another. Worldwide, the virus kills about 600,000 children each year, mostly in developing countries. Left untreated, rotavirus-induced diarrhea can become severe and lead to dehydration, which can be fatal. Rotavirus spreads through poor hygiene and sanitation practices.

ESCHERICHIA COLI 0157:H7 This potentially deadly strain of *E. coli,* transmitted in contaminated food, can cause bloody diarrhea and kidney damage. In 2012 an outbreak reported in nine states was traced to contaminated romaine lettuce. Other outbreaks have been linked to ground beef, alfalfa sprouts, unpasteurized juice, petting zoos, and contaminated public swimming pools. An estimated 70,000 cases of *E. coli* 0157:H7 infection and 61 deaths occur in the United States each year.

HANTAVIRUS Since hantavirus pulmonary syndrome (HPS) was first recognized in 1993, over 300 cases have been reported in the United States. HPS is caused by the rodent-borne Sin Nombre virus (SNV) and is spread primarily through airborne viral particles from rodent urine, droppings, or saliva. It is characterized by a dangerous fluid buildup in the lungs and is fatal in about 45% of cases. In 2012, an outbreak of hantavirus caused the death of at least three campers in Yosemite National Park.

EBOLA The 2014 outbreak in West Africa is the largest and most complex Ebola outbreak since the Ebola virus was first discovered in 1976. At the time of writing, a total of 9,911 confirmed or probable cases, and 4,868 deaths have been reported in Guinea, Sierra Leone, and Liberia. The CDC and the WHO report that at least 17 cases of Ebola have been treated in Europe and the United States. Most were health workers who contracted Ebola in West Africa and were transported back to their home country for treatment.

Ebola is often a fatal disease spread through direct contact with bodily fluids. Ebola on dry surfaces, such as doorknobs and countertops, can survive for several hours. Some countries have limited or even banned entrance to international travelers at risk for Ebola. Nigeria has successfully rid the country of all cases through treatment and containment.

Factors Contributing to Emerging Infections
What's behind this rising tide of infectious diseases?

One factor is drug resistance. New or increasing drug resistance has been found in organisms that cause malaria, tuberculosis, gonorrhea, influenza, AIDS, and pneumococcal and staphylococcal infections. Some bacterial strains now appear to be resistant to all available antibiotics. Another factor is poverty. More than 1 billion people live in extreme poverty, and half the world's population has no regular access to essential drugs. Population growth, urbanization, overcrowding, and migration (including the movement of refugees) also spread infectious diseases. A poor public health infrastructure is often associated with poverty and social upheaval, but problems such as contaminated water supplies can occur even in industrial countries. Inadequate vaccination has led to the reemergence of diseases such as diphtheria and pertussis. Natural disasters such as hurricanes also disrupt the public health infrastructure, leaving survivors with contaminated water and food supplies and no shelter from disease-carrying insects.

> Some bacterial strains now appear to be **resistant to all available antibiotics.**

Travel and commerce, and mass food production and distribution also contribute, as do human behaviors. More than 500 million travelers cross national borders each year, and international tourism and trade open the world to infectious agents. SARS was quickly spread throughout the world by infected air travelers.

Food now travels long distances to our table, and microbes are transmitted along with it. Mass production of food increases the likelihood that a chance contamination can lead to mass illness.

The widespread use of injectable drugs rapidly transmits HIV infection and hepatitis. Changes in sexual behavior over the past 40 years have led to a proliferation of old and new STDs. The use of day care facilities for children has led to increases in the incidence of several infections that cause diarrhea.

Immune Disorders

Considering the complexity of the immune system, it is not surprising that the system sometimes fails to operate properly, resulting in disease.

When the immune system breaks down and has lost the ability to recognize body cells and tissues as "self," the result is an autoimmune disease. In most autoimmune diseases, the immune system targets or destroys specific tissues. For example, in type 1 diabetes, the insulin-producing cells of the pancreas are destroyed. In multiple sclerosis, the protective coating around nerves is targeted and destroyed. In rheumatoid arthritis, the membranes lining the joints are destroyed. The causes of autoimmune diseases are not well understood. The rates of many of these diseases are much higher in women than in men, which may reflect the fact that in general females have more robust immune responses—this hypothesis is currently under investigation. The role of estrogen is also under investigation as a contributing factor in this discrepancy.

Sometimes the immune system looses its detect cells that have recently become abnormal, as in the case of cancerous mutations. This can happen when people get older, when they have certain immune disorders (like HIV infection), or when the immune system is suppressed by chemotherapy and other drugs. Cancer cells may multiply uncontrollably before the immune system is able to respond sufficiently. In recent years, conventional cancer treatments have been augmented with a treatment known as immunotherapy. Cancer-specific vaccines are also under development.

SUPPORTING YOUR IMMUNE SYSTEM

You can help ensure the optimal functioning of your immune system by choosing healthy behaviors, for example:

- Eat a balanced diet and maintain a healthy weight.

- Get enough sleep. People who sleep fewer than six hours per night tend to have compromised immune function. In addition, quality sleep is as important as sufficient sleep.

- Exercise, but not when you're sick.

- Don't smoke.

- If you drink alcohol, do so only in moderation.

- Make sure you get enough Vitamin D. Vitamin D is made in the skin upon exposure to sunlight. It is not always possible to get sufficient sunlight exposure.

- Wash your hands frequently. When soap and water are not available, use hand sanitizer.

- Avoid contact with people who are contagious with an infectious disease.

- Make sure you drink water only from clean sources.

- Avoid contact with disease carriers such as rodents, mosquitoes, and ticks.

- Practice safer sex, do not use injectable drugs.

- Make sure you have received all your recommended vaccinations, and keep them up-to-date.

THE MAJOR STIs

Sexually transmitted infections (STIs)—also still called **sexually transmitted diseases (STDs)**—spread from person to person mainly through sexual activity. STIs are a particularly insidious group of illnesses because a person can be infected and able to transmit the disease, yet not look or feel sick.

The following seven STIs pose major health threats:

- HIV/AIDS
- Chlamydia
- Gonorrhea
- Human papillomavirus (HPV)
- Herpes
- Hepatitis
- Syphilis

These diseases are considered major threats because they are serious in themselves, cause grave complications if left untreated, and pose risks to a fetus or newborn. STIs often result in long-term consequences, including chronic pain, infertility, stillbirths, genital cancers, and death.

The United States has the highest or near highest rate of STIs of any industrialized nation. The Centers for Disease Control and Prevention (CDC) estimated that, in 2013, 110 million Americans were infected with an STI. Young people ages 15–24 account for half of STI cases in the United States. Over 19 million Americans become newly infected with an STI each year.

HIV Infection and AIDS

The **human immunodeficiency virus (HIV)** causes **acquired immunodeficiency syndrome (AIDS)**. Due to advancements in HIV treatment, the life expectancy for individuals receiving highly active **antiretroviral** treatment may approach that of individuals who are not infected with HIV. Worldwide for most people infected with HIV, adequate treatment is not available, contributing to a high degree of illness and mortality. Untreated HIV infection may advance to AIDS within 8–10 years of diagnosis. This stage of HIV infection is defined by a severely compromised immune system and the presence of opportunistic infections.

Many experts believe that the global HIV epidemic peaked in the late 1990s, at about 3.5 million new infections per year, compared with an estimated 2.3 million new infections in 2012. Despite a slowing of the epidemic, however, AIDS remains a primary cause of death in Africa and continues to be a major cause of mortality around the world.

---

sexually transmitted disease (STD) or sexually transmitted infection (STI) TERMS An infection that is mainly transmitted by sexual contact; some can also be transmitted by other means.

human immunodeficiency virus (HIV) The virus that causes HIV infection and AIDS.

acquired immunodeficiency syndrome (AIDS) An advanced stage of HIV infection.

antiretrovirals drugs that suppress retroviruses like HIV.

In 2011, the world marked the 30th year since AIDS, a fatal acquired immunodeficiency disease, made its debut in the homosexual communities of California and New York. A year later, similar cases were being described in hemophiliacs, individuals who had received blood transfusions, injection drug users, and infected women and their newborn infants. With this change in demographics came the knowledge and awareness that AIDS was not just a disease of gay men. AIDS is now a worldwide scourge. Currently, 75 million people are infected and more than 36 million have died from AIDS-related illness since the epidemic began.

The vast majority of cases have occurred in economically emerging countries, where heterosexual contact is the primary means of transmission. HIV continues to be a disease that disproportionately affects ethnic minorities and the poor.

Worldwide, women are the fastest-growing group of newly infected people. In 2012, just over half of adults living with HIV were women. In sub-Saharan Africa, the region most heavily burdened with HIV, 57% of adults living with HIV are women. Globally, certain subsets of women such as female sex workers and transgender women are at even greater risk of HIV infection. These populations have HIV prevalence of 12–30% and 19%, respectively.

Despite the ongoing tragedy of the HIV epidemic, strides have been made in treatment and prevention measures. By the end of 2012, an estimated 9.7 million people living in low- and middle-income countries were receiving antiretrovirals (drugs that suppress retroviruses like HIV). Due to these scaled-up preventive efforts, the annual number of newly infected children has continued to decline along with overall AIDS-related deaths. Treating HIV with effective drugs not only prolongs life and decreases suffering, it also has a major impact in reducing the spread of the virus because treated individuals are generally much less infectious than untreated people.

HIV rates of new infections have remained steady or have even dropped in many regions. Though sub-Saharan Africa remains the hardest-hit area of the world, the number of new infections dropped from 2.2 million in 2001 to 1.6 million in 2012. The expanded availability of antiretroviral medications to this region has contributed significantly to this decline, with a 32% drop in AIDS-related deaths between 2005 and 2011 alone. Still, over two-thirds of all HIV-infected people in the world live in sub-Saharan Africa, and nearly three-quarters of all deaths due to AIDS in 2012 occurred there.

Eastern Europe and parts of Asia have also been hit hard by HIV. In many of these areas, HIV infection is seen in intravenous drug users and their sexual partners.

Efforts to combat AIDS are complicated by political, economic, and cultural barriers. Education and prevention programs are often hampered by resistance from social and religious institutions and by the taboo on openly discussing sexual issues. Condoms are not commonly used in many countries, and women in many societies do not have control over sexual situations to demand that men use condoms. Empowering women is a crucial priority in reducing the spread of HIV. In particular, reducing sexual violence against women, promoting financial independence, and increasing women's education and employment opportunities are essential.

Successful prevention approaches include STI treatment and education, public education campaigns about safer sex, and syringe exchange programs for injection drug users. Efforts are ongoing to improve access to barrier protective devices such as condoms. Other measures have included male circumcision, which has been shown to reduce HIV transmission in some studies.

In industrialized nations such as the United States, new drugs are easing AIDS symptoms and lowering viral levels dramatically for some patients. In the past few years, a growing number of people

---

In the United States about 1.1 million people have been infected with HIV. The incidence of HIV has leveled off at about 50,000 new infections annually. More than 659,000 Americans with an AIDS diagnosis have died since the start of the epidemic in 1981. Today, nearly 20% of Americans are unaware of their HIV status.

> **HIV infection** A chronic, progressive viral infection that damages the immune system.
>
> **TERMS**
>
> **CD4 T cell** A type of white blood cell that helps coordinate the activity of the immune system; the primary target of HIV infection. A decrease in the number of these cells correlates with the severity of HIV-related illness.

> **QUICK STATS**
>
> The incidence of HIV in the United States has leveled off, with about **50,000** new infections annually.
> —CDC, 2013

What Is HIV Infection? **HIV infection** is a chronic disease that progressively damages the body's immune system, making an otherwise healthy person less able to resist a variety of infections and disorders. Normally, when a virus or other pathogen enters the body, it is targeted and destroyed by the immune system. But HIV attacks the immune system itself, invading and taking over **CD4 T cells** (white blood cells that fight infection), macrophages, and other essential elements of the immune system. HIV enters a human cell and converts its own genetic material, RNA, into DNA. It then inserts this DNA into the chromosomes of the host cell. The viral DNA is not only instrumental in producing new copies of HIV, but seriously reduces immune functions.

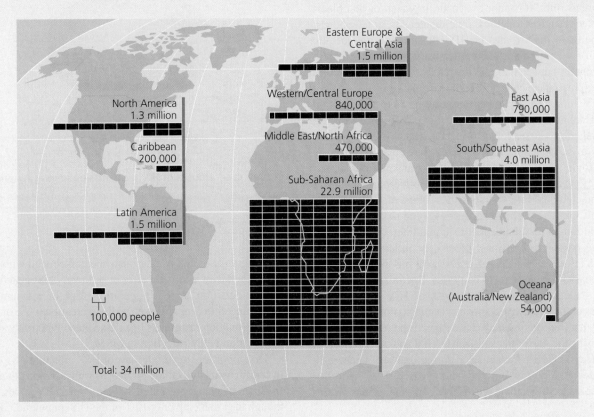

Approximate number of people living with HIV/AIDS in 2011.

SOURCE: Joint United Nations Programme on HIV/AIDS. 2013. *UNAIDS Report on the Global AIDS Epidemic, 2013.* Geneva: UNAIDS.

in poor countries have gained access to antiretroviral drugs because of the introduction of inexpensive generic drugs and increased international funding for HIV treatment. Still, far too many people with HIV remain untreated, and far too many new infections are occurring.

Immediately following infection with HIV, billions of infectious particles are produced every day. For a time, the immune system keeps pace, also producing billions of new cells. Unlike the virus, however, the immune system cannot make new cells indefinitely; as long as the virus keeps replicating, it wins in the end. The destruction of the immune system is signaled by the loss of CD4 T cells. As CD4 cells decline, an infected person may begin to experience mild to moderately severe symptoms. A person is diagnosed with AIDS when the number of CD4 cells in the blood drops below a certain level (200/µl). People with AIDS are vulnerable to a number of serious **opportunistic (secondary) infections**.

The first weeks after being infected with HIV are called the *primary infection* phase. People have large amounts of HIV in the bloodstream and genital fluids, making it easier to transmit the virus. Several months later, infected people develop antibodies to the virus, so commonly available tests will show a positive result. The next phase of HIV infection is the chronic **asymptomatic** (symptom-free) stage, also called the *latency* phase. This period can last from 2 to 20 years, averaging 11 years in untreated adults. During this time, the virus progressively infects and destroys the cells of the immune system. Even if they are symptom-free, people infected with HIV can transmit the disease to others.

> **opportunistic (secondary) infection** An infection caused when organisms take the opportunity presented by a primary (initial) infection to multiply and cause a new, different infection.
>
> **asymptomatic** Showing no signs or symptoms of a disease.

Transmitting the Virus   HIV lives only within cells and body fluids, not outside the body. It is transmitted by blood and blood products, semen, vaginal and cervical secretions, and breast milk. It cannot live in air, in water, or on objects or surfaces such as toilet seats, eating utensils, or telephones.

The three main routes of HIV transmission are specific kinds of sexual contact, direct exposure to infected blood, and contact between an HIV-infected woman and her child during pregnancy, childbirth, or breastfeeding.

HIV is more likely to be transmitted by unprotected anal or vaginal intercourse than by other sexual activities. During vaginal intercourse, male-to-female transmission is more likely to occur than female-to-male transmission. HIV has been found in preejaculatory fluid, so transmission can occur before ejaculation. Being the receptive partner during unprotected anal intercourse is the riskiest of all sexual activities. Oral–genital contact carries some risk of transmission, although less than anal or vaginal intercourse.

The presence of lesions, blisters, or inflammation from other STIs in the genital, anal, or oral areas makes it two to nine times easier for the virus to be passed. Spermicides may also cause irritation and increase the risk of HIV transmission. Studies of the widely used spermicide nonoxynol-9 (N-9) have found that frequent use may cause vaginal and rectal irritation, increasing the risk of transmission of HIV and other STIs.

The risk of HIV transmission during oral sex is generally considered to be low but may be increased if a person has oral sores or other damage to the gums or tissues in the mouth.

Studies in economically emerging nations with high rates of HIV infection have found that circumcised males have a lower risk of HIV infection than uncircumcised males.

Direct contact with the blood of an infected person is another major route of HIV transmission. Needles and syringes used to inject drugs (including heroin, cocaine, and anabolic steroids) are usually contaminated with the user's blood.

In the past, before effective screening was available, some people were infected with HIV through blood transfusions and other medical procedures involving blood products. All blood in licensed U.S. blood banks and plasma centers is now thoroughly screened for HIV.

The final major route of HIV transmission is mother-to-child, also called *vertical* or *perinatal transmission*, which can occur during pregnancy, childbirth, or breastfeeding. Without intervention, the likelihood of HIV transmission from mother to child is 20–45%; however, testing and treatment can dramatically lower this incidence.

Populations of Special Concern for HIV Infection

Among Americans with AIDS, the most common means of HIV exposure is sexual activity between men (Figure 13.3). Each year the largest number of new cases of HIV infections is among men who have sex with men (MSM). Only 67% of sexually active MSM reported getting an HIV test in the past year. In 2010 this group accounted for 63% of all HIV infections, even though they are estimated to represent just 2% of the population.

* MSM = Men who have sex with men
  IDU = Injection drug users

FIGURE 13.3   **Routes of HIV transmission among Americans.**
SOURCE: Centers for Disease Control and Prevention. 2013. *HIV in the United States: At a Glance.* Atlanta: CDC (http://www.cdc.gov/hiv/statistics/basics/ataglance.html).

Drug and alcohol use has also been associated with risky sexual behavior and is directly or indirectly associated with HIV acquisition in this population. Use of methamphetamine and club drugs, as well as the recreational use of erectile dysfunction drugs, has been associated with risky sexual behavior and HIV infection in MSM.

Disproportionately high rates of HIV infection also occur in certain racial and ethnic groups, as well as among the poor. In 2010 blacks represented 44% of new HIV cases even though they make up only 12% of the U.S. population. Black women accounted for 64% of new HIV infections among women; most were infected through heterosexual sex. Hispanics accounted for 21% of all new HIV infections. These patterns of HIV infection reflect complex social, economic, and behavioral factors. Reducing the rates of HIV transmission and AIDS death in minorities, women, and high-risk groups requires addressing problems of poverty, discrimination, and drug abuse.

Symptoms

Within a few days or weeks of infection with HIV, most people will develop symptoms of primary (also called acute) HIV infection. These symptoms can include fever, fatigue, rashes, headache, swollen lymph nodes, body aches, night sweats, sore throat, nausea, and ulcers in the mouth.

Diagnosis of HIV at this very early stage of infection is extremely beneficial. People with early-stage HIV can make lifestyle changes to improve their overall health during this period. They can also protect their partners during this phase, when viral levels are very high.

Other than the initial flulike symptoms, most people have few if any symptoms in the first months or years of HIV infection. As the immune system weakens, however, a variety of symptoms can develop—persistent swollen lymph nodes; lumps, rashes, sores, or other growths on or under the skin or on the mucous membranes; persistent yeast infections; unexplained weight loss; fever and drenching night sweats; dry cough and shortness of breath; persistent diarrhea; easy bruising and unexplained bleeding; profound fatigue; memory loss; difficulty with balance; tremors or seizures; changes in vision, hearing, taste, or smell; changes in mood and other psychological symptoms; and persistent or recurrent pain. Many of these symptoms can also occur with a variety of other illnesses.

People with HIV infection are highly susceptible to opportunistic infections. The infection most often seen in the United States among people with HIV is *Pneumocystis pneumonia*, a fungal infection. **Kaposi's sarcoma**, a previously rare form of cancer, is common in HIV-infected men. Women with HIV infection often have frequent and difficult-to-treat vaginal yeast infections. Cases of tuberculosis (TB) are increasingly being reported in people with HIV.

Diagnosis   The most commonly used screening tests for HIV are **HIV antibody tests**. Standard testing involves an initial test called an **ELISA**; if it is positive, a second test—either a **Western blot** or immunofluorescence assay—is done to confirm the results (see the box "Getting an HIV Test").

Antibodies may not appear in the blood for weeks or months after infection, so people who are newly infected are likely to have a negative antibody test. In its early stages, the infection can be detected with an **HIV RNA assay**, which directly measures the presence of the virus in the blood.

If a person is diagnosed as **HIV positive**, the next step is to determine the disease's severity to plan appropriate treatment. The status of the immune system can be gauged by taking CD4 T cell measurements every few months. The infection itself can be monitored by tracking the viral load (the amount of virus in the body) through the HIV RNA assay.

Periodic routine testing is the best way for anyone to find out if he or she is infected with HIV. The CDC recommends universal HIV testing as part of routine medical care for everyone aged 13–64. People at greater risk should be tested periodically.

A diagnosis of AIDS, the most severe form of HIV infection, is given if a person is HIV positive and either has developed an infection defined as an AIDS indicator or has a severely damaged immune system (as measured by CD4 T-cell counts).

In the United States, every state has laws that require doctors, clinics, and laboratories to report all diagnosed cases of HIV and AIDS to public health authorities, who use this information to track the spread of the disease. A new blood test makes it possible to estimate the length of time a person has been infected with HIV, so the CDC is now able to get a fairly accurate picture of the HIV epidemic in the United States. Despite efforts to safeguard confidentiality and prohibit discrimination, mandatory reporting of HIV infection remains controversial. If people believe they are risking their jobs, friends, or social acceptability, they may be less likely to get tested. The CDC recommends that states continue to provide opportunities for people to be tested anonymously, including via home tests.

> In many people, combination therapies can **reduce HIV in the blood to undetectable levels.**

Treatment   Although there is no known cure for HIV infection, medications can significantly alter the course of the disease and extend life. The drop in the number of U.S. AIDS deaths that has occurred since 1996 is in large part due to the increasing use of combinations of new drugs.

The main types of antiviral drugs used against HIV/AIDS are reverse transcriptase inhibitors, protease inhibitors, integrase inhibitors, and entry inhibitors. These drugs either block HIV from replicating itself or prevent it from infecting other cells. Research has shown that using combinations of antiviral drugs can sometimes reduce HIV in the blood to undetectable levels. More than 30 drugs are now available to treat HIV, including three once-a-day tablets (containing a combination of HIV medications). However, people on antiviral drugs can still transmit the infection, and concerns are growing that even these very aggressive treatments are starting to fail and that drug-resistant strains of HIV are developing rapidly. In addition to antiviral drugs, most patients with low CD4 T cell counts take a variety of antibiotics to help prevent opportunistic infections such as pneumonia, tuberculosis, and other bacterial and fungal infections.

In some cases medications are used to prevent infection in people who have been exposed to HIV, such as victims of sexual assault and health care workers with potential exposure to HIV-infected blood or body fluids. This type of treatment, called postexposure prophylaxis (PEP), should begin as soon as possible after exposure, but always within 72 hours. PEP treatment usually lasts 28 days.

The cost of treatment for HIV continues to be an area of major concern. Costs are tremendous even for relatively wealthy countries, but 95% of people with HIV infection live in poor countries, where treatments are unlikely to be

TERMS

***Pneumocystis* pneumonia**   A fungal infection common in people infected with HIV.

Kaposi's sarcoma   A form of cancer characterized by purple or brownish lesions that are generally painless and occur anywhere on the skin; usually appears in men infected with HIV.

HIV antibody test   A blood test to determine whether a person has been infected by HIV; becomes positive within weeks or months of exposure.

ELISA (enzyme-linked immunosorbent assay)   A blood test that detects the presence of antibodies to HIV.

Western blot   A blood test that detects the presence of HIV antibodies; a more accurate and more expensive test used to confirm positive results from an ELISA test.

HIV RNA assay   A test used to determine the viral load (the amount of HIV in the blood).

HIV positive   A diagnosis resulting from the presence of HIV in the bloodstream; also referred to as *seropositive*.

CRITICAL CONSUMER
Getting an HIV Test

You should strongly consider being tested if any of the following apply to you or any past or current sexual partners:

- You have had unprotected sex (vaginal, anal, or oral) with more than one partner or with a partner who was not in a mutually monogamous relationship with you.

- You have used or shared needles, syringes, or other paraphernalia for injecting drugs (including steroids).

- You have exchanged sex for drugs or money.

- You received a transfusion of blood or blood products between 1978 and 1985.

- You have ever been diagnosed with hepatitis, tuberculosis, or an STI.

If you decide to be tested, you can have the test done by a health care provider or you can take a home test.

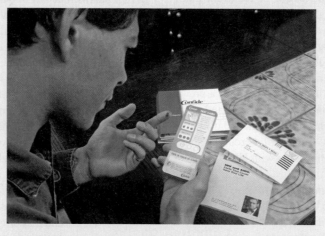

Physician or Clinic Testing

Your physician, student health clinic, Planned Parenthood, public health department, or local AIDS association can arrange your HIV test. Testing usually costs $50–$100, but public clinics often charge little or nothing. The standard test involves drawing a sample of blood that is sent to a lab, where it is checked for antibodies. If the first stage of testing is positive, a confirming test is done. This standard test takes one to two weeks, and you'll be asked to phone or come in personally to obtain your results, which should also include appropriate counseling.

Alternative tests are available at some clinics. The Orasure test uses oral fluid, which is collected by swabbing the inside of the mouth. Urine tests are also available. New rapid tests are now also available at some locations. These tests involve the use of blood or oral fluid and can provide results in as little as 20 minutes. If a rapid test is positive for HIV infection, a confirming test will be performed.

Before you get an HIV test, be sure you understand what will be done with the results. Results from confidential tests may still become part of your medical record and be reported to state and federal public health agencies. If you decide you want to be tested anonymously, ask your physician about an anonymous test, or use a home test.

Home Testing

Home test kits for HIV cost $40–$70. Avoid test kits sold on the Internet that are not FDA-approved. As of this printing, there were two HIV home-testing devices approved by the U.S. FDA: Home Access and OraQuick. Positive results with either test kit need to be confirmed with follow-up testing. To use the Home Access test, you prick a finger with a supplied lancet, blot a few drops of blood onto blotting paper, and mail it to the company's laboratory. In about a week (or within three business days for more expensive "express" tests), you call a toll-free number to find out your results. Anyone testing positive is routed to a trained counselor, who can provide emotional and medical support. The OraQuick HIV test, manufactured by Orasure, was approved in September 2013 by the FDA. This home test is the first rapid HIV test approved for home use. Like the Orasure test available to clinics, the OraQuick home test uses a sample taken from the mouth and returns results in 20 minutes. The results of home test kits are completely anonymous. Anyone testing positive should call their medical doctor or the OraQuick Consumer Support Center so that they can be counseled and routed to care.

Understanding the Results

A negative test result means that no antibodies were found in your sample. However, as noted in the text, it usually takes at least a month after exposure to HIV (and possibly as long as six months in some people) for antibodies to appear. Therefore, an infected person may get a false-negative result. If you test negative but your risk of infection is high, ask about obtaining an HIV RNA assay, which allows very early diagnosis.

A positive result means that you are infected. It is important to seek medical care and counseling immediately. Rapid progress is being made in treating HIV, and treatments are potentially much more successful when started early. For more information about testing, visit the CDC National HIV and STI Testing Resources website (www.hivtest.org).

available to anyone except the wealthiest few. Pharmaceutical companies, the World Bank, and the international community are working to lower drug costs and provide aid for developing regions. HIV treatment is also challenging because taking the combination drugs is complicated, and the drugs have short-term side effects that may cause people to stop taking them. The drugs can also have long-term side effects, including serious health problems. The National Institutes of Health (NIH) has issued guidelines for HIV treatment that help patients and their doctors with decisions about treatment.

Prevention Research on the development of a safe, effective, and inexpensive vaccine to stop the spread of HIV worldwide has been ongoing.

Approaches to prevention include abstinence, consistent condom use with all sexual acts, and needle exchange programs for persons who use intravenous drugs. The FDA has approved a drug to be taken by people who do not have HIV but are at high risk for it. It is called a pre-exposure prophylaxis (PrEP), meaning that it is a prevention method intended to be used with other methods for reducing HIV risk.

How Can You Protect Yourself? Although AIDS cannot be cured, infection can be prevented. You can protect yourself by avoiding behaviors that may bring you into contact with HIV.

In a sexual relationship, the current and past behaviors of you and your partner determine the amount of risk involved. If you are uninfected and in a mutually monogamous relationship with another uninfected person, you are not at risk for HIV. For anyone not involved in a long-term, mutually monogamous relationship, abstinence from any sexual activity that involves the exchange of body fluids is the only sure way to prevent HIV infection (Figure 13.4).

People who inject drugs should avoid sharing needles, syringes, filters, or anything that might have blood on it. Needles can be decontaminated with a solution of bleach and water, but this is not a foolproof procedure, and HIV can survive in a syringe for a month or longer. HIV can also survive boiling. For more guidelines and tips, see the box "Preventing STI Infection".

Chlamydia

Chlamydia trachomatis causes **chlamydia,** the most prevalent bacterial STI in the United States. Both men and women are susceptible to chlamydia, but, as with most STIs, women bear the greater burden because of possible complications and consequences of the disease. For women, the highest rates of infection occur among 15- to 24-year-olds. For men, the highest rates occur among 20- to 24-year-olds.

> **chlamydia** An STI transmitted by the bacterium *Chlamydia trachomatis.*
>
> TERMS

High Risk

Unprotected anal sex is the riskiest sexual behavior, especially for the receptive partner.

Unprotected vaginal intercourse is the next riskiest, especially for women, who are much more likely to be infected by an infected male partner than vice versa.

Oral sex is probably considerably less risky than anal and vaginal intercourse but can still result in HIV transmission.

Sharing of sex toys can be risky because they can carry blood, semen, or vaginal fluid.

Use of a condom reduces risk considerably but not completely for any type of intercourse. Anal sex with a condom is riskier than vaginal sex with a condom; oral sex with a condom is less risky, especially if the man does not ejaculate.

Hand-genital contact and deep kissing are less risky but could still theoretically transmit HIV; the presence of cuts or sores increases risk.

Sex with only one uninfected and totally faithful partner is without risk, but effective only if both partners are uninfected and completely monogamous.

Activities that don't involve the exchange of body fluids carry no risk: hugging, massage, closed-mouth kissing, masturbation, phone sex, and fantasy.

Abstinence is completely without risk. For many people, it can be an effective and reasonable method of avoiding HIV infection and other STDs during certain periods of life.

No Risk

FIGURE 13.4 **What's risky and what's not: The approximate relative risk of HIV transmission of various sexual activities.**

Accurate information about HIV/AIDS is available from many sources, including college health clinics, health professionals, and community organizations.

TAKE CHARGE
Preventing STI Infection

Before you begin a sexual relationship with someone, talk with your potential partner about HIV, safer sex, and condom use. The following guidelines may help you avoid infection:

- Don't drink alcohol or use drugs in sexual situations. Mood-altering drugs can affect your judgment and make you more likely to take risks.

- Limit the number of partners. Avoid sexual contact with people who have HIV or an STI or who have engaged in risky behaviors in the past.

- Use condoms during every act of intercourse including oral sex. Condoms do not provide perfect protection, but they greatly reduce your risk of contracting an infection.

- Use condoms properly for maximum protection.

- Avoid sexual contact that could cause cuts or tears in the skin or tissue.

- Get periodic screening tests for STIs and HIV. Sexually active young women and MSM should be tested for STIs at least annually or more frequently depending on risk behaviors.

Women should have a Pap test at age 21 and every three years thereafter.

- Get vaccinated. All sexually active men and women should be vaccinated against hepatitis B. All MSM should be vaccinated against hepatitis A. Young men and women aged 26 years and younger should consider getting vaccinated against HPV.

- Get prompt treatment for any STIs you contract. Make sure your partner gets tested and treated, too. Don't have sex until both of you have completed your treatment.

- If you inject drugs of any kind, don't share needles, syringes, or anything that might have blood on it. If your community has a syringe exchange program, use it. Seek treatment.

- If you are at risk for HIV infection, don't donate blood, sperm, or body organs. Don't have unprotected sex or share needles or syringes. Consider talking to your provider to see if PrEP is right for you. Get tested for HIV soon, and get treated. HIV-infected people who get early treatment generally feel better and live longer than those who delay.

If left untreated, chlamyida can lead to pelvic inflammatory disease (PID). It also greatly increases a woman's risk for infertility and ectopic (tubal) pregnancy. The CDC currently recommends annual chlamydia testing for all sexually active women aged 25 or younger and for older women who are at increased risk (such as those who have multiple sex partners).

Chlamydia can also lead to infertility in men, although not as often as in women. In men under age 35, chlamydia is the most common cause of epididymitis, which is inflammation of the sperm-carrying ducts. In men, up to half of all cases of **urethritis,** inflammation of the urethra, are caused by chlamydia.

Infants of infected mothers can acquire the infection through contact with the pathogen in the birth canal during delivery.

Symptoms   Most people experience few or no symptoms from chlamydia infection, increasing the likelihood that they will inadvertently spread the infection to their partners. In men, chlamydia symptoms can include painful urination, a slight watery discharge from the penis, and sometimes pain around

the testicles. Women may notice increased vaginal discharge, burning with urination, pain or bleeding with intercourse, and lower abdominal pain. The exact time from chlamydia infection to symptomatic disease is unknown, though it may range 12 weeks.

Diagnosis and Treatment   Chlamydia is diagnosed through laboratory tests on a urine sample or a small amount of fluid from the urethra, cervix, rectum, or vagina. Once chlamydia has been diagnosed, the infected person and his or her partner(s) are given antibiotics—usually doxycycline for a week or azithromycin, which can cure infection in one dose. Testing and treatment of partners is important. When it is unlikely that a partner will seek medical treatment, the CDC recommends that an extra prescription for antibiotics be provided to the patient or medications provided to give to his or her partner. This strategy, called *expedited partner therapy*, is legal and encouraged in some states under certain circumstances.

Gonorrhea

Gonorrhea is caused by the bacterium *Neisseria gonorrhoeae*. More than 320,000 new cases of gonorrhea were reported to the CDC in 2011, a slight increase from the previous year. The highest incidence is among 15- to 24-year-olds. Like chlamydia, untreated gonorrhea can cause PID in women and urethritis and epididymitis in men. An infant passing through the birth canal of an infected

---

urethritis   Inflammation of the tube that carries urine from the bladder to the outside opening.

gonorrhea   A sexually transmitted bacterial infection caused by bacterium *Neisseria gonorrhoeae* that usually affects mucous membranes.

TERMS

mother may contract *gonococcal conjunctivitis,* an infection in the eyes that can cause blindness if not treated.

Symptoms   In males the first symptoms are due to urethritis, which causes urinary discomfort and a thick, yellowish white or yellowish green discharge from the penis. Up to half of males have very minor symptoms or none at all. Most females with gonorrhea are asymptomatic. Those who have symptoms often experience pain with urination, increased vaginal discharge, and severe menstrual cramps. Gonorrhea can also infect the throat or rectum of people who engage in oral or anal sex.

Diagnosis and Treatment   Gonorrhea is detectable through several tests; depending on the test, samples of urine or cervical, urethral, throat, or rectal fluids may be collected. Antibiotics are used to treat gonorrhea, but increasing drug resistance is a major concern. As such, the recommended treatment is a combination of ceftriaxone (an injectable cephalosporin) along with either a single dose of azithromycin or seven days of doxycycline regardless of chlamydia testing results.

Pelvic Inflammatory Disease

Pelvic inflammatory disease (PID) is a major complication in 10–40% of women who have been infected with either gonorrhea or chlamydia and have not received treatment. PID occurs when the initial infection travels upward beyond the cervix into the uterus, oviducts, ovaries, and pelvic cavity. PID may be serious enough to require hospitalization and sometimes surgery. Even if the disease is treated successfully, about 25% of affected women will have long-term problems, such as a continuing susceptibility to infection, ectopic pregnancy, infertility, and chronic pelvic pain.

PID is the leading cause of infertility in young women, often going undetected until the inability to become pregnant leads to further evaluation.

As with all STIs, the more sex partners a woman has had, the greater her risk of PID. Smokers have twice the risk of PID as nonsmokers. Using IUDs for contraception increases the risk of PID, although this risk is greatly reduced for women with only one uninfected sexual partner.

Symptoms   Symptoms of PID vary greatly. Some women may be asymptomatic; others may have abdominal pain, fever, chills, nausea, and vomiting. Early symptoms are essentially the same as those described for chlamydia and

gonorrhea. Symptoms often begin or worsen during or soon after a woman's menstrual period. Many women have abnormal vaginal bleeding—either bleeding between periods or heavy and painful menstrual bleeding.

Diagnosis and Treatment   Diagnosis of PID is made on the basis of symptoms, physical examination, ultrasound, and laboratory tests. **Laparoscopy** may be used to confirm the diagnosis and obtain material for cultures.

Antibiotics are usually started immediately; in severe cases, the woman may be hospitalized and antibiotics given intravenously. It is especially important that an infected woman's partners be treated. As many as 60% of the male contacts of women with PID are infected but asymptomatic.

Human Papillomavirus

Human papillomavirus (HPV) infection causes several diseases, including common warts, **genital warts,** and genital cancers. HPV causes virtually all cervical cancers, as well anal, penile vulvar, vaginal, and some forms of oropharyngeal cancers (the oropharynx includes the back of the mouth and the throat). Genital HPV is usually spread through sexual activity, including oral sex. HPV is the most common STI in the United States. About 6.2 million Americans become infected with HPV each year. In all, more than 80% of sexually active people will have been infected with HPV by the age of 50. HPV is especially common in young people, with some of the highest infection rates among college students (see the box "College Students and STIs"). Many young women contract HPV infection within three months of becoming sexually active.

Why Do College Students Have High Rates of STIs?

Risky sexual behavior is common. One study of college students found that fewer than half used condoms consistently and one-third had had 10 or more sex partners. Another study found that 19% of male students and 33% of female students had consented to sexual intercourse simply because they felt awkward refusing.

- College students underestimate their risk of STIs. Although students may have considerable knowledge about STIs, they often feel the risks do not apply to them—a dangerous assumption. One study of students with a history of STIs showed that more than half had unprotected sex while they were infected, and 25% of them continued to have sex without ever informing their partner(s).

- Many students are infected but don't know it. A 2006 study of asymptomatic college women revealed that nearly 10% were infected with chlamydia.

What Effect Does Alcohol or Drug Use Have on My Likelihood of Getting an STI?

- Between one-third and one-half of college students report participating in sexual activity as a direct result of being intoxicated. All too often, sexual activity while intoxicated leads to unprotected intercourse.

- Students who binge-drink are more likely to have multiple partners, use condoms inconsistently, and delay seeking treatment for STIs than are students who drink little or no alcohol. Sexual assaults occur more frequently when either the perpetrator or the victim has been drinking.

What Can Students Do to Protect Themselves against STIs?

- Limit the number of sex partners. Even people who are always in a monogamous relationship can end up with extensive potential exposure to STIs if, over the years, they have numerous relationships.

- Use condoms consistently, and don't assume it's safe to stop after you've been with a partner for several months. HIV infection, HPV infection, herpes, and chlamydia can be asymptomatic for months or years and can be transmitted at any time. If you haven't been using condoms with your current partner, start now.

- Enjoy sexuality on your own terms. Don't let the expectations of friends and partners cause you to ignore your own feelings. Let your own wellness be your first priority. If you choose to be sexually active, learn about safer sex practices.

- Get to know your partner, and talk to him or her before becoming intimate. Be honest about yourself, and encourage your partner to do the same. But practice safer sex no matter what.

There are more than 100 different strains of HPV, and different strains cause different types of infection. More than 30 types are likely to cause genital infection. Types 6 and 11 cause 90% of visible genital warts. There are at least 12 other HPV strains including 16 and 18, which are considered high-risk strains for cancer and most often implicated in anogenital cancers (anal, cervical, penile, vaginal, and vulvar cancers).

Two HPV vaccines—Gardasil and Cervarix—have been approved by the FDA. Gardasil protects against four types of HPV virus that together account for 90% of genital warts and 70% of cervical cancers and most anal cancers. Gardasil has also been shown to prevent cancers of the vagina, vulva, and anus. Cervarix protects against two types of HPV but not against the type that causes genital warts. Gardasil was originally approved for girls and women, but in 2009 it was also approved for boys and men aged 9–26. Given the low vaccination rates in females, many experts believe that it makes sense to routinely vaccinate young males against HPV. The CDC recommends the vaccine for all girls 11 and 12 with either HPV vaccine and boys aged 11 and 12 with Gardasil. This age was chosen because the vaccine is most effective when given prior to exposure to genital HPV, and this virus is so common that many young people will be exposed to it shortly after becoming sexually active. Catch-up vaccination is recommended for individuals 13–26 years old, including those most at risk such as MSM and immunocompromised individuals.

Symptoms Most people infected with HPV have no visible warts or other symptoms and are not aware that they are infected and contagious to others. The good news is that the immune system usually clears the virus on its own, and infection disappears without any treatment. But in some cases, the infection persists and causes genital warts or cancers.

The types of HPV that cause cervical cancer do not produce any visible changes on the external genitals. The types that cause genital warts can produce anything from a small bump to a large, warty growth. Untreated warts can grow together to form a cauliflower-like mass. In males, they appear on the penis and often involve the urethra, appearing first at the opening and then spreading inside. In women, warts may appear on the labia or vulva and may spread to the *perineum,* the area between the vagina and the rectum. They may also appear on the cervix.

Diagnosis and Treatment Genital warts are usually diagnosed based on the appearance of the lesions. HPV infection of the cervix is often detected on routine Pap tests. Special tests are now available to detect the presence of HPV infection and to distinguish among the more common strains of HPV, including those that cause most cases of cervical cancer.

Treatment of genital warts focuses on reducing the number and size of warts, through cryosurgery (freezing), electrocautery (burning), or laser surgery. Even after treatment and the disappearance of visible warts, the individual may continue to carry HPV in healthy-looking tissue and can probably still infect others. Cervical abnormalities that are cancerous or precancerous are treated surgically or with other techniques such as electrical excision, freezing, and laser.

Anyone who has ever had HPV infection should inform all partners and use condoms, even though they do not provide total protection. Whether or not they have had the vaccine, all women should have regular pelvic exams and Pap tests.

Genital Herpes

Up to one in five adults in the United States has **genital herpes**. Worldwide, genital herpes is extremely common, and it is a major factor in HIV transmission.

Two types of herpes simplex viruses, HSV 1 and HSV 2, cause genital herpes and oral–labial herpes (cold sores). Infection with HSV is generally lifelong. After infection, the virus lies dormant in nerve cells and can reactivate at any time.

HSV 1 infection is so common that 50–80% of U.S. adults have antibodies to it (indicating previous exposure to the virus); most were exposed to HSV 1 during childhood. HSV 2 infection usually occurs during adolescence and early adulthood, often between ages 18 and 25.

HSV 2 is almost always sexually transmitted including during oral sex. The infection spreads readily whether people have active sores or are completely asymptomatic. Because HSV is asymptomatic in 80–90% of people, the infection is often acquired from a person who does not know that he or she is infected. Transmission is more likely from an infected female to her male partner than from an infected male to his female partner.

If you have ever had an outbreak of genital herpes, you should consider yourself always contagious and inform your partners. Avoid intimate contact when any sores are present, and use condoms during all sexual contact. One study showed that using condoms for every act of intercourse results in a 30% decrease in the transmission of herpes compared with no condom use. Condoms are more effective in preventing the transmission of other STIs than herpes, but this study shows that they can make a significant difference in preventing the spread of genital herpes.

Newborns can occasionally be infected with HSV, usually during passage through the birth canal of an infected mother. Without treatment, 65% of newborns with HSV will die, and most who survive will have some degree of brain damage.

Pregnant women who have been exposed to genital herpes should inform their physicians so that appropriate precautions can be taken to protect their babies from infection.

Symptoms Up to 90% of people who are infected with HSV have no symptoms. Those who develop symptoms often first notice them within 2–20 days of having sex with an infected partner. (However, it is not unusual for the first outbreak to occur months or even years after initial exposure.) The first episode of genital herpes frequently causes flulike symptoms in addition to genital lesions. The lesions tend to be painful or itchy and can occur anywhere on the genitals, inner thighs, or anal area. Depending on their location, they can cause considerable pain with urination. Lymph nodes in the groin may become swollen and tender. The sores usually heal within three weeks.

On average, newly diagnosed people will experience five to eight outbreaks per year, with a decrease in the frequency of outbreaks over time. Recurrent episodes are usually less severe than the initial one, with fewer and less painful sores that heal more quickly. Outbreaks can be triggered by stress, illness, fatigue, sun exposure, sexual intercourse, and menstruation.

Diagnosis and Treatment Genital herpes can be diagnosed on the basis of symptoms, but laboratory testing is helpful if there is any question about the diagnosis. Several blood tests can detect the presence of HSV antibodies in the blood.

There is no cure for herpes. Once infected, a person carries the virus for life. Antiviral drugs such as acyclovir can be taken at the beginning of an outbreak to shorten the severity and duration of symptoms. Support groups are available to help people learn to cope with herpes. There is no vaccine to prevent herpes, but research is ongoing.

Hepatitis B

Hepatitis (inflammation of the liver) can cause serious and sometimes permanent damage to the liver, which can result in death in severe cases. One of the many types of hepatitis

TERMS

genital herpes A sexually transmitted infection caused by the herpes simplex virus.

hepatitis Inflammation of the liver, which can be caused by infection, drugs, or toxins; some forms of infectious hepatitis can be transmitted sexually.

Hepatitis B is a highly contagious STI that can easily spread among people who live in close contact with one another. Vaccination against hepatitis B is recommended for all college students.

is caused by hepatitis B virus (HBV). Like HIV, HBV is found in most body fluids, including blood and blood products, semen, saliva, urine, and vaginal secretions. HBV is much more contagious than HIV. It is easily transmitted through any sexual activity that involves the exchange of body fluids. The primary risk factors for HBV are sexual exposure and injection drug use; having multiple sex partners greatly increases risk. HBV can also be transmitted through nonsexual close contact, including the use of contaminated needles, razor blades, toothbrushes, and eating utensils. Because of crowded living conditions in many college settings, vaccination against HBV is recommended for incoming college students.

Other forms of viral hepatitis can also be sexually transmitted. Hepatitis A is of particular concern for people who engage in anal sex; a vaccine is available and is recommended for all people at risk. Large population-based studies have demonstrated an association between hepatitis C virus (HCV) and individuals who engage in high-risk sexual encounters. Over the past few years there has been a surge of safe and effective treatments to cure HCV; thus testing and managing the care of infected individuals may assist in curbing this problem.

Symptoms Many people infected with HBV never develop symptoms; they have what are known as silent infections. Mild cases of hepatitis cause flulike symptoms such as fever, body aches, chills, and loss of appetite. As the illness progresses, there may be nausea, vomiting, dark-colored urine, abdominal pain, and jaundice.

Most adults who have acute hepatitis B recover completely within a few weeks or months. But about 5% of adults who are infected with HBV become chronic carriers

of the virus, capable of infecting others for the rest of their life. Some chronic carriers remain asymptomatic, while others develop chronic liver disease. Chronic hepatitis can cause cirrhosis, liver failure, and a deadly form of liver cancer.

Diagnosis and Treatment Hepatitis is diagnosed by blood tests used to analyze liver function, detect the infecting organism, and detect antibodies to the virus. There is no cure for HBV and no specific treatment for acute infections; antiviral drugs and immune system modulators may be used for chronic HBV infection. Vaccination against HBV is recommended for all infants and children as well as previously unvaccinated adults.

Syphilis

Syphilis, a disease that once caused death and disability for millions, can now be effectively treated with antibiotics.

Syphilis rates in 2011 were unchanged from the previous year in that they were lower than they had been in the previous 10 years. However, rates in young men who have sex with men were rising; rates of co-infection with HIV were also high in this group. Studies have found an association between syphilis infection and the use of the Internet as a means to meet sex partners among MSM. Another trend is an increase in the proportion of cases of syphilis transmitted through oral sex.

Syphilis is caused by a spirochete called *Treponema pallidum,* a thin, corkscrew-shaped bacterium. The disease is usually acquired through sexual contact, although infected pregnant women can transmit it to their fetuses. The pathogen passes through any break or opening in the skin or mucous membranes and can be transmitted by kissing, vaginal or anal intercourse, or oral–genital contact.

Symptoms Syphilis progresses through several stages. *Primary syphilis* is characterized by an ulcer called a **chancre** that appears within 10–90 days after exposure. The chancre is usually found at the site where the organism entered the body, such as the genital area, but it may also appear in other sites such as the mouth, breasts, or fingers. Chancres contain large numbers of bacteria and make the disease highly contagious when present; they are often painless and typically heal on their own within a few weeks. If the disease is not treated during the primary stage, about a third of infected individuals progress to chronic stages of infections.

Secondary syphilis is usually characterized by a skin rash that appears three to six weeks after the chancre. The rash may cover the entire body or only a few areas, but the palms of the hands and soles of the feet are usually involved. Areas of skin affected by the rash are highly contagious but usually heal within several weeks or months.

If the disease remains untreated, the symptoms of secondary syphilis may recur over a period of several years; affected individuals may then lapse into an asymptomatic latent stage in which they experience no further consequences of infection. However, in about one-third of cases of

syphilis A sexually transmitted bacterial infection caused by the spirochete *Treponema pallidum*.

TERMS

chancre The sore produced by syphilis in its earliest stage.

untreated secondary syphilis, the individual develops *late,* or *tertiary syphilis.* Late syphilis can damage many organs of the body, possibly causing severe dementia, cardiovascular damage, blindness, and death.

In infected pregnant women, the syphilis bacterium can cross the placenta. If the mother is not treated, the probable result is stillbirth, prematurity, or congenital deformity. In many cases the infant is also born infected *(congenital syphilis)* and requires treatment.

Diagnosis and Treatment   Syphilis is diagnosed by examination of infected tissues and with blood tests. All stages can be treated with antibiotics, but damage from late syphilis can be permanent.

Other STIs

Trichomoniasis (often called *trich*) is a common STI among young women. The single-celled organism that causes trich, *Trichomonas vaginalis,* thrives in warm, moist conditions, making women particularly susceptible to these infections in the vagina. Women who become symptomatic with trich develop a greenish, foul-smelling vaginal discharge and severe itching and pain in the vagina. Men usually have no symptoms, but may have mild irritation after urinating, or a slight discharge. Prompt treatment with metronidazole (Flagyl) is important because studies suggest that trich may increase the risk of HIV transmission and, in pregnant women, premature delivery.

Bacterial vaginosis (BV) is the most common cause of abnormal vaginal discharge in women of reproductive age. BV occurs when healthful bacteria that normally inhabit the vagina become displaced by unhealthful species. BV is generally not considered a sexually transmitted infection, but may be associated with sexual activity—for example, change in partners, multiple partners, and female same-sex relationships. Symptoms of BV include vaginal discharge with a fishy odor and sometimes vaginal irritation. BV is treated with topical and oral antibiotics.

Lymphogranuloma venereum (LGV) is an infection of the lymphatic system caused by three strains of the bacteria *Chlamydia trachomatis* (not the same strain that causes the genital STI chlamydia). The incidence of LGV in the United States is unknown; however, outbreaks have occurred in the Netherlands and other European countries among men who have sex with men. LGV is more common in men than in women; the main risk factor is being HIV positive. The first symptom is an ulcer at the site of sexual penetration that appears 3–30 days after exposure; there may also be swollen glands in the genital area. Among those who practice anal receptive intercourse, symptoms may include rectal ulcers, bleeding, and pain. If the infection is untreated, chronic symptoms may develop, so individuals with symptoms should see a physician.

Pubic lice (commonly known as *crabs*) and **scabies** are highly contagious parasitic infections. They are usually treated with topical medicines, but oral medications are sometimes needed as well.

WHAT YOU CAN DO ABOUT STIs

You can take responsibility for your health and contribute to a general reduction in the incidence of STIs in three major areas: education, diagnosis and treatment, and prevention.

Education

Educational campaigns about HIV/AIDS and other STIs have paid off in changing attitudes and sexual behaviors. Levels of awareness about HIV infection among the general population are quite high, although some segments of the population are harder to reach and continue to engage in very high-risk behaviors. Learning about STIs is still up to every person individually, as is applying that knowledge to personal situations.

Diagnosis and Treatment

Early diagnosis and treatment of STIs can help you avoid complications and help prevent the spread of infection.

- *Be alert for symptoms.* If you are sexually active, be alert for any sign or symptom of disease, such as a rash, a discharge, sores, or pain. Although only a physician can make a proper diagnosis of an STI, you can perform a genital self-examination between check-ups to look for early warning signs of disease, such as bumps, sores, blisters, or warts.

- *Get vaccinated.* Every young, sexually active person should be vaccinated against hepatitis B. Men who have sex with men should be vaccinated against hepatitis A, and men and women aged 9–26 should be vaccinated against HPV.

- *Get tested.* The CDC recommends that everyone between the ages of 13 and 64 be tested for HIV at least once during routine medical care. If you are sexually active, be sure to get periodic STI checks, even if you have no symptoms. If you have a risky sexual encounter, see a physician as soon as possible.

---

trichomoniasis   A protozoal infection caused by *Trichomonas vaginalis,* transmitted sexually and externally.

bacterial vaginosis (BV)   A condition that may be linked to sexual activity; caused by an overgrowth of certain bacteria inhabiting the vagina.

lymphogranuloma venereum (LGV)   An infection of the lymphatic system caused by three strains of the bacterium *Chlamydia trachomatis,* transmitted sexually.

pubic lice   Parasites that infest the hair of the pubic region, commonly called crabs.

scabies   A contagious skin disease caused by a type of burrowing parasitic mite.

TERMS

- **Inform your partners.** Telling a partner that you have exposed him or her to an STI isn't easy. Despite the awkwardness and difficulty, it is crucial that your sex partner or partners be informed and urged to seek testing and/or treatment as quickly as possible.

- **Get treated.** With the exception of AIDS treatments, treatments for STIs are safe and generally inexpensive. If you are being treated, follow instructions carefully and complete all the medication as prescribed. Don't stop taking the medication just because you feel better or your symptoms have disappeared.

Connect to Your Choices

Have you ever thought about where you get your behaviors and habits related to STIs? Many factors can influence our behaviors and habits, some not as obvious as others. Was your family conscientious about making sure you got all the recommended vaccinations when you were growing up? Did you have comprehensive sex education in high school? Do the significant people in your peer group use condoms and practice safer sex? Does your campus health clinic promote HIV/AIDS awareness?

What are the external factors that influence your choices about sexually transmitted diseases? What are your inner motivations and core values, and how do they affect your choices? Based on what you learned in this chapter, will you make some different choices in the future? If so, what will they be?

Go online to Connect to complete this activity: www.mcgraw-hillconnect.com

TIPS FOR TODAY AND THE FUTURE

Your immune system is a remarkable germ-fighting network, but it needs your help to work at its best.

RIGHT NOW YOU CAN:

- Move your bedtime up 15 minutes, starting tonight.
- Make an appointment with your health care provider if you are worried about possible STI infection.
- Resolve to discuss condom use with your partner if you are sexually active and are not already using condoms.

IN THE FUTURE YOU CAN:

- Learn how to communicate effectively with a partner who resists safer sex practices or is reluctant to discuss his or her sexual history. Support groups and educational classes can help.
- Make sure all your vaccinations are up-to-date; ask your doctor if you should be vaccinated against hepatitis A or B, HPV, or any other STIs.

Prevention

If you choose to be sexually active, think about prevention *before* you have a sexual encounter and plan accordingly. By thinking and talking about responsible sexual behavior, you are expressing a sense of caring for yourself, your potential partner, and your future children.

SUMMARY

- The immune system includes both surface barriers and the cells that mount the immune response. Physical and chemical barriers to microorganisms include skin, mucous membranes, and the cilia lining the respiratory tract.

- The immune response is carried out by white blood cells that are continuously produced in the bone marrow. Cells of the innate immune system include neutrophils, eosinophils, macrophages, dendritic cells, and natural killer cells. Cells of the adaptive immune system are lymphocytes—in particular, T cells and B cells.

- The immune response has four stages: recognition of the invading pathogen; rapid replication of killer T cells and B cells; attack by killer T cells and macrophages; and suppression of the immune response.

- Immunization is based on the body's ability to remember previously encountered organisms.

- Allergic reactions occur when the immune system responds to harmless substances as if they were dangerous pathogens.

- The step-by-step process by which infections are transmitted from one person to another involves a pathogen, its reservoir, a portal of exit, a means of transmission, a portal of entry, and a new host. Infection can be prevented by breaking the chain at any point.

- The spread of disease may result in epidemics or pandemics.

- Bacteria are single-celled organisms; some cause disease in humans. Significant bacterial infections include pneumonia, meningitis, strep throat, toxic shock syndrome, MRSA, tuberculosis, Lyme disease, and ulcers.

- Most antibiotics work by interrupting the production of new bacteria; they do not work against viruses. Bacteria can become resistant to antibiotics.

- Viruses cannot grow or reproduce themselves; different viruses cause the common cold, influenza, measles, mumps, rubella, chicken pox, cold sores, mononucleosis, encephalitis, hepatitis, polio, and warts.

- Other infectious diseases are caused by certain types of fungi, protozoa, and parasitic worms.

- Autoimmune diseases occur when the body identifies its own cells as foreign. A healthy immune system can destroy mutant cells that may become cancerous. The immune system needs little help other than adequate nutrition and rest, and protection from excessive stress. Vaccinations also help protect against disease.

- HIV affects the immune system, making an otherwise healthy person less able to resist a variety of infections. HIV is carried in blood and blood products, semen, vaginal and cervical secretions, and breast milk. HIV is transmitted through the exchange of these fluids.

- There is currently no cure or vaccine for HIV infection. Drugs have been developed to slow the course of the disease and to prevent or treat certain secondary infections.

- Chlamydia causes epididymitis and urethritis in men; in women, it can lead to PID and infertility if untreated.

- Untreated gonorrhea can cause PID in women and epididymitis in men, leading to infertility. In infants, untreated gonorrhea can cause blindness.

- Pelvic inflammatory disease (PID), usually a complication of untreated gonorrhea or chlamydia, is an infection of the uterus and oviducts that may extend to the ovaries and pelvic cavity. It can lead to infertility, ectopic pregnancy, and chronic pelvic pain.

- Human papillomavirus (HPV) causes genital warts and cervical cancer. The virus can be transmitted by asymptomatic people. Even after treatment, a person may continue to carry the virus in healthy-looking tissue. The immune system often clears HPV on its own.

- Genital herpes is a common viral infection that can cause painful blisters on the genitals. The virus remains in the body for life and causes recurrent outbreaks.

- Hepatitis B is an inflammation of the liver caused by one of the many types of hepatitis viruses. It is transmitted through both sexual and nonsexual contact.

- Syphilis is a highly contagious bacterial infection that can be treated with antibiotics. If left untreated, it can lead to deterioration of the central nervous system and death.

- Other diseases that can be transmitted sexually or are linked to sexual activity include trichomoniasis, bacterial vaginosis, lymphogranuloma venereum (LGV), pubic lice, and scabies. Any STI that causes sores or inflammation can increase the risk of HIV transmission.

- Individuals can contribute to a reduction in the incidence of STIs by educating themselves, being diagnosed and treated for any infections, and practicing preventive strategies.

FOR MORE INFORMATION

BOOKS

Blaser, M. J. 2014. *Missing Microbes: How the Overuse of Antibiotics Is Fueling Our Modern Plagues.* New York: Holt, Henry & Company, Inc.

Handsfield, H. H. 2011. *Color Atlas & Synopsis of Sexually Transmitted Diseases,* 3rd ed. New York: McGraw-Hill.

Pepin, J. 2011. *The Origin of AIDS.* Cambridge, UK: Cambridge University Press. *A highly readable investigation into the perplexing evolutionary origin and early epidemiology of the AIDS virus.*

Reid, E. 2012. *The Thriving Child: Parenting Successfully through Allergies, Asthma, and Other Common Challenges.* New York: Center Street. *A mother's description of raising two children with allergies and asthma in New York City and developing a healthy environment for her family.*

Shilts, R. 2007. *And the Band Played On: Politics, People, and the AIDS Epidemic, 20th Anniversary Edition.* New York: St. Martin's Griffin. *Originally published in 1987, this landmark book chronicles the early years of the AIDS epidemic, tracing the political, medical, and social forces that facilitated the spread of the epidemic.*

Sompayrac, L. M. 2012. *How the Immune System Works,* 4th ed. Malden, MA: Blackwell Science. *A highly readable overview of basic concepts of immunity.*

Wellings, Kaye, et al., eds. 2012. *Sexual Health: A Public Health Perspective.* Berkshire, UK: Open University Press.

ORGANIZATIONS, HOTLINES, AND WEBSITES

Alliance for the Prudent Use of Antibiotics. Provides information about the proper use of antibiotics and tips for avoiding infections.

http://www.tufts.edu/med/apua

American Academy of Allergy, Asthma, and Immunology. Provides information and publications; pollen counts are available from the website.

http://www.aaaai.org

American Autoimmune-Related Diseases Association. Provides background information, coping tips, and an online knowledge quiz about autoimmune diseases.

http://www.aarda.org

American Social Health Association (ASHA). Provides written information on STDs and referrals for those infected; sponsors support groups for people with herpes and HPV.

http://www.ashastd.org

Black AIDS Institute. Provides public health information about a variety of topics including testing, treatment, vaccines, and health care access; focuses on black people and the black community.

http://www.blackaids.org

CDC National Center for Emerging and Zoonotic Infectious Diseases. Provides extensive information on a wide variety of infectious diseases.

http://www.cdc.gov/ncezid/

CDC National Prevention Information Network. Provides extensive information and links for HIV/AIDS and other STDs.

http://www.cdcnpin.org

CDC National STD and AIDS Hotlines. Callers can obtain information, counseling, and referrals for testing and treatment. The hotlines offer information on more than 20 STDs and include Spanish and TTY service.

800-342-AIDS *or* 800-227-8922

800-344-SIDA (Spanish)

800-243-7889 (TTY, deaf access)

CDC: Vaccines. Information and answers to frequently asked questions about immunizations.

http://www.cdc.gov/vaccines/

HIV InSite: Gateway to AIDS Knowledge. Provides information about prevention, education, treatment, statistics, clinical trials, and new developments; from the University of California, San Francisco.

http://hivinsite.ucsf.edu

Joint United Nations Programme on HIV/AIDS (UNAIDS). Provides statistics and information on the international HIV/AIDS situation.

http://www.unaids.org

MedlinePlus: Sexually Transmitted Diseases. Maintained by the CDC, a clearinghouse of links and information on STIs and other sexual health topics.

http://www.nlm.nih.gov/medlineplus/sexuallytransmitteddiseases
.html

http://www.nlm.nih.gov/medlineplus/sexualhealthissues.html

National Foundation for Infectious Diseases. Provides information about a variety of diseases and disease issues.

http://www.nfid.org

National Institute of Allergy and Infectious Diseases. Includes fact sheets about many topics relating to allergies and infectious diseases, including tuberculosis and STIs.

http://www.niaid.nih.gov

The NAMES Project Foundation, AIDS Memorial Quilt. Includes the story behind the quilt, images of quilt panels, and information and links relating to HIV infection.

http://www.aidsquilt.org

Planned Parenthood Federation of America. Provides information about STDs, family planning, and contraception.

http://www.plannedparenthood.org

World Health Organization (WHO): Sexually Transmitted Infections. Provides information on international statistics and prevention efforts.

http://www.who.int/topics/sexually_transmitted_infections/en

World Health Organization, World Malaria Report 2013. The report summarizes information on malaria-endemic countries, updates the analyses presented in the 2012 report, highlights the progress made toward global malaria targets set for 2015, and describes challenges for global control and elimination of malaria.

http://www.who.int/malaria/publications/world_malaria
_report_2013/en/index.html

SELECTED BIBLIOGRAPHY

AIDS.gov. 2012. *Sexual Risk Factors* (http://aids.gov/hiv-aids-basics/prevention/reduce-your-risk/sexual-risk-factors/).

AIDS.gov. 2013. *Pre-Exposure Prophylaxis (PrEP)* (http://aids.gov/hiv-aids-basics/prevention/reduce-your-risk/pre-exposure-prophylaxis/).

American Association of Blood Banks. 2014. *Blood FAQ* (http://www.aabb.org/resources/bct/Pages/bloodfaq.aspx).

American College Health Association. 2013. *American College Health Association–National College Health Assessment II: Reference Group Executive Summary Spring 2013*. Linthicum, MD: ACHA.

American Social Health Association. 2014. *Herpes Testing Toolkit* (http://www.ashasexualhealth.org/healthcare-providers/educational-resources/herpes-testing-toolkit.html).

Blaser, M. 2011. Antibiotic overuse: Stop the killing of beneficial bacteria. *Nature* 476: 393–394.

Bradley H., et al.2014. Seroprevalence of herpes simplex virus types 1 and 2—United States, 1999–2010. *Journal of Infectious Diseases* 209(3): 325–333.

Butler, D., and H. Ledford. 2012. U.S. biosecurity board revises stance on mutant-flu studies. *Nature,* 30 March (http://www.nature.com/news/us-biosecurity-board-revises-stance-on-mutant-flu-studies-1.10369).

Centers for Disease Control and Prevention. 2011. CDC Grand Rounds: Chlamydia prevention: Challenges and strategies for reducing disease burden and sequelae. *Morbidity and Mortality Weekly Report* 60(12): 370–373.

Centers for Disease Control and Prevention. 2011. Recommendations on the use of quadrivalent human papillomavirus vaccine in males—Advisory Committee on Immunization Practices (ACIP), 2011. *Morbidity and Mortality Weekly Report* 60(50): 1705–1708.

Centers for Disease Control and Prevention. 2011. *Sexually Transmitted Disease Surveillance, 2012*. Atlanta: U.S. Department of Health and Human Services.

Centers for Disease Control and Prevention. 2013. Disease burden from viral hepatitis A, B, and C in the United States," from *Viral Hepatitis Statistics & Surveillance*. Atlanta: U.S. Department of Health and Human Services (http://www.cdc.gov/hepatitis/Statistics/index.htm).

Centers for Disease Control and Prevention. 2013. *Expedited Partner Therapy* (http://www.cdc.gov/std/ept/).

Centers for Disease Control and Prevention. 2013. HIV Testing and Risk Behaviors Among Gay, Bisexual, and Other Men Who Have Sex with Men—United States. *Morbidity and Mortality Weekly Report* 62(47): 958-962.

Centers for Disease Control and Prevention. 2013. Incidence, Prevalence, and Cost of Sexually Transmitted Infections in the United States (http://www.cdc.gov//stats/STI-Estimates-Fact-Sheet-Feb-2013.pdf).

Centers for Disease Control and Prevention. 2014. *CDC's National Asthma Control Program* (http://www.cdc.gov/nceh/information/asthma.htm).

Centers for Disease Control and Prevention. 2014. *Methicillin-resistant Staphylococcus aureus (MRSA) infections* (http://www.cdc.gov/mrsa/community/).

Centers for Disease Control and Prevention. 2014. *Pertussis (Whooping Cough).* (http://www.cdc.gov/pertussis/).

Centers for Disease Control and Prevention. 2014. *Seasonal influenza (flu)* (http://www.cdc.gov/flu/).

Centers for Disease Control and Prevention. 2014. *Trends in Tuberculosis—United States, 2012* (http://www.cdc.gov/tb/publications/factsheets/statistics/TBTrends.htm).

Centers for Disease Control and Prevention. 2014. *Adolescent and Adult Vaccine Quiz: What Vaccines Do You Need?* (http://www2a.cdc.gov/nip/adultimmsched/).

Centers for Disease Control and Prevention, National Center for HIV/AIDS, Viral Hepatitis, STD and TB prevention, Division of HIV/AIDS Prevention. 2013. *HIV in the United States: At a Glance*. (http://www.cdc.gov/hiv/pdf/policies_NationalProgressReport.pdf).

Chandra, A., et al. 2011. Sexual behavior, sexual attraction, and sexual identity in the United States: Data from the 2006–2008 National Survey of Family Growth. *National Health Statistics Report*, No. 36.

Chhabra, N., et al. 2012. Pharmacotherapy for multidrug resistant tuberculosis. *Journal of Pharmacology and Pharmacotherapy* 3(2): 98–104.

Choopanya K., et al. 2013. Antiretroviral prophylaxis for HIV infection in injecting drug users in Bangkok, Thailand (the Bangkok Tenofovir Study): A randomized, double-blind, placebo-controlled phase 3 trial. *Lancet* 381: 20832090.

Cohen, S, et al. 2009. Sleep habits and susceptibility to the common cold. *Archives of Internal Medicine* 169: 62–67.

Do Prado, M. F., et al. 2012. Antimicrobial efficacy of alcohol-based gels with a 30-s application. *Letters in Applied Microbiology* 54(6): 564–567.

Frieri, M, and A. Valluri. 2011. Vitamin D deficiency as a risk factor for allergic disorders and immune mechanisms. *Allergy Asthma Proceedings* 32(6): 438–444.

Ginocchio, C. C., et al. 2012. Prevalence of *Trichomonas vaginalis* and coinfection with Chlamydia trachomatis and Neisseria gonorrhoeae in the United States as determined by the Aptima *Trichomonas vaginalis* nucleic acid amplification assay. *Journal of Clinical Microbiology*, 23 May (epub ahead of print).

Gradison, M. 2012. Pelvic inflammatory disease. *American Family Physician* 85(8): 791–796.

Harmon, K. 2011. What will the next influenza pandemic look like? *Scientific American,* 19 September.

The Henry J. Kaiser Family Foundation. 2013. *The HIV/AIDS epidemic in the United States.*

The Henry J. Kaiser Family Foundation. 2013. *HIV testing in the United States.*

Hutton, H. E., et al. 2013. Alcohol use, anal sex, and other risky sexual behaviors among HIV-infected women and men. *AIDS and Behavior* 17(5): 1694.

Irwin, M. R., 2012. Sleep and infectious disease risk. *Sleep* 35(8): 1025–1026.

Jemal, A et al. 2013. Annual report to the nation on the status of cancer, 1975–2009, featuring the burden and trends in human papillomavirus (HPV)–associated cancers and HPV vaccination coverage levels. *Journal of the National Cancer Institute* 105: 175–201.

Joint United Nations Programme on HIV/AIDS (UNAIDS). 2012. *UNAIDS World AIDS Day Report*. Geneva: UNAIDS.

Lam, C. B., and E. S. Lefkowitz. 2012. Risky sexual behaviors in emerging adults: Longitudinal changes and within-person variations. *Archives of Sexual Behaviors*, 11 May (epub ahead of print).

Lamb, A. K., et al. 2011. Reducing asthma disparities by addressing environmental inequities: A case study of Regional Asthma Management and Prevention's advocacy efforts. *Family & Community Health* 34: S54–S62.

Ledford, H. 2014. HIV rebound dashes hope of 'Mississippi baby' cure. *Nature*, 10 July.

Lehtinen, M., et al. 2012. Overall efficacy of HPV-16/18 AS04-adjuvanted vaccine against grade 3 or greater cervical intraepithelial neoplasia: 4-year end-of-study analysis of the randomised, double-blind PATRICIA trial. *Lancet Oncology* 13(1): 89–99.

Markowitz, L. E., et al. 2013. Reduction in human papillomavirus (HPV) prevalence among young women following HPV vaccine introduction in the United States, National Health and Nutrition Examination Surveys, 2003–2010. *The Journal of Infectious Diseases* 208(3): 385–393.

McRee, A. L., et al. 2012. Human papillomavirus vaccine discussions: An opportunity for mothers to talk with their daughters about sexual health. *Sexually Transmitted Diseases* 29(5): 394–401.

National Institutes of Health. 2013. *The HIV Life Cycle* (http://aidsinfo.nih.gov/education-materials/fact-sheets/19/73/the-hiv-life-cycle).

Oswalt, S., and T. Wyatt. 2013. Sexual health behaviors and sexual orientation in a U.S. national sample of college students. *Archives of Sexual Behavior* 42(8): 1561–1572.

Patel, P., et al. 2012. Prevalence and risk factors associated with herpes simplex virus-2 in a contemporary cohort of HIV-infected persons in the United States. *Sexually Transmitted Diseases* 3(2): 154–160.

Perillo, R. P., and J. W. Ward. 2012. *A Silent Epidemic: Why Chronic Hepatitis B Matters*. Web video. Medscape Education Family Medicine (http://www.medscape.org/viewarticle/759762).

Pennell, L. M., et al. 2012. Sex affects immunity. *Journal of Autoimmunity* 38(2): 1282–1291.

Piot, P., and T. Quinn. 2013. The AIDS Pandemic—A Global Health Paradigm. *New England Journal of Medicine* 368(23): 2210–2218.

Porkka-Heiskanen, T., et al. 2013. Sleep, its regulation and possible mechanisms of sleep disturbances. *Acta Physiologica (Oxford)* 208(4): 311–328.

Rashid, H., et al. 2012. Vaccination and herd immunity: What more do we know? *Current Opinion in Infectious Diseases* 25(3): 243–249.

Satterwhite, C. L., et al. 2013. Sexually transmitted infections among U.S. women and men: Prevalence and incidence estimates, 2008. *Sexually Transmitted Diseases* 40(3).

Tohme, R., and S. D. Holmberg. 2012. Transmission of hepatitis C virus infection through tattooing and piercing: A critical review. *Clinical Infectious Diseases* 54(8): 1167–1178.

U.S. Food and Drug Administration. 2013. *First Rapid Home-Use HIV Kit Approved for Self-Testing* (http://www.fda.gov/forconsumers/consumerupdates/ucm310545.htm).

U.S. Preventive Services Task Force. 2012. *Screening for Cervical Cancer* (http://www.uspreventiveservicestaskforce.org/uspstf/uspscerv.htm).

U.S. Preventive Services Task Force. 2013. *Screening for Hepatitis C Virus Infection in Adults* (http://www.uspreventiveservicestaskforce.org/uspstf12/hepc/hepcfinalrs.htm#summary).

Workowski, W. A. 2012. Sexually transmitted infections and HIV: Diagnosis and treatment. *Topics in Antiviral Medicine* 20(1): 11–16.

World Health Organization. 2013. *Global report: UNAIDS report on the global AIDS epidemic 2013*. Geneva: World Health Organization.

World Health Organization. 2013. *Pneumonia Still Responsible for One-Fifth of Child Deaths* (http://who.int/mediacentre/news/releases/2013/world-pneumonia-day-20131112/en/index.html).

World Health Organization. 2014. *Ebola virus disease: Fact sheet no. 103*. Media Centre, September, 2014.

BEHAVIOR CHANGE STRATEGY
Talking about Condoms and Safer Sex

The time to talk about safer sex is before you begin a sexual relationship. But even if you've been having unprotected sex with your partner, you can still start practicing safer sex now.

There are many ways to bring up the subject of safer sex and condom use with your partner. Be honest about your concerns and stress that protection against STIs means that you care about yourself and your partner. You may find that your partner shares your concerns and also wants to use condoms. He or she may be happy and relieved that you have brought up the subject of safer sex.

However, if he or she resists the idea of using condoms, you may need to negotiate (see the dialogue suggestions). Stress that you both deserve to be protected and that sex will be more enjoyable when you aren't worrying about STIs. If you and your partner haven't used condoms before, buy some and familiarize yourselves with how to use them. Once you feel more comfortable handling condoms, you'll be able to use them correctly and incorporate them into your sexual activity. Consider trying the female condom as well.

If your partner still won't agree to use condoms, think carefully about whether you want to have a sexual relationship with this person. Maybe he or she is not the right partner for you.

IF YOUR PARTNER SAYS . . .	TRY SAYING . . .
"They're not romantic."	"Worrying about AIDS isn't romantic, and with condoms we won't have to worry." or "If we put one on together, a condom could be fun."
"I don't have any kind of disease! Don't you trust me?"	"Of course I trust you, but anyone can have an STI and not even know it. This is just a way to take care of both of us."
"I forgot to bring a condom, let's just do it without a condom this time."	"It only takes one time to get pregnant or to get an STI. I just can't have sex unless I know I'm as safe as I can be." or "I never have sex without a condom. Let's go get some." or "I have some, right here."
"I don't like sex as much with a rubber. It doesn't feel the same."	"This is the only way I feel comfortable having sex but believe me, it'll still be good even with protection! And it lets us both just focus on each other instead of worrying about all that other stuff.." or "They might feel different, but let's try." or "Sex won't feel good if we're worrying about diseases." or "How about trying the female condom?"
"But I love you."	"Being in love can't protect us from diseases." or "I love you, too. We still need to use condoms."
"But we've been having sex without condoms."	"I want to start using condoms now so we won't be at any more risk." or "We can still prevent infection or reinfection."
"I don't know how to use them."	"I can show you—want me to put it on for you?"
"No one else makes me use a condom!"	"This is for both of us . . . and I won't have sex without protection. Let me show you how good it can be—even with a condom."
"I'm [or you're] on the pill."	"But that doesn't protect us from STIs, so I still want to be safe, for both of us."

SOURCES: dialogue from San Francisco AIDS Foundation. 1998. *Condoms for Couples* (Accessed at http://www.thebody.com/content/art2492.html#romantic). Reprinted with permission.

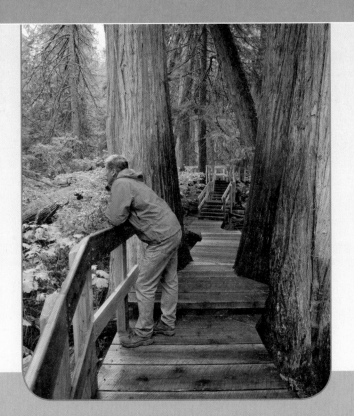

CHAPTER OBJECTIVES

- Explain how population growth affects the earth's environment and contributes to pollution and climate change

- Discuss the causes and effects of air and water pollution, and describe strategies that people can take to protect these resources

- Discuss the issue of solid waste disposal and the impact it has on the environment and human health

- Identify some key sources of chemical and radiation pollution, and discuss methods for preventing such pollution

- Explain how energy use affects the environment, and describe steps everyone can take to use energy more efficiently

CHAPTER 14

Environmental Health

We are constantly reminded of our intimate relationship with everything that surrounds us—our **environment.** Although the planet provides us with food, water, air, and everything else that sustains life, it also provides us with natural occurrences—earthquakes, tsunamis, hurricanes, drought, climate changes—that destroy life and disrupt society. Humans have always had to struggle against the environment to survive. Today, in addition to dealing with natural disasters, we also have to find ways to protect the environment from the by-products of our way of life.

This chapter introduces the concept of environmental health and explains how the environment affects us. The chapter also discusses the ways humans affect the planet and its resources, and describes steps you can take to improve your personal environmental health while reducing your impact on the earth.

ENVIRONMENTAL HEALTH DEFINED

The field of **environmental health** grew out of efforts to control communicable diseases. These efforts led to systematic garbage collection, sewage treatment, filtration and chlorination of drinking water, food inspection, and the establishment of public health enforcement agencies.

Cleaning up the environment changed the health profile of the industrialized world, reducing or eliminating deaths from diseases like cholera and typhoid fever. Unfortunately, infectious diseases have not been eradicated worldwide.

In the United States a huge, complex public health system is constantly at work behind the scenes. Every time the system is disrupted, danger recurs. After any disaster that damages a community's public health system prompt restoration of basic health services becomes crucial to human survival. Every time we venture beyond the boundaries of our everyday world, whether traveling to a poorer country or camping in a wilderness area, we are reminded of the importance of these basics: clean water, sanitary waste disposal, safe food, and insect and rodent control.

> **TERMS**
>
> **environment**   The natural and human-made surroundings in which we spend our lives.
>
> **environmental health**   The collective interactions of humans with the environment and the short-term and long-term health consequences of those interactions.

Natural events—such as Typhoon Haiyan, which killed more than 5,000 people in the Philippines in 2013—can wipe out whole villages and essential services, polluting water and facilitating the spread of disease.

Ask Yourself

QUESTIONS FOR CRITICAL THINKING AND REFLECTION

How often do you think about the environment's impact on your personal health? In what ways do your immediate surroundings (your home, neighborhood, school, workplace) affect your well-being? In what ways do you influence the health of your personal environment?

Over the past few decades, the focus of environmental health has expanded and become more complex, for several reasons. We now recognize that environmental pollutants contribute not only to infectious diseases and immediate symptoms but to many chronic diseases as well. In addition, technological advances have increased our ability to affect and damage the environment. Further, rapid population growth (more than doubling in the past 50 years), which has resulted partly from past environmental improvements, means that ever more people are consuming and competing for resources, increasing human environmental impact.

Environmental health encompasses all the interactions of humans with their environment and the health consequences of these interactions. Fundamental to this definition is a recognition that we hold the world in trust for future life on Earth. Our responsibility is to pass on a world no worse, and preferably better, than the one we live in today. Although many environmental problems are complex and seem beyond the control of the individual, there are ways that every person can make a difference to the future of the planet.

POPULATION GROWTH AND CONTROL

Throughout most of history, humans have been a minor pressure on the planet. About 300 million people were alive in the year 1 CE (Common Era); by the time Europeans were settling in the Americas 1,600 years later, the world population had increased gradually to a little over half a billion. But then it began rising exponentially—zooming to 1 billion by about 1800, more than doubling by 1930, and then doubling again in just 40 years (Figure 14.1).

The average number of children per woman fell from 5 in 1950 to half that (2.6) in 2010. This decline in fertility has been happening in Western countries for decades and is now also happening in many of today's poor countries.

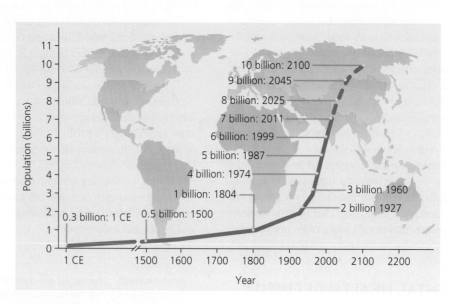

FIGURE 14.1 **World population growth.** The United Nations estimates that the world's population will continue to increase dramatically until it stabilizes above 10 billion people in 2100.

sources: United Nations Population Division. 2011. *World Population Prospects: The 2010 Revision.* New York: United Nations (http://esa.un.org/unpd/wpp/); U.S. Bureau of the Census.

Changes are also projected for the world's age distribution: For the first time in history, there are more older people than young children. By 2050 there will be 3.4 times the number of people age 60 and over than of children age 4 and under.

This rapid expansion of population is generally believed to be responsible for most of the stress humans put on the environment. It is also a driving force behind many of the relatively more recent environmental health concerns, including chemical pollution, global climate change, and the thinning of the atmosphere's ozone layer.

No one knows how many people the world can support, but most scientists agree that there is a limit. A 2011 report from the United Nation's Convention on Biological Diversity states that the population's demand for resources already exceeds the earth's capacity by 20%. The primary factors that may eventually put a cap on human population are likely to be the limits of the earth's resources—food, water, land, and energy.

The mass media have exposed the entire world to the American lifestyle and raised people's expectations of living at a comparable level. But such a lifestyle is supported by levels of energy consumption that the earth cannot support indefinitely. The United States has about 5% of the world's population but uses 25% of the world's energy.

Although it is apparent that population growth must be controlled, population trends are difficult to influence and manage. A variety of interconnecting factors fuel the current population explosion, including high fertility rates, lack of family planning resources, and low death rates.

To be successful, population management policies must change the condition of people's lives, especially poverty, to remove the pressures to have large families. Research indicates that the combination of improved health, better education, and increased literacy and employment opportunities for women work together with family planning to decrease birth rates.

AIR QUALITY AND POLLUTION

Air pollution is not a human invention or even a new problem. The air is polluted naturally with every forest fire, pollen bloom, and dust storm, as well as with countless other natural pollutants. To these natural sources, humans have always contributed the by-products of our activities.

Air pollution is linked to a wide range of health problems, and the very young and the elderly are among the most susceptible to air pollution's effects.

The United States has about 5% of the world's population but uses 25% of the world's energy.

Air Quality and Smog

The U.S. Environmental Protection Agency (EPA) uses a measure called the **Air Quality Index (AQI)** to indicate whether air pollution levels pose a health concern. The AQI is used for five major air pollutants: carbon monoxide (CO), sulfur dioxide (SO_2), nitrogen dioxide (NO_2), particulate matter (PM), and ground-level ozone.

A major source of these pollutants is the burning of **fossil fuels** in vehicles and industrial processes. AQI values run from 0 to 500; the higher the AQI, the greater the level of pollution and associated health danger. Local AQI information is often available in newspapers, on television and radio, on the Internet, and from state and local telephone hotlines.

The term **smog** was first used in the early 1900s in London to describe the combination of smoke and fog. What we typically call *smog* today is a mixture of pollutants, with ground-level ozone being the key ingredient. Major smog occurrences are linked to the combination of several factors: Heavy motor vehicle traffic, high temperatures, and sunny weather can increase the production of ozone. Pollutants are also more likely to build up in areas with little wind or where a topographic feature such as a mountain range or valley prevents the wind from pushing out stagnant air.

The Greenhouse Effect and Global Warming

The temperature of the earth's atmosphere depends on the balance between the amount of energy the planet absorbs from the sun (mainly as high-energy ultraviolet radiation) and the amount of energy radiated back into space as lower-energy infrared radiation. Key components of temperature regulation are carbon dioxide, water vapor, methane, and other **greenhouse gases**—so

Air Quality Index (AQI)   A measure of local air quality and what it means for health. TERMS

fossil fuels   Buried deposits of decayed animals and plants that are converted into carbon-rich fuels by exposure to heat and pressure over millions of years; oil, coal, and natural gas are fossil fuels.

smog   Hazy atmospheric conditions resulting from increased concentrations of ground-level ozone and other pollutants.

greenhouse gas   A gas (such as carbon dioxide) or vapor that traps infrared radiation instead of allowing it to escape through the atmosphere, resulting in a warming of the earth (the *greenhouse effect*).

named because, like the glass panes in a greenhouse, they let through visible light from the sun but trap some of the resulting infrared radiation and reradiate it back to the earth's surface. This reradiation causes a buildup of heat that raises the temperature of the lower atmosphere, a natural process known as the **greenhouse effect.** (See page T1-5 of the color transparency insert "Touring Lifestyle Behaviors" in Chapter 10.) Without it, earth's atmosphere would be far cooler and much more hostile to life.

There is scientific consensus that human activity is causing **global warming** or *climate change.* The concentration of greenhouse gases is increasing because of human activity, especially the combustion of fossil fuels. Carbon dioxide levels in the atmosphere have increased rapidly in recent decades and currently stand at 396.18 parts per million. The use of fossil fuels pumps more than 20 billion tons of carbon dioxide into the atmosphere every year. Deforestation, often by burning, also sends carbon dioxide into the atmosphere and reduces the number of trees available to convert carbon dioxide into oxygen.

The 12-month period between May 2011 and April 2012 was the warmest period on record since record keeping began in 1895, and the 10 warmest periods have all occurred since June 1999. The average global temperature has risen more than 1.4 degrees Fahrenheit in the past century. Most scientists agree that temperatures will continue to rise, although estimates vary as to how much they will change. If global warming persists, experts say the impact may be devastating. Possible consequences include increased rainfall and flooding in some regions, and increased drought in others; increased mortality from heat stress, urban air pollution, and tropical diseases; a poleward shift of about 50–350 miles (150–550 km) in the location of vegetation zones, affecting crop yields, irrigation demands, and forest productivity; alterations of ecosystems, resulting in possible species extinction; and increasingly rapid and drastic melting of the earth's polar ice caps.

At the 2011 United Nations Climate Change Conference in Durban, South Africa, some groups endorsed the current scientific consensus that keeping the increase in global temperature below 2°C is necessary to stave off the worst effects of climate change.

> **Without the ozone layer to absorb the sun's UV radiation, life on earth would be impossible.**

---

greenhouse effect   A warming of the earth due to a buildup of greenhouse gases in the atmosphere.

global warming   An increase in the earth's atmospheric temperature when averaged across seasons and geographical regions; also called *climate change.*

ozone layer   A layer of ozone molecules (O_3) in the upper atmosphere that screens out UV rays from the sun.

chlorofluorocarbons (CFCs)   Chemicals used as spray can propellants, refrigerants, and industrial solvents, which have been implicated in the destruction of the ozone layer.

TERMS

Thinning of the Ozone Layer

Another air pollution problem is the thinning of the **ozone layer** of the atmosphere, a fragile, invisible layer about 10–30 miles above the earth's surface that shields the planet from the sun's hazardous ultraviolet (UV) rays. Since the mid-1980s scientists have observed the seasonal appearance and growth of a hole in the ozone layer over Antarctica. More recently thinning over other areas has been noted.

The ozone layer is being destroyed primarily by **chlorofluorocarbons (CFCs)**, industrial chemicals that rise into the atmosphere and release chlorine atoms, which destroy ozone.

The largest and deepest ozone hole on record occurred on September 6, 2000, measured at 11.5 million square miles (29.9 million square kilometers). In 2012, the maximum size of the ozone hole was 8.2 million square miles (21.2 million square kilometers), or the area of the United States, Canada, and Mexico combined. The Antarctic ozone layer likely will not return to its early 1980s state until about 2065. Because of an international agreement that regulates the production of ozone-depleting chemicals, overall atmospheric ozone is no longer decreasing. The gradual recovery is masked by annual variations caused by weather fluctuations over Antarctica.

Without the ozone layer to absorb the sun's UV radiation, life on earth would be impossible. (UV radiation levels under the Antarctic hole were high enough to cause sunburn within seven minutes.) The potential effects of increased long-term exposure to UV light for humans include skin cancer, wrinkling and aging of the skin, cataracts and blindness, and reduced immune response. The United Nations Environment Programme predicts that a drop of 10% in overall ozone levels would cause a 26% rise in the incidence of nonmelanoma skin cancers. Some scientists already blame ozone loss for many cases of melanoma.

Energy Use and Air Pollution

Americans are now the second biggest energy consumers in the world; Chinese are first. We use energy to create electricity, transport us, power our industries, and run our homes. About 83% of the energy we use comes from fossil fuels—oil, coal, and natural gas. The remainder comes from nuclear power and renewable energy sources such as hydroelectric, wind, and solar power.

Energy consumption is at the root of many environmental problems, especially those relating to air pollution. Automobile exhaust and the burning of oil and coal by industry and by electric power plants are primary causes of smog, acid precipitation, and the greenhouse effect. The mining of coal and the extraction and transportation of oil and natural gas cause pollution on land and in the water.

Nuclear power generation creates hazardous wastes and carries the risk of dangerous releases of radiation.

Despite increases in U.S. consumer gas prices, more than 70% of commuters drive alone to work, and low-fuel-economy sport utility vehicles (SUVs) remain popular. Every gallon of gas burned puts about 20 pounds of carbon dioxide into the atmosphere. Two key strategies for controlling energy use are conservation and the development of nonpolluting, renewable energy sources.

Environmental Threats of Extreme Energy Sources

As the worldwide demand for energy rises and supplies of easily accessible oil dwindle, some energy companies have turned to what are often called "extreme energy sources." This term describes fossil fuels that are relatively difficult to access and extract from the environment. Examples include deepwater oil rigs, tar sands oil extraction, and drilling and hydrofracking of natural gas.

The Deepwater Horizon oil rig that exploded in April 2011 in the Gulf of Mexico was a deepwater rig. As oil gushed into the waters of the Gulf at an estimated rate of 60,000 barrels a day, it became clear that BP, the company that owned the rig, did not know how to stop it. It took BP three months to plug the leak, after nearly 5 million barrels of oil were released into the Gulf. The disaster killed thousands of birds, hundreds of endangered sea turtles, and many dolphins and other marine mammals, and the long-term health effects to the remaining wildlife are not known. The Gulf's ecosystems may need generations to recover fully, and some parts of it may never recover.

Tar sands (or oil sands) are sand deposits that are saturated with a dense form of petroleum called bitumen. The largest deposits are found in Canada, Kazakhstan, and Russia. Making liquid fuel from the oil in tar sands is a very energy-intensive process. When used as fuel, the resulting molasses-like product produces two to four times the amount of greenhouse gases per barrel compared to other conventional oils. In addition, Canada's tar sands oil will need to travel through thousands of miles of leak-prone pipelines across pristine wildlife habitats in both Canada and the United States.

Hydraulic fracturing, or "fracking," uses pressurized mixes of fluids to create cracks in rock formations deep underground, releasing natural gas. The term fracking is commonly used to describe both the drilling and fracturing processes in natural gas extraction. Critics have raised concerns about the safety of the technique, especially since many of these wells are in residential areas, near homes and schools. The specific chemicals used have not been publicly disclosed by energy companies using this technique, and reports of groundwater contamination have been verified by independent third parties.

Renewable Energy

Renewable energy sources are those sources that are naturally replenished and essentially inexhaustible, such as wind and sunlight. Together with technologies that improve energy efficiency, renewable energy sources contribute to sustainability—the capacity of natural or human systems to endure and maintain well-being over time. A common definition of *sustainable development* is development that meets society's present needs without compromising the ability of future generations to meet their needs.

Renewable energy sources include wind power, solar power, water and wave power, geothermal power, and biomass and biofuels from renewable sources, among others. Energy efficiency is not a power source, but it affects our energy future and has been called by some "the fifth fuel."

Worldwide, renewable energy sources were providing one-quarter of power capacity from all sources and 19% of the global electricity supply in 2011, and 118 countries had enacted some type of policy target or promotion policy related to renewable energy. Many of these targets call for 15–25% of energy or electricity to be provided by renewable sources by 2020.

Alternative Fuels

The U.S. Department of Energy (DOE) is encouraging researchers and automobile manufacturers to produce vehicles that can handle alternative fuels such as ethanol. Ethanol, a form of alcohol, is a renewable and largely domestic transportation fuel produced from fermenting plant sugars such as corn, sugarcane, and other starchy agricultural products. Ethanol use reduces the amount of imported oil required to produce gasoline, reduces overall greenhouse gas emissions from automobiles, and supports the U.S. agricultural industry. Ethanol can be used alone or mixed with gasoline.

Ethanol, however, has its critics, who say the alternative fuel may do more harm than good. For one thing, some

Wind power, generated from turbines, is a clean and renewable source of energy.

reports show that corn-based ethanol requires more energy to produce than it yields when burned as fuel.

In addition, the production of ethanol diverts corn crops from the food supply and may be a factor in food shortages around the world. The food-related concerns prompted the United Nations to call for a moratorium on food-based ethanol production until nonfood sources of alternative fuels could be developed.

Another alternative fuel is biodiesel, a fuel made primarily from vegetable oils, fats, or greases. It is the fastest-growing alternative fuel in the United States, is biodegradable, and produces lower levels of most air pollutants than petroleum-based products. Biodiesel, like ethanol, can be problematic depending on its material source. If it is produced from waste animal fat and grease or as a by-product of other agricultural processes, it can be carbon-neutral. But in some parts of the world natural vegetation and forests have been cleared and burned to grow soybeans and palm oil trees to make biodiesel, and these negative environmental and social effects can outweigh any benefit.

Hybrid and Electric Vehicles   Hybrid electric vehicles (HEVs) use two or more distinct power sources to propel the vehicle, such as a battery and an internal combustion engine. The hybrid vehicle typically realizes greater fuel economy than a conventional car does and produces fewer polluting emissions. Hybrids also tend to run with less noise than conventional vehicles. Hybrids are gaining credibility and popularity with consumers and are being more commonly used in both corporate and government vehicle fleets. A new generation of all-electric vehicles (EVs) has recently been introduced to consumer markets, taking advantage of better battery storage performance, "quick-charging station" infrastructure, and changing consumer perceptions of trip use and distance. Researchers hope that hybrid and battery technologies can be extended to all classes of vehicles.

A new generation of electric vehicles is taking advantage of the development of infrastructure to power its use.

Indoor Air Quality (IAQ)

Although most people associate air pollution with the outdoors, buildings may also harbor potentially dangerous pollutants. Some of these compounds trigger allergic responses, and others have been linked to cancer. Common indoor pollutants include the following: environmental tobacco smoke (ETS); carbon monoxide and other combustion by-products from woodstoves, fireplaces, kerosene heaters and lamps, and gas ranges; volatile organic compounds (VOCs), gases emitted from paints, lacquers, cleaning supplies, aerosols, building materials, furnishings, and office equipment; and biological pollutants like bacteria, dust mites, mold, and animal dander, which can cause health problems when inhaled, especially for people with asthma and other respiratory conditions.

Preventing Air Pollution

You can do a great deal to reduce air pollution. Here are a few ideas:

- Cut back on driving. Ride your bike, walk, use public transportation, or carpool in a fuel-efficient vehicle.

- Keep your car tuned up and well maintained. Keep your tires inflated at recommended pressures. To save energy when driving, avoid quick starts, stay within the speed limit, limit the use of air conditioning, and don't let your car idle unless absolutely necessary.

- Buy energy-efficient appliances and use them only when you have full loads. Do laundry in warm or cold water instead of hot. Clean refrigerator coils and clothes dryer lint screens frequently.

- Replace incandescent bulbs with light-emitting diode (LED) and compact fluorescent bulbs (not fluorescent tubes).

- Make sure your home is well-insulated with ozone-safe agents; use insulating shades and curtains to keep heat in during winter and out during summer.

- Plant and care for trees in your yard and neighborhood. They recycle carbon dioxide, so trees work against global warming. They also provide shade and cool the air so less air conditioning is needed.

- Before discarding a refrigerator, air conditioner, or humidifier, check with the waste hauler or your local government to ensure that ozone-depleting refrigerants will be removed prior to disposal.

- Keep paints, cleaning agents, and other chemical products tightly sealed in their original containers.

- Clean and inspect chimneys, furnaces, and other appliances regularly. Install carbon monoxide detectors.

- Always use an outside-venting hood when cooking.

WATER QUALITY AND POLLUTION

Few parts of the world have enough safe, clean drinking water, and yet few things are as important to human health.

Water Contamination and Treatment

Many cities rely at least in part on wells that tap local groundwater, but often it is necessary to tap lakes and rivers to supplement wells. Because such surface water is more likely to be contaminated with both organic matter and pathogenic microorganisms, it is purified in water treatment plants before being piped into the community. **Fluoridation,** a water treatment process that reduces tooth decay by 15–40%, has been used successfully in the United States for more than 60 years.

In most areas of the United States, water systems have adequate, dependable supplies, are able to control waterborne disease, and provide water with acceptable color, odor, and taste. However, problems occur. The CDC estimate that 1 million Americans become ill and 900–1000 die each year from microbial illnesses from drinking water.

Water Shortages

Water shortages are a growing concern in many regions of the world. Some parts of the United States, such as the desert West, are experiencing rapid population growth that outstrips the ability of local systems to provide adequate water to all.

Groundwater pumping and the diversion of water from lakes and rivers for irrigation are further reducing the amount of water available to local communities.

Sewage

Most cities have sewage treatment systems that separate fecal matter from water in huge tanks and ponds and stabilize it so that it cannot transmit infectious diseases. After it is treated and biologically safe, the water is released back into the environment. The sludge that remains behind is often contaminated with **heavy metals** and is handled as

Ask Yourself

QUESTIONS FOR CRITICAL THINKING AND REFLECTION

How would you describe the quality of the water where you live? Are there lakes or streams where you can safely swim or fish? What local information sources can you find about water quality in your area?

hazardous waste. If not contaminated, sludge may be used as fertilizer, although this practice is being discouraged by scientists and some government agencies, and is not permitted in organic agriculture.

Many cities have expanded sewage treatment measures to remove heavy metals and other hazardous chemicals. This action has resulted from many studies linking exposure to chemicals such as mercury, lead, and **polychlorinated biphenyls (PCBs)** with long-term health consequences, including cancer and damage to the central nervous system.

Protecting the Water Supply

By reducing your own water use, you help preserve your community's valuable supply. By taking steps to keep the water supply clean, you reduce pollution overall and help protect the land, wildlife, and other people from illness. Here are some simple steps you can take:

- Take showers, not baths, to minimize your water consumption. Don't let water run when you're not actively using it while brushing your teeth, shaving, or hand-washing clothes.

- Install sink faucet aerators and water-efficient showerheads, which use two to five times less water with no noticeable decrease in performance. Purchase a water-saving toilet, or put a displacement device in your toilet tank to reduce the amount of water used with each flush.

- Fix any leaky faucets in your home. Leaks can waste thousands of gallons of water per year.

- Don't pour toxic materials such as cleaning solvents, bleach, or motor oil down the drain. Store them until you can take them to a hazardous waste collection center.

> **Less than 1% of the world's fresh water is readily accessible for human use.**

TERMS

fluoridation The addition of fluoride to the water supply to reduce tooth decay.

heavy metal A metal with a high specific gravity, such as lead, copper, or tin.

polychlorinated biphenyl (PCB) An industrial chemical used as an insulator in electrical transformers and linked to certain human cancers; banned worldwide since 1977 but persistent in the environment.

- Don't pour old medicines down the drain or flush them down the toilet. Some pharmacies will take back unused or expired medications for disposal, and many communities have drop-off days for these drugs.

SOLID WASTE POLLUTION

Humans living in the industrialized world generate huge amounts of waste, which must be handled appropriately to ensure environmental safety.

Solid Waste

The bulk of the organic food garbage produced in American kitchens is now dumped in the sewage system by way of the mechanical garbage disposal. The garbage that remains is not hazardous from the standpoint of infectious disease because there is very little food waste in it, but it does represent an enormous disposal and contamination problem.

What's in Our Garbage? The biggest single component of household trash by weight is paper products, including junk mail, glossy mail-order catalogs, and computer printouts (Figure 14.2). About 1% of the solid waste is toxic; a new source of toxic waste is the disposal of computer components in both household and commercial waste. Burning, as opposed

QUICK STATS

The average American generates **4.4 pounds** of trash per day; about 1.5 pounds of this is recycled.

—Environmental Protection Agency, 2014

TERMS

sanitary landfill A disposal site where solid wastes are buried.

biodegradation The process by which organic substances break down naturally and disappear back into the environment.

recycling The use of waste materials as raw materials in the production of new products.

---

to burial, reduces the bulk of solid waste, but it can release hazardous material into the air, depending on what is being burned.

Manufacturing, mining, and other industries all produce large amounts of potentially dangerous materials that cannot simply be dumped.

Disposing of Solid Waste Since the 1960s, billions of tons of solid waste have been buried in **sanitary landfill** disposal sites. Sometimes protective liners are used around the site, and nearby monitoring wells are now required in most states. Layers of solid waste are regularly covered with thin layers of dirt until the site is filled. Some communities then plant grass and trees and convert the site into a park. Landfill is relatively stable; almost no decomposition occurs in the solidly packed waste. Much of this waste contains chemicals, ranging from leftover pesticides to paints and oils, that should not be released into the environment. Despite precautions, buried contaminants sometimes leak into the surrounding soil and groundwater. Burial is also expensive and requires huge amounts of space.

Biodegradation is the process by which organic substances are broken down naturally by living organisms. Items that are biodegradable can break down naturally, safely, and quickly into the raw materials of nature, then disappear back into the environment. Table 14.1 shows the amount of time required for different types of material to biodegrade.

Recycling In **recycling,** many kinds of waste materials are collected and used as raw materials in the production of new products. Recycling is a good idea because it reduces the amount of solid waste sitting in landfills, some of which takes decades to decay naturally.

Discarded Technology: eWaste Americans scrap about 400 million consumer electronic devices each year. This "e-waste" is the fastest-growing portion of our waste

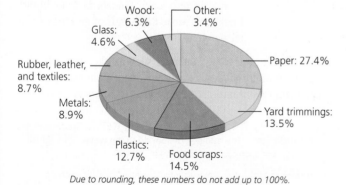

Wood: 6.3%
Other: 3.4%
Glass: 4.6%
Rubber, leather, and textiles: 8.7%
Metals: 8.9%
Plastics: 12.7%
Food scraps: 14.5%
Yard trimmings: 13.5%
Paper: 27.4%

Due to rounding, these numbers do not add up to 100%.

FIGURE 14.2 Components of municipal solid waste, by weight, before recycling.

SOURCE: Environmental Protection Agency. 2014. *Municipal Solid Waste Generation, Recycling and Disposal in the United States: Facts and Figures for 2012.* Washington, DC: EPA. Pub. No. EPA-530-F-14-001.

Table 14.1	Biodegrading Times of Different Objects
ITEM	**TIME REQUIRED TO BIODEGRADE**
Banana peel	2–10 days
Paper	2–5 months
Rope	3–14 months
Orange peel	6 months
Wool sock	1–5 years
Cigarette butt	1–12 years
Plastic-coated milk carton	5 years
Aluminum can	80–100 years
Plastic six-pack holder ring	450 years
Glass bottle	1 million years
Plastic bottle	Forever

stream. Junked electronic devices are toxic because they contain varying amounts of lead, mercury, and other heavy metals. Many components of electronic devices are valuable, however, and can be recycled and reused. Local and state e-waste recycling programs are becoming more common, and private companies are also getting into the e-waste recycling business. If you recycle your electronic devices, look for a "green" program or one that is certified by e-stewards, an organization that advocates for responsible e-waste recycling (www.e-stewards.org).

Reducing Solid Waste

By reducing your consumption, recycling more, and throwing away less, you can conserve landfill space and put more reusable items back into service. Here are some ideas to help you reduce solid waste:

- Buy products with the least amount of packaging you can, or buy products in bulk or packaged in recyclable containers.

- Buy recycled or recyclable products. Avoid disposables; instead use long-lasting or reusable products such as refillable pens and rechargeable batteries.

- Avoid using foam or paper cups and plastic stirrers by bringing your own ceramic coffee mug and metal spoon to work or wherever you drink coffee or tea. Pack your lunch in reusable containers.

- To store food, use glass jars and reusable plastic containers rather than foil and plastic wrap.

- Recycle your newspapers, glass, cans, paper, and other recyclables. If you receive something packaged with foam pellets, take them to a commercial mailing center that accepts them for recycling.

- Do not throw electronic items, batteries, or fluorescent lights into the trash. Take these to state-approved recycling centers.

- Start a compost pile for your organic garbage (non-animal food and yard waste) if you have a yard. If you live in an apartment, you can take your organic wastes to a community-composting center. Many communities now offer curbside collection of kitchen scraps for recycling into compost, which is sold to farms and wineries.

Ask Yourself

QUESTIONS FOR CRITICAL THINKING AND REFLECTION

What are your own waste disposal habits like? Do you recycle everything you possibly can? Do you get rid of items that are still usable? Even if you are conscientious about the way you deal with waste, how could you improve your habits?

CHEMICAL POLLUTION AND HAZARDOUS WASTE

New chemical substances are constantly being introduced into the environment as pesticides, herbicides, solvents, and hundreds of other products. More people and wildlife are exposed to them than ever before.

Asbestos

A mineral-based compound, asbestos was widely used for fire protection and insulation in buildings until the late 1960s. Microscopic asbestos fibers can be released into the air when this material is applied or when it later deteriorates or is damaged. These fibers can lodge in the lungs, causing **asbestosis,** lung cancer, and other serious lung diseases. Similar conditions expose workers to risk in the coal mining industry, from coal and silica dust (black lung disease), and in the textile industry, from cotton fibers (brown lung disease).

Lead

Thanks to better preventive efforts, lead poisoning is not as serious a problem today as it was in the past. Still, the CDC estimates that about 435,000 children under age 6 may have unsafe lead levels in their blood; the actual number could be much higher. Many of these children live in poor, inner-city areas (see the box "Poverty, Gender, and Environmental Health"). When lead is ingested or inhaled, it can damage the central nervous system, cause mental impairment, hinder oxygen transport in the blood, and create digestive problems. Severe lead poisoning may cause coma or even death. Neurological damage can be permanent. Lead exposure has been linked to attention deficit hyperactivity disorder (ADHD) in children.

Lead-based paints are the chief culprit in lead poisoning of children. They were banned from residential use in 1978, but as many as 57 million American homes still contain lead paint. New guidelines requiring contractors to take special lead containment measures when doing renovations, repairs, or painting in certain buildings were implemented in April 2010. The use of lead in plumbing is now also banned, but some old pipes and faucets contain lead.

Pesticides

Pesticides are used to prevent the spread of insect-borne diseases and to maximize food production by killing insects that eat crops. Both uses have risks as well as benefits. For

asbestosis A lung condition caused by inhalation TERMS of microscopic asbestos fibers, which inflame the lung and can lead to lung cancer.

pesticides Chemicals used to prevent the spread of diseases transmitted by insects and to maximize food production by killing insects that eat crops.

Residents of poor and minority communities are often exposed to more environmental toxins than residents of wealthier communities are, and they are more likely to suffer from health problems caused or aggravated by pollutants.

Poor neighborhoods are often located near highways and industrial areas that have high levels of air and noise pollution; they are also common sites for hazardous waste production and disposal. Residents of substandard housing are more likely to come into contact with lead, asbestos, carbon monoxide, pesticides, and other hazardous pollutants associated with peeling paint, old plumbing, and poorly maintained insulation and heating equipment.

In addition, poor people are more likely to have jobs that expose them to asbestos, silica dust, and pesticides, and they are more likely to catch and consume fish contaminated with PCBs, mercury, and other toxins.

The most thoroughly researched and documented link among poverty, the environment, and health is lead poisoning in children. One 2013 study showed that whether they lived in a rural or urban environment, black, non-Hispanic Latinos were more likely exposed to soil lead concentrations than nonminorities were.

The CDC and the American Academy of Pediatrics recommend annual testing of blood lead levels for all children under age 6, with more frequent testing for children at special risk.

Asthma is another health threat that appears to be linked with both environmental and socioeconomic factors. The number of Americans with asthma has grown dramatically in the past 20 years; most of the increase has occurred in children from poor families. Researchers are not sure what accounts for this increase, but suspects include household pollutants, pesticides, air pollution, cigarette smoke, and allergens like cockroaches. These risk factors are likely to cluster in poor urban areas where inadequate health care may worsen asthma's effects.

Gender also influences exposure to environmental hazards. In many societies, women are more often involved in day- to-day activities associated with the environment, including food preparation, agricultural work, and tasks around the home. These activities can expose women to indoor air pollution, water pollution, foodborne pathogens, agricultural chemicals, and waste contamination. Indoor pollutants, especially soot from burning wood, charcoal, and other solid fuels used for home heating and cooking, are a particular risk. Exposure to this particulate pollution increases the risk of respiratory diseases, lung cancer, and reproductive problems.

All humans are exposed to chemicals in air, food, and drinking water, and we all carry a body load of chemicals. Some of these chemicals bioaccumulate in our bones, blood, or fatty tissues. Women are smaller than men, on average, and have a higher percentage of body fat, so chemicals that accumulate in fatty tissue may pose a relatively greater risk for women. On the other hand, men may be more likely to work in industries that involve significant occupational exposures to disease-related toxins. For example, coal miners have an increased risk of lung cancer (black lung disease).

Although any chemical exposure can be a concern for health, women face the added risk of passing pollutants to a developing fetus during pregnancy or to an infant through breastfeeding. Even relatively low exposure to pollutants can result in a significant chemical body load in an infant or young child because of their small body size. And because infants and children are still developing, the effects of chemical exposure can be significant and devastating. It is not unusual for dangerous toxin exposures to be first recognized through noticeable effects on infants or children.

example, DDT was extremely effective in controlling insect-borne diseases in tropical countries and in increasing crop yields throughout the world, but it was found to disrupt the life cycles of birds, fish, and reptiles and was banned in the United States in 1972. DDT also builds up in the food chain, increasing in concentration as larger animals eat smaller ones—a process known as **biomagnification** or *bioaccumulation*.

Mercury

A naturally occurring metal, mercury is a toxin that affects the nervous system and may damage the brain, kidneys, and gastrointestinal tract and increase blood pressure, heart rate, and heart attack risk. Mercury slows fetal and child development and causes irreversible deficits in brain function. Coal-fired power plants are the largest producers of mercury; other sources include mining and smelting operations and the disposal of consumer products containing mercury. Mercury persists in the environment and, like pesticides, it is bioaccumulative. In particular, large, long-lived fish may carry high levels of mercury. Chapter 9 includes information about safe fish consumption.

Other Chemical Pollutants

Hazardous wastes are commonly found in the home and should be handled and disposed of properly. They include automotive supplies (motor oil, antifreeze, transmission fluid), paint supplies (turpentine, paint thinner, mineral spirits), art and hobby supplies (oil-based paint, solvents, acids

> **biomagnification** The accumulation of a substance in a food chain; also known as *bioaccumulation*. **TERMS**

In the 1970s and 1980s, scientists began to document strange occurrences in wildlife: disrupted reproduction, birth defects, tumors, and behavioral changes in birds, fish, and reptiles. It was also becoming apparent that a drug given to pregnant women in the 1950s (a potent synthetic estrogen, DES) was causing infertility and rare reproductive cancers in their adult daughters. These effects were all stemming from exposure to man-made chemicals, known also as **endocrine disrupting chemicals (EDCs)**, which were disrupting the hormone systems of organisms. In the mid-1990s the term "endocrine disruption" was coined.

Low levels of EDCs can disrupt these systems by mimicking or blocking natural hormones, causing abnormal effects. EDC exposure before and after birth may cause lifelong effects, including fertility problems, cancers, cardiovascular diseases, obesity, and mental disorders. These effects have been proven in laboratory animals and supported by observational (epidemiological) studies in humans.

Various man-made chemicals, some in everyday products such as plastic, cosmetics, food packaging, flame-retardants, pesticides, and others, are proven EDCs.

Traditional methods of determining chemical toxicity usually test "gross" effects: death, deformities, and tumors. These methods typically do not test low (environmental) doses of chemicals; rather, they test at high doses and extrapolate down to find "safe" exposure levels. Often, EDCs have detrimental effects at low doses but not higher ones. Therefore, a new testing paradigm must be employed that addresses physiological effects at low doses. The modern environmental movement is very new, and as our scientific knowledge of these chemicals evolves and improves, so must government testing and policies surrounding the issues of EDCs, for the continued protection of human health.

What can you do?

- Educate yourself about the personal-care and household products you use.

- Eat organic foods. Eat lower on the food chain.

- Avoid plastic, especially in contact with food and drinks. Do not microwave plastic containers.

- Dust, vacuum, and wipe down surfaces often.

- Avoid nonstick cookware and products.

- Avoid flame-retardant clothes and furniture.

- Avoid handling cash-register receipts. If you must, use gloves.

- Be especially aware of potential exposure to pregnant women, infants, and children.

- Support legislation that will provide adequate testing and regulation of potential EDCs.

For more information and a list of EDCs visit www .endocrinedisruption.org.

> **endocrine disrupting chemicals (EDCs)**   TERMS
> Chemicals that disrupt the hormone systems of organisms.

and alkalis, aerosol sprays), insecticides, batteries, computer and electronic components, and household cleaners containing sodium hydroxide (lye) or ammonia. These chemicals are dangerous when inhaled or ingested, when they contact the skin or the eyes, or when they are burned or dumped. Many cities provide guidelines about approved disposal methods and have hazardous waste collection days.

Preventing Chemical Pollution

You can take steps to reduce the chemical pollution in your community.

- When buying products, read the labels, and try to buy the least toxic ones available. Choose nontoxic, nonpetrochemical cleansers, disinfectants, polishes, and other personal and household products.

- Dispose of your household hazardous wastes properly. If you are not sure whether something is hazardous or don't know how to dispose of it, contact your local environmental health office or health department.

Ask Yourself   ?

QUESTIONS FOR CRITICAL THINKING AND REFLECTION

Are there any hazardous chemicals in your home, such as cleaning products, solvents, paint, or batteries? Would you know what to do if one of these chemicals spilled? How would you clean it up?

- Buy organic produce and produce that has been grown locally.

- If you must use pesticides or toxic household products, store them in a locked place where children and pets can't get to them. Don't measure chemicals with food preparation utensils, and wear gloves whenever handling them.

- If you have your house fumigated for pest control, be sure to hire a licensed exterminator. Keep everyone, including pets, out of the house while the crew works and, if possible, for a few days after.

RADIATION POLLUTION

Radiation comes in different forms, such as ultraviolet rays, microwaves, or X-rays, and from different sources, such as the sun, electronics, uranium, and nuclear weapons.

Of most concern to health are gamma rays produced by radioactive sources such as nuclear weapons, nuclear energy plants, and radon gas. These high-energy waves are powerful enough to penetrate objects and break molecular bonds. Although gamma radiation cannot be seen or felt, its effects at high doses can include **radiation sickness** and death. At lower doses, chromosome damage, sterility, tissue damage, cataracts, and cancer can occur. Other types of radiation can also affect health. For example, exposure to UV radiation from the sun or from tanning salons can increase the risk of skin cancer. The effects of some sources of radiation, such as cell phones, remain controversial.

Nuclear Weapons and Nuclear Energy

Nuclear weapons pose a health risk of the most serious kind to all species. Reducing the stockpiles of nuclear weapons is a challenge and a goal for the 21st century. Power-generating plants that use nuclear fuel also pose health problems. When **nuclear power** was first developed as an alternative to oil and coal, it was promoted as clean, efficient, inexpensive, and safe. In general, these claims have proven to be the case. Power systems in several parts of the world rely on nuclear power plants. However, despite all the built-in safeguards and regulating agencies, accidents in nuclear power plants do happen, whether as a result of human error or following a natural disaster.

The 1986 fire and explosion at the Chernobyl nuclear power station in Ukraine caused hundreds of deaths and increased rates of genetic mutation and cancer in the surrounding population. The zone around Chernobyl has been sealed off to human habitation and could be unsafe for the next 24,000 years. In 2011, a 9.0 magnitude earthquake 15 miles below Japan's Honshu Island, followed by a powerful tsunami, rocked Japan's northern Fukushima Prefecture and severely damaged the

The 2011 Fukushima Daiichi nuclear disaster occurred when a tsunami, following a massive earthquake, flooded the low-lying rooms in which the plant's emergency generators were housed. The plant overheated, causing full meltdown in three of the six reactors.

> QUICK STATS
>
> There are **104 nuclear power plants** operating in the United States.
>
> —International Atomic Energy Agency, 2011

Fukushima Daiichi nuclear power plant complex. Seawater was used to cool the damaged reactors, and subsequently resulted in the largest release of radiation into the Pacific Ocean in history. All nuclear plants in Japan were shut down following this incident. Fisheries in the nearby area were also closed due to concern of exposure to radiation.

An additional enormous problem is disposing of the radioactive wastes these plants generate. To date, no storage method has been devised that can provide infallible, infinitely durable shielding for nuclear waste. Despite these problems, nuclear power is gaining favor again as an alternative to fossil fuels.

> **radiation** Energy transmitted in the form of rays, waves, or particles.
>
> **radiation sickness** An illness caused by excess radiation exposure, marked by low white blood cell counts and nausea; possibly fatal.
>
> **nuclear power** The use of controlled nuclear reactions to produce steam, which in turn drives turbines to produce electricity.
>
> TERMS

Medical Uses of Radiation

Another area of concern is the use of radiation in medicine, primarily in X-rays. Studies revealed that X-ray exposure is cumulative and that no level of exposure is absolutely safe.

From a personal health point of view, no one should ever have a "routine" X-ray examination; each such exam should have a definite purpose, and its benefits and risks should be carefully weighed.

Radiation in the Home and Workplace

Recently there has been concern about electromagnetic radiation associated with common modern devices such as microwave ovens, computer monitors, and even high-voltage power lines. These forms of radiation do have effects on health, but research results are inconclusive.

Another controversial issue today is the effect of radiation from cell phones on health. Cell phones use electromagnetic waves (radio frequency radiation) to send and receive signals. This radiation is not directional, meaning that it travels in all directions equally, including toward the user. Factors such as the type of digital signal coding in the network, the antenna and handset design, and the position of the phone relative to the head all determine how much radiation is absorbed by a user. Studies to date have not provided conclusive evidence that cell phone use actually exposes users to harmful levels of radiation.

Another area of concern is **radon,** a naturally occurring radioactive gas found in certain soils, rocks, and building materials.

Avoiding Radiation

•   Get only X-rays that you need, and keep a record of the date and location of every X-ray exam. Don't have a full-body CT scan for routine screening; the radiation dose of one full-body CT scan is nearly 100 times that of a typical mammogram.

•   Follow government recommendations for radon testing.

•   Use sunscreen to protect yourself from the sun's UV radiation.

NOISE POLLUTION

Loud or persistent noise in the environment can cause hearing loss and stress. Prolonged exposure to sounds above 80–85 **decibels** (a measure of the intensity of a sound wave) can cause permanent hearing loss. Hearing damage can occur after eight hours of exposure to sounds louder than 80 decibels. Regular exposure for longer than one minute to more than 100 decibels can cause permanent hearing loss. Children may suffer damage to their hearing at lower noise levels than those at which adults suffer damage.

Two common sources of excessive noise are the workplace and large gatherings of people at sporting events, rock concerts, and movie theaters. The Occupational Safety and Health Administration (OSHA) sets legal standards for noise in the workplace, but no laws exist regulating noise levels at concerts, which can be much louder than most workplaces. Here are some ways to avoid exposing yourself to excessive noise:

•   Wear ear protectors when working around noisy machinery.

•   When listening to music on a headset with a volume range of 1–10, keep the volume no louder than 6. Your headset is too loud if you are unable to hear people around you speaking in a normal tone of voice. Earmuff-style headphones may be easier on the ears than earbuds, which are inserted into the ear canal. Experts warn that earbuds should not be used more than 30 minutes a day unless the volume is set below 60% of maximum; headphones can be used up to one hour.

•   Avoid toys for children that make loud noise.

•   Avoid loud music. Don't sit or stand near speakers or amplifiers at a concert, and don't play a car radio or stereo so high that you can't hear the traffic.

---

radon   A naturally occurring radioactive gas emitted from rocks and natural building materials that can become concentrated in insulated homes, causing lung cancer.

decibel   A unit for expressing the relative intensity of sounds on a scale from 0 for the average least perceptible sound to about 120 for the average pain threshold.

TERMS

---

connect™

Connect to Your Choices

Have you ever thought about where you get your behaviors and habits related to the environment? Many factors can influence our behaviors and habits, some not as obvious as others. When you were growing up, was your family aware of environmental issues and respectful of the environment? Do people in your peer group dispose of their trash when they're outdoors, or do they leave trash behind? Does your school promote environmental awareness and action, such as by participating in the green campus movement, providing for the proper recycling of old computers, cell phones, and other e-waste, and celebrating Earth Day in meaningful ways?

What are the external factors that influence your choices about the environment? What are your inner motivations and core values, and how do they affect your choices? Based on what you learned in this chapter, will you make some different choices in the future? If so, what will they be?

Go online to Connect to complete this activity: www.mcgraw-hillconnect.com

Environmental health involves protecting ourselves from environmental dangers and protecting the environment from the dangers created by humans.

RIGHT NOW YOU CAN:

- Turn off the lights, televisions, and stereos in any unoccupied rooms.
- Turn off power strips when not in use.
- Turn down the heat a few degrees and put on a sweater, or turn off the air conditioner and change into cooler clothes.
- Check your trash for recyclable items and take them out for recycling. If your town does not provide curbside pickup for recyclable items, find out where the nearest community recycling center is.

IN THE FUTURE YOU CAN:

- As your existing lightbulbs burn out, replace them with LED or compact fluorescent lightbulbs.
- Have your car checked to make sure it runs as well as it can and puts out the lowest amount of polluting emissions possible.
- Go online and find one of the many calculators available that can help you estimate your environmental footprint. After calculating your footprint, figure out ways to reduce it.

SUMMARY

- Environmental health encompasses all the interactions of humans with their environment and the health consequences of those interactions.

- The world's population is increasing rapidly, especially in the developing world. Factors that may eventually limit human population are food, availability of land and water, energy, and a minimum acceptable standard of living.

- Increased amounts of air pollutants are especially dangerous for children, older adults, and people with chronic health problems.

- Factors contributing to the development of smog include heavy motor vehicle traffic, hot weather, and stagnant air.

- Carbon dioxide and other natural gases act as a greenhouse around the earth, increasing the temperature of the atmosphere. Levels of these gases are rising through human activity; as a result, the world's climate could change.

- Environmental damage from energy use can be limited through energy conservation and the development of nonpolluting, renewable sources of energy.

- Indoor pollutants can trigger allergies and illness in the short term and chronic disease in the long term.

- Concerns with water quality focus on pathogenic organisms and hazardous chemicals from industry and households, as well as on water shortages.

- Sewage treatment prevents pathogens from contaminating drinking water; it often must also deal with heavy metals and hazardous chemicals.

- The amount of garbage is growing all the time; paper is the biggest component. Recycling can help reduce solid waste disposal problems.

- Potentially hazardous chemical pollutants include asbestos, lead, pesticides, mercury, and many household products. Proper handling and disposal are critical.

- Radiation can cause radiation sickness, chromosome damage, and cancer, among other health problems.

- Loud or persistent noise can lead to hearing loss and/or stress; two common sources of excessive noise are the workplace and rock concerts.

FOR MORE INFORMATION

BOOKS

Ingram, L. B., and F. Malamud-Roam. 2013. *The West Without Water: What Past Floods, Droughts, and Other Climatic Clues Tell Us about Tomorrow.* Oakland, CA: University of California Press.

Kolbert, E. 2014. *The Sixth Extinction: An Unnatural History.* New York: Henry Holt & Company.

Nadakavukaren, A. 2011. *Our Global Environment: A Health Perspective,* 7th ed. Prospect Heights, IL: Waveland Press. *A broad survey of major environmental issues and their effects on personal and community health.*

Wright, R. T. 2010. *Environmental Science: Toward a Sustainable Future.* New York: Pearson. *An easy-to-read introduction to the realm of environmental science and its importance to our future.*

ORGANIZATIONS, HOTLINES, AND WEBSITES

Breathing Earth. Provides CO_2 emissions, birth rate and death rate simulation.

   http://www.breathingearth.net/

CDC National Center for Environmental Health. Provides brochures and fact sheets about a variety of environmental issues.

   http://www.cdc.gov/nceh/default.htm

Earth Times. An international online newspaper devoted to global environmental issues.

   http://www.earthtimes.org

Ecological Footprint. Calculates your personal ecological footprint based on your diet, transportation patterns, and living arrangements.

   http://www.myfootprint.org

Indoor Air Quality Information Hotline. Answers questions, provides publications, and makes referrals.

   800-438-4318

National Lead Information Center. Provides information packets and specialist advice.

http://www2.epa.gov/lead

National Oceanic and Atmospheric Administration (NOAA): Climate. Provides information about a variety of issues related to climate, including global warming, drought, and El Niño and La Niña.

http://www.noaa.gov/climate.html

National Safety Council. Provides information about lead, radon, indoor air quality, hazardous chemicals, and other environmental issues.

http://www.nsc.org/pages/home.aspx

Student Environmental Action Coalition (SEAC). A coalition of student and youth environmental groups; the website has contact information for local groups.

http://www.seac.org

TEDX, The Endocrine Disruption Exchange. Information about endocrine disrupting chemicals, the prenatal origins of diseases, natural gas extraction, and pesticides.

http://endocrinedisruption.org/

Woods Hole Oceanographic Institute. FAQs: Radiation from Fukushima.

https://www.whoi.edu/page.do?pid=83397&tid=3622&cid=94989

United Nations. Several U.N. programs are devoted to environmental problems on a global scale; the websites provide information about current and projected trends and about international treaties developed to deal with environmental issues.

http://www.un.org/popin (Population Information Network)

http://www.unep.org (Environment Programme)

U.S. Department of Energy: Energy Efficiency and Renewable Energy (EERE). Provides information about alternative fuels and tips for saving energy at home and in your car.

http://www.eere.energy.gov/

U.S. Environmental Protection Agency (EPA). Provides information about EPA activities and many consumer-oriented materials. The website includes special sites devoted to global warming, ozone loss, pesticides, and other areas of concern.

http://www.epa.gov

Worldwatch Institute. A public policy research organization focusing on emerging global environmental problems and the links between the world economy and the environment.

http://www.worldwatch.org

Yale Environment 360. An online magazine offering opinion, analysis, reporting and debate on global environmental issues.

http://e360.yale.edu/

There are many national and international organizations working on environmental health problems. A few of the largest and best known are listed below:

Greenpeace: 800-326-0959; http://www.greenpeace.org
National Audubon Society: 212-979-3000; http://www.audubon.org
National Resources Defense Council: (212) 727-2700; http://www.nrdc.org
National Wildlife Federation: 800-822-9919; http://www.nwf.org
Nature Conservancy: 800-628-6860; http://www.nature.org
Sierra Club: 415-977-5500; http://www.sierraclub.org

U.S. Green Building Council: 800-795-1747; http://www.usgbc.org;
World Wildlife Fund—U.S.: 800-960-0993; http://www.worldwildlife.org

SELECTED BIBLIOGRAPHY

Aelion, C. M, et al. 2013. Associations between soil lead concentrations and populations by race/ethnicity and income-to-poverty ratio in urban and rural areas. *Environmental Geochemistry and Health* 35(1): 1–12.

Brown, M. J., et al. 2012. Lead in drinking water and human blood lead levels in the United States. *Morbidity and Mortality Weekly Report* 61: 1–9.

CDC National Center for Environmental Health. 2013. *Lead* (http://www.cdc.gov/nceh/lead/).

Centers for Disease Control and Prevention. 2011. Surveillance for waterborne disease outbreaks and other health events associated with recreational water—United States, 2007–2008. *Morbidity and Mortality Weekly Report, Surveillance Summaries* 60(2212): 1–32.

Centers for Disease Control and Prevention. 2013. Blood Lead Levels in Children Aged 1–5 Years—United States, 1999–2010. *Morbidity and Mortality Weekly Report* 62(13): 245–248.

Chew, G. L. 2012. Assessment of environmental cockroach allergen exposure.*Current Allergy and Asthma Reports* 12(5): 456–464.

Chouinard, Yvon. 2014. Tear down deadbeat dams. *New York Times,* 8 May.

Cohen, J. E. 2010. Population and climate change. *Proceedings of the American Philosophical Society* 154(2): 158–182.

De Coster, S., and N. vanLarebeke, 2012. Endocrine-disrupting chemicals: Associated disorders and mechanisms of action. *Journal of Environmental and Public Health,* 6 September. (epub ahead of print).

Delamater, Paul L., et al. 2012. An analysis of asthma hospitalizations, air pollution, and weather conditions in Los Angeles County, California. *Science of the Total Environment* 425: 110–118.

Franchini, M. et al. 2012. Air pollution, vascular disease and thrombosis: Linking clinical data and pathogenic mechanisms. *Journal of Thrombosis and Haemostasis,* 25 September (epub ahead of print).

Grasso, M. et al. 2012. The health effects of climate change: A survey of recent quantitative research. *International Journal of Environmental Research and Public Health* 9(5): 1523–1547.

Griffith, G. P., et al. 2012. Predicting interactions among fishing, ocean warming, and ocean acidification in a marine system with whole-ecosystem models. *Conservation Biology, 25* September (epub ahead of print).

Hegarty, M. J. 2012. Invasion of the hybrids.*Molecular Ecology* 21(19): 4669–4671.

Energy Information Agency. 2012. *Gasoline and Diesel Fuel Update* (http://www.eia.gov/petroleum/gasdiesel/).

Environmental Protection Agency. 2014. *Municipal Solid Waste* (http://www.epa.gov/waste/nonhaz/municipal/index.htm).

Moynihan, T. 2014. Is there any link cellphones and cancer? Mayo Clinic (http://www.mayoclinic.org/healthy-living/adult-health/expert-answers/cell-phones-and-cancer/faq-20057798?footprints=mine).

Pennisi, E. 2012. Water reclamation going green. *Science* 337(6095): 674–676.

REN21. 2011. *Renewables 2011 Global Status Report.* Paris: REN21 Secretariat.

United Nations Population Division. 2011. *World Population Prospects: The 2010 Revision.* New York: United Nations.

World Health Organization. 2010. Cholera, 2010. *Weekly Epidemiological Record* 85(13): 1177–1128.

World Health Organization. 2014. Water Sanitation and Health (WSH) (http://www.who.int/water_sanitation_health/mdg1/en/, accessed June 9, 2014).

Worldwatch Institute. 2012. *Vital Signs 2012.* New York: Norton (http://vitalsigns.worldwatch.org/).

CHAPTER OBJECTIVES

- Explain the self-care decision-making process and discuss options for self-treatment
- Describe the advantages of the Affordable Care Act
- Describe the basic premises, practices, and providers of complementary and alternative medicine
- Explain how to communicate effectively with health care providers and use their input to evaluate different types of treatment
- Discuss different types of health insurance plans

CHAPTER **15**

Conventional and Complementary Medicine

Today people are becoming more empowered and confident in their ability to solve personal health problems on their own. People who manage their own health care gather information and learn skills from a variety of resources. They solicit opinions and advice in order to practice safe, effective self-care, and to make decisions about seeking professional medical care—whether conventional Western medicine, or complementary and alternative medicine.

This chapter will help you develop skills to identify and manage medical problems and to make the health care system work effectively for you.

SELF-CARE

Effectively managing medical problems involves developing several skills. First, you need to learn to be a good observer of your own body and assess your symptoms. You also must be able to decide when to seek professional advice and when you can safely deal with a problem on your own. You need to know how to safely and effectively self-treat common medical problems. Finally, you need to know how to develop a partnership with physicians and other health care providers and how to implement treatment plans.

Self-Assessment

Symptoms are often an expression of the body's attempt to heal itself. For example, the pain and swelling that occur after an ankle injury immobilize the injured joint so healing can take place. A fever may be an attempt to inhibit the growth and reproduction of infectious agents. A cough can help clear the airways and protect the lungs.

Carefully observing symptoms also helps you identify signals that indicate you need professional help. You should begin by noting when a symptom begins, how often and when it occurs, what makes it worse, what makes it better, and whether you have any associated symptoms or illnesses. You can also monitor your body's vital signs, such as temperature and heart rate. Medical self-tests for blood pressure, blood sugar, pregnancy detection, and urinary tract infections can also help you make a more informed decision about when to seek medical help and when to self-treat.

Knowing When to See a Physician

In general, you should see a physician for symptoms that you would describe as follows:

1. **Severe.** If the symptom is very severe or intense, medical assistance is advised. Examples include severe pains, major injuries, and other emergencies.
2. **Unusual.** If the symptom is peculiar and unfamiliar, it is wise to check it out with your physician. Examples include unexplained lumps, changes in a mole, problems with vision, difficulty swallowing, numbness, weakness, unexplained weight loss, and blood in the sputum, urine, or stool.
3. **Persistent.** If the symptom lasts longer than expected, seek medical advice. Examples in adults include fever for more than five days, a cough lasting longer than two weeks, a sore that doesn't heal within a month, and hoarseness lasting longer than three weeks.
4. **Recurrent.** If a symptom returns again and again, medical evaluation is advised. Examples include recurrent headaches, abdominal pain, and backache.

Sometimes a single symptom is not a cause for concern, but when the symptom is accompanied by other symptoms, the combination suggests a more serious problem. For example, a fever accompanied by neck pain can suggest meningitis.

If you think that you need professional help, you must decide how urgent the problem is. If it is a true emergency, you should go (or ask someone to take you) to the nearest hospital emergency department. Emergencies include the following:

- Major trauma or injury especially to the head, a suspected broken bone, deep wound, severe burn, eye injury, or animal bite
- Uncontrollable bleeding or internal bleeding, as indicated by blood in the sputum, vomit, or stool
- Intolerable and uncontrollable pain or severe chest pain
- Severe shortness of breath
- Persistent abdominal pain, especially if associated with nausea and vomiting
- Poisoning or drug overdose
- Sudden numbness, weakness or loss of function involving an arm or leg, speech difficulty, or drooping of the face
- Loss of consciousness or seizure
- Stupor, drowsiness, or disorientation that cannot be explained
- Severe or worsening reaction to an insect bite or sting, or to a medication or food, especially if breathing becomes difficult

If your problem is not an emergency but still requires medical attention, call your physician's office. Often you can be given medical advice over the phone without needing a visit to the clinic.

Self-Treatment

In most cases, your body itself can relieve your symptoms and heal the disorder. Patience and careful self-observation are often the best choices in self-treatment.

Nondrug Options   Nondrug options are often easy, inexpensive, safe, and highly effective. For example, ice packs, massage, gentle yoga stretching, and neck exercises may at times be more helpful than drugs in relieving headaches and other pains. Getting adequate rest, increasing exercise, drinking more water, eating more or less of certain foods, using humidifiers, changes in ergonomics when working at a desk, and similar remedies are just some of the hundreds of nondrug options for preventing or relieving many common health problems. For a variety of disorders caused or aggravated by stress, the treatment of choice may be relaxation or other stress management strategies.

Self-Medication   Self-treatment with nonprescription medications is an important part of health care. Nonprescription, or **over-the-counter (OTC), medications**, are medicines that the Food and Drug Administration (FDA) has determined are safe for use without a prescription. There are more than 100,000 OTC drugs on the market; about 60% of all medications are sold over the counter.

Hundreds of products sold over-the-counter today use ingredients or dosage strengths that were available only by prescription 20 years ago. With this increased consumer choice, however, comes increased consumer responsibility for using OTC drugs safely.

Although many OTC products are effective, others are unnecessary or divert attention from better ways of coping. Many ingredients in OTC drugs—an estimated 70%—have not been proven to be effective, a fact the FDA does not dispute. And any drug may have risks and side effects.

Follow these simple guidelines to self-medicate safely:

1. Always read labels and follow directions carefully. The information on most OTC drug labels now appears in a standard format developed by the FDA (Figure 15.1). Ingredients, directions for safe use, and warnings are clearly indicated. If you have any question, ask a pharmacist or a qualified health care provider before using a product.

> **Many ingredients in OTC drugs have not proved effective,** a fact the FDA does not dispute.

---

over-the-counter (OTC) medication   A medication or product that can be purchased by a consumer without a prescription.   TERMS

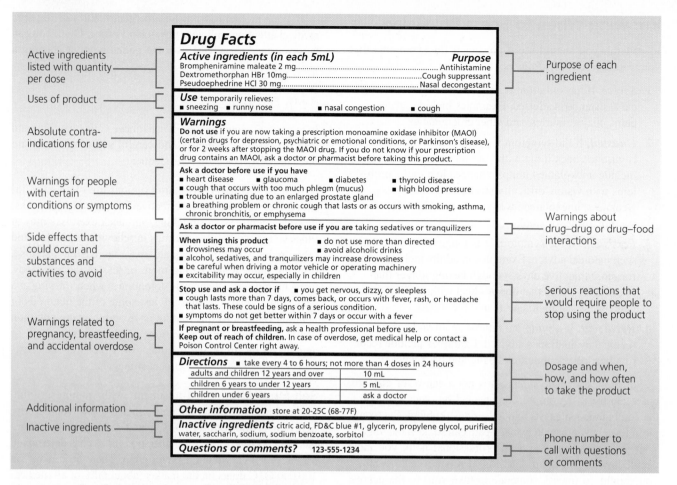

Active ingredients listed with quantity per dose

Uses of product

Absolute contra-indications for use

Warnings for people with certain conditions or symptoms

Side effects that could occur and substances and activities to avoid

Warnings related to pregnancy, breastfeeding, and accidental overdose

Additional information

Inactive ingredients

Drug Facts

Active ingredients (in each 5mL)   **Purpose**
Brompheniramine maleate 2 mg...Antihistamine
Dextromethorphan HBr 10mg...Cough suppressant
Pseudoephedrine HCl 30 mg...Nasal decongestant

Use temporarily relieves:
■ sneezing ■ runny nose   ■ nasal congestion   ■ cough

Warnings
Do not use if you are now taking a prescription monoamine oxidase inhibitor (MAOI) (certain drugs for depression, psychiatric or emotional conditions, or Parkinson's disease), or for 2 weeks after stopping the MAOI drug. If you do not know if your prescription drug contains an MAOI, ask a doctor or pharmacist before taking this product.

Ask a doctor before use if you have
■ heart disease   ■ glaucoma   ■ diabetes   ■ thyroid disease
■ cough that occurs with too much phlegm (mucus)   ■ high blood pressure
■ trouble urinating due to an enlarged prostate gland
■ a breathing problem or chronic cough that lasts or as occurs with smoking, asthma, chronic bronchitis, or emphysema

Ask a doctor or pharmacist before use if you are taking sedatives or tranquilizers

When using this product   ■ do not use more than directed
■ drowsiness may occur   ■ avoid alcoholic drinks
■ alcohol, sedatives, and tranquilizers may increase drowsiness
■ be careful when driving a motor vehicle or operating machinery
■ excitability may occur, especially in children

Stop use and ask a doctor if   ■ you get nervous, dizzy, or sleepless
■ cough lasts more than 7 days, comes back, or occurs with fever, rash, or headache that lasts. These could be signs of a serious condition.
■ symptoms do not get better within 7 days or occur with a fever

If pregnant or breastfeeding, ask a health professional before use.
Keep out of reach of children. In case of overdose, get medical help or contact a Poison Control Center right away.

Directions ■ take every 4 to 6 hours; not more than 4 doses in 24 hours

adults and children 12 years and over	10 mL
children 6 years to under 12 years	5 mL
children under 6 years	ask a doctor

Other information store at 20-25C (68-77F)

Inactive ingredients citric acid, FD&C blue #1, glycerin, propylene glycol, purified water, saccharin, sodium, sodium benzoate, sorbitol

Questions or comments?   123-555-1234

Purpose of each ingredient

Warnings about drug–drug or drug–food interactions

Serious reactions that would require people to stop using the product

Dosage and when, how, and how often to take the product

Phone number to call with questions or comments

FIGURE 15.1   **Reading and understanding OTC drug labels.**

SOURCE: Food and Drug Administration. 1999. Over-the-counter human drugs: Labeling requirements: Final rule. *Federal Register* 64(51), 17 March, 13254–13303.

2. Do not exceed the recommended dosage or length of treatment unless you discuss this with your health care provider.

3. Use caution if you are taking other medications or supplements because OTC drugs and herbal supplements can interact with some prescription drugs. If you have questions about drug interactions, ask your health care provider or pharmacist *before* you take medicines in combination.

4. Try to select medications with one active ingredient rather than a combination. A product with multiple ingredients is likely to include drugs for symptoms you don't have as well as added side effects.

5. When choosing medications, try to buy **generic drugs,** which contain the same active ingredient as brand-name products but generally at a much lower cost.

6. Never take or give a drug from an unlabeled container or when you can't read the label.

7. If you are pregnant or nursing or have a chronic condition such as kidney or liver disease, consult your health care provider before self-medicating.

8. The expiration date marked on many medications is an estimate of how long the medication is likely to be safe and effective. However, an extensive study by the FDA found that 90% of all prescription and OTC medications are potent for several years after their stated expiration date. Exceptions include tetracycline and other antibiotics, nitroglycerine, and insulin. Expiration dates are very conservative. If you have any question about a medicine's expiration date, ask a pharmacist.

9. Store your medications in a cool, dry place that is out of the reach of children.

10. Use special caution with aspirin. Because of an association with a rare but serious problem known as Reye's syndrome, aspirin should not be used by children or adolescents who may have the flu, chicken pox, or any other viral illness.

generic drug   A drug that is not registered or protected by a commercial trademark; a drug that does not have an exclusive brand name.

TERMS

Do you often self-medicate for common medical problems, such as headaches or colds? If so, how careful are you about reading product labels and following directions? For example, would you know if you were taking two OTC medications that contained the same ingredient (such as ibuprofen) at the same time?

PROFESSIONAL CARE

When self-care is not appropriate or sufficient, you need to seek professional medical care, whether by going to a hospital emergency department, or by scheduling an appointment by phone or online with your physician or another conventional health care provider. In recent years the majority of Americans have also sought health care from practitioners of **complementary and alternative medicine (CAM)**—defined as those therapies and practices that do not form part of **conventional medicine,** which is defined as mainstream health care and medical practices taught in most U.S. medical schools and offered in most U.S. hospitals. The most frequently used CAM therapies are nonvitamin, nonmineral natural products; chiropractic care; deep breathing exercises; meditation; massage; and yoga (Table 15.1). Use of acupuncture, deep breathing exercises, massage therapy, meditation, naturopathy, and yoga, among others, has increased over the past two decades, as has the use of CAM overall. Among Americans who use CAM, 92% use it together with conventional medicine, not in place of it.

The term CAM includes both the terms **complementary** and **alternative medicine**: "Complementary" means an approach that combines nonmainstream and conventional medicine. "Alternative" refers to an approach that replaces conventional medicine.

Another term, **integrative medicine,** is when unconventional methods are *added* to conventional ones (such as internal medicine, physical therapy, or dentistry). In integrative medicine it is understood that conventional methods are considered first, and unconventional medicine may be included if it may have additional benefits.

Consumers turn to integrative medicine or CAM for a variety of purposes related to health and well-being, such as boosting their immune systems, lowering their cholesterol levels, losing weight, quitting smoking, or enhancing their memory. Despite their growing popularity, many CAM practices remain controversial, and consumers need to be critically aware of safety issues. The National Center for Complementary and Alternative Medicine (NCCAM), a branch of the National Institutes of Health (NIH), was established in 1992 to apply rigorous scientific methodology

Table 15.1	Use of Complementary and Alternative Therapies by Adults

TYPE OF THERAPY	PERCENTAGE WHO USED THERAPY IN LAST 12 MONTHS
Natural products (nonvitamin, nonmineral)	17.7
Deep breathing exercises	12.7
Meditation	9.4
Chiropractic care	8.6
Massage	8.3
Yoga	6.1
Diet-based therapies	3.6
Progressive relaxation	2.9
Guided imagery	2.2
Homeopathic treatment	1.8
Acupuncture	1.4
Tai chi	1.0
Energy healing therapy/Reiki	0.5
Biofeedback	0.2
Hypnosis	0.2
Any therapy	38.3

SOURCE: Barnes, P. M., et al. 2008. Complementary and alternative medicine use among adults and children: United States, 2007. *CDC National Health Statistics Report #12.* Hyattsville, MD: National Center for Health Statistics.

and standards for proving or disproving the safety and effectiveness of CAM.

The following sections examine the principles and providers of both conventional medicine—the dominant medical system in the United States and Europe, also referred to as standard *Western medicine* or *biomedicine*—and integrative medicine and CAM, with particular attention to consumer issues.

complementary and alternative medicine (CAM) Health care practices and products that are not considered part of conventional, mainstream medical practice as taught in most U.S. medical schools and are not available at most U.S. health care facilities; examples of CAM practices include acupuncture and herbal remedies.

conventional medicine A system of medicine based on the application of the scientific method; diseases are thought to be caused by identifiable physical factors and characterized by a representative set of signs and symptoms; also called *biomedicine* or *standard Western medicine.*

complementary medicine Unconventional medical practices that are used together with conventional ones.

alternative medicine Unconventional medical practices that are used instead of conventional methods.

integrative medicine Conventional health care practice that is sometimes augmented by adding unconventional (CAM) modalities if they may benefit the patient.

TERMS

Ask Yourself

QUESTIONS FOR CRITICAL THINKING
AND REFLECTION

?

What are your views about the use of CAM treatments and therapies? What events or information have shaped those views? Would you consider using complementary or alternative medicine?

CONVENTIONAL MEDICINE

Referring to conventional medicine as "standard Western medicine" draws attention to the fact that it differs from the various medical systems that have developed in China, Japan, India, and other parts of the world. Calling it "biomedicine" reflects conventional medicine's foundation in the biological and physical sciences.

Premises and Assumptions of Conventional Medicine

One of the important characteristics of Western medicine is the belief that disease is caused by identifiable physical factors. Western medicine identifies the causes of disease as pathogens (such as bacteria and viruses), physical factors (such as trauma or toxins), genetic factors, or unhealthy lifestyles that result in changes at the cellular and molecular levels. In most cases, the focus is primarily on the physical causes of illness rather than mental or spiritual imbalance.

Another feature that distinguishes Western biomedicine from other medical systems is the concept that almost every disease is defined by a certain set of signs (objective physical manifestations) and symptoms (the subjective effects perceived by an individual), and that they are similar in most patients suffering from the disease. Western medicine tends to treat diseases as biological disturbances occurring in a patient rather than the result of mind, body, and spirit interactions.

A disease can be caused by either internal or external factors. Internal factors include anatomic or physiologic abnormalities, and defective genetic, hormonal, and immune mechanisms. External causes include infections by bacteria and viruses, and some cases of traumatic injury. The public health measures of the 19th and 20th centuries—chlorination of drinking water, sewage disposal, food safety regulations, vaccination programs, education about hygiene, and so on—were an outgrowth of this orientation.

The implementation of public health measures is one way to control diseases; others include preventive lifestyle measures and the use of drugs and surgery. The discovery and development of sulfa drugs, antibiotics, and steroids in the 20th century, along with advances in chemistry that made it possible to identify the active ingredients in common

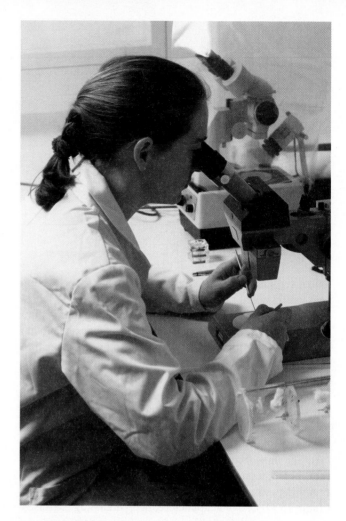

Conventional Western medicine is grounded in scientific explanations resulting from the application of the scientific method or through observable outcomes in randomized controlled studies.

plant-derived remedies, paved the way for the current close identification of Western medicine with **pharmaceuticals** (medical drugs, both prescription and over-the-counter). Western medicine also relies heavily on surgery and on advanced medical technology to discover the physical cause of an individual's disease and to correct, remove, or destroy it.

Further, Western medicine is based on the scientific method for obtaining knowledge and explaining health-related phenomena using scientific explanations that have these characteristics:

- *Empirical*—They are based on the evidence of the senses and on objective and systematic observation, often carried out under carefully controlled conditions; they must be capable of verification by other observers or through the use of technology (such as lab tests and physical measurement, such as blood pressure).

pharmaceuticals   Medical drugs, both prescription and over-the-counter.   TERMS

- *Rational*—They follow the rules of logic and are consistent with known facts.

- *Testable*—Either they are verifiable through direct observation or they lead to predictions about what should occur under conditions not yet observed.

- *Parsimonious*—They explain phenomena with the fewest causes.

- *General*—They have broad explanatory power.

- *Rigorously evaluated*—They are constantly evaluated for consistency with the evidence and known principles, for parsimony, and for generality.

- *Tentative*—Scientists are willing to entertain the possibility that their explanations are faulty, based on new, better, or connected evidence.

Western medicine translates the scientific method in health care practice by applying the research process, a highly refined and well-established approach to exploring the causes of disease and ensuring the safety and efficacy of treatments. Research ranges from case studies—descriptions of a single patient's illness and treatment—to randomized controlled trials (RTCs) conducted on large populations; RTCs are considered the highest level of scientific medical research. Drugs are developed and tested through an elaborate course that typically begins with preliminary research in a laboratory and continues through trials with human participants, review and approval by the FDA, and monitoring of the drug's effects even after it is on the market. The process may take several years or more, and only about 20% of drugs are eventually approved for marketing. The FDA now has new tracks to speed up the approval process, but the time for approval varies vastly, including clinical trials.

When results of research studies are published in medical journals, the community of scientists, physicians, researchers, and scholars has the opportunity to share the findings and enter a dialogue about the subject. Publication of research often prompts further research designed to replicate and confirm the findings, challenge the conclusions, or pursue related lines of thought or experimentation. (For guidelines on how to interpret research when it is reported in the popular media, see the box "Evaluating Health News.")

Pharmaceuticals and the Placebo Effect

A placebo is a chemically inactive substance that a patient believes is an effective therapy for his or her condition. (For procedures that don't involve drugs, such as surgery or acupuncture, a *sham* procedure is used.) By comparing the effects of the actual treatment with the effects of the placebo or sham, researchers can judge whether the treatment is effective.

The *placebo effect* occurs when a patient improves after receiving a placebo. In such cases, the effect of the placebo on the patient cannot be attributed to the specific actions or properties of the drug or procedure. Researchers have consistently found that 30–40% of all patients given a placebo show some improvement. This result has been observed for a wide variety of conditions or symptoms, including coughing, seasickness, depression, migraines, and angina. Placebos are particularly effective when they are administered by someone whom the patient likes and believes in.

Researchers hypothesize that the patients' positive expectations of the medication's effects may have resulted in changes in nerve activity and muscle activity or in electrical or chemical activity in the brain.

A positive aspect of the placebo effect can add to the benefits of the treatment. Psychoneuroimmunology (PNI) is a scientific discipline that investigates physiologic mechanisms for explaining placebo effects. Getting well, like getting sick, is a complex process. Anatomy, physiology, emotions, hope, beliefs, and expectations all contribute to the way the body reacts to medical treatments and utilizes its own healing mechanisms.

The Providers of Conventional Medicine

Conventional medicine is practiced by a wide range of health care professionals in the United States. Several kinds of professionals are permitted to practice specific fields of medicine independently, including medical doctors, osteopaths, dentists, podiatrists, and optometrists.

- **Medical doctors** are practitioners who hold a doctor of medicine (MD) degree from an accredited medical school. In the United States, becoming a practicing physician involves three to eight years of graduate medical study beyond undergraduate premedical training, and includes a residency and possibly a specialty fellowship.

- **Doctors of osteopathic medicine** (DO) receive formal premedical education to earn a bachelor's degree and further education and training at an osteopathic medical school. Osteopathic education emphasizes structural and functional relationships and a whole-person approach to medicine. Osteopathic physicians practice in all of the medical and surgical specialties and subspecialties, but may also practice and specialize in osteopathic manipulative therapy (OMT).

TERMS

medical doctor   A physician who holds the doctor of medicine (MD) degree from an accredited medical school; an *allopathic* physician.

doctor of osteopathic medicine   A physician who holds the doctor of osteopathy (DO) degree from an accredited osteopathic medical school; osteopathy incorporates the theories and practices of scientific medicine and includes osteopathic manual therapy.

TAKE CHARGE
Evaluating Health News

Health-related research published in scientific medical journals is often summarized for the public in the popular media, which may oversimplify, exaggerate, or sensationalize the results. The following questions can help you evaluate scientific health advice presented in popular media:

1. *Is the report based on scientific studies?* Information or advice based on carefully designed research studies has more validity than opinions or casual observations.

2. *What is the source of the information?* A study published in a respected peer-reviewed scientific journal has been examined by editors and researchers who are professionally prepared to evaluate the merits of a study and its results and its application to actual patients. Most journals include information on the funding source and the authors' affiliations that may introduce a bias or conflict of interest. Studies sponsored by drug companies or other commercial groups are suspect. Sources sponsored by universities, government agencies, professional groups (such as WebMD), and others that are rigorously peer-reviewed normally base their reports on scientific information and are considered more valid than commercial websites. Wikipedia is not considered a scientifically valid resource. When health information is critical, the consumer should review the original reference rather than rely solely on secondary interpretations.

3. *How many subjects were included in the study?* A study involving many subjects is more likely to yield reliable results than a study involving only a few subjects. Most quality studies include a "statistical power analysis" section that specifies how many subjects were necessary. Too few subjects are suspect; too many subjects above the number specified in the power analysis may inflate the practical usefulness of the results even though "statistical significance" was achieved. (Statistical significance is usually reported as a p-value; when it is less than or equal to 0.05 or 5%, it is considered "statistically significant.")

4. *Who were the subjects?* Research findings are more likely to apply to you if you share important characteristics with the participants in the study.

5. *What kind of study was it?* Randomized controlled trials and meta-analyses are considered the most valid. Epidemiological studies (which involve noncontrolled observations) may *suggest* useful information, but they cannot always establish cause-and-effect relationships. Consider the following when deciding whether a study's results should be considered significant:

- *Were the treatment group results compared to those of a control group or an already accepted therapy?*

- *Were the subjects randomly assigned to the experimental groups?*

- *Was the study blinded (to the subjects, the experimenters /evaluators, or both)?*

- *Was it a multicenter study?* A few high-quality randomized controlled trials are multicenter studies. The results of several studies conducted in different places at different times can be mathematically combined as a "meta-analysis." A well-conducted meta-analysis is considered one of the most valid study designs.

6. *What do the statistics really say?* Are the results statistically significant (meaning there is a 5% or lower probability (p-value) that the findings resulted by chance alone)? Does the study have the required number of subjects according to a statistical power analysis? Some studies report the effect size instead of or in addition to a p-value. Most of the time the effect size is more revealing than the p-value.

7. *Is new health advice being offered?* If the media report new guidelines for health behavior or medical treatment, examine the source. Be suspicious of absolutes and overstated claims that use words such as "certainty," "always," and "never." Scientifically accurate reports use words such as "results show," "for many people," and "the evidence suggests." Reliable information sources should present the limitations of a study's results and consider a great deal of evidence before offering health advice. Above all, use common sense, and check with your physician before making a major change in your health habits based on news reports.

connect
ACTIVITY
DO IT ONLINE

---

dentist A practitioner who holds a doctor of medical dentistry (DMD) or doctor of dental surgery (DDS) degree and whose practice includes the diagnosis, treatment, and prevention of diseases and injuries of the teeth, mouth, and jaws.

TERMS

podiatrist A practitioner who holds a doctor of podiatric medicine (DPM) degree and specializes in the medical and surgical care of the feet.

optometrist A practitioner who holds a doctor of optometry (OD) degree and is trained to examine the eyes, detect eye diseases, and prescribe corrective lenses.

- **Dentists** focus on the care of the teeth and mouth. They are graduates of four-year dental schools and hold the doctor of dental surgery (DDS) or doctor of medical dentistry (DMD) degree.

- **Podiatrists** are practitioners who specialize in the medical and surgical care of the feet. They hold a doctor of podiatric medicine (DPM) degree.

- **Optometrists** are practitioners trained to examine the eyes, detect eye diseases, and treat certain vision problems most often through the use of corrective lenses. They hold a doctor of optometry (OD) degree.

- **Nurses** or *registered nurses* (*RNs*) are practitioners concerned with the diagnosis and treatment of human responses to actual or potential health problems. They may receive advanced education to become a nurse practitioner (NP), certified registered nurse anesthetist (CRNA), or a certified nurse midwife (CNM).

- **Physician assistants** are healthcare professionals who are licensed to practice medicine as part of a team with physicians.

In addition to these practitioners, there are millions of other highly educated health care professionals: physical therapists (PTs or DPTs), pharmacists (PharmDs), medical social workers (MSWs), and registered dieticians (RDs).

Choosing a Primary Care Physician

Most experts believe it is best to have a primary care physician (PCP) who gets to know you, coordinates your medical care, and refers you to specialists when you need them. The primary care disciplines include family practice, internal medicine, pediatrics, and gynecology.

Many physicians coordinate your care through highly trained medical professionals such as physician assistants and nurse practitioners, who perform many services that have traditionally been provided by physicians, including prescribing medications and performing minor surgery. They work as part of a team with your doctor and are frequently able to spend more time to provide patient education and answer detailed questions about your concerns, preventive measures, and lifestyle choices.

To select a physician, begin by making a list of possible choices. If your insurance limits the health care providers you can see, check the plan's list first. If your health plan lets you choose a physician, ask for recommendations from family, friends, coworkers, local medical societies, and the physician referral service at a local clinic or hospital.

Once you have the names of a few physicians, you might want to check online or call their offices to find out information such as the following:

- Is the physician covered by your health plan and accepting new patients?

> The image of the all-knowing physician and the passive patient is fading. **What is emerging is a physician–patient partnership.**

- What are the office hours, and when is the physician or office staff available?
- What do patients do if they need urgent care or have an emergency?
- Which hospitals does the physician use?
- How many other physicians are available to cover when he or she isn't available, and who are they?
- How long does it usually take to get a routine appointment?
- Does the office send reminders about preventive services and tests such as Pap tests?
- Does the physician (or a nurse or physician assistant) give advice online or over the phone for common problems and continued care of a diagnosed problem?

A physician's practice philosophy is another important factor to consider. Schedule a first visit to get a sense of how well matched you are and how well he or she might meet your medical needs.

Getting the Most Out of Your Medical Care

The key to making the health care system work for you lies in good communication with your physician and other members of the health care team.

The Physician–Patient Partnership The image of the all-knowing physician and the passive patient is fading. What is emerging is a physician–patient *partnership* in which the physician acts more like a consultant and the patient participates more actively (see the box "Creating Your Own Health Record"). You should expect your physician to be attentive, caring, and able to listen and clearly explain health care matters to you. You also must do your part. You need to be assertive in a firm but nonaggressive manner. You need to express your feelings and concerns, ask questions and, if necessary, be persistent. If your physician is unable to communicate clearly with you despite your best efforts, you probably need to change physicians.

Your Physician Appointments You may be offered the opportunity to see a physician assistant or nurse practitioner who works with your physician.

nurse A health provider (RN) who is concerned with the diagnosis and treatment of human responses to actual or potential health problems and acts to promote, maintain or restore health. **TERMS**

physician assistant A healthcare professional who is licensed to practice medicine as part of a team with physicians.

We each need to be responsible for compiling our important medical records and keeping them safe and easily available to us or a caretaker in case we need the records for an emergency, or when traveling, moving, or looking for a new primary care provider. College is a good time to start doing this for yourself.

Some personal computerized health record systems can be purchased online, or one can be devised individually. Whether purchased or created individually, here's what it should contain:

• Your name, emergency contact, birth date, blood type, religious preference (if any), and the date this record was compiled or updated.

• All known allergies (including medications).

• A list of all chronic conditions and the date of their diagnosis (diabetes, high blood pressure, asthma, emphysema, etc.)

• Any hereditary diseases.

• The names and dosages of all medications you are taking and reasons for taking them.

• The results of tests or procedures such as blood pressure, cholesterol, vision and others.

• The dates and reasons for all past hospitalizations and operations. If the reasons were serious or may affect future treatments (for example, major organ involvement, surgical prostheses), a hospital discharge summary should be included.

• The date of physical exams and any major findings.

• Vaccination schedules.

• A print-out of all laboratory test results, and a written report of any imaging studies (X-rays, CAT scans, MRIs, etc.),

electrocardiograms (ECGs), and special tests such as audiograms and exercise stress tests. Check to verify that dates are included.

You may view or request a copy of your medical records or a summary of the information. To request copies, you should ask for an "authorization for the release of information form." Any fee should include only the cost of copying and postage (if you request mailing). If after receiving your medical record you believe any information about you is incorrect or incomplete, you can request an amendment through your physician or a medical information professional, and you have the right for your amendment to be permanently included in your record.

SOURCES: MedlinePlus. *Personal Health Records* (www.nlm.nih.gov/medlineplus /personalhealthrecords.html); AHIMA Foundation. *myPHR* (www.myphr.com).

connect
ACTIVITY
DO IT ONLINE

Present your concerns at the beginning of the visit to set the agenda. Be specific and concise about your symptoms, and be open and honest about your concerns. Let your physician know if you are taking any drugs, are allergic to any medications, are breast-feeding, or may be pregnant. At the end of the visit, briefly repeat the physician's diagnosis, prognosis, the purpose of any tests, and instructions you have received to make sure you understand your next steps.

The Diagnostic Process   The first step in the diagnostic process is the medical history, which includes your primary reason for the visit, your current symptoms, your past medical history, and your social history (job, family life,

major stressors, living conditions, and health habits). Keeping up-to-date records of your medical history can help you provide your physician with key facts about your health.

The next step is usually the physical exam, which begins with a review of vital signs: blood pressure, heart rate (pulse), breathing rate, and temperature. Depending on your primary complaint, your physician may give you a complete physical, or the exam may be directed to specific areas, such as your ears, nose, and throat.

Additionally, your physician may order medical tests to complete the diagnosis. Diagnostic testing provides a wealth of information to help solve medical problems. Physicians can order imaging studies (such as X-rays, MRIs, or CAT scans), biopsies, blood and urine tests, and **endoscopies** to view, probe, or analyze almost any part of the body.

If your physician orders a test for you, be sure you know why you need it, what the risks and benefits of the test are for you, how you should prepare for it (for example, by fasting

endoscopy   A medical procedure in which a viewing instrument is inserted into a body cavity or opening.

TERMS

or discontinuing medications or herbal remedies), and what the test will involve. Also ask what the test results mean because no test is 100% accurate—**false positives** and **false negatives** can occur—and interpretation of some tests is subjective.

Medical and Surgical Treatments

Many conditions can be treated in a variety of ways; in some cases, lifestyle changes are sufficient. In other cases, the physician may prescribe a medication.

Thousands of lives are saved each year by antibiotics, insulin, and other drugs, but we pay a price for having such powerful tools. A report from the Institute of Medicine (IOM) estimates that 1.5 million prescription drug-related errors—called *adverse drug events,* or ADEs—occur each year in the United States. ADEs happen for several reasons:

- *Medication errors:* Physicians may overprescribe drugs, sometimes in response to pressure by patients. Adverse drug effects (ADEs) can occur if a physician prescribes the wrong drug or a dangerous combination of drugs. Such problems are especially prevalent among older adults, who typically take multiple medications. At the pharmacy, patients may receive the wrong drug or may not be given complete information about drug risks, side effects, and interactions.

- *Off-label drug use:* Once a drug is approved by the FDA for one purpose, it can legally be prescribed (although not marketed) for purposes not listed on the label. Many off-label uses are safe and supported by some research, but both consumers and health care providers need to take special care with off-label use.

- *Online pharmacies:* Although convenient, some online pharmacies may sell products or engage in practices that are illegal in the offline world, putting consumers at risk for receiving adulterated, expired, ineffective, or counterfeit drugs. The FDA recommends that consumers avoid sites that prescribe drugs for the first time without a physical exam, sell prescription drugs without a prescription, or sell medications not approved by the FDA. You should also avoid sites that do not provide access to a registered pharmacist to answer questions or that do not provide a U.S. address and phone number to contact if there's a problem. The National Association of Boards of Pharmacy sponsors a voluntary certification program for Internet pharmacies. To be certified, a pharmacy must have a state license and allow regular inspections.

- *Costs:* Spending on prescription drugs is rising faster than the rate of inflation and is now the fastest-growing portion of U.S. health care spending. Consumers may be able to lower their drug costs by using generic versions of medications; by joining a drug discount program sponsored by a company,

organization, or local pharmacy; and by investigating mail-order or Internet pharmacies.

Importing lower-cost drugs from Canada is controversial and problematic. Canada imports U.S. drugs and regulates Canadian-produced drugs, so safety should theoretically not be a concern for drugs from Canada. However, companies in Canada may make drugs for export only, thus avoiding regulation, and online pharmacies may claim they are operating in Canada but may be located in another country where there is little or no regulation. U.S. regulators have found online sites advertising Canadian drugs but shipping fake or substandard versions of medications. In addition, shipping costs can be high, and U.S. generic drugs are often less expensive than Canadian drugs.

Patients share responsibility for their use of prescription drugs. Many people don't take their medications properly, skipping doses, taking incorrect doses, stopping too soon, or not taking the medication at all. An estimated 30–50% of the more than 3 billion prescriptions dispensed annually in the United States are not taken correctly and thus do not produce the desired results. Consumers can increase the safety and effectiveness of their treatment by carefully reading any prescription's label and fact sheets or brochures that come with the medication. Whenever you are given a prescription, ask the following questions:

- Are there nondrug alternatives?
- What is the name of the medication, and what is it supposed to do, within what period of time?
- Can I take a generic drug rather than a brand-name one?
- Is there written information about the medication?

If written information is provided, check it for the following information:

- How and when do I take the medication, how much do I take, and for how long? What should I do if I miss a dose?
- What medications, foods, drinks, or activities should I avoid when taking this drug?
- What are the side effects, and what do I do if they occur?

Surgery is another staple of Western medical treatment. Each year more than 70 million operations and related procedures are performed. About 20% are in response to an emergency such as a severe injury, and 80% are

TERMS

false positive A test result that incorrectly detects a disorder or condition in a person who does not have the disorder or condition.

false negative A test result that fails to correctly detect a disease or condition.

elective surgeries, meaning the patient can generally choose when and where to have the operation, if at all. Many elective surgeries can be done on an **outpatient** basis, so the patient does not have to be admitted to a hospital for the procedure.

If a health care provider suggests surgery for any reason, ask the following questions:

- Why do I need surgery at this time?
- Is a wait-and-see approach possible or advisable? If so, what are the risks?
- Are any nonsurgical options available, such as medicine or physical therapy?
- What are the risks and complications of the surgery?
- Can the operation be done on an outpatient basis?
- What can I expect before, during, and after surgery?

INTEGRATIVE MEDICINE AND CAM

Increasingly more conventional Western medical providers are receptive to integrative medicine, and they may approve or recommend safe and effective CAM to conventional treatment. Whereas conventional Western medicine tends to focus on the body, on the physical causes of disease, and on ways to eradicate pathogens in order to restore health, CAM tends to focus on the mind, body, and spirit in seeking ways to prevent diseases and restore the whole person to balance so that he or she can regain health. This is referred to as **holistic health care**—considering the whole person as a mind–body–spirit entity when diagnosing, treating, or preventing any illness or disorder. The opposite of *holistic* is *dualistic,* which refers to treating the mind and body separately.

CAM therapies are steadily gaining momentum in the United States. More than 42% of hospitals offer one or more CAM therapies, and 46 major American universities have added integrative medical centers to their facilities. In addition, nearly all medical schools have curricular offerings on integrative therapies. Although research studies on CAM modalities have been relatively small in size and conservative in their conclusions, some of their results are considered promising.

For example, a 2010 study tracked the symptoms of two groups of fibromyalgia patients: one that learned a variety of tai chi movements and another that practiced stretching exercises and received wellness counseling. Over the course of the study, the patients who practiced tai chi reported significantly less pain than the other group, and the benefits lasted well beyond the study's end.

Another 2010 study showed that about 6% of adult Americans who suffer back pain have tried at least one CAM therapy. The therapies most commonly used for back pain are chiropractic, massage, yoga, tai chi, qigong, and acupuncture. Nearly two-thirds said they experienced significantly reduced pain as a result of CAM therapy.

NCCAM places CAM practices into several broad categories: alternative medical systems, mind–body medicine, natural products, manipulative and body-based practices, and other CAM practices. What follows is a general introduction to types of CAM available and a brief description of some of the more widely used ones.

Alternative Medical Systems

Many cultures formed complete systems of medical philosophy, theory, and practice long before the current Western biomedical approach was developed. The complete systems that are best known in the United States include traditional Chinese medicine (TCM), also known as traditional Oriental medicine, and homeopathy. Traditional medical systems have also been developed in many other regions of the world, including North, Central, and South America; the Middle East; India; Tibet; and Australia. In many countries, these medical approaches continue to be used today—frequently alongside Western medicine and quite often by physicians trained in Western medicine.

Alternative medical systems tend to have concepts in common. For example, the concept of life force or energy exists in many cultures. In traditional Chinese medicine, the life force contained in all living things is called *qi* (sometimes spelled chi). Most traditional medical systems think of disease as a disturbance or imbalance not just of physical processes but also of forces or energies within the body, the mind, and the spirit. Treatment aims at reestablishing equilibrium, balance, and harmony.

Because the whole patient, rather than an isolated body part or disease, is treated in most comprehensive alternative medical systems, it is rare that only a single treatment approach is used. Most commonly, multiple remedies and techniques are employed together and are adjusted according to the changes in the patient's health status.

Traditional Chinese Medicine In **traditional Chinese medicine (TCM)** the free and harmonious flow of qi defines health—a positive feeling of well being and vitality in body, mind, and spirit. TCM works to restore and balance the flow of blocked qi; the goal is not only to treat

---

elective surgery A nonemergency operation that the patient can choose to schedule.

TERMS

outpatient A person receiving medical attention without being admitted to the hospital.

holistic health care Practice that takes into account the whole person—body, mind, and spirit—when assessing, treating, and preventing illnesses and maintaining health.

traditional Chinese medicine (TCM) The traditional medical system of China, which views illness as the result of a problem in the quality, quantity, or flow of qi, the life force; therapies include acupuncture, herbal medicine, and massage.

illnesses but also to increase energy, prevent disease, and support immunity.

Two of the primary treatment methods in TCM are **herbal remedies** and **acupuncture.** Chinese herbal remedies number about 5800. In addition to herbs, plant products, fungi (mushrooms), animal parts, and minerals may be used. The use of a single medicinal substance is rare in Chinese herbal medicine; rather, several different substances are combined in precise proportions, often to make a tea or soup.

Acupuncture is used to correct disturbances in the flow of qi through the insertion of thin needles through the skin at appropriate sites. Qi is believed to flow through the body along several meridians, or pathways, and there are hundreds of acupuncture points located along these meridians. The points chosen for acupuncture are highly individualized for each patient, and they change during treatment as the patient's health status changes.

The World Health Organization has compiled a list of more than 40 conditions for which acupuncture may be beneficial. At a conference called by the NIH, a panel of experts found that acupuncture was effective in relieving nausea and vomiting after chemotherapy, and pain after surgery, including dental surgery. Newer studies show that acupuncture may help relieve the painful symptoms of fibromyalgia and reduce the joint pain and stiffness of osteoarthritis. There is not yet enough evidence to show conclusively that acupuncture is effective for menstrual cramps, tennis elbow, carpal tunnel syndrome, asthma, or certain other conditions.

Few side effects have been reported with acupuncture. The FDA regulates acupuncture needles like other standard medical devices and requires that they be sterile. Most states require licensing for acupuncture practitioners, but requirements vary widely.

Homeopathy As a CAM system of medical practice that has unconventional Western origins, **homeopathy** involves treating an individual with highly diluted substances, hoping to trigger the body's natural system of healing. Based on a patient's specific signs and symptoms, a homeopathic practitioner determines the most appropriate treatment. A primary principle of homeopathy is "like cures like." This principle states that a substance that produces the symptoms of an illness can help cure or prevent the illness when given in very diluted, minute quantities. Homeopathic training is offered on the Internet, in brief courses, and through correspondence courses. Some states require homeopaths to be licensed and fulfill certain requirements before they are permitted to practice.

Naturopathy **Naturopathy** is based on the premise that the body has the ability to restore and maintain optimal health. Naturopathic physicians focus on removing barriers to good health and creating healing internal and external environments. They use nutritional counseling, acupuncture, herbology, homeopathic medicine, and other holistic approaches to treatment. The most frequently treated conditions include allergies, chronic pain, obesity, heart disease, fertility problems, and cancer. Naturopaths work in hospitals, clinics, and community health centers. They are licensed in several states.

Mind–Body Medicine

Mind–body interventions make use of the integral connection between mind and body and the effect each can have on the other. They include many of the stress management techniques discussed in Chapter 2, including meditation, yoga, visualization, tai chi chuan, and biofeedback. Psychotherapy, support groups, prayer, and music and art therapy are mind–body interventions. The placebo effect is one of the most widely known examples of mind–body interdependence.

Hypnotherapy is considered to be a CAM modality, although its use for certain conditions was accepted more than 40 years ago by the American Medical Association (AMA).

Hypnotherapy involves the induction of a state of deep relaxation during which the patient is more likely to accept suggestions to influence health and overcome conditions such as chronic pain, pain during surgery or childbirth, unhealthy habits, and anxiety and phobias. The therapist helps the patient change unwanted behavior or deal with pain and other symptoms. A number of NIH-sponsored reports found strong evidence for the effectiveness of hypnosis in reducing chronic pain stemming from a variety of medical conditions.

Health professionals who are properly trained in hypnotherapy use this modality to augment their conventional treatments. Many states require hypnotherapists to be licensed, but the requirements for licensing vary substantially.

> The World Health Organization lists **more than 40 conditions that may benefit from acupuncture treatment.**

TERMS

herbal remedy A medicine prepared from plants.

acupuncture Insertion of thin needles through the skin at points along meridians—pathways through which qi is believed to flow.

homeopathy An alternative, unconventional medical system that uses a holistic approach to diagnosis, and treatments that involve administering very small doses of remedies that would produce symptoms like those of the illness.

naturopathy An alternative medical system based on supporting the body's ability to heal itself and maintain optimal health by removing barriers and creating a healing internal and external environment.

hypnotherapy A mind–body technique that uses relaxation and imagery to help a patient imagine specific health outcomes and establish a belief that they can be achieved; commonly used for managing pain, phobias, and addictions.

Natural Products

Natural products, also known as *biologically based therapies,* include substances derived from plant or animal sources. They consist primarily of herbal therapies or remedies, botanicals, and extracts from animal tissues (such as shark cartilage). Herbal remedies are a major component of all indigenous forms of medicine. Prior to the development of pharmaceuticals at the end of the 19th century, people everywhere in the world relied on materials from nature for pain relief, wound healing, and treatment of a variety of ailments. Much of the **pharmacopoeia** of present-day scientific medicine originated in the folk medicine of native people, and many prescription drugs used today have been derived from plants.

Most natural products are sold in the United States as dietary supplements and are therefore largely unregulated by the FDA. Like foods, dietary supplements must carry ingredient labels, and manufacturers are responsible for ensuring that their dietary supplements are safe and properly labeled for marketing. The FDA is responsible for monitoring the labeling and accompanying literature of dietary supplements and for overseeing their safety once they are on the market.

Well-designed clinical studies have been conducted on a number of natural products. A few commonly used herbals, their uses, and the evidence supporting their efficacy are presented in Table 15.2. Participants in clinical trials with herbals such as St. John's wort, ginkgo biloba, and echinacea experienced only minor adverse effects. New studies are also evaluating the effects of varying dosages and their interactions with conventional drugs.

Although most drug–herb interactions are relatively minor compared to conventional drug–drug interactions, some can be potentially serious. Because of reports of bleeding, a popular herb, ginkgo biloba, although generally well tolerated, should be used cautiously in people suffering from clotting disorders or taking blood thinners, or prior to some surgical or dental procedures. St. John's wort interacts with drugs used to treat HIV infection and heart disease, and the herb may also reduce the effectiveness of oral contraceptives, antirejection drugs used in patients receiving organ transplants, and some medications used to treat infections, depression, asthma, and seizure disorders. Supplements containing kava kava have been linked to liver damage, and anyone who has liver problems, drinks large amounts of alcohol, or takes medications that can affect the liver is advised to consult a physician or pharmacist before using kava kava–containing supplements.

Another potential problem is the possibility of contaminants. Some herbal medicine products have been found to contain potentially harmful levels of lead, mercury, or arsenic. The content of herbal preparations is also variable.

Studies have shown that most people do not reveal their use of CAM therapies to their conventional health care providers, a problem that can have significant health consequences. Any herbs that are used in combination with conventional drugs should be evaluated for safety by a knowledgeable health care provider such as a pharmacist.

Manipulative and Body-Based Practices

Touch and body manipulation are long-standing forms of health care. Manual healing techniques include the concept that misalignment or dysfunction in one part of the body can cause pain or dysfunction in that or another part. Correcting these misalignments can help restore optimal health.

Many manipulative and body-based practices are integral components of physical therapy and osteopathic medicine, although certain techniques fit the definition of CAM because they are not a part of conventional health care practice. The most commonly used CAM manual healing method is **chiropractic,** a method that focuses on the relationship between structure and function, primarily of the spine, joints, muscles, and the nervous system, to maintain or restore health. An important therapeutic procedure is the manipulation of joints, particularly those of the spinal column. However, chiropractors also use a variety of other techniques, including exercise, patient education and lifestyle modification, nutritional supplements, and orthotics (mechanical supports and braces) to treat patients.

Chiropractors, or doctors of chiropractic, are trained for a minimum of four years at accredited chiropractic colleges and can go on to postgraduate training in many countries. Although specifically listed by NCCAM as one of the manipulative and body-based practices of CAM, chiropractic is accepted by many health care and health insurance providers to a far greater extent than the other types of CAM therapies. Based on research showing the efficacy of chiropractic management in acute low-back pain, spinal manipulation has been included in the federal guidelines for the treatment of this condition, and electrodiagnostic tests show that chiropractic is effective in controlling back pain. Promising results have also been reported with the use of chiropractic techniques in neck pain and headaches.

A word of caution is in order: Spinal manipulation must be performed only by a properly trained professional such as a chiropractor, osteopathic physician, or physical therapist who is specially trained and certified in orthopedic manual physical therapy (OMPT).

---

natural products CAM therapies that include biologically based interventions and products; examples include herbal remedies, extracts from animal tissues, and dietary supplements.

pharmacopoeia A collection of descriptions and formulas for drugs and medicinal preparations.

chiropractic A CAM manipulative, body-based practice that focuses on disorders of the spine, and musculoskeletal and nervous systems, and the effects of these disorders on general health; the primary treatment is manipulation of the spine and other joints.

Table 15.2 — Commonly Used Herbals, Their Uses, Evidence for Their Effectiveness, and Contraindications

BOTANICAL	USE	EVIDENCE	EXAMPLES OF ADVERSE EFFECTS AND INTERACTIONS
Cranberry (*Vaccinium macrocarpon*)	Prevention or treatment of urinary tract infections	Effective for treating certain bladder infections	None known
Dandelion (*Taraxacum officinale*)	As a "tonic" against liver or kidney ailments	None yet	May cause diarrhea in some users; people with gallbladder or bile duct problems should not take dandelion
Echinacea (*Echinacea purpurea, E. angustifolia, E. pallida*)	Stimulation of immune functions; to prevent colds and flulike diseases; to lessen symptoms of colds and flu	Some trials showed that it prevents colds and flu and helps patients recover faster from colds	Might cause liver damage if taken over long periods of time (more than 8 weeks); because it is an immune stimulant, it is not advisable to take it with immune suppressants (e.g., corticosteroids) or during chemotherapy
Evening primrose oil (*Oenothera biennis L.*)	Reduction of inflammation	Long-term supplementation effective in reducing symptoms of rheumatoid arthritis	None known
Feverfew (*Tanacetum parthenium*)	Prevention of headaches and migraines	Most trials indicate that it is more effective than placebo	Should not be used by people allergic to other members of the aster family; has the potential to increase the effects of warfarin and other anticoagulants
Garlic (*Allium sativum*)	Reduction of cholesterol	Short-term studies have found a modest effect	May interact with some medications, including anticoagulants, cyclosporine, and oral contraceptives
Ginkgo (*Ginkgo biloba*)	Improvement of circulation and memory	Improves cerebral insufficiency and slows progression of senile dementia in some patients; improves blood flow in legs	Could increase bleeding time; should not be taken with nonsteroidal anti-inflammatory drugs (e.g., NSAIDs, acetaminophen) or anticoagulants; gastrointestinal disturbance
Ginseng (*Panax ginseng*)	Improvement of physical performance, memory, immune function, and glycemic control in diabetes; treatment of herpes simplex 2	No conclusive evidence exists for any of these uses	Interacts with warfarin and alcohol in mice and rats, so should probably not be used with these drugs; may cause liver damage
St. John's wort (*Hypericum perforatum*)	Treatment of depression	There is evidence that it is significantly more effective than placebo, is as effective as some standard antidepressants for mild to moderate depression, and causes fewer adverse effects	Known to interact with a variety of pharmaceuticals and should not be taken together with digoxin, theophylline, cyclosporine, indinavir, and serotonin reuptake inhibitors
Saw palmetto (*Serenoa repens*)	Improvement of benign prostatic hypertrophy	Studies show that saw palmetto may reduce mild prostate enlargement	Has no known interactions with drugs, but should probably not be taken with hormonal therapies
Valerian (*Valeriana officinalis*)	Treatment of insomnia	May help with some sleep disorders	Interacts with thiopental and pentobarbital and should not be used with these drugs

Exercise for health maintenance, promotion, and disease prevention currently fits the definition of a CAM modality. However, the American College of Sports Medicine (ACSM) and the American Medical Association (AMA) are actively trying to move exercise into the medical mainstream. A study has found that 65% of Americans would be more interested in exercising for staying healthy if advised to do so by their physicians.

A new program, Exercise Is Medicine™, encourages physicians to record a patient's exercise level as a routine vital sign during clinical visits, along with pulse, respiratory rate, temperature, and blood pressure. Those who are able will be advised to exercise for 30 minutes and to stretch and engage in light muscle training for an additional 10 minutes five days each week. The Exercise Is Medicine website (www.exerciseismedicine.org) advises physicians, other health care providers, medical educators, and the public about the benefits of exercise. Through efforts such as this, exercise is likely to transition from a CAM modality to a conventional modality and to be taught in more American medical schools, and recommended and used as a treatment in American health care institutions.

Other CAM Practices

CAM practices also include movement therapies, traditional healing practices, and energy therapies. Movement therapies, such as the Feldenkrais method, the Alexander technique, and Pilates, promote physical, mental, emotional, and spiritual well-being. Traditional healers may rely on touch as well as other senses, for example, sound—the shamanic clanging of a bell or the quality of a singing voice. These healers may incorporate psychological or religious therapy in addition to prescribing herbal remedies.

Energy therapies are forms of treatment that use energy originating from the patient's or therapist's body or from other sources such as therapeutic magnets. Energy therapies are based on the concept that energy surrounds and penetrates the body and can be influenced by movement, touch, pressure, or the placement of hands in or through the fields. **Qigong,** a component of traditional Chinese medicine, combines movement, meditation, and regulation of breathing to enhance the flow of qi to improve blood circulation and enhance immune function. **Therapeutic touch** is derived from ancient techniques involving using the hands to detect and transmit energy (electromagnetic energy). It is based on the premise that healers can identify and correct energy imbalances by passing their hands over the patient's body. **Reiki** is another example of energy therapy; it is intended to correct disturbances in the flow of life energy (*ki* in the Japanese tradition) and enhance the body's healing powers through the use of specific hand positions on or near the patient's body to promote balance.

Bioelectromagnetics is the study of interactions between living organisms and electromagnetic fields, both those produced by the organism itself and those produced by outside sources. The recognition that the body produces electromagnetic fields has led to the development of many diagnostic procedures in Western medicine, including electroencephalography (EEG), electrocardiography (ECG), and nuclear magnetic resonance imaging (MRI).

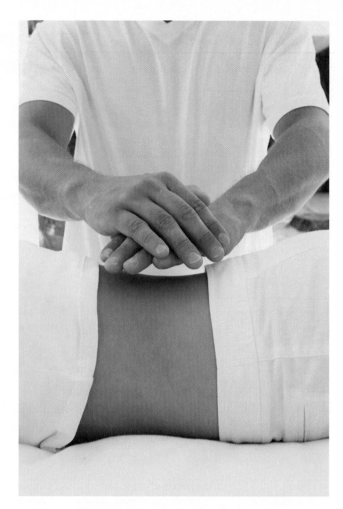

One of several energy medicine therapies, Reiki has bioenergetic and physical components.

Bioelectromagnetic-based therapies include the use of electromagnetic fields to manage pain, increase blood flow, and treat conditions such as arthritic pain.

Evaluating Complementary and Alternative Therapies

Compared to conventional medical therapies, CAM has less scientific information available about it and less regulation of associated products and providers. Therefore it is important for consumers to take an active role when they are thinking about using CAM.

Working with Your Physician When a health issue might be serious, the NCCAM advises consumers not to seek complementary therapies without first consulting a conventional health care provider. It's usually best to become informed and discuss conventional treatments that have been shown to be beneficial for your condition. If you are thinking of trying any complementary or alternative therapies, it is important to discuss these with your physician, pharmacist, or other conventional provider who is knowledgeable about

---

energy therapies Forms of CAM treatment that use energy fields originating either within the body or from outside sources to promote health and healing.

qigong A component of traditional Chinese medicine that combines movement, meditation, and regulation of breathing to increase the flow of qi, hoping to improve blood circulation, and enhance immune function.

therapeutic touch A CAM practice based on the premise that healers can identify and correct energy imbalances by passing their hands over the patient's body.

Reiki A CAM practice intended to correct disturbances in the flow of life energy and enhance the body's healing powers through the use of various hand positions on the patient.

bioelectromagnetic-based therapies CAM therapies based on the notion that electromagnetic fields can be used to promote healing and manage pain.

TERMS

your health status and is also informed about CAM or is willing to learn by consulting proper resources. If they are not informed about CAM, it may be helpful to bring information from reliable, evidence-based sources with you. Areas to discuss with your physician or pharmacist include the safety of the treatment; evidence for its effectiveness, if any; issues of timing; and likely cost.

If appropriate, schedule a follow-up visit with your physician to assess your condition and your progress after a certain amount of time using a complementary therapy. Keep a symptom diary to track your symptoms and gauge your progress. (Symptoms such as pain and fatigue are difficult to recall with accuracy, so an ongoing symptom diary is an important tool.) If you plan to pursue a therapy against your physician's advice, you need to tell him or her.

For supplements, particularly botanicals, pharmacists can also be an excellent source of information; they should be informed about any other unconventional or conventional medications you are taking.

Questioning the CAM Practitioner You can also get information from individual practitioners, educational programs, professional organizations, and state licensing boards. Ask about education, training, licensing, and certification. If appropriate, check with local or state regulatory agencies or the consumer affairs department to determine if any complaints have been lodged against the practitioner. Some guidelines for talking with a CAM practitioner include the following:

- Ask the practitioner why he or she thinks the therapy will be beneficial for your condition. Ask for a full description of the therapy and any potential side effects. In all cases, demand an evidence-based approach.

- Describe in detail any conventional treatments you are receiving or plan to receive.

- Ask how long the therapy should continue before it can be determined if it is beneficial.

- Ask about the expected cost of the treatment. Does it seem reasonable? Will your health insurance pay some or all of the costs?

> NCCAM advises consumers not to seek CAM treatment **without talking to their usual health care providers first.**

If anything an unconventional practitioner says or recommends directly conflicts with advice from your physician, discuss it with your physician before making any major changes in your current treatment regimen or lifestyle.

PAYING FOR HEALTH CARE

The American health care system is one of the most advanced and comprehensive in the world, but it is also the most expensive (Figure 15.2). In 2012 Americans spent $2.7 trillion on health care, or more than $9000 per person. Many factors contribute to the high cost of health care in the United States, including the cost of advanced equipment and new technology, expensive treatments for some illnesses, aging of the population, and the demand for profits by many commercial health enterprises.

The Current System

Because of expanding health care costs and an increasing difficulty for some Americans to pay for them, Congress passed the **Affordable Care Act** in 2009 (ACA). The bill was signed into law by President Barack Obama in 2010. The ACA's main aims are to control costs and provide more regulation to the way insurance companies cover medical expenses. Two key provisions of the ACA are that it increases preventive services and forbids insurance companies to discriminate on the basis of preexisting medical conditions.

Health care is financed by a combination of private and public insurance plans, patient out-of-pocket payments, and government assistance. Before the ACA, private insurance and individual patients paid about 55% of the total; the government paid the rest, mainly through Medicare and Medicaid. Most nonelderly Americans receive health insurance through their employers, but as medical costs increase, the number of Americans with private insurance has decreased by approximately 10% over the past two decades.

By some estimates, as many as 50 million Americans—the vast majority of them employed—had no health insurance at all prior to the ACA. Many more were underinsured, meaning they may be uninsured for periods of time, have health insurance that does not cover all needed services, and/or have high-out-of-pocket costs. New and extended government health insurance programs for children reduced the number of Americans under age 18 who lack health insurance; still, 9.8 million American children were uninsured in 2010 before the ACA was available.

Ask Yourself

QUESTIONS FOR CRITICAL THINKING AND REFLECTION

Have you ever considered using a complementary or alternative treatment? If so, was it in addition to conventional treatment or instead of it? What kind of research did you do before having the treatment? What advice did your primary health care provider give you about it?

Affordable Care Act A U.S. law intended to reform medical care by requiring nearly all Americans to have health insurance coverage and by making health care more affordable for individuals and families. **TERMS**

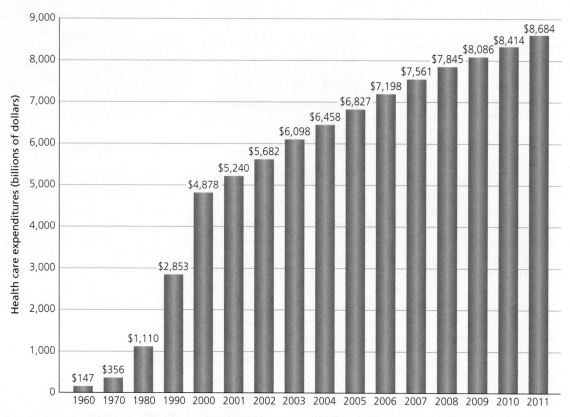

FIGURE 15.2 **National health care expenditures (public and private), 1960–2011.**

SOURCE: National Center for Health Statistics. 2013. *Health, United States: 2012*. Hyattsville, MD: National Center for Health Statistics.

Health Insurance

Health insurance as required under the ACA protects you against losses incurred for medical expenses due to illness or injury. Depending on the policy, coverage may also include preventive services such as yearly exams; other physician services; medications; hospital stays; emergency department visits; physical, occupational, and speech therapy; vision care; dental coverage; and other expenses. Some insurance policies provide riders for specific CAM coverage for an additional charge. Policies differ based on the services covered, the amount of the deductible and the copayment, and the limit of coverage. Of course, with many plans, the more services you add to a policy, the higher the premium. Coverage may be provided as an employment benefit or through a government-sponsored plan such as Medicaid (for certain disabled and low-income individuals) or Medicare (typically individuals aged 65 or older and those with certain illnesses).

Health insurance enables people to receive health care they might not otherwise be able to afford.

The plans are either fee-for-service (indemnity) or managed care. With both types, the individual or the employer pays a basic premium, usually on a monthly basis. As part of the ACA, states now provide interactive online exchanges that supply information about various insurance plans, which can be adapted to fit an individual's needs and income level. Most insurance is provided by and can be purchased from private companies using the online exchanges.

Traditional Fee-for-Service (Indemnity) Plans In a fee-for-service, or indemnity, plan, you can use any physician or hospital you choose. You or the provider sends the bill to your insurance company, which pays part of it. Usually you have to pay a deductible amount each year, and then the plan will pay a percentage—often 80%—of what it considers the "usual and customary" charge for covered services. You pay the remaining 20%, which is known as coinsurance.

Managed Care Plans **Managed care plans** have agreements with a network of specified physicians, hospitals, and health care providers to offer a range of services to plan members at reduced cost. In general, you have lower out-of-pocket costs and less paperwork with a managed care plan than with an indemnity plan, but you also have less freedom in choosing your health care providers. Most Americans with

> **managed care plan** A health care program that integrates the financing and delivery of services by using designated providers, utilization review, and incentives for following the plan's policies; HMOs, PPOs, and POS plans are managed care plans.
>
> TERMS

Overview

The Affordable Care Act (ACA) was signed into law on March 23, 2010. Many of the changes mandated by the act were implemented in 2014. Here is a brief summary of additional changes enacted by the new law.

Coverage

• *Ends preexisting condition exclusions:* Beginning January 1, 2014, health plans can no longer deny or limit benefits due to a pre-existing condition.

• *Keeps young adults covered:* If you are under 26, you may be eligible to be covered under your parents' health plan.

• *Ends arbitrary withdrawals of insurance coverage:* Insurers can no longer cancel your coverage because of honest mistakes in your application.

• *Guarantees the right to appeal:* You now have the right to ask that your plan reconsider its denial of payment.

Costs

• *Ends lifetime limits on coverage:* Lifetime dollar limits on most benefits you receive are not permitted.

• *Reviews premium increases:* Insurance companies must now publicly justify rate hikes.

• *Helps you get the most from your premium dollars:* Your premium dollars must be spent primarily on health care—not administrative costs.

Care

• *Covers preventive care at no cost to you:* Recommended preventive health services are covered with no copayment.

• *Protects your choice of doctors:* From your plan's network, you can choose the primary care doctor you want.

• *Removes insurance company barriers to emergency services:* You can seek emergency care at a hospital outside your health plan's network.

Finding a Plan

Under the ACA, a health insurance marketplace, also called health exchanges, facilitates the purchase of health insurance in every state. The health exchanges provide a selection of government-regulated health care plans that students and others may choose from. Those who are below minimum income requirements are eligible for federal subsidies to help cover the cost of the premiums.

Benefits to College Students

Students can now stay on their parents' health insurance plan until age 26—even if they are married or have coverage through an employer. Beginning in 2014, college students, like others, have to abide by the "individual mandate" in the ACA. Students who aren't on their parents' plan and don't want to purchase insurance through their school can review and purchase plans through the health insurance marketplace.

Students whose income is below a certain level could qualify for Medicaid. Check with your state to see if you're eligible.

Individuals with nonimmigrant status, which includes worker visas and student visas, qualify for insurance coverage through the exchanges.

For more information, check out HealthCare.gov.

---

job-based insurance are covered by managed care plans, which may follow several different models:

• **Health maintenance organizations (HMOs)** offer members a range of services for a set monthly fee. You choose a primary care physician who manages your care and refers you to specialists if you need them.

• **Preferred provider organizations (PPOs)** have arrangements with physicians and other providers who have agreed to accept lower fees.

• **Point-of-service (POS) plans** are options offered by many HMOs in which you can see a physician outside the plan and still be partially covered.

health maintenance organization (HMO) A prepaid health insurance plan that offers health care from designated providers.

preferred provider organization (PPO) A prepaid health insurance plan in which providers agree to deliver services for discounted fees; patients can go to any provider, but using nonparticipating providers results in higher costs to the patient.

point-of-service (POS) plan A combination of the HMO and PPO plans: Although you can seek out-of-network treatment, you will pay most of the cost unless you are referred by your PCP.

TERMS

Many managed care plans try to reduce costs over the long term by paying for routine preventive care, such as regular checkups and screening tests and prenatal care; they may also encourage prevention by offering health education and lifestyle modification programs for members.

Government Programs   Americans who are 65 or older and younger people with certain disabilities can be covered by **Medicare,** a federal health insurance program that helps pay for hospitalization, physician services, and prescription drugs. **Medicaid** is a joint federal–state health insurance program that covers some low-income people, especially children, pregnant women, and people with certain disabilities. These government programs will be affected and face changes with the full implementation of the ACA.

Medicare   A federal health insurance program for people 65 or older and for younger people with certain disabilities.

Medicaid   A federally subsidized state-run plan of health care for people with low income.

TERMS

SUMMARY

- Informed self-care requires knowing how to evaluate symptoms. It's necessary to see a physician if symptoms are severe, unusual, persistent, or recurrent.

- Self-treatment doesn't necessarily require medication, but OTC drugs can be a helpful part of self-care.

- Conventional medicine is characterized by a focus on the physical causes of disease; the identification of signs and symptoms; the use of drugs and surgery for treatment; and the use of scientific thinking and research to understand diseases.

- Conventional practitioners include medical doctors, doctors of osteopathic medicine, podiatrists, optometrists, and dentists, as well as other highly trained professionals.

- The diagnostic process involves a medical history, a physical exam, and medical tests. Patients should ask questions about tests and treatments recommended by their provider.

- Safe use of prescription drugs requires knowledge of what the medication is supposed to do, how and when to take it, and the possible side effects.

- All surgical procedures carry risk; patients should ask about alternatives and get a second opinion from another physician.

- Complementary and alternative medicine (CAM) is defined as those therapies and practices that do not form part of conventional health care and medical practice as taught in most U.S. medical schools and offered in most U.S. hospitals.

- Integrative medicine is a term used when CAM methods are *added* to conventional practice—conventional methods are considered first, and CAM may be included if it may have additional benefits.

- CAM is characterized by a view of health as a balance and integration of body, mind, and spirit and a body of knowledge based on the accumulated observations and experience of practitioners.

- Alternative medical systems such as traditional Chinese medicine and homeopathy are complete systems of medical philosophy, theory, and practice.

- Mind–body medicine includes meditation, biofeedback, group support, hypnosis, and prayer.

- Natural products include herbal remedies, botanicals, animal tissue products, and dietary supplements.

- Manipulative and body-based practices include massage and other healing techniques; the most frequently used is chiropractic.

- Other CAM practices include movement therapies, traditional healing practices, and energy therapies.

- Because there is presently less information available about CAM and less regulation of its providers and modalities, consumers must be proactive in researching and choosing treatments, using critical thinking skills.

- The Affordable Care Act and other recent government reforms of the health care system (particularly the insurance industry) aim to make affordable health insurance coverage available to more Americans.

- Health insurance plans are usually described as either fee-for-service (indemnity) or managed care plans. Indemnity plans allow consumers more choice in medical providers, but managed care plans are less expensive.

- Government programs include Medicaid for the poor, and Medicare for those aged 65 and over or chronically disabled.

FOR MORE INFORMATION

BOOKS

American College of Physicians. 2009. *The ACP Evidence-Based Guide to Complementary and Alternative Medicine.* Washington, DC: American College of Physicians. *Highly regarded manual of CAM practices and evidence supporting them.*

Micozzi, M. S. 2011. *Fundamentals of Complementary and Alternative Medicine,* 4th ed. New York: Saunders. *Detailed descriptions of the CAM modalities, with evidence supporting specific therapies for certain conditions.*

Physicians' Desk Reference. 2014. *PDR for Nonprescription Drugs,* 35th ed. Montvale, NJ: Thomson Healthcare. *A reference covering the safety and efficacy of over-the-counter medications and herbals.*

ORGANIZATIONS, HOTLINES, AND WEBSITES

American Board of Medical Specialties. Provides information about board certification, including information about specific physicians.

http://www.abms.org

American Chiropractic Association. Provides information about chiropractic care, consumer tips, and a searchable directory of certified chiropractors.

http://www.acatoday.org

American Medical Association (AMA). Provides information about physicians, including their training, licensure, and board certification.

http://www.ama-assn.org

American Osteopathic Association. Provides information about osteopathic physicians, including board certification.

http://www.osteopathic.org/Pages/default.aspx

ExerciseIsMedicine.org. Rationale to make exercise the next physical exam "vital sign" along with temperature, pulse, respiration, and blood pressure, and to strengthen the science and evidence for the efficacy of exercise prescription in health care settings.

www.exerciseismedicine.org

Food and Drug Administration: Information for Consumers. Provides materials about dietary supplements, foods, prescription and OTC drugs, and other FDA-regulated products.

http://www.fda.gov/ForConsumers/default.htm

National Center for Complementary and Alternative Medicine (NCCAM). Provides general information packets, answers to frequently asked questions about CAM, consumer advice for safer use of CAM, research abstracts, and bibliographies.

http://nccam.nih.gov

SELECTED BIBLIOGRAPHY

Abd Jalil, M. A., A. N. Shui, and N. Muhammed. 2012. Role of medicinal plants and natural products on osteoporotic fracture healing. *Evidence-Based Complementary and Alternative Medicine, 2* September (epub ahead of print).

American Academy of Family Physicians. 2014. *Patient Protection and Affordable Care Act (ACA)* (http://www.aafp.org/advocacy/informed/coverage/aca.html).

American Board of Medical Specialties. 2014. *Specialties & Subspecialties.* (www.abms.org/who_we_help/physicians/specialties.aspx).

Ayers, S. L., and J. J. Kronenfeld. 2012. Delays in seeking conventional medical care and complementary and alternative medicine utilization. *Health Services Research* 47(5): 2081–2096.

Baer, H. A. et al. 2012. A dialogue between naturopathy and critical medical anthropology: What constitutes holistic health? *Medical Anthropology Quarterly* 26(2): 241–256.

Bryan, S., G. P. Zipp, and R. Parasher. 2012. The effects of yoga on psychosocial variables and exercise adherence: A randomized, controlled pilot study. *Alternative Therapies in Health and Medicine* 18(5): 50–59.

Clear Bankruptcy. 2014. *10 Leading Causes of Bankruptcy* (http://www.clearbankruptcy.com/financial-literacy/10-leading-causes-of-bankruptcy.aspx).

Cramer, H., et al. 2012. Mindfulness-based stress reduction for low back pain: A systematic review. *BMC Complementary and Alternative Medicine* 12(1): 162.

Del Prete, A., et al. 2012 herbal products: Benefits, limits and applications in chronic liver disease. *Evidence-Based Complementary and Alternative Medicine,* 6 September (epub ahead of print).

D'Silva, S. et al. 2012. Mind–body medicine therapies for a range of depression severity: A systematic review. *Psychosomatics* 53(5): 407–423.

Fava, M. 2010. Using complementary and alternative medicines for depression. *Journal of Clinical Psychiatry* 71(9): e24.

Fronstin, P. 2012. Employment-based health benefits: Recent trends and future outlook. *Inquiry* 49(2): 101–115.

Gahche, J., et al. 2011. Dietary supplement use among U.S. adults has increased since NHANES III (1988–1994). *NCHS Data Brief,* no. 61. Hyattsville, MD: National Center for Health Statistics.

Harris, P., et al. 2012. Prevalence of complementary and alternative medicine (CAM) use by the general population: A systematic review and update. *International Journal of Clinical Practice* 66(10): 924–939.

Jahnke, R., et al. 2010. A comprehensive review of health benefits of qigong and tai chi. *American Journal of Health Promotion* 24(6): e1–e25.

Kanodia, A. K., et al. 2010. Perceived benefit of complementary and alternative medicine (CAM) for back pain: A national survey. *Journal of the American Board of Family Medicine* 23(3): 354–362.

Litscher, G., et al. 2012. High-tech acupuncture and integrative laser medicine. *Evidence-Based Complementary and Alternative Medicine,* 4 September (epub ahead of print).

Millet, J. D. 2010. Progress in complementary and alternative medicine research: Yale Research Symposium on Complementary and Integrative Medicine. *Yale Journal of Biology and Medicine* 83(3): 127–129.

O'Malley, P. A. 2012. Preventing and reporting adverse drug events: Pharmacovigilance for the clinical nurse specialist. *Clinical Nurse Specialist* 26(3): 136–137.

Sarris, J., et al. 2012. Complementary medicine, exercise, meditation, diet, and lifestyle modification for anxiety disorders: A review of current evidence. *Evidence-Based Complementary and Alternative Medicine,* 27 August (epub ahead of print).

Sasson, C. et al. 2012. The changing landscape of America's health care system and the value of emergency medicine. *Academy of Emergency Medicine,* 20 September (epub ahead of print).

Shen, P. F., et al. 2012. Acupuncture intervention in ischemic stroke: A randomized controlled prospective study. *American Journal of Chinese Medicine* 40(4): 685–693.

Society of Homeopaths. 2014. *What Is Homeopathy?* (http://www.homeopathy-soh.org/about-homeopathy/what-is-homeopathy/).

Spears, W., et al. 2012. Parents' perspectives on their children's health insurance: Plight of the underinsured. *Journal of Pediatrics,* 22 August (epub ahead of print).

Textbookdollars.com. 2014. *What Does Obamacare Mean for College Students?* (www.textbookdollars.com/blog/obamacare-college-students/).

Wahbeh, H., S. M. Elsas, and B. S. Oken. 2008. Mind–body interventions: Applications in neurology. *Neurology* 70(24): 2321–2328.

Wang, C., et al. 2010. A randomized trial of tai chi for fibromyalgia. *New England Journal of Medicine* 363(8): 743–754.

Young Invincibles. 2014. *Health Care.* (http://younginvincibles.org/issues/health-care/).

Zhao, X. F., et al. 2012. Mortality and recurrence of vascular disease among stroke patients treated with combined TCM therapy. *Journal of Traditional Chinese Medicine* 32(2): 173–178.

Zhuang, L. X., et al. 2012. An effectiveness study comparing acupuncture, physiotherapy, and their combination in poststroke rehabilitation: A multicentered, randomized, controlled clinical trial. *Alternative Therapies in Health and Medicine* 18(3): 8–14.

Personal Safety

CHAPTER **16**

CHAPTER OBJECTIVES

- Identify factors that contribute to unintentional injuries
- List the most common types of unintentional injuries and strategies for preventing them
- Describe factors that contribute to violence and intentional injuries
- Discuss different forms of violence and how to protect yourself from intentional injuries
- List strategies for helping others in an emergency situation

Each year more than 180,000 Americans die from injuries and many more are temporarily or permanently disabled. The economic cost of injuries is high, with over $750 billion spent each year for medical care and rehabilitation of injured people. Injuries also cause emotional suffering for injured people and their families, friends, and colleagues.

Engineering strategies such as safety belts can help lower injury rates, as can the passage and enforcement of safety-related laws, such as those requiring tamper-proof containers for OTC medications. Public education campaigns about risky behaviors such as driving under the influence of alcohol or smoking in bed can also help prevent injuries. Ultimately, though, it is up to each person to take responsibility for his or her actions and make wise choices about safety behaviors.

DIFFERENTIATING INJURIES

An **intentional injury** is one that is purposely inflicted by yourself or by another person. If an injury occurs when no harm is intended, it is considered an **unintentional injury.**

Motor vehicle crashes, falls, and fires often result in unintentional injuries. (Public health officials prefer not to use the word *accidents* to describe unintentional injuries because it suggests events beyond human control. *Injuries* are predictable outcomes of factors that can be controlled or prevented.)

Although Americans tend to express more concern about intentional injuries, unintentional injuries are actually far more common. Unintentional injuries are the fifth leading cause of death among all Americans and the leading cause of death among children and young adults. Because unintentional injuries are so common, they account for more **years of potential life lost** than any other cause of death.

TERMS

intentional injury An injury that is purposely inflicted by either yourself or another person.

unintentional injury An injury that occurs without harm being intended.

years of potential life lost The difference between an individual's life expectancy and his or her age at death.

UNINTENTIONAL INJURIES

Injury situations are generally categorized into four general classes, based on where they occur: motor vehicle injuries, home injuries, leisure injuries, and work injuries. The greatest number of disabling injuries occur in the home (Table 16.1).

What Causes an Injury?

Most injuries are caused by a combination of human and environmental factors. Human factors are inner conditions or attitudes that lead to an unsafe state, whether physical, emotional, or psychological. Environmental factors are external conditions and circumstances, such as poor road conditions, a slippery surface, or the undertow of the ocean at the beach.

A common human factor that leads to injuries is risk-taking behavior. People vary in the amount of risk they tend to take in life, but young men are especially prone to taking risks (see the box "Injuries among Young Men"). Alcohol and drug use is another common risk factor that leads to many injuries and deaths.

Psychological and emotional factors can also play a role in injuries. People sometimes act on the basis of inadequate or inaccurate beliefs about what is safe or unsafe. However, many people who have accurate information still decide to engage in risky behavior. Young people often have unsafe attitudes, such as "I won't get hurt" or "It won't happen to me." Such attitudes can lead to risk taking and ultimately to injuries.

Environmental factors leading to injury may be natural (weather conditions), social (a drunk driver), work-related (defective equipment), or home-related (faulty wiring). Making the environment safer is an important aspect of safety. Laws are often passed to try to make our environment safer. Examples include speed limits on highways and workplace safety requirements.

Motor Vehicle Injuries

According to the National Safety Council (NSC), nearly 35,000 Americans were killed and nearly 3.7 million injured in motor vehicle crashes in 2011. Motor vehicle deaths in this country have decreased by 24% in the last decade. Worldwide, motor vehicle crashes kill 1.3 million and injure up to 50 million people each year, making motor vehicle injuries the 11th leading cause of death overall. **Motor vehicle injuries** also result in the majority of cases of paralysis due to spinal injuries, and they are the leading cause of severe brain injury in the United States.

Factors Contributing to Motor Vehicle Injuries
Common causes of motor vehicle injuries are speeding, aggressive driving, fatigue, inexperience, the use of cell phones, handheld devices, and other distractions, the use of alcohol and other drugs, and the incorrect use of safety belts and other safety devices.

TERMS

motor vehicle injuries Unintentional injuries and deaths involving motor vehicles in motion, both on and off the highway or street; incidents causing motor vehicle injuries include collisions between vehicles and collisions with objects or pedestrians.

Table 16.1	Unintentional Injuries in the United States (2009)	
	DEATHS	DISABLING INJURIES
Home	60,600	18.8 million
Motor vehicle	34,600	3.7 million
Leisure	25,500	9.7 million
Work	3,909	5.0 million
All classes*	122,900	37.0 million

*Deaths and injuries for the four separate classes total more than the "All classes" figures because of rounding and because some deaths and injuries are included in more than one class.

SOURCE: National Safety Council. 2013. *Injury Facts, 2013 Edition.* Itasca, IL: National Safety Council.

VITAL STATISTICS

Table 16.2	Lifetime Odds of Death Due to Injury
Motor vehicle	1 in 108
Suicide	1 in 109
Poisoning	1 in 123
Fall	1 in 158
Homicide (assault by firearm)	1 in 340
Car occupant	1 in 415
Pedestrian	1 in 749
Drowning	1 in 1,112
Fire	1 in 1,419
Choking from inhalation and ingestion of food	1 in 3,842
Exposure to excessive natural cold	1 in 6,349
Firearm discharge	1 in 7,059
Electric current	1 in 12,146
Exposure to natural heat	1 in 11,111
Hornet/bee/wasp sting	1 in 71,107
Lightning	1 in 126,158

SOURCE: National Safety Council. 2013. *Lifetime Odds of Deaths for Selected Causes, U.S.* Itasca, IL: National Safety Council.

Overall, rates of injury are highest among young adults and seniors over age 75. Except among the oldest group of adults, the nonfatal injury rate is substantially higher in males than in females—and it peaks among young adult males (see figure). Males also significantly outnumber females in injury deaths, whether unintentional or intentional.

Why do men, especially young men, have such high rates of injury? Gender roles may be a key factor: Traditional gender roles for males may associate masculinity with risk-taking behavior and a disregard for pain and injury, and risk-taking behavior may be particularly common among young men. Men are more likely to drive dangerously, drink and drive, binge-drink, and use aggressive behavior to control situations—all of which can lead to higher rates of fatal and nonfatal injury. Men may also have a lower perception of risk of dangerous behaviors compared with women.

Traditional gender roles may also make it more difficult for men to admit to injury or emotional vulnerability. Physical injuries may worsen or become chronic if care is not sought promptly. Untreated depression can lead to suicide.

In addition, men may have greater exposure to some injury situations. Compared with women, men may drive more miles, have greater access to

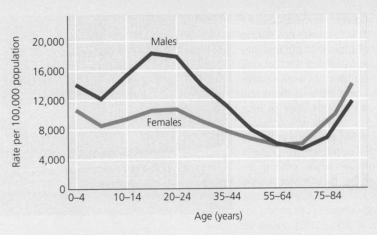

Nonfatal injury rate by age and sex.

firearms, and be more likely to ride motorcycles, operate machinery, and have jobs associated with high rates of workplace injuries. They may be more likely to engage in sports and other recreational activities that are associated with high rates of injuries. Greater access to and use of firearms plays a role in higher rates of deaths among men from assault and suicide. As described in Chapter 3, women are more likely than men to attempt suicide, but men are much more likely to succeed, primarily because they are more likely to use firearms.

Some researchers suggest that the male hormone testosterone may play a role in risky and aggressive behavior.

Differences in brain structure and activity may also influence how men and women respond to stressors and how quickly and to what degree they become verbally or physically aggressive in response to anger.

SOURCES: Centers for Disease Control and Prevention. 2004. Surveillance for fatal and nonfatal injuries—United States, 2001. *MMWR Surveillance Summaries* 53(SS07): 1–57; World Health Organization. 2002. *Gender and Road Traffic Injuries.* Geneva: WHO; Courtenay, W. 1998. College men's health: An overview and a call to action. *Journal of American College Health* 46(6): 279–290.

SPEEDING Nearly two-thirds of all motor vehicle crashes are caused by bad driving behaviors, especially speeding. As speed increases, momentum and the force of impact increase, and the time allowed for the driver to react (reaction time) decreases. Speed limits are posted to establish the safest maximum speed limit for a given area under ideal conditions; if visibility is limited or the road is wet, the safe maximum speed may be considerably lower.

AGGRESSIVE DRIVING Aggressive driving includes frequent, erratic, and abrupt lane changes; tailgating; running red lights or stop signs; passing on the shoulder; and blocking other cars trying to change lanes or pass. Aggressive drivers increase the risk of crashes for themselves and others. Injuries may also occur if aggressive drivers stop their vehicles and confront each other following an incident.

FATIGUE AND SLEEPINESS Driving requires mental alertness and attentiveness. Studies have shown that sleepiness causes slower reaction times, reduced coordination and vigilance, and delayed information processing. Research shows that even mild sleep deprivation causes deterioration in driving ability comparable to that caused by a 0.05% blood alcohol concentration—a level considered hazardous when driving.

CELL PHONES, HANDHELD DEVICES, AND OTHER DISTRACTIONS Anything that distracts a driver can increase the risk of a motor vehicle injury. Common distractions include talking to someone on a cell phone or in the vehicle, texting, eating, smoking, and reaching for controls in the car. Objects and activities outside the vehicle are sources of distraction as well. More than a dozen U.S. cities have banned digital billboards because of their potential to distract drivers. Several common causes of crashes, such as disregarding stop signs,

Cell Phones, Texting, and Distracted Driving

At any given moment, about 1 out of 11 U.S. drivers are talking on a cell phone. To put that into perspective, a recent telephone survey of 18- to 24-year-olds revealed over 50% of them use their cell phones daily or several times a week while driving.

Available evidence indicates that the distraction of using a cell phone while driving increases the risk of motor vehicle crashes. In a study using a driver training simulator, cell phone users were about 20% slower to respond to sudden hazards than were other drivers, and they were about twice as likely to rear-end a braking car in front of them. Among young adult drivers who used cell phones, reaction time was reduced to the level of a 70-year-old driver who was not using a phone.

More people are now being observed texting while driving, which is potentially more dangerous because most individuals need to look directly at the screen of their handheld devices to send and read messages. Results of a study of college-aged students texting while operating a driving simulator revealed their risk of crashing was multiplied by a factor of 8 (compared to a group of college-aged students talking on their cell phone whose risk had increased by a factor of 4).

Several states have banned the use of cell phones while driving and even more prohibit the use of devices to text message or e-mail. Although using your phone for calling or texting while driving is legal in some states, your safest strategy is not to use your phone for either while driving. For people who live where cell phone use is legal while driving and who choose to use a phone, the following strategies may help increase safety:

- Be familiar with your phone and its functions, especially speed dial and redial.

- Store frequently called numbers on speed dial so you can place calls without looking at the phone.

- If your phone has voice-activated dialing, use it.

- Use a hands-free device so you can keep both hands on the steering wheel.

- Let the person you are speaking with know you are driving and be prepared to end the call at any time.

- Don't place or answer calls in heavy traffic or hazardous weather conditions.

- Don't take notes or look up phone numbers while driving.

- Time calls so you can place them when you are at a stop.

SOURCES: AAA Foundation for Traffic Safety. 2009. *Safety Culture: Text Messaging and Cell Phone Use While Driving* (www.aaafoundation.org/pdf/TextingFS091012.pdf); TXTResponsibly. 2012. *Gauging Your Distraction* (www.txtresponsibly.org/resources/tools/); National Safety Council. 2012. *Distracted Driving* (www.nsc.org/safety_road/Distracted_Driving/Pages/distracted_driving.aspx).

have been linked to driver distraction. Distraction is a contributing factor in 25–50% of all crashes. About 70% of distracted driver crashes involve noncollision (single-vehicle) or rear-end crashes.

Cell phones are a widely documented source of distraction for drivers. One highly regarded study showed that drivers who use cell phones are four times as likely to be involved in a crash as drivers who don't, primarily because the distraction increases reaction times. Estimates provided by the NSC attribute 1.3 million traffic crashes (about 24% of all crashes) to the use of cell phones and text messaging. So far, 12 states (California, Connecticut, Delaware, Hawaii, Illinois, Maryland, New Jersey, Nevada, New York, Oregon, Washington, and West Virginia), the District of Columbia, Guam, Puerto Rico, and the U.S. Virgin Islands have banned the use of handheld phones while driving. Other states are considering similar legislation. In 37 states and the District of Columbia, novice drivers are banned from using either handheld or hands-free cell phones while driving (see the box "Cell Phones, Texting, and Distracted Driving"). Currently 41 states, the District of Columbia, and Guam now ban all drivers from text messaging while driving; another six states have no-texting laws that apply specifically to novice drivers. Given increasing concerns about distractions when driving, the National Transportation Safety Board (NTSB) recommended, in December 2011, a full ban on use of portable electronic devices (including cell phones) while driving. Drivers could still use their GPS navigation systems and their cell phones in emergency situations.

ALCOHOL AND OTHER DRUGS Alcohol is involved in about 3 out of 10 fatal crashes. Alcohol-impaired driving is illegal in all states and the District of Columbia. The legal limit for blood alcohol concentration (BAC) is 0.08%, but people can be impaired at much lower BACs. Because alcohol affects reason and judgment as well as the ability to make fast, accurate, and coordinated movements, a person who has been drinking will be less likely to recognize that he or she is impaired.

Use of many over-the-counter and all psychoactive drugs is potentially dangerous if you plan to drive.

SAFETY BELTS, AIRBAGS, AND CHILD SAFETY SEATS   Although mandatory safety belt laws are in effect in 49 states (excluding New Hampshire) and the District of Columbia, only 86% of motor vehicle occupants used safety belts in 2012, even though they are the single most effective way to reduce the risk of crash-related death. Combination lap and shoulder belts are even more effective in improving survival rates.

Some people think that if they are involved in a crash they are better off being thrown free of their vehicle. In fact, the chances of being killed are 25 times greater if you are thrown from a vehicle, whether it is due to injuries caused by hitting a tree or the pavement or by being hit by another vehicle. Safety belts not only prevent you from being thrown from the car at the time of the crash but also provide protection from second collisions: If a car is traveling at 65 mph and hits another vehicle, the car stops first; then the occupants stop because they, too, are traveling at 65 mph. Second collisions occur when occupants hit something inside the car, such as the dashboard or windshield. Safety belts stop these second collisions from occurring and spread the first collisions' force over the occupants' bodies.

Since 1998 all new cars and light trucks have been equipped with dual airbags—one for the driver and one for the front passenger. Many vehicles also offer side airbags, which further reduce the risk of injury. Advanced airbag systems include risk reduction technologies such as sensors to detect crash severity, seat position, passenger size, and whether a passenger is wearing a safety belt. Although airbags provide supplementary protection in the event of a collision, most are useful only in head-on collisions. They also deflate immediately after inflating and therefore do not provide protection in collisions involving multiple impacts. Airbags are not a replacement for safety belts; everyone in a vehicle should buckle up.

Airbags deploy forcefully and can injure a child or short adult who is improperly restrained or sitting too close to the dashboard, although second-generation airbags are somewhat safer for children than older devices. To ensure that airbags work safely, always follow these basic guidelines: Place infants in rear-facing infant seats in the back seat, transport children aged 12 and under in the back seat, always use safety belts and appropriate safety seats, and keep 10 inches between the airbag cover and the breastbone of the driver or passenger. If necessary, adjust the steering wheel or use seat cushions to ensure that an inflating airbag will hit a person in the chest and not in the face. Children who have outgrown child safety seats but are still too small for adult safety belts alone (usually aged 4–8). These children should be secured using booster seats that ensure that the safety belt is positioned low across the waist.

Preventing Motor Vehicle Injuries   About 75% of all motor vehicle collisions occur within 25 miles of home and at speeds lower than 40 mph. Strategies for preventing motor vehicle injuries include the following:

- Obey the speed limit.
- Always wear a safety belt.
- Never drive under the influence of alcohol or other drugs, and never ride with a driver who is.
- Keep your car in good working order.
- Always allow enough following distance. Use the three-second rule: When the vehicle ahead passes a reference point, count out three seconds. If you pass the reference point before you finish counting, drop back and allow more following distance. This rule works well at slower speeds when roads are dry and weather conditions are good. When traveling on highways or in poor weather conditions, allow four seconds.
- Choose interstate highways rather than rural roads. Highways are much safer because of better visibility, wider lanes, fewer surprises, and other factors.
- Always signal when turning or changing lanes.
- Stop completely at stop signs. Follow all traffic laws.
- Take special care at intersections. Look left, right, and then left again. Make sure you have time to complete your maneuver in the intersection.
- Don't pass on two-lane roads unless you're in a designated passing area and have a clear view ahead.

> Airbags are **not a replacement for safety belts;** everyone in a vehicle should buckle up.

Motorcycles and Motorized Scooters   About one out of every seven traffic fatalities among people aged 15–34 involves someone riding a motorcycle. The data also reveal that motorcycle riders are 35 times more likely to die in a crash than occupants of a car or other motor vehicle. Injuries from motorcycle collisions are generally more severe than those involving automobiles because motorcycles provide little, if any, protection.

People riding motorized scooters face additional challenges. Such vehicles usually have a maximum speed of 30–35 mph and have less power for maneuverability, especially in an emergency.

Strategies for preventing motorcycle and motor scooter injuries include the following:

- Wear light-colored clothing, drive with your headlights on, and correctly position yourself in traffic.
- Develop the necessary skills. Lack of skill is a major factor in motorcycle and motor scooter injuries.

CRITICAL CONSUMER
Choosing a Bicycle Helmet

Wearing a bicycle helmet can help you avoid serious head injury, brain damage, or even death in the event of a collision or fall. Helmets have a layer of stiff foam, which absorbs shock and cushions a blow to your head, covered by a thin plastic shell that will skid along the ground. For maximum protection, it's important to select a correctly fitting helmet. When you go shopping, remember the four S's: size, strap, straight, and sticker.

• *Size:* Try on several different sizes before making your selection; it may take several tries before you find the most comfortable fit. The helmet should be very snug but not overly tight on your head. Pads are usually provided to help adjust the fit. A good salesperson can also help you get the right fit. When the helmet is strapped onto your head, it should not move more than an inch in any direction, and you should not be able to pull or twist it off no matter how hard you try.

• *Strap:* Be sure that the chinstrap fits snugly under your chin and that the V in the strap meets under your ear. Avoid thin straps, which can be uncomfortable. Be sure that the buckle is strong and won't pop open and that the straps are sturdy.

• *Straight:* The helmet should sit straight on your head, not tilted back or forward. A rule of thumb is that the rim should be about two finger widths above your eyebrows (depending on the height of your forehead).

• *Sticker:* Helmets sold in the United States must meet uniform safety standards established by the U.S. Consumer Product Safety Commission (CPSC). Look for a sticker or label that says the helmet meets the CPSC standard. If a helmet does not have one, it does not meet federal safety standards and should not be used.

You are more likely to wear your helmet if it is comfortable, so be sure that vents on the helmet provide airflow to promote cooling and sweat control. You will be safer with a brightly colored helmet that makes you more visible to drivers, especially in rainy, foggy, or dark conditions. Reflective tape will also increase your visibility. Finally, a helmet is a good place to put emergency information (your name, address, and phone number, plus any emergency medical conditions and an emergency contact).

If you are involved in a crash, replace your helmet. Even if the helmet doesn't have any visible signs of damage, its ability to protect your head may be compromised.

sources: Bicycle Helmet Safety Institute. 2010. *A Buyer's Guide to Bicycle Helmets* (www.helmets .org/guide.htm); Bicycle Helmet Safety Institute. 2010. *How to Fit a Bicycle Helmet* (www .helmets.org/fit.htm).

Skidding from improper braking is the most common cause of loss of control.

• Wear a helmet. Helmets should be marked with the DOT symbol, certifying that they conform to federal safety standards established by the U.S. Department of Transportation. Helmet use is required by law in most states.

• Protect your eyes with goggles, a face shield, or a windshield.

• Drive defensively, particularly when changing lanes and at intersections, and never assume that other drivers can see you.

Bicycles Bicycle injuries result primarily from riders not knowing or understanding the rules of the road, failing to follow traffic laws, not having sufficient skill or experience to handle traffic conditions, or being intoxicated. Bicycles are considered vehicles; bicyclists must obey all traffic laws that apply to automobile drivers, including stopping at traffic lights and stop signs.

Head injuries are involved in about three out of four bicycle-related deaths. Wearing a helmet reduces the risk of head injury by 66% to 88% (see the box "Choosing a Bicycle Helmet"). Safe cycling strategies include the following:

• Wear safety equipment, including a helmet, eye protection, gloves, and proper footwear. Secure the bottom of your pant legs with clips, and secure your shoelaces so they don't get tangled in the chain.

• Wear light-colored, reflective clothing. Equip your bike with reflectors, and use lights, especially at night or when riding in wooded or other dark areas.

• Ride with the flow of traffic, not against it, and follow all traffic laws. Use bike paths when they are available.

• Ride defensively; never assume that drivers have seen you. Be especially careful when turning or crossing at corners and intersections. Watch for cars turning right.

• Stop at all traffic lights and stop signs. Know and use hand signals.

Pedestrians About one in seven motor vehicle deaths involves pedestrians, and more than 160,000 pedestrians are injured each year. The highest rates of death and injury occur among the very young and the elderly. About 4 out of 10 pedestrian deaths occur when people cross or enter the roadway between intersectins. Alcohol intoxication plays a significant role in up to half of all adult pedestrian fatalities. Walkers and runners should face traffic and cross only at marked crosswalks and intersections.

Home Injuries

The most common fatal **home injuries** are the result of falls, fires, poisoning, choking, drowning, and unintentional shootings.

Falls Most deaths occurring from falls involve falling on stairs or steps or from one level to another. Falls also occur on the same level, from tripping, slipping, or stumbling. Alcohol is a contributing factor in many falls. Strategies for preventing falls include the following:

- Install handrails and nonslip surfaces in the shower and bathtub.
- Keep floors, stairs, and outside areas clear of objects or conditions that could cause slipping or tripping, such as ice, snow, electrical cords, and toys.
- Put a light switch by the door of every room so no one has to walk across a room to turn on a light. Use night lights in bedrooms, halls, stairs, and bathrooms.
- When climbing a ladder, use both hands. Never stand higher than the third step from the top. When using a stepladder, make sure the spreader brace is in the locked position. With straight ladders, set the base out one foot for every four feet of height.
- Don't use chairs to reach things.
- If there are small children in the home, place gates at the top and bottom of stairs. Never leave a baby unattended on a bed or table. Install window guards to prevent children from falling out of windows.

Fires Most fires begin in the kitchen, living room, or bedroom. Cooking is now the leading cause of home fire injuries; careless smoking is the leading cause of fire deaths, followed by problems with heating equipment and arson. To prevent fires, it's important to dispose of all cigarettes in ashtrays and to never smoke in bed. Other strategies include proper maintenance of fireplaces, furnaces, heaters, chimneys, and electrical outlets, cords, and appliances. If you use a portable heater, keep it at least three feet away from curtains, bedding, or anything else that might catch fire. Never leave heaters on unattended.

It's important to be adequately prepared to handle fire-related situations. Plan at least two escape routes out of each room, and designate a location outside the home as a meeting place. For practice, stage a home fire drill; do this at night because that's when most deadly fires occur.

Data show that about three out of five home fire deaths occur in homes with no working smoke alarms. Install smoke detectors on every level of your home. Your risk of dying in a fire is almost twice as high if you do not use them.

These strategies can help prevent injuries in a fire:

- Get out as quickly as possible, and go to the designated meeting place. Don't stop for a keepsake or a pet. Never hide in a closet or under a bed. Once outside, count heads to see if everyone is out. If you think someone is still inside the burning building, tell the firefighters. Never go back inside a burning building.
- If you're trapped in a room, feel the door. If it is hot or if smoke is coming in through the cracks, don't open it; use the alternative escape route. If you can't get out, go to the window and shout for help.
- Smoke inhalation is the largest cause of death and injury in fires. To avoid inhaling smoke, crawl along the floor away from the heat and smoke. Cover your mouth and nose, ideally with a wet cloth, and take short, shallow breaths.
- If your clothes catch fire, don't run. Drop to the ground, cover your face, and roll back and forth to smother the flames. Remember: stop–drop–roll.

Poisoning More than 2.5 million poisonings and over 35,000 poison-related deaths occur every year in the United States. Most poison exposures are unintentional. Poisonous substances include cleaning agents, petroleum-based products, insecticides and herbicides, cosmetics, nail polish and remover, and many houseplants. Drug overdoses, whether from prescription drugs, recreational drugs, or combinations of drugs and alcohol, are classified as poisonings. All potentially poisonous substances should be used only as directed and stored out of the reach of children.

The most common type of poisoning by gases is carbon monoxide poisoning. Carbon monoxide gas is emitted by motor vehicle exhaust and some types of heating equipment. The effects of exposure to this colorless, odorless gas include headache, blurred vision, and shortness of breath, followed by dizziness, vomiting, and unconsciousness. Carbon monoxide detectors (similar to smoke detectors) are available for home use; they should be used according to the manufacturer's instructions. To prevent poisoning by gases, never operate a vehicle in an enclosed space, have your furnace inspected yearly, and use caution with any substance or device that produces potentially toxic fumes.

Keep the national poison control hotline number (800-222-1222) in a convenient location. A call to the national hotline will be routed to a local poison control center, which

> **home injuries** Unintentional injuries and deaths that occur in the home and on home premises to occupants, guests, domestic servants, and trespassers; falls, burns, poisonings, suffocations, unintentional shootings, drownings, and electrical shocks are examples. **TERMS**

provides expert emergency advice 24 hours a day. If a poisoning occurs, it's important that you act quickly. Remove the poison from contact with the victim's eyes, skin, or mouth, or move the victim away from contact with poisonous gases. Call the poison control center immediately for instructions; do not follow the emergency instructions on product labels because they may be incorrect. Depending on the situation, you may be instructed to give the victim water to drink, or to flush affected parts of the skin or eyes with water. Do not induce vomiting. If you are advised to go to a hospital emergency department, take the poisonous substance or container with you.

Suffocation and Choking Suffocation and choking account for over 6,000 deaths annually. Children can suffocate if they put small items in their mouth, get tangled in their crib bedding, or get trapped in airtight appliances like old refrigerators. Keep small objects out of reach of children under age 3, and don't give them raw carrots, hot dogs, popcorn, gum, or hard candy. Examine toys carefully for small parts that could come loose. Don't give plastic bags or balloons to small children.

Adults can also become choking victims, especially if they fail to chew food properly, eat hurriedly, or try to talk and eat at the same time. Many choking victims can be saved with the **Heimlich maneuver.** The American Red Cross recommends abdominal thrusts as the easiest and safest thing to do when an adult is choking. Back blows in conjunction with abdominal thrusts are an acceptable procedure for dislodging an object from the throat of an infant.

Firearms Over one-third of all unintended firearm deaths and nonfatal injuries involve children and young adults under 25 years of age. People who use firearms should remember the following:

- Always treat a gun as though it were loaded, even if you know it isn't.

- Never point a gun—loaded or unloaded—at anything you do not intend to shoot.

- Always unload a gun before storing it. Store unloaded firearms under lock and key, in a place separate from the ammunition.

- Always inspect firearms carefully before handling.

Heimlich maneuver A maneuver developed by
Henry J. Heimlich, M.D., to help force an obstruction
from the airway.

TERMS

leisure injuries Unintentional injuries and deaths that occur in public places, or places used in a public way, not involving motor vehicles; include most sports and recreation deaths and injuries; examples are falls, drownings, burns, and heat and cold stress.

personal flotation device A device designed to save a person from drowning by buoying up the body while in the water.

- If you ever plan to handle a gun, take a firearms safety course first.

- If you own a gun, buy and use a gun lock designed specifically for that weapon.

Proper storage is critical. Do not assume that young children cannot fire a gun. Every year, over 100 Americans are unintentionally shot to death by children under 6.

If you plan to handle a gun, avoid alcohol and drugs, which affect judgment and coordination.

Leisure Injuries

Leisure activities encompass a large part of our free time, so it is not surprising that **leisure injuries** are a significant health-related problem in the United States. Specific safety strategies for activities associated with leisure injuries include the following:

- Don't swim alone, in unsupervised places, under the influence of alcohol, or for an unusual length of time. Use caution when swimming in unfamiliar surroundings or in water colder than 70°F. Check the depth of water before diving. Make sure that residential pools are fenced and that children are never allowed to swim unsupervised.

- Always use a **personal flotation device** (also known as a life jacket) when on a boat.

- For all sports and recreational activities, make sure facilities are safe, follow the rules, and practice good sportsmanship. Develop adequate skill in the activity, and use proper safety equipment, including, where appropriate, a helmet, eye protection, correct footwear, and knee, elbow, and wrist pads.

- If using equipment such as skateboards, snowboards, mountain bikes, or all-terrain vehicles, wear a helmet and other safety equipment, and avoid excessive speeds and unsafe stunts. Playground equipment should be used only for those activities for which it is designed.

- If you are active in excessively hot and humid weather, drink plenty of fluids, rest frequently in the shade, and slow down or stop if you feel uncomfortable. Danger signals of heat stress include excessive perspiration, dizziness, headache, muscle cramps, nausea, weakness, rapid pulse, and disorientation.

- Do not use alcohol or other drugs during recreational activities—such activities require coordination and sound judgment.

Weather-Related Injuries

Even though conditions may seem harmless at times, they can become very dangerous.

- *Heat:* Extreme heat is the leading weather-related killer in the United States, according to the National Weather Service. Heat-related illness such as heat stroke and heat exhaustion can be fatal, especially for children, older adults, and people who are dehydrated. The best way to deal with excessive heat is to stay indoors as much as possible, with a fan or air conditioner on. Wear lightweight, light-colored clothing, drink plenty of water to stay hydrated, and avoid heavy meals.

- *Cold:* Conditions such as hypothermia (low body temperature) and frostbite (frozen skin or flesh) can be deadly. If you must go outdoors in very cold weather, dress in layers and cover your face, fingers, and ears to protect them from frostbite. Make sure your home and car are prepared with plenty of fuel, drinking water, warm clothes and blankets, batteries, and other emergency supplies.

- *Wind:* In extremely windy conditions, take cover in a sturdy shelter, preferably a permanent structure with a foundation. In a severe storm such as a tornado, move to the lowest portion of the building or to a small interior room away from windows. If you're outdoors when a severe storm or tornado strikes, lie flat in a low spot or ditch. Don't stay inside a car or hide under an open-sided structure such as a bridge; such structures can act as a funnel and make wind more intense.

- *Lightning:* About 400 Americans are struck by lightning every year, and about 10% of them die. When conditions are right for lightning, go indoors. Stay out of water, even indoors, because water pipes can conduct electricity. Don't use corded telephones or appliances because their wiring can also conduct the power from a lightning strike.

- *Flooding:* If you're near rapidly rising water, move to higher ground and call for help. Don't attempt to drive or walk through flooded streets, and don't traverse a bridge if it is being pounded by high, fast-moving water.

Work Injuries

The Bureau of Labor Statistics estimates that over 3 million Americans suffered injuries on the job in 2012. More than half of those injuries resulted in days away from work, job transfer, or some kind of restriction. Certain types of **work injuries,** including skin disorders and repetitive strain injuries, are increasing. Although laborers make up less than half of the workforce, they account for more than 75% of all

> Laborers constitute less than half of the American workforce but **suffer 75% of all work-related injuries.**

work-related injuries and illnesses. Most fatal occupational injuries involve crushing injuries, severe lacerations, burns, and electrocutions. In November 2013, OSHA proposed a new rule to improve tracking of workplace injuries and illnesses through electronic submission of data on a quarterly basis.

Back problems accounted for over 225,000 work injuries in 2011; Many back injuries that occur on the job could be prevented through proper lifting technique.

- Avoid bending at the waist. Remain in an upright position and crouch down if you need to lower yourself to grasp the object. Bend at the knees and hips.
- Place feet securely about shoulder-width apart; grip the object firmly.
- Lift gradually, with straight arms. Avoid quick, jerky motions. Lift by standing up or pushing with your leg muscles. Keep the object close to your body.
- If you have to turn, change the position of your feet. Twisting is a common and dangerous cause of injury. Plan ahead so that your pathway is clear and turning can be minimized.
- Put the object down gently, reversing the steps for lifting.

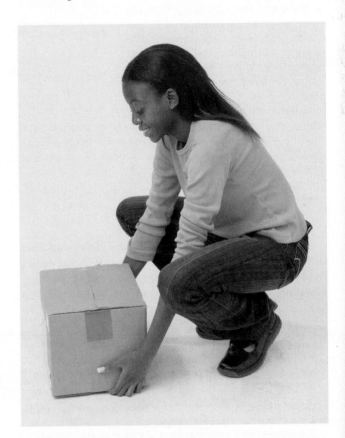

The correct lifting technique is to stay upright, bending at the knees and hips.

TAKE CHARGE
Repetitive Strain Injury

Repetitive strain injuries (RSIs) impact the musculoskeletal and nervous systems of the body and affect many people around the world. Other terms to describe this condition include *repetitive motion disorder (RMD), cumulative trauma disorder (CTD),* and *occupational overuse syndrome (OOS).*

An RSI can be caused by a combination of physical and psychosocial stressors, but the injury typically involves some kind of repetitive action or forceful exertion on the body over time. Pain in the extremities as well as the back and shoulders is commonly cited and tends to worsen with extended activity.

The task associated with an RSI may be something relatively simple and nonexertive like typing, writing, or clicking a computer mouse. One of the most common work-related injuries is *carpal tunnel syndrome (CTS),* which is characterized by pressure on the median nerve in the wrist that also affects tendons and ligaments in the forearm. Symptoms of CTS include numbness, tingling, burning, and/or aching in the hand, particularly in the thumb and the first three fingers. The pain may worsen at night and may shoot up from the hand as far as the shoulder. If it does not clear up on its own, immobilization of the joint at night can be helpful; other options may involve anti-inflammatory drugs or even surgery in extreme cases.

In terms of physical activity by an athlete, examples include conditions commonly referred to as "golfer's elbow" or "tennis elbow," where the joints are continually exposed to extreme stress in order to complete an action accurately with speed and force.

With new technologies being introduced every day, another type of RSI is now being recognized. Many people who use their thumbs to text are suffering from a condition referred to as "Blackberry thumb." Similarly, people who spend countless hours using handheld controls to play video games are experiencing "gamer's thumb."

In all cases, research indicates the primary risk factors are usually associated with poor posture, improper techniques for completing an activity, and overuse of a certain part of the body. The good news is that a person can make adjustments to reduce the risk of an RSI, either in what is being done or through modification of the environment. Warm up your wrists before you begin any repetitive motion activity, and take frequent breaks to stretch and flex your wrists and hands:

- Extend your arms out in front of you and stretch your wrists by pointing your fingers to the ceiling; hold for a count of five. Then straighten your wrists and relax your fingers for a count of five.

- With arms extended, make a tight fist with both hands and then bend your wrists so your knuckles are pointed toward the floor; hold for a count of five. Then straighten your wrists and relax your fingers for a count of five.

Repeat these stretches several times, and finish by letting your arms hang loosely at your sides and shaking them gently for several seconds. It's also important to maintain a physically active lifestyle, take plenty of breaks to avoid hours of sedentary activity, continue stretching during an activity, apply proper ergonomic principles, and try to minimize other stress factors.

Carpal tunnel

Ligament

Tendon sheath

Tendons

Median nerve

Carpals

Musculoskeletal injuries and disorders in the workplace include **repetitive strain injuries (RSIs).** RSIs are caused by repeated strain on a particular part of the body. Twisting, vibrations, awkward postures, and other stressors may contribute to RSIs. **Carpal tunnel syndrome** is one type of RSI that has increased in recent years due to increased use of computers, both at work and in the home (see the box "Repetitive Strain Injury" for more information).

repetitive strain injury (RSI) A musculoskeletal injury or disorder caused by repeated strain on the hand, arm, wrist, or other part of the body; also called *cumulative trauma disorder (CTD).*

carpal tunnel syndrome Compression of the median nerve in the wrist, often caused by repetitive use of the hands, such as in computer use; characterized by numbness, tingling, and pain in the hands and fingers; can cause nerve damage.

TERMS

Ask Yourself

QUESTIONS FOR CRITICAL THINKING AND REFLECTION

Think of one injury you have suffered. What were you doing when you were injured? Thinking back on the injury, was there anything you could have done to avoid or minimize it? How did the experience change your attitudes or behaviors?

VIOLENCE AND INTENTIONAL INJURIES

Violence—the use of physical force with the intent to inflict harm, injury, or death upon yourself or another—is a major public health concern in the United States. According to the Federal Bureau of Investigation (FBI), over 1.2 million violent crimes occurred in the United States in 2012. Examples of violence are assault, homicide, sexual assault, domestic violence, suicide, and child abuse. In comparison to other industrialized countries, U.S. rates of violence are unusually high in only two areas—homicide and firearm-related deaths.

Factors Contributing to Violence

Most intentional injuries and deaths are associated with an argument or the committing of another crime. However, there are many forms of violence, and no single factor can explain all of them.

Social Factors Rates of violence are not the same throughout society; they vary by geographic region, neighborhood, socioeconomic level, and many other factors. According to the FBI, violence was highest in the South in 2012, followed by the Midwest region of the country. Neighborhoods that are disadvantaged in status, power, and economic resources are typically the ones with the most violence. Rates of violence are highest among young people and minorities, groups that have relatively little power. In 2012 people under age 25 accounted for 4 out of 10 arrests for violent crime in the United States and nearly half (48%) of the arrests for property crime.

People who feel a part of society (have strong family and social ties), who are economically integrated (have a reasonable chance at getting a decent job), and who grow up in areas where there is a feeling of community (good schools, parks, and neighborhoods) are significantly less likely to engage in violence.

Studies have shown that the environment on some college campuses can contribute to violence. Because college campuses are transitory communities some people may have less incentive to cooperate and coexist amicably.

Violence in the Media The mass media play a major role in exposing audiences of all ages to violence as an acceptable and effective means of solving problems. On the average, children in the United States watch about four hours of television daily and may view as many as 10,000 violent acts on television and in movies each year. Computer and video games also include many violent acts, leading to concern that children's exposure to violence will make them more accepting or tolerant of it. The consequences of violence are depicted much less frequently.

Researchers have found that exposure to media violence at least temporarily increases aggressive feelings in children, making them more likely to engage in violent or fearful behavior; the direct, short-term effects on teens and adults are less clear. Parents should monitor the TV shows, movies, video games, music, and other forms of media to which children are exposed. Watching programs with children gives parents the opportunity to talk to children about violence and its consequences, to explain that violence is not the best way to resolve conflicts or solve problems, and to point out examples of positive behaviors such as kindness and cooperation.

Gender In most cases, violence is committed by men (Figure 16.1). Males are nine times more likely than females to commit murder, and three times more likely than females to be murdered. Male college students are twice as likely to be the victim of violence as female students.

Women do commit acts of violence, including a small but substantial proportion of murders of spouses. This fact has been used to argue that women have the same capacity to commit violence as men, but most researchers note substantial differences. Men often kill their wives as the culmination of years of violence or after stalking them; they may kill their entire families and themselves at the same time. Women virtually never kill in such circumstances; rather, they kill their husbands after repeated victimization or while being beaten.

Interpersonal Factors Although most people fear attack from strangers, the majority of victims are acquainted with their attacker. More than half of murders of women and three-fourths of sexual assaults are committed by someone the woman knows. Crime victims and violent criminals tend to share many characteristics—that is, they are likely to be young, male, in a minority, and poor.

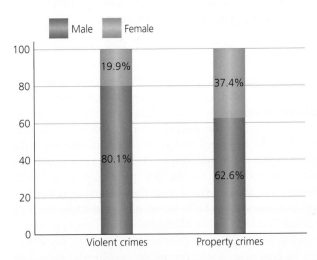

FIGURE 16.1 Arrests in the United States, 2012. Males were arrested significantly more often than females for both violent and property crimes.

SOURCE: Federal Bureau of Investigation. 2012. *Crime in the United States 2012.* Washington, DC: U.S. Department of Justice (www.fbi.gov/about-us/cjis/ucr/crime-in-the-u.s/2012/crime-in-the-u.s.-2012/tables/42tabledatadecoverviewpdf).

Alcohol and Other Drugs Substance misuse and dependence are consistently associated with interpersonal violence and suicide. Intoxication affects judgment and may increase aggression in some people, causing a small argument to escalate into a serious physical confrontation. On college campuses, alcohol is involved in about 95% of all violent crimes.

Firearms Many criminologists feel that the high rate of homicide in the United States is directly related to the fact that we are the only industrialized country in which handguns are widespread and easily available. The use of a handgun can change a suicide attempt to a completed suicide and a violent assault to a murder.

Over 100,000 deaths and injuries occur in the United States each year as a result of the use of firearms. Firearms are used in more than two-thirds of homicides, and studies reveal a strong correlation between the incidence of gun ownership and homicide rates for a given area of the country. Over half of all suicides involve a firearm, and people living in households in which guns are kept have a risk of suicide that is four or more times greater than that of people living in households without guns.

Assault

Assault is the use of physical force by a person or people to inflict injury or death on another. Homicide, aggravated assault, and robbery are examples of assault. Research indicates that the victims of assaultive injuries and their perpetrators tend to resemble one another in terms of ethnicity, educational background, psychological profile, and reliance on weapons. In many cases, the victim actually magnifies the confrontation through the use of a weapon.

Homicide

The FBI estimates that nearly 13,000 Americans were murdered in 2012. Men, teenagers, young adults, and members of minority groups, particularly African Americans and Latinos, are most likely to be murder victims. Although homicide rates for African Americans have declined dramatically in the past 25 years, the murder rate for black males is several times higher than the rate for the U.S. population as a whole. Poverty and unemployment have been identified as key factors in homicide, and these factors may account for the high rates of homicide among blacks and other minority groups.

Most homicides are committed with a firearm, occur during an argument, and occur among people who know one another. Intrafamilial homicide, where the perpetrator and victim are related, accounts for about one out of every eight homicides. About 40% of family homicides are committed by spouses, usually following a history of physical and emotional abuse directed at the woman.

QUICK STATS

In 2011, **21%** of aggravated assaults involved the use of a firearm.

—FBI, 2012

Gang-Related Violence

Gangs are most frequently associated with large cities, but gang activity also extends to the suburbs and even to rural areas. It is estimated that more than 1 million Americans belong to gangs. The average age for joining a gang is 14, so 40% of gang members are less than 18 years of age.

Gangs are more common in areas that are poor and suffer from high unemployment, population density, and crime. In these areas, a young person may feel that his or her hope of legitimate success in life is out of reach and knows that involvement in the drug market makes some gang members rich. Often gangs serve as a mechanism for companionship, self-esteem, support, and security. Indeed, in some areas gang membership may be viewed as the only possible means of survival.

Hate Crimes

When bias against another person's race or ethnicity, national origin, religion, sexual orientation, or disability motivates a criminal act, the offense is classified as a hate crime. Hate crimes may be committed against people or property. Those committed against people may include intimidation, assault, and even rape or murder. Crimes against property most frequently involve graffiti, the desecration of churches or synagogues, cross burnings, and other acts of vandalism or property damage.

Over 6,200 hate crimes were reported in 2011; many more go unreported. Crimes against people made up about 60% of all incidents; intimidation and assault are the most common offenses. Racial or ethnic bias was cited as a motivation in nearly half of the hate crimes reported in 2011. National origin or ethnicity was cited in 12% of cases, religion in 20%, and sexual orientation in 21%.

Research indicates that a substantial number of hate crimes are committed by males under age 20. Hate crimes are frequently, but not always, associated with fringe groups that have extremist ideologies, such as the Ku Klux Klan and neo-Nazi groups. The rapid growth of hate sites on the Internet is another area of concern.

School Violence

According to the National School Safety Center, over 300 school-associated violent deaths of students, faculty, and administrators occurred in the last decade. Most of these deaths occurred in urban areas or at high schools and involved use of a firearm. As with other types of violence, both victims and offenders were predominantly young men. Homicide and suicide are the most serious but least common types of violence in schools; an estimated 400,000 less serious incidents of violence and crime occur each year, including theft, vandalism, and fights not involving weapons.

Children are actually much safer at school than away from it. Fewer than 1% of all homicides among youths aged 5–19 occur at school, and 90% of schools report no incidents of serious violence. Children and adolescents are far more likely to be killed by an adult in their own homes or away from school than they are to die as a result of school-associated violence. According to the National Institute of Justice (NIJ), the overall number of violent incidents has decreased steadily over the past two decades; however, the number of multiple-victim events may have increased.

Although schools are basically safe places overall, steps can be taken to identify at-risk youths and improve safety for all students. General characteristics of youths who have caused violent deaths in schools include uncontrollable angry outbursts, violent and abusive language and behavior, isolation from peers, depression and irritability, access to and preoccupation with weapons, and lack of support and supervision from adults.

Being a victim of teasing, bullying, or social exclusion (rejection) may lead to aggressive behavior or violence.

Recommendations for reducing school violence include offering classroom training in anger management, social skills, and improved self-control; providing mental health and social services for students in need; developing after-school programs that help students build self-esteem and make friends; and keeping guns out of the hands of children and out of schools. Tragic incidents like the shooting that took place at Sandy Hook Elementary School in Newtown, Connecticut, in 2012 have also resulted in installation of security and surveillance systems in schools throughout the country, as well as new protocols for entry into school buildings.

> Being a victim of teasing, bullying, or rejection may lead to **aggressive behavior or violence.**

Workplace Violence

Data show that workplace violence has decreased by 35% in the past decade, yet OSHA still reports that nearly 2 million American workers are victims of workplace violence each year, including about 500 homicides. In about 60% of cases, workplace violence is committed by strangers; acquaintances account for nearly 40% of cases; and intimates account for 1%. Most of the perpetrators of workplace violence are white males over age 21. Women's leading cause of death in the workplace is homicide. Firearms are used in nearly 80% of workplace homicides, and the majority of these homicides occur during the commission of a robbery or other crime.

Police and corrections officers have the most dangerous jobs, followed by taxi drivers, security guards, bartenders, mental health professionals, and workers at gas stations and convenience and liquor stores. According to the Department of Labor, workers in state government offices experience more workplace violence of all types than do workers in local government or private industry.

General crime prevention strategies, including use of surveillance cameras and silent alarms and limiting the amount of cash on hand, can help reduce workplace violence related to robberies. A highly stressed workplace is a risk factor in cases of violence between acquaintances or coworkers; clear guidelines about acceptable behavior and prompt action after any threats or incidents of violence can help control this type of workplace violence.

Terrorism

In 2001 more Americans died as a result of terrorism than in any year before or since; the attacks on September 11 killed more than 3000 people, including citizens of 78 countries. The FBI defines *terrorism* as the unlawful use of force or violence against people or property to intimidate or coerce a government, the civilian population, or any segment thereof in furtherance of political or social objectives. Terrorism can be either domestic, carried out by groups based in the United States, or international. It comes in many forms, including biological, chemical, nuclear, and cyber. Its intent is to promote helplessness by instilling fear of harm or destruction.

Terrorism prevention activities occur at all levels of government. U.S. government efforts include close work with the diplomatic, law enforcement, intelligence, economic, and military communities. The mission of the U.S. Department of Homeland Security is to help prevent, protect against, and respond to acts of terrorism on U.S. territory. It coordinates efforts to protect electric and water supply systems, transportation, gas and oil, emergency services, the computer infrastructure, and other systems.

Individuals have a role in preventing terrorism by making sure they are prepared in case of a terrorist attack or a disaster. They can also be proactive by reporting anything they see or hear that is suspicious or threatening. The best approach is taking personal responsibility and not letting the fear of terrorism immobilize or impede your ability to act.

Family and Intimate-Partner Violence

Family violence generally refers to any rough and illegitimate use of physical force, aggression, or verbal abuse by one family member toward another. Once referred to as domestic violence, the term **"intimate-partner violence" (IPV)** is now used to describe physical, social, or psychological harm imposed by a current partner or spouse. Based on reported cases, an estimated 6–8 million women and children in the United States are victimized each year as a result of IPV. Nearly five children die every day as a result of abuse and neglect.

> **Intimate-partner violence (IPV)** Physical, sexual, or psychological harm by a current or former partner or spouse.
>
> TERMS

TAKE CHARGE
Recognizing the Potential for Abusiveness in a Partner

There are no sure ways to tell whether someone will become abusive or violent toward an intimate partner, but there are warning signs that you can look for. (Remember that, although most abusive relationships involve male violence directed at a woman, women can also be abusive, as can partners in a same-sex relationship. Because most abusers are male, the following material refers to the abuser as "he." If you are concerned that a person you are involved with has the potential for violence, observe his or her behavior, and ask yourself these questions:

• What is this person's attitude toward women? How does he treat his mother and his sister? How does he work with female students, female colleagues, or a female boss? How does he treat your women friends?

• What is his attitude toward your autonomy? Does he respect the work you do and the way you do it? Or does he mock it, tell you how to do it better, or encourage you to give it up? Does he tell you he'll take care of you?

• How self-centered is he? Does he want to spend leisure time on your interests or his?

• Is he possessive or jealous? Does he want to spend every minute with you? Does he cross-examine you about things you do when you're not with him?

• What happens when things don't go the way he wants them to? Does he always have to get his way?

• Is he moody, mocking, critical, or bossy? Do you feel as if you're walking on eggshells when you're with him?

• Do you feel you have to avoid arguing with him?

• Does he drink too much or use drugs?

• Does he refuse to use condoms or take other precautions for safer sex?

Listen to your own uneasiness, and stay away from any man who disrespects women, who wants or needs you intensely and exclusively, and who has a knack for getting his own way almost all the time.

If you are in a serious relationship with a controlling person, you may already have experienced abuse. Consider the following questions:

• Does your partner constantly criticize you, blame you for things that are not your fault, or verbally degrade you?

• Does he humiliate you in front of others?

• Is he suspicious or jealous? Does he accuse you of being unfaithful or monitor your mail or phone calls?

• Does he track all your time? Does he discourage you from seeing friends and family?

• Does he prevent you from getting or keeping a job or attending school? Does he control your shared resources or restrict your access to money?

• Has he ever pushed, pulled, slapped, hit, kicked, bitten, or restrained you? Thrown an object at you? Used a weapon on you?

• Has he ever destroyed or damaged your personal property or sentimental items, or threatened to do so?

• Has he ever forced you to have sex or to do something sexually you didn't want to do?

• Does he anger easily when drinking or taking drugs?

• Has he ever threatened to harm you or your children, friends, pets, or property?

• Has he ever threatened to blackmail you if you leave?

If you answered yes to one or more of these questions, you may be experiencing domestic abuse. If you believe you or your children are in imminent danger, look in your local telephone directory for a women's shelter, or call 911. If you want information, referrals to a program in your area, or assistance, contact one of the organizations listed in the For More Information section at the end of the chapter.

Battering Studies reveal that over 85% of domestic violence victims are women. Violence against wives or intimate partners as a result of battering occurs at every level of society, although it is more common at lower socioeconomic levels. It occurs more frequently in relationships with a high degree of conflict—an apparent inability to resolve arguments through negotiation and compromise. Over 25% of women report having been physically assaulted or raped by an intimate partner, and more than 50% report having experienced some type of abuse—physical or psychological—in a relationship. In more than 10% of cases, the domestic violence continues for 20 years or longer. The problem of intimate violence is apparent even among young people; each year, 1.5 million high school students are victims of physical violence while on a date.

At the root of much of this abusive behavior is the need to control another person. Abusive partners are controlling partners. They not only want to have power over another person, but also believe they are entitled to it, no matter what the cost to the other person (see the box "Recognizing the Potential for Abusiveness in a Partner").

In abusive relationships, the abuser (in most cases a man) usually has a history of violent behavior, traditional beliefs about gender roles, and problems with alcohol abuse. He has low self-esteem and seeks to raise it by dominating and imposing his will on another person. Research has revealed a three-phase cycle of battering, consisting of a period of increasing tension, a violent explosion and loss of control, and a period of contriteness in which the man begs forgiveness and promises it will never happen again. The batterer is drawn back to this cycle over and over again, but he never succeeds in changing his feelings about himself.

Battered women often stay in violent relationships for years. They may be economically dependent on their partners, feel trapped or fear retaliation if they leave, believe their children need a father, or have low self-esteem themselves. They may love or pity their husband, or they may believe they'll eventually be able to stop the violence. They usually leave the relationship only when they become determined that the violence must end. Battered women's shelters offer physical protection, counseling, support, and other assistance.

Stalking and Cyberstalking Battering is closely associated with **stalking,** characterized by harassing behaviors such as following or spying on a person and making verbal, written, or implied threats. In the United States it is estimated that 7 million women and men are stalked each year; about two-thirds of stalkers are men. About three out of four female victims are stalked by current or former intimate partners; of these, over two-thirds had been physically or sexually assaulted by that partner during the relationship. Weapons are used to threaten or harm victims in one out of five cases. Stalking of female college students may be greater than that experienced by the general population. A stalker's goal may be to control or scare the victim or to keep her or him in a relationship. Most stalking episodes last a year or less.

The use of the Internet, e-mail, chat rooms, Facebook, Instagram, and other electronic means to stalk another person is known as **cyberstalking.** As with offline stalking, the majority of cyberstalkers are men, and the majority of victims are women, although there have been same-sex cyberstalking incidents.

Cyberstalkers may send harassing or threatening messages to the victim, or they may encourage others to harass the victim—for example, by impersonating the victim and posting inflammatory messages and personal information on bulletin boards or in chat rooms. Guidelines for staying safe online include the following:

- Avoid using your real name on the Internet. Select an age- and gender-neutral identity.

- Avoid filling out profiles for accounts with information that could be used to identify you.

- Do not share personal information in public spaces anywhere online or give it to strangers.

- Learn how to filter unwanted e-mail messages.

- Always use passwords that are unique and contain many characters—preferably an alphanumeric combination to make it more difficult for someone to hack into your account.

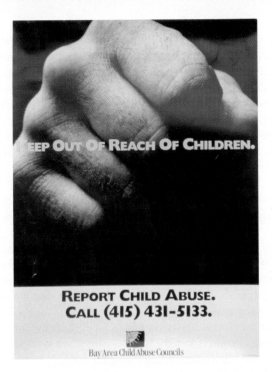

REPORT CHILD ABUSE. CALL (415) 431-5133.

Bay Area Child Abuse Councils

Education, counseling, and support can help the victims of family violence.

- If you use a social networking site, it is best to set your profile to "private" if that is an option.

- If you experience harassment online, do not respond to the harasser. Log off or go to a different site. If harassment continues, contact the harasser's Internet service provider (ISP) by identifying the domain of the stalker's account (after the "@" sign); most ISPs have an e-mail address for complaints. Often an ISP can try to stop the conduct by direct contact with the harasser or by closing his or her account. Save all communications for evidence, and contact your ISP and your local police department. Many states have laws against cyberstalking.

Violence against Children In 2011 there were more than 3 million reports of alleged child abuse and neglect in the United States, with the number of children involved being near 6 million. Nearly 1 million of the cases (about one out of six) involved physical abuse, and over 4.5 million (about three out of four) were a result of neglect. Parents who abuse children tend to have low self-esteem, to believe in physical punishment, to have a poor marital relationship,

stalking Repeatedly harassing or threatening a person through behaviors such as following a person, appearing at a person's residence or workplace, leaving written messages or objects, making harassing phone calls, or vandalizing property; frequently directed at a former intimate partner.   TERMS

cyberstalking The use of e-mail, chat rooms, bulletin boards, or other electronic communication devices to stalk another person.

and to have been abused themselves (although many people who were abused as children do not grow up to abuse their own children). Poverty, unemployment, and social isolation are characteristics of families in which children are abused. External stressors related to socioeconomic and environmental factors are most closely associated with neglect, whereas stressors related to interpersonal issues are more closely associated with physical abuse. Single parents, both men and women, are at especially high risk for abusing their children.

Elder Abuse   Each year over 4 million older adults are abused, exploited, or mistreated by someone who is supposed to be giving them care and protection; only one in 24 incidents is reported. Most abusers are family members who are serving as caregivers. Elder abuse can take different forms: physical, sexual, or emotional abuse; financial exploitation; neglect; or abandonment. Neglect accounts for about three out of five reported cases. Physical abuse accounts for about one out of six reported cases, and financial exploitation for about one out of eight reported cases.

Abuse often occurs when caring for a dependent adult becomes too stressful for the caregiver. Many believe that the solution to elder abuse is support in the form of greater social and financial assistance, such as adult day care centers and education and public care programs.

Sexual Violence

The use of force and coercion in sexual interactions is one of the most serious problems in human relationships. The most extreme manifestation of sexual coercion—forcing a person to submit to another's sexual desires—is rape, but sexual coercion occurs in many subtler forms, including sexual harassment.

Sexual Assault: Rape   Sexual coercion that relies on the threat and use of physical force or takes advantage of circumstances that render a person incapable of giving consent (such as being drunk) constitutes **sexual assault** or **rape**. When the victim is younger than the legally defined age of consent, the act constitutes **statutory rape,**

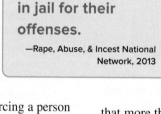

QUICK STATS

Only **3%** of rapists ever spend a day in jail for their offenses.

—Rape, Abuse, & Incest National Network, 2013

Most rape victims are **assaulted by someone they know,** not by a stranger.

whether or not coercion is involved. Coerced sexual activity in which the victim knows or is dating the rapist is often referred to as **date rape,** or *acquaintance rape.* Most victims know their assailants, but fewer than 40% of all sexual crimes are reported.

Any woman—or man—can be a rape victim. Over 200,000 cases of rape are reported each year. It is estimated that at least 500,000 more women are raped each year, but those incidents are unreported. Research shows that 1 in 5 women and 1 in 71 men have experienced an attempted or completed rape at some point in their lives. A study of college students also found that between 1 in 4 and 1 in 5 college women experience a completed or attempted rape during their college years. Most male-on-male rapes do not occur in prison.

WHO COMMITS RAPE?   Men who commit rape may be any age and come from any socioeconomic group. Some rapists are exploiters in the sense that they rape on the spur of the moment and mainly want immediate gratification. Some attempt to compensate for feelings of sexual inadequacy and an inability to obtain satisfaction otherwise. Others are more hostile and sadistic and are primarily interested in hurting and humiliating a particular woman or women in general. Often the rapist is more interested in dominance, control, and power than in sexual satisfaction.

Most women are in much less danger of being raped by a stranger than of being sexually assaulted by a man they know or date. Surveys suggest that as many as 25% of women have had experiences in which the men they were dating persisted in trying to force sex despite pleading, crying, screaming, or resisting. Surveys have also found that more than 60% of all rape victims were raped by a current or former spouse, boyfriend, or date.

Most cases of date rape are never reported to the police, partly because of the subtlety of the crime. Usually no weapons are involved, and direct verbal threats may not have been made. Victims of date rape tend to shoulder much of the responsibility for the incident, questioning their own judgment and behavior rather than blaming the aggressor.

Strong evidence suggests that 15% of American women who have ever married have been raped by their husbands or ex-husbands; as many as 60% of battered women may have been raped by their husbands. A charge of spousal rape can now be taken to court in all states.

FACTORS CONTRIBUTING TO DATE RAPE   Men and women tend to differ in their perception of romantic encounters and signals. In one study, researchers found that men interpreted women's actions on dates, such as smiling or talking in a low voice, as indicating an interest in having sex, whereas the

sexual assault *or* **rape**   The use of force to have **TERMS** sex with someone against that person's will.

statutory rape   Sexual interaction with someone under the legal age of consent.

date rape   Sexual assault by someone the victim knows or is dating; also called *acquaintance rape.*

Guidelines for Women

• Believe in your right to control what you do. Set limits, and communicate these limits clearly, firmly, and early. Say no when you mean no.

• Be assertive with someone who is sexually pressuring you. Men sometimes interpret passivity as permission.

• If you are unsure of a new acquaintance, go on a group date or double date. If possible, provide your own transportation.

• Remember that some men assume sexy dress and a flirtatious manner mean a desire for sex.

• Remember that alcohol and drugs interfere with clear communication about sex.

• Use the statement that has proven most effective in stopping date rape: "This is rape, and I'm calling the police."

Guidelines for Men

• Be aware of social pressure. It's OK to not score.

• Understand that no means no. Don't continue making advances when your date resists or tells you she wants to stop. Remember that she has the right to refuse sex.

• Don't assume sexy dress and a flirtatious manner are invitations to sex, that previous permission for sex applies to the current situation, or that your date's relationships with other men constitute sexual permission for you.

• Remember that alcohol and drugs interfere with clear communication about sex.

---

women interpreted the same actions as just being friendly. Men who rape their dates tend to have certain attributes, including hostility toward women, a belief that dominance alone is a valid motive for sex, and an acceptance of sexual violence.

DATE-RAPE DRUGS About 5% of DFSA victims are given date-rape drugs. Also called predator drugs, the drugs include flunitrazepam (Rohypnol), gamma hydroxybutyrate (GHB), and ketamine ("Special K"). Rohypnol is not legal in the United States, but ketamine and GHB can be legally obtained because they are used for legitimate medical purposes.

These drugs have a variety of effects, including sedation; if slipped surreptitiously into a drink, they can incapacitate a person within about 20 minutes and make her or him more vulnerable to assault. Rohypnol, GHB, and other drugs also often cause anterograde amnesia, meaning victims have little memory of what happened while they were under the influence of the drug. The Drug-Induced Rape Prevention and Punishment Act of 1996 adds up to 20 years to the prison sentence of any rapist who uses a drug to incapacitate a victim.

Strategies such as the following can help ensure that your drink is not tampered with at a bar or party:

• Drink moderately and responsibly. Avoid group drinking and drinking games.

• Be wary of opened beverages—alcoholic or nonalcoholic—offered by strangers. When at an unfamiliar bar, watch the bartender pour your drink.

• If an opened beverage tastes, looks, or smells strange, do not drink it. If you leave your drink unattended,

> If a woman chooses not to resist, **it does not mean** that she has not been raped.

such as when you dance or use the restroom, get a fresh drink when you return to your table.

• If you go to a party, club, or bar, go with friends. Have a prearranged plan for checking on each other visually and verbally. If you feel giddy or light-headed, get assistance.

Both males and females can take actions that will reduce the incidence of acquaintance rape; see the box "Preventing Date Rape" for specific suggestions.

DEALING WITH A SEXUAL ASSAULT Each situation is unique, and a woman should respond in whatever way she thinks best. If you are threatened by a rapist and decide to fight back, here is what Women Organized Against Rape (WOAR) recommends:

• Trust your gut feeling. If you feel you are in danger, don't hesitate to run and scream. It is better to feel foolish than to be raped.

• Yell—and keep yelling. It will clear your head and start your adrenaline going; it may scare your attacker and also bring help.

• If an attacker grabs you from behind, use your elbows for striking his neck, his sides, or his stomach.

• Try kicking. Your legs are the strongest part of your body, and your kick is longer than his reach. Kick with the foot that is further back. Aim low to avoid losing your balance.

• His most vulnerable spot is his knee; it's low, difficult to protect, and easily knocked out of place. Don't try to kick a rapist in the crotch; he has been protecting this area all his life and will have better protective reflexes there than at his knees.

- Once you start fighting, keep it up. Your objective is to get away as soon as you can.

- Remember that ordinary rules of behavior don't apply. It's OK to vomit, act crazy, or claim to have a sexually transmitted disease.

If you are raped, tell what happened to the first friendly person you meet. Call the police, tell them you were raped, and give your location. Try to remember as many facts as you can about your attacker; write down a description as soon as possible. Don't wash or change your clothes, or you may destroy important evidence. The police will take you to a hospital for a complete exam; show the physician any injuries. Tell the police simply, but exactly, what happened. If you decide that you don't want to report the rape to the police, be sure to see a physician as soon as possible. You need to be checked for pregnancy and STIs.

THE EFFECTS OF RAPE Rape victims suffer both physical and psychological injury. For most, physical wounds heal within a few weeks. Psychological pain may endure and be substantial. Even the most physically and mentally strong are likely to experience shock, anxiety, depression, shame, and a host of psychosomatic symptoms after being victimized. Some victims experience rape trauma syndrome, which is characterized by fear, nightmares, fatigue, crying spells, and digestive upset. Self-blame is very likely; society has contributed to this tendency by perpetuating the myths that women can actually defend themselves and that no one can be raped if she doesn't want to be. Fortunately these false beliefs are dissolving in the face of evidence to the contrary.

Many organizations offer counseling and support to rape victims. Look in the telephone directory under Rape or Rape Crisis Center for a hotline number to call. Your campus may have counseling services or a support group.

Child Sexual Abuse   Child sexual abuse is any sexual contact between an adult and a child who is below the legal age of consent. Adults and older adolescents are able to coerce children into sexual activity because of their authority and power over them. Threats, force, or the promise of friendship or material rewards may be used to manipulate a child. Sexual contacts are typically brief and consist of genital manipulation; genital intercourse is much less common.

Sexual abusers are usually male, heterosexual, and known to the victim. The abuser may be a relative, a friend, a neighbor, or another trusted adult acquaintance. Child abusers are often pedophiles, people who are sexually attracted to children. They may have poor interpersonal and sexual relationships with other adults and feel socially inadequate and inferior. One highly traumatic form of sexual abuse is **incest:** sexual activity between people too closely related to legally marry.

Child sexual abuse is often unreported. Surveys suggest that as many as 27% of women and 16% of men were sexually abused as children. An estimated 150,000–200,000 new cases of child sexual abuse occur each year. It can leave lasting scars; victims are more likely to suffer as adults from low self-esteem, depression, anxiety, eating disorders, self-destructive tendencies, sexual problems, and difficulties in intimate relationships.

If you were a victim of sexual abuse as a child and feel it may be interfering with your functioning today, you may want to address the problem. A variety of approaches can help, such as joining a support group of people who have had similar experiences, confiding in a partner or friend, or seeking professional help.

Sexual Harassment   Unwelcome sexual advances, requests for sexual favors, and other verbal, visual, or physical conduct of a sexual nature constitute **sexual harassment** if such conduct explicitly or implicitly affects academic or employment decisions or evaluations; interferes with an individual's academic or work performance; or creates an intimidating, hostile, or offensive academic, work, or student living environment.

Extreme cases of sexual harassment occur when a manager, professor, or other person in authority uses his or her ability to control or influence jobs or grades to coerce people into having sex or to punish them if they refuse.

---

incest   Sexual activity between close relatives, such as siblings or parents and their children.

sexual harassment   Unwelcome sexual advances, requests for sexual favors, and other conduct of a sexual nature that affects academic or employment decisions or evaluations; interferes with an individual's academic or work performance; or creates an intimidating, hostile, or offensive academic, work, or student living environment.

TERMS

Ask Yourself

QUESTIONS FOR CRITICAL THINKING AND REFLECTION

Have you or has anyone you know ever been the victim of a violent act? If so, what were the circumstances surrounding the event? What was the outcome? How did the event affect your life? In hindsight, what steps could have been taken to avoid or prevent the incident?

College campuses can be the site of criminal activity and violence just as any other environment or living situation can be—and so they require the same level of caution and awareness that you would use in other situations. Two key points to remember: 80% of campus crimes are committed by one student against another, and alcohol or drug use is involved in 90% of campus felonies. Drinking or drug use can affect judgment and lower inhibitions, so be aware if you or another person is under the influence. Here are some suggestions for keeping yourself safe on campus:

• Don't travel alone after dark. Many campuses have shuttle buses that run from spots on campus such as the library and the dining hall to residence halls and other locations. Escorts are often available to walk with you at night.

• Be familiar with well-lit and frequently traveled routes around campus if you do need to walk alone.

• If you have a car, follow the usual precautions about parking in well-lit areas, keeping the doors locked as you are driving, and never picking up hitchhikers.

• Always have your keys ready as you approach your residence hall, room, and car. Don't lend your keys to others.

• Let friends and family members know your schedule of classes and activities to create a sort of buddy system.

• Be sure the doors and windows of your dorm room have sturdy locks, and use them.

• Don't prop open doors or hold doors open for nonstudents or nonresidents trying to enter your dorm. Be aware of nonresidents around your dorm. If someone says that he or she is meeting a friend inside, that person should be able to call the friend from outside the building.

• Keep valuables and anything containing personal information—credit cards, wallets, jewelry, and so on—hidden. Secure expensive computer and stereo equipment with cables so that it can't be easily stolen. Use a quality U-shaped lock whenever you leave a bicycle unattended.

• Be alert when using an ATM, and don't display large amounts of cash.

• Stay alert and trust your instincts. Don't hesitate to call the police or campus security if something doesn't seem or feel right.

The Jeanne Clery Disclosure of Campus Security Policy and Campus Crime Statistics Act, named for a Lehigh University student who was murdered in her residence hall in 1986, requires colleges and universities to collect and report campus crime statistics. You can now review this information online at the Crime Statistics website of the U.S. Department of Education's Office of Postsecondary Education (ope.ed.gov/security/Search.asp).

A hostile environment can be created by conduct such as sexual gestures, display of sexually suggestive objects or pictures, derogatory comments and jokes, sexual remarks about clothing or appearance, obscene letters, and unnecessary touching.

If you have been the victim of sexual harassment, you can take action to stop it. Be assertive with anyone who uses language or actions you find inappropriate. If possible, confront your harasser and tell him or her that the situation is unacceptable to you and you want the harassment to stop. If assertive communication doesn't work, assemble a file or log documenting the harassment, noting the details of each incident and information about any witnesses who may be able to support your claims. You may discover others who have been harassed by the same person, which will strengthen your case. Then file a grievance with the harasser's supervisor or employer.

If your attempts to deal with the harassment internally are not successful, you can file an official complaint with your city or state Human Rights Commission or Fair Employment Practices Agency, or with the federal Equal Employment Opportunity Commission. You may also wish to pursue legal action under the Civil Rights Act or under local laws prohibiting employment discrimination. Often the threat of a lawsuit or other legal action is enough to stop the harasser.

What You Can Do about Violence

Violence in our society is a serious threat to our collective health and well-being. This is especially true on college campuses (see the box "Staying Safe on Campus"). Schools are now providing training for conflict resolution and are educating people about the diverse nature of our society, thereby encouraging tolerance and understanding.

Reducing gun-related injuries may require changes in the availability, possession, and lethality of the 10–14 million firearms sold legally in the United States each year. As part of the Brady gun control law, computerized instant background checks are performed for most gun sales to prevent purchases by convicted felons, people with a history of mental instability, and certain other groups. In some states, waiting periods are required in addition to the background checks. Some groups advocate a complete and universal federal ban on the sale of all handguns.

PROVIDING EMERGENCY CARE

A course in **first aid** can help you respond appropriately when someone is injured. One important benefit of first aid training is learning what *not* to do in certain situations. For example, a person with a suspected neck or back injury should not be moved unless there are other life-threatening conditions. A trained person can assess emergency situations accurately before acting.

Emergency rescue techniques can save the lives of people who are choking, who have stopped breathing, or whose hearts have stopped beating. As described earlier, the Heimlich maneuver is used when a victim is choking. Pulmonary resuscitation (also known as rescue breathing, artificial respiration, or mouth-to-mouth resuscitation) is used when a person is not breathing. Cardiopulmonary resuscitation

(CPR) is used when a pulse cannot be found. In 2010 the American Heart Association made significant changes in its CPR guidelines for laypersons. Previous guidelines were to clear the airway, check for breathing, and begin chest compressions (ABC). The new guidelines are to begin chest compressions, clear the airway, and check for breathing (CAB). Starting with compressions gets the blood circulating, which is critical to keeping the person alive until help arrives. Compressions should be delivered fast, about 100 times a minute. Courses in first aid and CPR are offered by the American Heart Association and the American Red Cross.

A new feature of some of these courses is training in the use of automated external defibrillators (AEDs), which monitor the heart's rhythm and, if appropriate, deliver an electrical shock to restart the heart. Because of the importance of early use of defibrillators in saving heart attack victims, these devices are being installed in public places, including casinos, airports, and many office buildings.

As a person providing assistance, you are the first link in the **emergency medical services (EMS) system,** a system designed to network community resources for providing emergency care.

Ask Yourself

QUESTIONS FOR CRITICAL THINKING AND REFLECTION

What kinds of emergency training have you had? What kinds of skills do you have that would enable you to help someone who was hurt, was trapped, or needed some other kind of assistance?

connect™

Connect to Your Choices

Have you ever thought about where you get your behaviors and habits related to your personal safety? Many factors can influence our behaviors and habits, some not as obvious as others. Does your social circle include people who are risk takers, who think they're invincible, or who drink excessively? Are there unsafe places in your community, such as swimming pools or waterways without lifeguards? Does your residence have smoke alarms or sprinklers? Does your school have an emergency warning system in case of a terrorist attack or a dangerous situation on campus?

What are the external factors that influence your choices about personal safety? What are your inner motivations and core values, and how do they affect your choices? Based on what you learned in this chapter, will you make some different choices in the future? If so, what will they be?

Go online to Connect to complete this activity: www.mcgraw-hillconnect.com

---

first aid   Emergency care given to an ill or injured person until medical care can be obtained.   TERMS

emergency medical services (EMS) system   A system designed to network community resources for providing emergency care.

TIPS FOR TODAY AND THE FUTURE

Protecting yourself from injuries means taking sensible safety precautions every day, and preparing yourself to deal with an emergency.

RIGHT NOW YOU CAN:

- Check your home for any object or situation that could cause an injury, such as a tripping hazard, top-heavy shelves, and so on.
- Test the batteries in your home's smoke detectors, and change them if necessary. Test the detectors to make sure they work properly.
- If you ride a bike, check your helmet to ensure that it fits properly and will protect you in a crash. If you have any doubts, throw it away and buy a new one.

IN THE FUTURE YOU CAN:

- Get trained in CPR, rescue breathing, and the use of an automated external defibrillator. If you have already had such training, take a refresher course.
- Be watchful for hazardous situations at your school and workplace. If you notice anything suspicious, report it to an appropriate person right away.
- Prepare for a poisoning emergency by putting the number of your local poison control hotline in a conspicuous place.

SUMMARY

- Injuries are caused by a dynamic interaction of human and environmental factors. Risk-taking behavior is associated with a high rate of injury.

- Key factors in motor vehicle injuries include aggressive driving, speeding, a failure to wear safety belts, alcohol and drug intoxication, fatigue, and distraction.

- Motorcycle, motor scooter, and bicycle injuries can be prevented by developing appropriate skills, driving or riding defensively, and wearing proper safety equipment, especially a helmet.

- Most fall-related injuries are a result of falls at floor level, but stairs, chairs, and ladders are also involved in a significant number of falls.

- Careless smoking and problems with cooking or heating equipment are common causes of home fires. Being prepared for fire emergencies means planning escape routes and installing smoke detectors.

- The home can contain many poisonous substances, including medications, cleaning agents, plants, and fumes from cars and appliances.

- Performing the Heimlich maneuver can prevent someone from dying from choking.

- The proper storage and handling of firearms can help prevent injuries; assume that any gun is loaded.

- Many injuries during leisure activities result from the misuse of equipment, lack of experience, use of alcohol, and a failure to wear proper safety equipment.

- Most work-related injuries involve extensive manual labor; back problems and repetitive strain injuries are most common.

- Factors contributing to violence include poverty, the absence of strong social ties, the influence of the mass media, cultural attitudes about gender roles, problems in interpersonal relationships, alcohol and drug abuse, and the availability of firearms.

- Types of violence include assault, homicide, gang-related violence, hate crimes, school violence, workplace violence, and terrorism.

- Battering and child abuse occur at every socioeconomic level. The core issue is the abuser's need to control other people.

- Most rape victims are women, and most know their attackers. Factors in date rape include different standards of appropriate sexual behavior for men and women and different perceptions of actions.

- Child sexual abuse often results in serious trauma; usually the abuser is a trusted adult.

- Sexual harassment is unwelcome sexual advances or other conduct of a sexual nature that affects academic or employment performance or evaluations or that creates an intimidating, hostile, or offensive academic, work, or student living environment.

- Strategies for reducing violence include conflict resolution training, social skills development, and education programs that foster tolerance and understanding among diverse groups.

- Steps in giving emergency care include making sure the scene is safe for you and the injured person, conducting a quick examination of the victim, calling for help, and providing emergency first aid.

FOR MORE INFORMATION

BOOKS

Carr, B., and E. Wondolowski. 2011. *The Prepper's Pocket Guide: 101 Easy Things You Can Do to Ready Your Home for a Disaster.* Berkeley, CA: Ulysses Press. *A practical guide to help prepare for potential disasters, both personal and environmental.*

Jones, S. A. 2011. *First Aid, Survival, and CPR: Home and Field Pocket Guide.* Philadelphia: F. A. Davis Company. A portable, waterproof guide for all kinds of first aid and survival emergencies; includes a section on pet first aid.

World Health Organization. 2010. *Preventing Intimate Partner and Sexual Violence against Women: Taking Action and Generating Evidence.* Geneva: World Health Organization. *The latest volume in a series of publications addressing the varying types of violence affecting our global society.*

ORGANIZATIONS, HOTLINES, AND WEBSITES

American Association of Poison Control Centers. Provides free, confidential, and expert advice related to poisoning. 800-222-1222

http://www.aapcc.org

American Automobile Association Foundation for Traffic Safety. Provides consumer information about all aspects of traffic safety; the website has online quizzes and extensive links.

http://www.aaafoundation.org/home

American Bar Association: Domestic Violence. Provides information about statistics, research, and laws relating to domestic violence.

http://www.americanbar.org/groups/domestic_violence
/resources/statistics.html

CyberAngels Internet Safety Program. Provides information about online safety and help and advice for victims of cyberstalking.

http://www.cyberangels.org

Governor's Highway Safety Association. Provides up-to-date information about cell phone and texting laws, as well as general information and publications related to traffic safety.

http://www.ghsa.org/html/stateinfo/laws/cellphone_laws.html

Insurance Institute for Highway Safety. Provides information about crashes on the nation's highways, as well as reports on topics such as speeding and crashworthiness of vehicles.

http://www.iihs.org

National Center for Health Statistics (Centers for Disease Control and Prevention). Monitors the health of the United States and provides up-to-date information and statistical data to the public and professionals.

http://www.cdc.gov/nchs/

National Center for Injury Prevention and Control. Provides consumer-oriented information about unintentional injuries and violence.

http://www.cdc.gov/injury

National Center for Victims of Crime. An advocacy group for crime victims; provides statistics, news, safety strategies, tips on finding local assistance, and links to related sites.

http://www.victimsofcrime.org

National Highway Traffic Safety Administration. Supplies materials about reducing deaths, injuries, and economic losses from motor vehicle crashes.

http://www.nhtsa.gov

National Safety Council. Provides information and statistics about preventing unintentional injuries.

http://www.nsc.org

National Violence Hotlines. Provide information, referral services, and crisis intervention.

800-799-SAFE (-7233) (domestic violence), http://www
.thehotline.org

800-422-4453 (child abuse), http://www.childhelp.org

800-656-HOPE (-4673) (sexual assault), http://www.rainn.org

Occupational Safety and Health Administration. Provides information about topics related to health and safety issues in the workplace.

http://www.osha.gov

Prevent Child Abuse America. Provides statistics, information, and publications relating to child abuse, including parenting tips.

http://www.preventchildabuse.org

Rape, Abuse, and Incest National Network (RAINN). Provides guidelines for preventing and dealing with sexual assault and abuse.

http://www.rainn.org

Tolerance.Org. Offers suggestions for fighting hate and promoting tolerance; sponsored by the Southern Poverty Law Center.

http://www.tolerance.org

World Health Organization: Violence and Injury Prevention and Disability. Provides statistics and information about the consequences of intentional and unintentional injuries worldwide.

http://www.who.int/violence_injury_prevention

The following sites provide statistics and background information about violence and crime in the United States:

Bureau of Justice Statistics: http://bjs.ojp.usdoj.gov

Federal Bureau of Investigation: http://www.fbi.gov

National Criminal Justice Reference Service: http://www.ncjrs
.gov/

SELECTED BIBLIOGRAPHY

Arnowitz, T. 2013. How safe are college campuses? *Journal of American College Health* 61(2): 57–59.

Burgess, M., and S. Burpo. 2012. The effect of music videos on college students' perceptions of rape. *College Student Journal* 46(4): 748–763.

Centers for Disease Control and Prevention. 2010. *Unintentional Drug Poisoning in the United States.* Atlanta, GA: CDC.

Cramer, R., et al. 2013. An examination of sexual orientation and transgender-based hate crimes in the post-Matthew Shepard era. *Psychology, Public Policy, and Law* 19(3): 355–368.

FIA Foundation for the Automobile and Society. 2010. *U.N. Decade of Action for Road Safety, 2011–2020* (www.fiafoundation.org/publications /Documents/decade_is_action_booklet.pdf).

Glascoff, M., M. Wallen, and J. Shrader. 2012. College student utilization of designated drivers after drug or alcohol use. *Chronicle for Driver Education Professionals* 59: 14–17.

Iqbal, S. et al. 2012. National carbon monoxide poisoning surveillance framework and recent estimates. *Public Health Reports* 127(5): 486–496.

Kleisen, L. 2013. A positive view on road safety: Can 'car karma' contribute to safe driving styles? *Accident Analysis and Prevention* 50: 605–712.

Levinson, A. A., B. Lannert, and M. Yalch. 2012. The effects of intimate partner violence on women and children survivors: An attachment perspective. *Psychodynamic Psychiatry* 40(3): 397–433.

Liu, Y. C., and Y. K. Ou. 2011. Effects of age and the use of hands-free cellular phones on driving behavior and task performance. *Traffic Injury Prevention* 12(6): 550–558.

Mendez, C., and B. Dillon. 2012. Workplace violence: Impact, causes, and prevention. *WORK* 42(1): 15–20.

Narang, P., et al. 2010. Do guns provide safety? At what cost? *Southern Medical Journal* 103(2): 151–153.

National Center for Health Statistics. 2012. Deaths: Preliminary data for 2010. *National Vital Statistics Reports* 64(4): 1–51.

National Highway Traffic Safety Administration. 2012. High visibility enforcement demonstration programs in Connecticut and New York reduce hand-held phone use. *Annals of Emergency Medicine* 59(2): 141–142.

National Safety Council. 2013. *Injury Facts 2013 Edition.* Itasca, IL: National Safety Council.

National School Safety Center. 2010. *School Associated Violent Deaths.* Oak Park, CA: National School Safety Center.

National Weather Service. 2013. *Weather Safety* (http://www.weather.gov /safety.php).

Palfrey, J., and S. Palfrey. 2013. Preventing gun deaths in children. *New England Journal of Medicine* 368: 401–403.

Reyns, B., B. Henson, and B. Fisher. 2012. Stalking in the twilight zone: Extent of cyberstalking victimization and offending among college students. *Deviant Behavior* 33(1): 1–25.

Ross, T., et al. 2010. The bicycle helmet attitudes scale: Using the Health Belief Model to predict helmet use among undergraduates. *Journal of American College Health* 59(1): 29–36.

Roudsari, B., et al. 2009. Ethnicity, age, and trends in alcohol-related driver fatalities in the United States. *Traffic Injury Prevention* 10(5): 410–414.

Sansone, R., and L. Sansone. 2010. Road rage: What's driving it? *Psychiatry (Edgmont)* 7(7): 14–18.

Swogger, M. T., et al. 2012. Self-reported childhood physical abuse and perpetration of intimate partner violence: The moderating role of psychopathic traits. *Criminal Justice and Behavior* 39(7): 910–922.

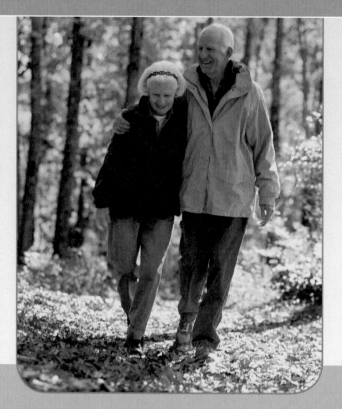

CHAPTER OBJECTIVES

- List strategies for healthy aging

- Identify key physical, social, and mental changes that may accompany aging and explain how people can best confront these changes

- Describe practical considerations for older adults and caregivers, including housing, finances, health care, communication, and transportation

- Describe the experience of living with a life-threatening illness and list ways to support a person who is dying

- Explain the grieving process and how support can be offered to adults and children who have experienced a loss

CHAPTER **17**

The Challenge of Aging

Aging is the process of becoming older, a process that is genetically determined but also profoundly affected by your environment. There is no specific point in life at which aging begins, and there is no precise age at which a person becomes "old." The satisfaction you will get from life is largely affected by your attitude toward aging and death, and how well you handle events that might be out of your control.

GENERATING VITALITY AS YOU AGE

Biological aging includes all the normal, progressive, irreversible changes to our bodies that begin at birth and continue until death. Psychological aging and social aging usually reflect more abrupt changes in circumstance and emotion: relocating, changing homes, losing a spouse and friends, retiring, having a lower income, and changing roles and social status. These changes represent opportunities for growth throughout life.

Successful aging requires preparation. People need to establish good health habits in their teens and twenties.

During their twenties and thirties, they usually develop important relationships and settle into a particular lifestyle. By their mid-forties, they generally know how much money they need to support the lifestyle they've chosen. At this point, they must assess their financial status and perhaps adjust their savings in order to continue enjoying that lifestyle after retirement. In their mid-fifties, they need to reevaluate their health insurance plans and may want to think about retirement housing. In their seventies and beyond, they need to consider ways of sharing their legacy with the next generation.

What Happens as You Age?

Many of the characteristics associated with aging are not due to aging at all. Rather, they result from the neglect and abuse of our bodies and minds. These assaults lay the

> **aging** A normal process of getting older, which includes physical, mental, and social changes, and a point past which there is a decline in function.   TERMS

foundation for later psychological problems and chronic conditions such as arthritis, heart disease, diabetes, hearing loss, vision problems, and hypertension.

Even with the healthiest behavior and environment, aging inevitably occurs. It results from genetic and biochemical processes we don't yet fully understand. The physiological changes in organ systems are caused by a combination of gradual aging and impairment from disease. Because of redundancy in most organ systems, the body's ability to function is not affected until damage is fairly extensive. Studies of healthy people indicate that functioning remains essentially constant until after age 70. Further research may help pinpoint the causes of aging and develop therapies to repair damage to aging organs.

Life-Enhancing Measures: Age-Proofing

You can prevent, delay, lessen, or even reverse some changes associated with aging through good habits. Simple, daily things can make a great difference to your level of energy and vitality—your overall wellness.

Challenge Your Mind Numerous studies show that older adults who stay mentally active have lower levels of the brain protein linked to Alzheimer's and dementia. Reading, writing, doing puzzles, learning language, and

Regular exercise is a key to successful, healthy aging.

studying music are good ways to stimulate the brain. The more complex the activity, the more protective it may be.

Develop Physical Fitness Exercise significantly enhances both psychological and physical health. A review of more than 70 scientific studies cited in the 2008 *Physical Activity Guidelines Advisory Committee Report* found that physically active people have about a 30% lower risk of dying prematurely compared with inactive people. Poor fitness and low physical activity levels were found to be better predictors of premature death than smoking, diabetes, or obesity. The committee found that about 150 minutes (2.5 hours) of physical activity per week is sufficient to decrease all causes of death and that it is the overall volume of energy expended, regardless of what kinds of activities produce the energy expenditure, that makes a difference in risk of premature death.

The positive effects of exercise include lower blood pressure and healthier cholesterol levels; better protection against heart attacks and an increased chance of survival should one occur; sustained or increased lung capacity; weight control through less accumulation of fat; maintenance of strength, flexibility, and balance; improved sleep; longer life expectancy; protection against osteoporosis and type 2 diabetes; increased effectiveness of the immune system; and maintenance of mental agility and flexibility, response time, memory, and hand–eye coordination.

The stimulus that exercise provides also seems to protect against the loss of **fluid intelligence,** which is the ability to find solutions to new problems. Fluid intelligence depends on rapidity of responsiveness, memory, and alertness. Individuals who exercise regularly are also less susceptible to depression and dementia.

Regular physical activity is essential for healthy aging, as it is throughout life. The *2008 Physical Activity Guidelines for Americans* include recommendations for older adults that are the same as for all adults:

•   All older adults should avoid inactivity. Some physical activity is better than none.

•   For substantial health benefits, older adults should do at least 150 minutes a week of moderate-intensity activity, or 75 minutes a week of vigorous-intensity activity, or a combination of both. For additional and more extensive health benefits, older adults should increase their aerobic physical activity to 300 minutes a week of moderate-intensity, or 150 minutes a week of vigorous-intensity, aerobic physical activity.

fluid intelligence   The ability to develop a solution when confronted with a new problem.

TERMS

TAKE CHARGE
Can Exercise Delay the Effects of Aging?

As people age, they often experience declines in functional health—the ability to perform the tasks of everyday life—and related declines in the quality of life. According to the CDC, more than 25% of Americans over age 65 report their health as only "fair" or "poor." Similarly, according to a Medicare survey, 31% of men and 42% of women aged 65–74 reported some sort of mobility limitation in 2003 (meaning they had difficulty walking one-quarter mile).

Can physical activity and exercise combat the degenerative effects of aging in middle-aged and older adults? The evidence indicates that they can. In reviewing the research, the U.S. government's Physical Activity Guidelines Advisory Committee concluded that physical activity can prevent or delay the onset of limitations and declines in functional health in older adults, can maintain or improve functional health in those who already have limitations, and can reduce the incidence of falls and fall-related injuries.

One mechanism by which physical activity prevents declines in functional health is through maintenance or improvement of the physiological capacities of the body, such as aerobic power, muscular strength, and balance—in other words, through improvements in physical fitness. Declines in these physiological capacities occur with biological aging and are often compounded by disease-related disability. But evidence shows that older adults who participate in regular aerobic exercise are 30% less likely than inactive individuals to develop functional limitations (such as a limited ability to walk or climb stairs) or role limitations (such as a limited ability to be the family grocery shopper). Although studies found that both physical activity and aerobic fitness were associated with reduced risk of functional limitations, aerobic fitness was associated with a greater reduction of risk. Evidence also suggests that regular physical activity is safe and beneficial for older adults who already have functional limitations.

Numerous studies have shown that regular exercise—particularly strength training, balance training, and flexibility exercises—can improve muscular strength, muscular endurance, and stability and provide some protection against falls. Aerobic activity, especially walking, also helps reduce risk of falls, and some evidence indicates that tai chi exercise programs are beneficial as well. Regular exercise not only reduces the incidence of falls but also greatly enhances mobility, allowing older people to live more independently and with greater confidence. Research also shows that regular physical activity can reduce anxiety and depression in older adults. Exercise stimulates blood flow to the brain and can even increase brain mass, helping the brain to function more efficiently and improving memory. There is some evidence that exercise may stave off mental decline and the occurrence of age-related dementia.

Current physical activity recommendations for older adults from the American Heart Association and the American College of Sports Medicine include moderate- to vigorous-intensity aerobic activity, strength training, and flexibility exercises, as well as balance exercises for older adults at risk for falls. Unfortunately more than 75% of Americans aged 65 and older do not get the recommended amounts of physical activity, and many get no exercise at all beyond the activities of daily living. Older adults are the least active group of Americans. Although it is important to exercise throughout life, the evidence indicates that older adults who become more active even late in life can experience improvements in physical fitness and functional health.

sources: Centers for Disease Control and Prevention. 2007. Prevalence of regular physical activity among adults—United States, 2001 and 2005. *Morbidity and Mortality Weekly Report* 56 (46): 1209–1212; Physical Activity Guidelines Advisory Committee. 2008. *Physical Activity Guidelines Advisory Committee Report, 2008.* Washington, DC: U.S. Department of Health and Human Services; Simonsick, E. M., et al. 2005. Just get out the door! Importance of walking outside the home for maintaining mobility: Findings from the Women's Health and Aging Study. *Journal of the American Geriatrics Society* 53(2): 198–203.

• Older adults should also do muscle-strengthening activities that are moderate or high intensity and involve all major muscle groups on two or more days a week because these activities provide additional health benefits.

There are also guidelines just for older adults:

• When older adults cannot do 150 minutes of moderate-intensity aerobic activity a week because of chronic conditions, they should be as physically active as their abilities and conditions allow.

• Older adults should do exercises that maintain or improve balance if they are at risk of falling.

• Older adults with chronic conditions should understand whether and how their conditions affect their ability to do regular physical activity safely.

• Older adults should perform flexibility exercises necessary for regular physical activity and activities of daily life.

For more about the beneficial effects of exercise for older adults, see the box "Can Exercise Delay the Effects of Aging?"

Eat Wisely Good health at any age is enhanced by eating a varied diet full of nutrient-rich foods. Special guidelines for older adults include the following:

• Get enough vitamin B-12 and extra vitamin D from fortified foods or supplements.

• Limit sodium intake to 1500 mg per day, and get enough potassium (4700 mg per day). Older adults tend to have higher blood pressure and to be salt-sensitive.

- Eat foods rich in dietary fiber and drink plenty of water to help prevent constipation.
- Pay special attention to food safety. Older adults are often more susceptible to foodborne illness.

Maintain a Healthy Weight   Weight management is especially difficult if you have been overweight most of your life. A sensible program of expending more calories through exercise, cutting calorie intake, or a combination of both will work for most people who want to lose weight, but there is no magic formula. Obesity is not physically healthy, and it leads to premature aging.

Control Drinking and Overdependence on Medications   Alcohol abuse ranks with depression as a common hidden mental health problem, affecting about 10% of older adults. (The ability to metabolize alcohol decreases with age.) The problem is often not identified because the effects of alcohol or drug dependence can mimic disease, such as Alzheimer's disease. Signs of potential alcohol or drug dependence include unexplained falls or frequent injuries, forgetfulness, depression, and malnutrition. Problems can be avoided by not using alcohol to relieve anxiety or emotional pain and not taking medication when safer forms of treatment are available.

Don't Smoke   The average pack-a-day smoker can expect to live about 13–14 fewer years than a nonsmoker. Furthermore, smokers suffer more illnesses that last longer, and they are subject to respiratory disabilities that limit their total vigor for many years before their death. Premature balding, skin wrinkling, and osteoporosis have been linked to cigarette smoking.

Schedule Physical Examinations to Detect Treatable Diseases   When detected early, many diseases, including hypertension, diabetes, and many types of cancer, can be successfully controlled by medication and lifestyle changes. Regular testing for glaucoma after age 40 can prevent blindness from this eye disease. Recommended screenings and immunizations can protect against preventable chronic and infectious diseases.

Recognize and Reduce Stress   Stress-induced physiological changes increase wear and tear on your body. Cut down on the stresses in your life. Don't wear yourself out through lack of sleep, substance abuse or misuse, or overwork. Practice relaxation using the techniques described in Chapter 2.

DEALING WITH THE CHANGES OF AGING

Just as you can act now to prevent or limit the physical changes of aging, you can also begin preparing yourself psychologically, socially, and financially for changes that may occur later in life.

Planning for Social Changes

Retirement marks a major change in the second half of life. As Americans' longevity has increased, people spend a larger proportion of their lives in retirement. By 2030, 18% of the population will be over age 65, up from 13% in 2010. In 2056, for the first time, the older population aged 65 and over is projected to outnumber the younger population aged 18 and under.

Changing Roles and Relationships   Changes in social roles are a major feature of life as we age. Children become young adults and leave home, putting an end to daily parenting. Parents experiencing this empty-nest syndrome must adapt to changes in their customary responsibilities and personal identities. And although retirement may be a desirable milestone for most people, it may also be viewed as a threat to prestige, purpose, and self-respect—the loss of a valued or customary role—and often requires some adjustment.

Retirement and the end of child rearing also bring about changes in the relationship between marriage partners. The amount of time a couple spends together will increase, and activities will change. Couples may need a period of adjustment in which they get to know each other as individuals again. Discussing what types of activities each partner enjoys can help couples set up a mutually satisfying routine of shared and independent activities.

Increased Leisure Time   Although retirement confers the advantages of leisure time and freedom from deadlines, competition, and stress, many people do not know how to enjoy their free time. If you have developed diverse interests, retirement can be a joyful and fulfilling period of your life. It can provide opportunities for expanding your horizons by giving you the chance to try new activities, take classes, and meet new people. Volunteering in your community can enhance self-esteem and allow you to be a contributing member of society.

The Economics of Retirement   Financial planning for retirement should begin early in life. People in their twenties and thirties should estimate how much money they need to support their standard of living, calculate their projected income, and begin a savings program. The earlier people begin such a program, the more money they will have at retirement.

Financial planning for retirement is especially critical for women. American women are much less likely than men to be covered by pension plans, reflecting the fact that many women have lower-paying jobs or work part-time during their childbearing years. They tend to have less money vested in other types of retirement plans as well. Although the gap is narrowing, women currently outlive men by about five to six years, and they are more likely to develop chronic conditions that impair their daily activities later in life. The net result of these factors is that older women are almost twice as likely as older men to live in poverty. Women should investigate their retirement plans and take charge of their finances to be sure they will be provided for as they get older.

Adapting to Physical Changes

Some changes in physical functioning are inevitable, and successful aging involves anticipating and accommodating these changes. Decreased energy and changes in health mean that older people have to develop priorities for how to use their energy. Rather than curtailing activities to conserve energy, they need to learn how to generate energy. Generating energy usually involves saying yes to enjoyable activities and paying close attention to the need for rest and sleep. Adapting, rather than giving up, favorite activities may be the best strategy for dealing with physical limitations. For example, if arthritis interferes with playing an instrument, a person can continue to enjoy music by taking up a different instrument or attending concerts.

Hearing Loss   The loss of hearing is a common physical change that can have a particularly strong effect on the lives of older adults. Hearing loss affects a person's ability to interact with others and can lead to a sense of isolation and depression. Hearing loss should be assessed and treated by a health care professional. In some cases hearing can be completely restored by dealing with the underlying cause of hearing loss. In other cases hearing aids may be prescribed.

Vision Changes   Vision usually declines with age. For some individuals this can be traced to conditions such as **glaucoma** or **age-related macular degeneration (AMD)** that can be treated medically. Glaucoma is caused by increased pressure within the eye due to built-up fluid. The optic nerve can be damaged by this increased pressure, resulting in a loss of side vision and, if untreated, blindness. Medication can relieve the pressure by decreasing the amount of fluid produced or by helping it drain more efficiently. Laser and conventional surgery are other options. Of the 4 million Americans with glaucoma, only half know that they have it; others lose the opportunity to control it and preserve their sight. People over 60, African Americans over 40, and anyone with a family history of glaucoma are at risk.

AMD is a slow disintegration of the *macula*—the tissue at the center of the retina where fine, straight-ahead detail is distinguished. AMD affects more than 1.5 million Americans over 40 and is the leading cause of blindness in people over age 75. Losing this vision makes it difficult to read, drive, or perform other close-up activities. Risk factors for AMD are age, gender (women may be at higher risk than men), smoking, elevated cholesterol levels, and family history. Some cases of AMD can be treated with laser surgery. Both glaucoma and AMD can be detected with regular screening.

By the time they reach their forties, many people have developed **presbyopia**—a gradual decline in the ability to focus on objects close to them. **Cataracts,** a clouding of the lens caused by lifelong oxidation damage (a by-product of normal body chemistry), may dim vision by the sixties.

Arthritis   An estimated 50 million American adults (about one of five) report having doctor-diagnosed **arthritis.** This degenerative disease causes joint inflammation leading to chronic pain, swelling, and loss of mobility.

There are more than 100 different types of arthritis; osteoarthritis (OA) is by far the most common. It most often affects the hands and weight-bearing joints of the body—the knees, ankles, and hips.

Strategies for reducing the risk of arthritis and, for those who already have OA, for managing it include exercise, weight management, and avoidance of heavy or repetitive muscle use. Exercise lubricates joints and strengthens the muscles around them, protecting them from further damage. Swimming, walking, cross-country skiing, cycling, and tai chi are good low-impact exercises.

Many people with OA take medication to relieve inflammation and reduce pain. Nonsteroidal anti-inflammatory drugs (NSAIDs) like ibuprofen can help but can irritate the digestive tract; prescription drugs that relieve pain without damaging the stomach may have other dangerous side effects. Acetaminophen can also reduce pain without upsetting the stomach, but exceeding the recommended dosage can cause liver damage.

glaucoma   An increase in pressure in the eye TERMS due to fluid buildup that can result in loss of side vision and, if left untreated, blindness.

age-related macular degeneration (AMD)   A deterioration of the macula (the central area of the retina) leading to blurred vision and sensitivity to glare; some cases can lead to blindness.

presbyopia   The inability of the eyes to focus sharply on nearby objects, caused by a loss of elasticity of the lens that occurs with advancing age.

cataracts   Opacity of the lens of the eye that impairs vision and can cause blindness.

arthritis   Inflammation and swelling of a joint or joints, causing pain and swelling.

Menopause   The natural process of menopause usually occurs during a woman's forties or fifties. The ovaries gradually stop functioning, estrogen levels drop, and eventually menstruation ceases. Several years before a woman stops menstruating, her periods usually become irregular, and she may experience hot flashes, vaginal dryness, sleep disturbances, and mood swings. This period, called *perimenopause,* can be troublesome for many women, some more than others.

Lifestyle strategies to reduce menopause-related problems include eating a healthy diet, exercising, losing weight, avoiding tobacco, and managing stress.

Sexual Functioning   The ability to enjoy sex can continue well into old age, particularly if people make the effort to understand and respond to the various changes that age brings to the natural pattern of sexual response. All too often, older people give up intercourse because they mistakenly interpret these changes as signs of impending impotence. Lovemaking may become a more leisurely affair as a couple gets older, but the benefits of maintaining the sexual aspect of the relationship into old age can be great.

Osteoporosis   As described in Chapter 9, **osteoporosis** is a condition in which bones become dangerously thin and fragile over time. Fractures are the most serious consequence of osteoporosis. Other problems associated with osteoporosis are loss of height and a stooped posture due to vertebral fractures, severe back and hip pain, and breathing problems caused by changes in the shape of the skeleton.

More than 40 million people in the United States either already have osteoporosis or are at high risk due to low bone mass. Women are at greater risk than men for osteoporosis because they have 10–25% less bone in their skeletons and because bone loss accelerates in women during the first 5–10 years after the onset of menopause due to the drop in estrogen production. Black or Latino women have higher bone density and fewer fractures than white or Asian women but may be at increased risk of osteoporosis due to lack of vitamin D (a condition caused by high levels of melatonin). Other risk factors include a family history of osteoporosis, early menopause (before age 45), abnormal or irregular menstruation, a history of anorexia, and a thin, small frame. Thyroid medication, corticosteroid drugs for arthritis or asthma, and long-term use of certain contraceptives can also have a negative effect on bone mass.

Preventing osteoporosis requires building as much bone as possible during your young years and then maintaining it as you age. Girls aged 9–18 are in their critical bone-building years,

and it is recommended that they eat more foods rich in calcium and vitamin D and get adequate exercise. Weight-bearing aerobic activities must be performed regularly throughout life to have lasting effects. Strength training improves bone density, muscle mass, strength, and balance, protecting against both bone loss and falls, a major cause of fractures. Even for people in their seventies, low-intensity strength training has been shown to improve bone density.

Two other lifelong strategies for reducing the effects of osteoporosis are avoiding tobacco use and managing depression and stress.

Bone mineral density testing can be used to gauge an individual's risk of fracture and help determine if any treatment is needed.

Handling Psychological and Mental Changes

Many older adults in good health remain mentally alert and retain their capacity to learn and remember new information. Many people become smarter as they become older and more experienced in life.

Dementia   **Dementia** is a loss of brain function that affects memory, thinking, language, judgment, and behavior. It affects about 1% of people aged 60–64 years and as many as 30–50% of people older than 85 years. Early symptoms of dementia include slight disturbances in a person's ability to grasp the situation he or she is in. As dementia progresses, memory failure becomes apparent, and the person may forget conversations, the events of the day, or how to perform simple tasks. It is important to have any symptoms evaluated by a health care professional because some of the over 50 known causes of dementia are treatable.

The most common forms of dementia among older people—Alzheimer's disease, and multi-infarct dementia—are irreversible. The most common, **Alzheimer's disease (AD),** is a progressive brain disorder

TERMS

osteoporosis   The loss of bone density, causing bones to become weak, porous, and more prone to fractures, usually at the hip, spine, or wrist.

dementia   Deterioration of mental functioning (including memory, concentration, and judgment) resulting from a brain disorder; often accompanied by emotional disturbances and personality changes.

Alzheimer's disease   A disease characterized by a progressive loss of mental functioning (dementia), caused by a degeneration of brain cells.

that damages and eventually destroys brain cells, leading to loss of memory, thinking, and other brain functions.

In 2013, an estimated 5.2 million Americans of all ages had Alzheimer's disease, which usually occurs in people over 60 but can occur in people as young as 40. By 2050, the number of people age 65 and older who currently have the disease may nearly triple from 5 million to a projected 13.8 million. Ultimately Alzheimer's is fatal, and currently there is no cure.

Multi-infarct dementia results from a series of small strokes or changes in the brain's blood supply that deprive the brain of oxygen and destroy brain tissue. Symptoms may appear suddenly and worsen with additional strokes; they include disorientation in familiar locations; walking with rapid, shuffling steps; incontinence; laughing or crying inappropriately; difficulty following instructions; and problems handling money. High blood pressure, cigarette smoking, and high cholesterol are some of the risk factors for stroke that may be controlled to prevent vascular dementia.

Grief Another psychological and emotional challenge of aging is dealing with grief and mourning. Aging is associated with loss—the loss of friends, family and spouse, peers, physical appearance, possessions, and health. Grief is the process of getting through the pain of loss, and it can be one of the loneliest and most emotionally intense times in a person's life. It can take years to completely come to terms with the loss of a loved one. Unresolved grief can have serious physical and psychological or emotional health consequences and may require professional help.

Depression and Suicide Unresolved grief can lead to depression, a common problem in older adults. If you notice the signs of depression in yourself or someone you know, consult a mental health professional. A marked loss of interest in usually pleasurable activities, decreased appetite, insomnia, fatigue, and feelings of worthlessness are signs of depression. Listen carefully when an older friend or relative complains about being depressed; it may be a request for help.

Although the elderly (age 65 and older) comprise about 13% of the U.S. population, they account for over 18% of all suicides. People aged 85 and older have the highest suicide rate of any age group. Older white men have a suicide rate almost six times that of the general population—more than women and minorities at any age.

Depression is probably the single most significant factor associated with suicidal behavior in older adults.

> There are many theories about aging, but **none fully explains all the changes** of the aging process.

LIFE IN AGING AMERICA

Life expectancy is the average length of time we can expect to live. It is calculated by averaging mortality statistics—the ages at death of a group of people over a certain period. In 2010 life expectancy for the total population was 78.7 years, but those who reach age 65 can expect to live even longer—20 more years. A man reaching age 65 today can expect to live, on average, until age 84. A woman turning age 65 today can expect to live, on average, until age 86. Women have a longer life expectancy than men do (see the box "Why Do Women Live Longer?"). Life expectancy also varies among ethnic groups; reasons for these differences include socioeconomic, genetic, and lifestyle factors.

As life expectancy increases, a larger proportion of Americans will be in their later years. This change will necessitate new government policies and changes in our general attitudes toward older adults.

America's Aging Minority

People over age 65 are a large minority in the American population—over 40.2 million people and about 14% of the total population in 2012. That number is expected to more than double by the year 2050.

The enormous increase in the over-65 population is markedly affecting our stereotypes of what it means to grow old. The misfortunes associated with aging—frailty, forgetfulness, poor health, isolation—occur in fewer people in their sixties and seventies and are shifting instead to burden the very old: those over age 85.

The homeownership rate exceeds 80% for those ages 65 to 84, declining slightly to about 76% for those older than 85. This rate is much higher than the homeownership rate for all households under age 65 (about 65%). Older people's living expenses are lower after retirement because they no longer support children and have fewer work-related expenses; they consume and buy less food. They are more likely to continue practicing their expertise for years after retirement: thousands of retired consultants, teachers, technicians, and craftspeople work until their middle and late seventies. They receive greater amounts of assistance, such as Medicare, pay proportionately lower taxes, and have greater net worth from lifetime savings.

As the aging population increases proportionately, however, the number of older people who are ill and dependent rises. Health care remains the largest expense for older adults. On average, they visit a physician 10–12 times a year, are hospitalized more frequently, and require twice as many prescription drugs as the general population. Most older Americans have at least one chronic condition; 77% have at least two.

Retirement finds many older people with their incomes reduced to subsistence levels. The majority of older

---

life expectancy The average length of time a person is expected to live.

TERMS

Women live longer than men in most countries around the world, even in places where maternal mortality rates are high. In the United States, women on average can expect to live about five years longer than men. Worldwide, women comprise 85% of the population that is more than 100 years old.

The reason for the gender gap in life expectancy is not entirely understood but may be influenced by biological, social, and lifestyle factors. Medical consensus used to be that estrogen contributed to women's longevity. Not only has this theory been disproved, but research indicates that estrogen supplements may be detrimental to postmenopausal women. However, estrogen production and other factors during a woman's younger years may protect her from early heart disease and from age-related declines in the heart's pumping power.

Another theory suggests that menstruation has contributed to women's longer life expectancy. Because women excrete excess iron during menstruation, it is thought that women tend to experience a later onset of cardiovascular disease than men do. Additionally, women may have lower rates of stress-related

illnesses because they cope more positively with stress.

The news for women is not all good, however, because not all their extra years are likely to be healthy years. They are more likely than men to suffer from chronic conditions like arthritis and osteoporosis. Women's longer life spans, combined with the facts that men tend to marry younger women and that

widowed men remarry more often than widowed women, mean there are many more single older women than men. Older men are more likely to live in family settings, whereas older women are more likely to live alone. Older women are also less likely to be covered by a pension or to have retirement savings, so they are more likely to be poor.

Social and behavioral factors may be more important than physiological causes in explaining the gender gap; for example, among the Amish, a religious sect that has strict rules against smoking and drinking, men usually live as long as women. This finding suggests that the longevity gap could be substantially narrowed through lifestyle changes. For example, men in general tend to take more risks than women—from driving more recklessly to using drugs and alcohol.

SOURCES: U.S. Census Bureau; National Center for Health Statistics. 2012. *Health, United States, 2012.* Hyattsville, MD: National Center for Health Statistics; World Health Organization. 2012. *Gender, Health, and Aging.* Geneva: World Health Organization.

connect ACTIVITY DO IT ONLINE

Americans live with fixed sources of income, such as pensions, that are eroded by inflation. **Social security** is the major source of income for most of the elderly. Social security was intended to serve as a supplement to personal savings and private pensions, not as a sole source of income. It is vital to plan for an adequate retirement income.

Family and Community Resources for Older Adults

With help from friends, family members, and community services, people in their later years can remain active and independent. Over half of noninstitutionalized older Americans live with a spouse; some live with a family member other than a spouse, and 30% live alone. Only 4% live in institutional settings, but among those over age 85, about 15% live in a nursing home.

QUICK STATS

The average American spends 20 years in retirement.

—U.S. Social Security Administration

In about three out of four cases, a spouse, a grown daughter, or a daughter-in-law assumes a caregiving role for elderly relatives.

Caregiving can be rewarding, but it is also hard work. If the experience is stressful and long-term, family members may become emotionally exhausted. Corporations are increasingly responsive to the needs of their employees who are family caregivers by providing services such as referrals, flexible schedules and leaves, and on-site adult care. Professional health care advice is another critical part of successful home care.

social security A government program that provides financial assistance to people who are unemployed, disabled, or retired (and over a certain age); financed through taxes on business and workers. **TERMS**

The best thing a family can do is talk honestly about the obligations, time, and commitment required by caregiving. Families should also explore community resources and professional assistance that may be available to reduce the stress in this difficult job.

Government Aid and Policies

The federal government helps older Americans through several programs, such as food stamps, housing subsidies, social security, Medicare, and Medicaid.

Medicare is a major health insurance program for older adults and disabled persons.

It provides basic health care coverage for acute episodes of illness that require skilled professional care. It pays for some preventive services. Medicare pays less than 2% of nursing home costs, and private insurers pay less than 1%, creating a tremendous financial burden for nursing home residents and their families. When their financial resources are exhausted, people may apply for Medicaid, which provides medical insurance to low-income people of any age.

Health care policy planners hope that rising medical costs for older adults will shrink dramatically through education and prevention. Health care professionals, including **gerontologists** and **geriatricians,** are beginning to practice preventive medicine, just as pediatricians do. They advise

TERMS

gerontologist   A scientist who studies the biological, psychological, and social phenomena associated with aging and old age.

geriatrician   A physician specializing in the diseases, disabilities, and care of older adults.

life support systems   Medical technologies, such as a ventilator, that allow vital body functions to be artificially sustained.

brain death   An irreversible cessation of brain activity indicated by various diagnostic criteria, including a flat EEG reading; this medical determination may be necessary when intensive hospital-based life support systems have been used to artificially sustain organ systems in the body.

electroencephalogram (EEG)   A record of the electrical activity of the brain (brain waves).

Ask Yourself

QUESTIONS FOR CRITICAL THINKING AND REFLECTION

What do you want your life to be like when you are old? Do you hope to retire, or keep working indefinitely? Where would you like to live? How much time do you spend thinking about these questions? What have you planned for your later years?

older people about how to avoid and, if necessary, how to manage disabilities.

WHAT IS DEATH?

Whether it is a mudslide in Washington State claiming dozens, or an explosion of a coal mine in Turkey killing hundreds, a man collapsing with a heart attack in a crowded restaurant, or a woman in her 90s dying peacefully with her family close by, images of death are easy to envision. Nevertheless, we rarely think about the inevitability of death in our own lives. Accepting and dealing with death are important tasks that present unique challenges to our sense of self, our relationships with others, and our understanding of the meaning of life itself.

Although pain and distress may accompany the dying process, facing death also presents an opportunity for growth as well as affirmation of the preciousness of simple aspects of our daily lives.

Questions about the meaning of death and what happens when we die are central concerns of the great religions and philosophies. Some promise a better life after death. Others teach that everyone is evolving toward perfection or divinity, a goal reached after successive rounds of death and rebirth. There are also those who suggest that it is not possible to know what—if anything—happens after death and that any judgment about life's worth must be made on the basis of satisfactions or rewards that we create for ourselves in our lifetimes.

Even in modern secular societies, religion plays a major role in shaping our attitudes and behaviors toward death. The mourning ceremonies associated with various religious practices ease the pangs of grief for many people. Dying and death are more than biological events; they have social and spiritual dimensions.

Defining Death

Traditionally death has been defined as cessation of the flow of vital body fluids. This cessation occurs when the heart stops beating and breathing ceases. These traditional signs are adequate for determining death in most cases. However, the use of ventilators, artificial heart pumps, and other **life support systems** allow many body functions to be artificially sustained. The concept of **brain death** was developed to determine whether a person is alive or dead when the traditional signs are inadequate because of supportive medical technology.

According to the standards published by a Harvard Medical School committee, brain death involves four characteristics: (1) lack of receptivity and response to external stimuli, (2) absence of spontaneous muscular movement and spontaneous breathing, (3) absence of observable reflexes, and (4) absence of brain activity, as signified by a flat **electroencephalogram (EEG).** The Harvard criteria require that a second set of tests be performed after 24 hours have elapsed, and they exclude cases of hypothermia (body temperature below 90°F) and situations involving central nervous system depressants, such as barbiturates.

In contrast to **clinical death,** which is determined by either the cessation of heartbeat and breathing or the criteria for establishing brain death, **cellular death** refers to a gradual process that occurs when heartbeat, respiration, and brain activity have stopped. It encompasses the breakdown of metabolic processes and results in complete nonfunctionality at the cellular level.

The way death is defined has potential legal and social consequences in a variety of areas, including criminal prosecution, inheritance, taxation, treatment of the corpse, and even mourning. It also affects the practice of organ transplantation because some organs—hearts, most obviously—must be harvested from a human being who is legally determined to be dead.

In Mexico, individuals publicly celebrate departed loved ones on the annual holiday, Día de los Muertos (Day of the Dead).

Learning about Death

Our understanding of death changes as we grow and mature, as do our attitudes toward it. Very young children view death as an interruption and an absence, but their lack of a mature time perspective means that they do not understand death as final and irreversible. A child's understanding of death evolves greatly from about age 6 to age 9. During this period, most children begin to understand that death is final, universal, and inevitable. A person who consciously recognizes these facts is said to possess a **mature understanding of death.**

It is important to add, however, that individuals who possess a mature understanding of death commonly hold nonempirical ideas about it as well. Such nonempirical ideas—that is, ideas not subject to scientific proof—deal mainly with the notion that human beings survive in some form beyond the death of the physical body. What happens to an individual's personality after he or she dies? Does the self or soul continue to exist after the death of the physical body? If so, what is the nature of this afterlife? Developing personally satisfying answers to such questions, which involve what Mark Speece and Sandor Brent term **noncorporeal continuity,** is also part of the process of acquiring a mature understanding of death.

> **Our understanding of death changes as we grow and mature,** as do our attitudes toward it.

Attitudes Toward Death

Our ability to find meaning and comfort in the face of mortality depends not only on our having an understanding of the facts of death, but also on our attitudes toward it. Many people seek to avoid any thought or mention of death. The sick and old are often isolated in hospitals and nursing homes. Relatively few Americans have been present at the death of a loved one. Where the reality of death is concerned, "out of sight, out of mind" often appears to be the rule of the day.

Although some commentators characterize the predominant attitude toward death in the United States as "death denying," others are reluctant to generalize so broadly. People often maintain conflicting or ambivalent attitudes toward death. Those who come to view death as a relief or release from insufferable pain may have at least a partial sense of welcoming death. Few people wholly avoid or wholly welcome death. In the past several decades, attitudes toward death in our culture have begun to slowly change, particularly as the hospice movement has grown.

Not all cultures are reluctant to publicly acknowledge death. For example, traditional Mexican culture honors the dead in an annual holiday known as Día de los Muertos (Day of the Dead), in which families celebrate their departed loved ones. Similar celebrations that honor the dead in a festive manner are common in many cultures throughout the world.

PLANNING FOR DEATH

Acknowledging the inevitability of death allows us to plan for it. Adequate planning can help ensure that a sudden, unexpected death is not made even more difficult for survivors. Even when

---

clinical death   The medical term defining when there is no longer blood flow in the body (the heart has stopped beating) and breathing has ceased; sufficient to determine death in most cases.

cellular death   The breakdown of metabolic processes at the level of the body's cells.

mature understanding of death   The recognition that death is universal and irreversible, that it involves the cessation of all physiological functioning, and that there are biological reasons for its occurrence.

noncorporeal continuity   The notion that human beings survive in some form after the death of the physical body.

TERMS

What situations or events make you think seriously about your own mortality? Is this something you consider now and then, or do you avoid thinking about death? What has influenced your willingness or reluctance to think about death?

death is not sudden, many decisions can be anticipated, considered, and discussed with close relatives and friends.

Making a Will

Surveys indicate that about 55% of Americans do not have a will. A **will** is a legal instrument expressing a person's intentions and wishes for the disposition of his or her property after death. It is a declaration of how your **estate**—that is, money, property, and other possessions—will be distributed after death. During the life of the **testator** (the person making the will), a will can be changed, replaced, or revoked. Upon the testator's death, it becomes a legal instrument governing the distribution of the testator's estate.

When a person dies **intestate**—that is, without having left a valid will—property is distributed according to rules set up by the state. If you haven't yet made a will, start thinking about how you'd like your property distributed in the case of your death. If you have a will, consider whether it needs to be updated in response to a key life event such as marriage, the birth of a child, or the purchase of a home.

You can also help your family members by completing a *testamentary letter.* This document includes information about your personal affairs, such as bank accounts, credit cards, the location of documents and keys, the names of your professional advisers, the names of people who should be notified of your death, and so on.

---

will A legal instrument expressing a person's intentions and wishes for the disposition of his or her property after death.

TERMS

estate The money, property, and other possessions belonging to a person.

testator The person who makes a will.

intestate Not having made a legal will.

hospice A system of palliative care specifically for patients that are likely to die within six months, often at home, to optimize the quality of life of dying patients and their families.

palliative care A collaborative, team-based approach to treatment that aims to prevent and relieve suffering in patients with serious or life-threatening illness.

persistent vegetative state A condition of profound unconsciousness in which a person lacks normal reflexes and is unresponsive to external stimuli, lasting for an extended period with no reasonable hope of improvement.

Considering Options for End-of-Life Care

An appropriate balance in end-of-life care may involve any combination of home care, hospital stays, nursing home care, and hospice care.

Home Care The majority of people express a preference for at-home care during the end of life. An obvious advantage of home care is the fact that the person is in a familiar setting, ideally in the company of family and friends. Family members may or may not be capable of providing the level of care that is needed, and skilled professional caregivers may have to be hired. Currently about 25% of Americans die at home.

Hospice Programs Terminally ill people who wish to die at home, in their assisted-living residence, or in a more peaceful hospital environment are often aided by **hospice** programs, which are widely available throughout the United States.

Hospice is a system of **palliative care,** a collaborative, team-based approach to treatment that aims to prevent and relieve suffering in patients with serious or life-threatening illness. The overarching goal of palliative care is to improve the quality of life for both the patient and family during this period in their lives.

About two-thirds of hospice patients receive care in the place they call "home," which is most frequently their private residence, but also can be a nursing home or a residential facility. Hospice care is also offered in hospitals and freestanding hospice facilities. Physicians, nurses, pharmacists, chaplains, social workers, home health aides, and trained volunteers make up the core of the hospice team.

More than 40% of people who died in the United States in 2012 were under the care of a hospice program. About 65% of hospice patients are over 75 years old, although hospice programs take care of patients of all ages, including children. In addition to helping patients achieve a good and peaceful death, an important gift of hospice care is the potential to help patients and families discover how much can be shared at the end of life through personal and spiritual connections.

Difficult Decisions at the End of Life

Modern medicine can sometimes keep the human organism alive despite the cessation of normal heart, brain, respiratory, or kidney function. But should a patient without any hope of recovery be kept alive by means of artificial life support? What if a patient has fallen into a **persistent vegetative state,** a state of profound unconsciousness, lacking any sign of normal reflexes and unresponsive to external stimuli, with no reasonable hope of improvement?

Ethical questions about a person's right to die have become prominent since the landmark case of Karen Ann Quinlan in 1975. At age 22 she was admitted in a comatose state to an intensive care unit, where her breathing was sustained by a mechanical ventilator. When she remained unresponsive, in a persistent vegetative state, her parents asked that the respirator be disconnected, but the medical staff responsible for Karen's care denied their request. The request to withdraw treatment eventually reached the New Jersey Supreme Court, which ruled that artificial respiration could be discontinued.

Since then courts have ruled on removing other types of life-sustaining treatment, including artificial feeding mechanisms that provide nutrition and hydration to permanently comatose patients who are able to breathe on their own. Notable was the case of Terri Schiavo in 2003. Terri had been diagnosed as being in a persistent vegetative state. Contending that she would not want to continue living on life support, Terri's husband requested that her feeding tube be removed. Terri's parents contested the request, and a series of legal actions ensued. Finally, in 2005, after intervention by the U.S. Supreme Court, physicians were allowed to remove the tube. Cases like this highlight the importance of expressing your wishes about life-sustaining treatment, in writing, before the need arises.

Withholding or Withdrawing Treatment   The right of a competent patient to refuse unwanted treatment is now generally established in both law and medical practice. The consensus is that there is no medical or ethical distinction between withholding (not starting) a treatment and withdrawing (stopping) a treatment once it has been started. The choice to forgo life-sustaining treatment involves refusing treatments that would be expected to extend life. The right to refuse treatment remains constitutionally protected even when a patient is unable to communicate. Although specific requirements vary, all states authorize some type of written advance directive to honor the decisions of individuals unable to speak for themselves but who have previously recorded their wishes in an appropriate legal document.

Physician-Assisted Suicide and Active Euthanasia
In contrast to withdrawing or withholding treatment, *physician-assisted suicide* and *active euthanasia* refer to practices that intentionally hasten the death of a person.

Physician-assisted suicide (PAS) which is legal in three states in the United States, occurs when a physician provides lethal drugs—at the patient's request—with the understanding that the patient plans to use them to end his or her life. The patient administers the fatal dose.

Oregon was the first state to legalize physician-assisted suicide following a citizens' initiative called the Death with Dignity Act, which was passed by the Oregon voters in 1994 and again in 1997. Even though PAS has been legally available in Oregon since 1994, the practice remains rare; in 2012 only 77 deaths occurred in Oregon as a result of physician-assisted suicide.

Another important Supreme Court ruling involved the concept of **double effect** in the medical management of pain. The doctrine of double effect states that a harmful effect of treatment, even if it results in death, is permissible if the harm is not intended and occurs as a side effect of a beneficial action. Sometimes the dosages of medication needed to relieve a patient's pain (especially those in the end stage of some diseases) must be increased to levels that can cause respiratory depression, which could hasten the patient's death. The doctrine of double effect allows physicians throughout the United States to do what is necessary to relieve pain, even if there is a chance that the medication may hasten death.

Unlike physician-assisted suicide, **active euthanasia** is the intentional act of killing someone who would otherwise suffer from an incurable and painful disease.

Voluntary euthanasia (also known as voluntary active euthanasia, or VAE) is the intentional termination of life at the patient's request. In practice, this generally means that a competent patient requests direct assistance to die, and he or she receives assistance from a qualified medical practitioner. Voluntary active euthanasia is legal under very strict guidelines in Belgium, Luxembourg, and the Netherlands, but is currently unlawful in the United States and the rest of the world. Taking active steps to end someone's life is a crime— even if the motive is mercy.

Completing an Advance Directive

To make your preferences known about medical treatment, you need to document them through a written **advance directive.**

physician-assisted suicide (PAS)   The practice TERMS of a physician intentionally providing, at the patient's request, lethal drugs or other means for a patient to hasten death with the understanding that the patient plans to use them to end his or her life. The patient administers the drug to himself or herself.

double effect   A situation in which a harmful effect occurs as an unintended side effect of a beneficial action, such as when medication intended to control a patient's pain has the unintended result of causing the patient's death.

active euthanasia   A deliberate act intended to end another person's life; voluntary active euthanasia involves the practice of a physician administering—at the request of a patient— medication or some other intervention that causes death.

advance directive   Any statement made by a competent person about his or her choices for medical treatment should he or she become unable to make such decisions or communicate them in the future.

Ask Yourself

Have you ever been involved in a funeral? What role did you play? Did you feel that the service reflected the values and beliefs of the deceased person? Did the experience cause you to think about your own funeral and what it should be like?

Two forms of advance directives are legally important. First is the **living will,** which enables individuals to provide instructions about the kind of medical care they wish to receive (or not receive) if they become incapacitated or otherwise unable to participate in treatment decisions.

The second important form of advance directive is the **health care proxy,** which is also known as a *durable power of attorney for health care.* This document makes it possible to appoint another person to make decisions about medical treatment if you become unable to do so. This decision maker may be a family member, close friend, or attorney with whom you have discussed your treatment preferences. The proxy is expected to act in accordance with your wishes as stated in an advance directive or as otherwise made known.

For advance directives to be of value, you must do more than merely complete the paperwork. Discuss your wishes ahead of time with caregivers and family members as well as with your physician.

Giving the Gift of Life

Each day about 79 people receive an organ transplant while another 18 people on the waiting lists die because not enough organs are available. As of January 2014, more than 121,000 Americans were waiting for organ transplants.

If you decide to become an organ donor, the first step is to indicate your wish by completing a **Uniform Donor Card** (Figure 17.1); alternatively, you can indicate your wish on

---

TERMS

living will   A type of advance directive that allows individuals to provide instructions about the kind of medical care they wish to receive, or not receive, if they become unable to participate in treatment decisions.

health care proxy   A type of advance directive that allows an individual to appoint another person as an agent in making health care decisions in the event he or she becomes unable to participate in treatment decisions; also known as a *durable power of attorney for health care.*

Uniform Donor Card   A consent form authorizing the use of the signer's body parts for transplantation or medical research upon his or her death.

embalming   The process of removing blood and other fluids and replacing them with chemicals to disinfect and temporarily retard deterioration of a corpse; some of the chemicals used, such as formaldehyde, are toxic.

 Organ/Tissue Donor Card

I wish to donate my organs and tissues. I wish to give:

☐ any needed organs and tissues

☐ only the following organs and tissues:

_____

Donor
Signature _____ Date _____

Witness _____

Witness _____

FIGURE 17.1   A sample organ/tissue donor card.

SOURCE: U.S. Department of Health and Human Services (http://www.organdonor.gov/index.html).

your driver's license in many states. Because relatives are called on to make decisions about organ and tissue donation at the time of a loved one's death, your second step is to discuss your decision with your family.

Planning a Funeral or Memorial Service

Funerals and memorial services are rites of passage that commemorate a person's life and acknowledge his or her passing from the community. Funerals and memorials allow survivors to support one another as they cope with their loss and express their grief. The presence of death rites in every human culture suggests that these ceremonies serve innate human needs.

Disposition of the Body   People generally have a preference about the final disposition of their body. For most Americans, the choice is either burial or cremation. *Burial* involves a grave dug into the soil or entombment in a mausoleum. If the family wishes that the body be viewed during a wake or in an open casket funeral, **embalming** is generally done.

Cremation involves subjecting a body to intense heat. Cremated remains can be buried, placed in a columbarium niche, put into an urn kept by the family or interred in an urn garden, or scattered at sea or on land. Cremation is now used in more than 40% of deaths in the United States, with the rate of cremation increasing rapidly in recent years.

Arranging a Service   A funeral or memorial service can be a healing experience that allows loved ones to share memories and support one another. The more the service fits the personality of the deceased person and meets the practical needs of the family, the better.

People who have a terminal illness sometimes find comfort and satisfaction in helping to plan for their own memorial services. A memorial service can be the joint creation of the dying person and family members who wish to be part of the project. Making at least some plans ahead of time can help ease the burden on survivors, who will undoubtedly face a great number of tasks and decisions when the death occurs (see the box "Tasks for Survivors").

A traditional funeral with a casket costs about $7000, and many funerals cost $10,000 or more. When no preplanning has been done, as often occurs, family members have to make decisions under time pressure and in the grip of strong feelings. As a result, they may make poor decisions and spend more than they need to. To avoid these problems, millions of consumers are now making funeral arrangements in advance, comparing prices and services so they can make well-informed purchasing decisions. Many people see funeral planning as an extension of will and estate planning.

Alternatives to traditional funerals exist. Cremation is a much less expensive alternative to a traditional burial and is rapidly becoming nearly as common. A direct cremation (no service or visitation at the funeral home) can cost as little as $600 in some cities. Cremated remains can be buried in a family plot or placed in a mausoleum, but many people choose to keep the ashes at home or scatter them in a beautiful location. Whole-body donation (usually to a medical school) is another option chosen by many people for altruistic reasons, as well as the fact that there is usually no cost. Another alternative to an expensive traditional funeral is a more personalized, "do-it-yourself" family-centered funeral, with minimal costs because most or all of the tasks needed to care for the deceased person are provided by family and friends.

To ensure that you make the best possible decisions when planning a funeral, follow these guidelines:

- Plan ahead. Think about what type of funeral you want, and ask your loved ones about their preferences.

- Shop around. If you are going to use a funeral home, look for one that belongs to the National Funeral Directors Association (NFDA), and compare prices from at least two funeral homes.

- Ask for a price list. The Funeral Rule requires funeral directors to give you an itemized price list when you ask either in person or over the telephone. Many funeral homes offer package funerals that cost less than individual items, but you may not need or want everything included in the package.

connect
ACTIVITY
DO IT ONLINE

- Decide on the goods and services you want. Basic services include planning the funeral and coordinating arrangements with the cemetery or crematory. Embalming is not necessary or legally required if the body is buried or cremated shortly after death. The casket is usually the single most expensive item; an average casket costs slightly more than $2000, but some caskets sell for as much as $10,000. You do not have to buy the casket from the funeral home you use. Many "big box" stores now sell caskets at much lower cost than funeral homes.

- Resist pressure to buy goods and services you don't really want or need. Funeral directors are required to inform you that you need buy only those goods and services you want. If you feel you are being pressured, go elsewhere.

- In choosing a cemetery, take into consideration its location; its religious affiliation, if any; the types of monuments allowed; and cost. Visit the cemetery ahead of time to make sure it's suitable. If cremation is chosen, use of a cemetery is optional.

- Once decisions have been made, put them in writing, give copies to family members, and keep a copy accessible. It's a good idea to review these decisions every few years and revise them if necessary.

COPING WITH DYING

There is no one right way to live with or die of a life-threatening illness. Every disease has its own set of problems and challenges, and each person copes with these problems and challenges in his or her own way. Much of the suffering experienced by people with a life-threatening illness comes from overwhelming feelings of loss on all levels.

Living with an illness that is life-threatening and incurable can be described as a living–dying experience. Hope and honesty are often delicately balanced—honesty to face reality as it is, and hope for a positive outcome. The early hope that the symptoms are not really serious gives way to hope that a cure is possible. When the illness is deemed incurable, there is hope for more time. As time begins to run out, one hopes for a pain-free death—a "good death."

The Tasks of Coping

In her groundbreaking 1969 book *On Death and Dying*, Elisabeth Kübler-Ross, a Swiss American psychiatrist and one of the first medical experts to focus on the topic of end

TAKE CHARGE
Tasks for Survivors

Some of the following tasks must be attended to soon after a death occurs, whereas others take weeks or months to complete. Many of these tasks, especially those that need to be dealt with in the first hours and days following the death, can be taken care of by friends and relatives of the immediate survivors. If the deceased person has been served by a hospice, the social worker has likely worked with the patient and family to make many of these plans ahead of time.

• Prepare a list of relatives, friends, and colleagues, and telephone them about the death as soon as possible. Friends can help with notifications.

• Find out if the deceased left instructions for disposition of the body or for a funeral or memorial service.

• If no prior plan exists, contact a funeral home, mortuary, or memorial society for help in making arrangements. Clergy, friends, and other family members can be asked to help decide what is most appropriate.

• If flowers are to be omitted from the funeral or memorial service, choose an appropriate charity or other memorial to which gifts can be made.

• Write the obituary. Consider including the deceased's age, birthplace, cause of death, occupation, academic degrees, memberships, military service, accomplishments, names and relationships of nearest survivors, and the time and place of the funeral or memorial service. If a small funeral is planned, and you are notifying people by phone or e-mail, you can wait to write the obituary later, or skip it entirely. You can also use an online obituary website, and even create an online memorial to a loved one.

• Ask friends to help coordinate the supplying of meals for the first few days following the death, as well as the management of other household tasks and child care, if necessary. You can also ask friends to coordinate a potluck or catered meal if you wish to have a gathering after the funeral. Simple snacks and drinks are fine, if you choose.

• If you have relatives and friends who will be coming from out of town for the funeral, ask a friend or family member to help with arrangements for lodging and transportation to and from the airport.

• If a funeral ceremony is planned, choose the individuals who are to be pallbearers, and notify them that you would like their participation.

• Gather photos or other mementos for a memory book, memory board, or memorial website.

• Do you want to have a small booklet with information about the deceased and perhaps a photo or poem to give to mourners at the funeral or memorial service? If so, get help from family members and friends to create the pamphlet and have it printed.

connect
ACTIVITY
DO IT ONLINE

---

of life, suggested that the response to an awareness of imminent death involves five psychological stages: denial, anger, bargaining, depression, and acceptance. Individuals go back and forth among the stages during the course of an illness, and different stages can occur simultaneously. Today the notion of stages has been deemphasized in favor of highlighting the tasks that require attention in order to cope well with a life-threatening illness. Psychologist and author Charles Corr, for example, distinguishes four primary dimensions in coping with dying:

1. *Physical:* Satisfying bodily needs and minimizing physical distress.

2. *Psychological:* Maximizing a sense of security, self-worth, autonomy, and richness in living.

3. *Social:* Sustaining significant relationships and addressing the social implications of dying.

4. *Spiritual:* Identifying, developing, or reaffirming sources of meaning and fostering hope.

People who apparently cope best with life-threatening illness often exhibit a fighting spirit that views the illness not only as a threat but also as a challenge. These people strive to inform themselves about their illness and take an active part in treatment decisions. They are optimistic and have a capacity to discover positive meaning in ordinary events. Holding to a positive outlook despite distressing circumstances involves creating a sense of meaning that is bigger than the threat. In the context of life-threatening illness, this creating of meaning encompasses a person's ability to comprehend the implications an illness has for the future, as well as for his or her ability to accomplish goals, maintain relationships, and sustain a sense of personal vitality, competence, and power.

Supporting a Person in the Last Phase of Life

People often feel uncomfortable in the presence of a person who is in the final stage of life. How should we act? What can we say? Perhaps the most important and comforting thing we can do for a dying person is to simply be present. Sitting quietly and listening carefully, we can take our cues from the person who is dying. If the person is capable of speaking, and wishes to talk, attentive listening is an act of great kindness. If the person doesn't wish to talk, or is not able to, physical touch such as holding hands or putting a hand on the person's shoulder can be the most effective way to express your love and concern.

As death is drawing near simple steps—such as repositioning the patient, covering him or her with a light blanket, dimming the room's lighting, playing soft favorite music, or holding hands—can provide great relief and reassurance in the last moments.

COPING WITH LOSS

Even if we have not experienced the death of someone close, we are all survivors of losses that occur in our lives because of changes and endings. The loss of a job, the ending of a relationship, transitions from one school or neighborhood to another—these are examples of the kinds of losses that occur in all our lives. Such losses are sometimes called little deaths, and in varying degrees they all involve grief.

Experiencing Grief

Grief is the reaction to loss. It encompasses thoughts and feelings as well as physical and behavioral responses. Mental distress may involve disbelief, confusion, anxiety, disorganization, and depression. The emotions that can be present in normal grief include not only sorrow and sadness, but also relief, anger, guilt, and self-pity, among others. Common behaviors associated with grief include crying, searching for the deceased, and talking repetitively about the deceased and the circumstances of the death. Bereaved people may be restless, as if not knowing what to do with themselves. Outward signs of grief may involve frequent sighing, crying, inappropriate laughter, insomnia, loss of appetite, and marked fatigue. Guilt is a common emotion after the death of a loved one. All such manifestations of grief can be present as part of our total response to **bereavement**—that is, the event of loss.

Mourning refers not so much to the *reaction* to loss but to the *process* by which a bereaved person adjusts to loss and incorporates it into his or her life. How this process is managed is determined, at least partly, by cultural and gender norms for the expression of grief.

The Course of Grief Grieving, like dying, is highly individual. In the first hours or days following a death, a bereaved person is likely to experience shock and numbness, as well as a sense of disbelief, especially if the death was unexpected. The cause or mode of death—natural, accidental, homicide, or suicide—influences how grief is experienced. Even when a death is anticipated, grief is not necessarily diminished when the loss becomes real.

The death of a loved one is frequently a severe physical as well as emotional stressor. Grieving people often have difficulty sleeping, may neglect to eat nourishing food, and may forget to take their usual medications. These factors add to the health risks associated with recent loss. People often report that they feel confused and have difficulty concentrating following a significant loss.

After the initial shock begins to fade, the course of grief is characterized by anxiety, apathy, and pining for the deceased. The pangs of grief are felt as the bereaved person deeply experiences the pain of separation. There is often a sense of despair as a person repeatedly goes over the events surrounding the loss, perhaps fantasizing that somehow everything could be undone and be as it was before.

As time goes on, the acute pain and emotional turmoil of grief begin to subside. Physical and mental balance are reestablished. The bereaved person becomes increasingly reintegrated into his or her social world. Sadness doesn't go away completely, but it recedes into the background much of the time. Although reminders of the loss stimulate waves of active grieving from time to time, the main focus is the present, not the past. Adjusting to loss may sometimes feel like a betrayal of the deceased loved one, but it is healthy to engage again in ongoing life and the future.

Social support for the bereaved is as critical during the later course of grief as it is during the first days after a loss. The first anniversary and major holidays following a significant loss can be times of renewed grieving when the support of others is important and appreciated. Knowing that others remember the loss and that they take time to connect is usually perceived as comforting.

Bereaved people may find it helpful to share their stories and concerns through organized support groups. Hospices provide bereavement support groups and counseling. Many online and in-person support groups are organized around specific types of bereavement, such as the loss of a child, the loss of a parent, or the loss of a loved one to suicide.

Supporting a Grieving Person

When a person finds out that a loved one has died, the initial reaction may be profound shock and overwhelming distress. Such a person may initially respond best to the physical comfort of hugging and holding. Later, simply listening may be the most effective way to help. Talking about a loss is an important way that many survivors cope with the changed reality, and they may need to tell their story over and over. The key to being a good listener is to avoid speaking too much, and to refrain from making judgments about whether the thoughts and feelings expressed by a survivor are right or wrong, good or bad.

> Grieving, like dying, is highly individual.

grief A person's reaction to loss as manifested physically, emotionally, mentally, and behaviorally.

bereavement The objective event of loss.

mourning The process whereby a person actively copes with grief in adjusting to a loss and integrating it into his or her life.

If a grieving friend or relative talks about suicide, or seems in danger of causing harm to himself or herself or others, seek professional help right away. The recent loss of a loved one is a major risk factor for suicide and self-harm. Be alert to signs that a grieving person is in serious danger.

When a Young Adult Loses a Friend

Among young people between the ages of 18 and 24 in the United States, the three leading causes of death tend to be sudden and unexpected: unintentional injuries, homicide, and suicide. Losing a close friend to an unexpected death can be particularly traumatic. There is usually an outpouring of sympathy and support toward the family of the deceased, but as a friend, you may feel left out and unsupported. Also, it is common to blame yourself in some way for your friend's death or feel that you should have somehow prevented the tragedy. If you lose a friend, be sure to look for support from friends, family, clergy, or health professionals, especially if the intense sadness or guilt feelings last for more than a few days or weeks. Friends can often help each other by working together to create their own way of celebrating the life of their lost friend.

Helping Children Cope with Loss

Children tend to cope with loss in a healthier fashion when they are included as part of their family's experience of grief and mourning. Although adults may be uncomfortable about sharing potentially disturbing or painful news with children, a child's natural curiosity usually negates the option of withholding information. Mounting evidence shows that it is best to include children from the beginning—as soon as a terminal prognosis is made, for example—to help them understand what is happening. Children should spend time with the dying person, if possible, to learn, share, and offer and receive comfort.

In talking about death with children, the most important guideline is to be honest. Set the explanation you are offering at the child's level of understanding. Find out what the child wants to know. In general, it's advisable to keep the explanation simple, stick to basics, and verify what the child has understood from your explanation.

COMING TO TERMS WITH DEATH

We may wish we could keep death out of view and not make a place for it in our lives. But this wish cannot be fulfilled. With the death of a beloved friend or relative, we are confronted with emotions and thoughts that relate not only to the immediate loss but also to our own mortality.

Our encounters with dying and death teach us that relationships are more important than things and that life offers no guarantees. In discovering the meaning of death in our own lives, we find that life is both precious and precarious.

Allowing ourselves to make room for death, we discover that it touches not only the dying or bereaved person and his or her family and friends but also the wider community of which we are all part. We recognize that dying and death offer opportunities for extraordinary growth in the midst of loss. Denying death, it turns out, results in denying life.

---

connect™

Connect to Your Choices

Have you ever thought about where you get your attitudes toward aging and death? Many factors can influence our attitudes, some not as obvious as others. Were your grandparents part of your life when you were growing up? Have your parents or grandparents talked with you about advance directives or their end-of-life wishes? How susceptible are you to ageism, and how strongly are you influenced by the youth orientation of the media? Have you gotten the idea from the mainstream culture that it's best not to think or talk about death?

What are the external factors that influence your attitudes toward aging? What are your inner motivations and core values, and how do they affect your choices? Based on what you learned in this chapter, will you make some different choices in the future? If so, what will they be?

Go online to Connect to complete this activity:
www.mcgraw-hillconnect.com

TIPS FOR TODAY AND THE FUTURE

The best way to ensure a high-quality life in later years is by cultivating healthy habits in your younger years.

RIGHT NOW YOU CAN:
- Think about any unhealthy habits you have and resolve to change them. Review the information in this text to devise strategies for change.
- Consider organ donation as a lasting gift of life to others. If you want to be an organ donor, make the appropriate arrangements now, as described in this chapter.

IN THE FUTURE YOU CAN:
- Learn a new skill, such as speaking a new language or playing a new instrument or game of strategy.
- Talk to your parents or grandparents about their wishes for the end of life. Let them know you care for them and want to be involved.

Ask Yourself

QUESTIONS FOR CRITICAL THINKING AND REFLECTION

Have you ever been in the position of being supportive to a bereaved person? What kind of support did he or she seem to appreciate most? Why do you think that was the case? How did the experience affect you?

- People who take charge of their health during their youth have greater control over the physical and mental aspects of aging.

- A lifetime of interests and hobbies helps maintain creativity and intelligence. Exercise and a healthful diet throughout life enhance physical and psychological health.

- Retirement can be a fulfilling and enjoyable time of life for those who adjust to their new roles, enjoy participating in a variety of activities, and have planned ahead for financial stability.

- Slight confusion and forgetfulness are not signs of a serious illness; however, severe symptoms may indicate Alzheimer's disease or another form of dementia.

- Resolving grief and mourning and dealing with depression are important tasks for older adults.

- People over age 65 form a large minority in the United States, and their status is improving. But older adults who are ill and dependent—often those who were already poor—experience major social and economic problems.

- Family and community resources can help older adults stay active and independent.

- Government aid to the elderly includes food stamps, housing subsidies, social security, Medicare, and Medicaid.

- Although death makes rational sense in terms of species survival and evolution, there may be no completely satisfying answer to the question of why death exists from a personal point of view.

- Dying and death are more than biological events; they have social and spiritual dimensions.

- The traditional criteria for determining death focus on vital signs such as breathing and heartbeat. Brain death is characterized by a lack of physical responses other than breathing and heartbeat, with absence of brain activity as signified by a flat electroencephalogram (EEG).

- Between ages 6 and 9, most children begin to develop an understanding that death is final, universal, and inevitable.

- A mature understanding of death can include ideas about the survival of the human personality or soul after death. Problems arise when avoidance or denial of death fosters the notion that it happens only to others.

- A will is a legal instrument that governs the distribution of a person's estate after death.

- End-of-life care may involve a combination of home care, hospital stays, and hospice or palliative care.

- Palliative care is a team-based approach to making dying patients comfortable by controlling pain and relieving suffering.

- Hospice programs are a type of palliative care specifically for patients that are likely to die within six months, often at home, to optimize the quality of life of dying patients and their families.

- Exercising choices about end-of-life care can involve making decisions about attempting to prolong life or choosing to allow natural death with comfort care.

- The right of a competent patient to refuse unwanted treatment is now generally established in both law and medical practice.

- Physician-assisted suicide occurs when a physician provides lethal drugs or other interventions, at a patient's request, with the understanding that the patient plans to use them to end his or her life. Voluntary active euthanasia refers to the intentional ending of a patient's life, at his or her request, by someone other than the patient.

- Advance directives, such as living wills, are used to express people's wishes about the use of life-sustaining treatment and how they wish to be treated if they cannot speak for themselves.

- People can donate their bodies or specific organs for transplantation and other medical uses after death. People of all ages can make their wishes to donate their organs known on their driver's license or other state forms. They also need to let their families know that they wish to be organ donors.

- For Americans, the decision about what to do with the body after death usually involves either burial or cremation.

- Bereaved people usually benefit from participating in a funeral or other type of memorial service to commemorate a loved one's life and death.

- Coping with dying involves physical, psychological, social, and spiritual dimensions.

- It is useful for patients and caregivers to understand the trajectory, or course, of dying.

- In offering support to a dying person, the gift of listening can be especially important.

- Grief encompasses thoughts and feelings as well as physical and behavioral responses.

- Mourning, the process by which a person integrates a loss into his or her life, is determined partly by social and cultural norms for expressing grief.

- Children tend to cope with death in a healthier fashion when they are included in their family's experience of grief and mourning.

- Dying and death offer opportunities for growth in the midst of loss.

FOR MORE INFORMATION

BOOKS

Bonanno, G. A. 2009. *The Other Side of Sadness: What the New Science of Bereavement Tells Us about Life after Loss.* New York: Basic Books. *Explains modern thinking about grief and resilience, with many vignettes. Very readable and encouraging—highly recommended for anyone who has experienced a recent loss.*

Callanan, M., and P. Kelley. 2012. *Final Gifts: Understanding the Special Awareness, Needs, and Communications of the Dying.*

New York: Simon & Schuster. *Real stories of the experience of dying people and their loved ones told by two hospice nurses.*

DeSpelder, L. A., and A. L. Strickland. 2011. *The Last Dance: Encountering Death and Dying,* 9th ed. New York: McGraw-Hill. *A comprehensive and readable text highlighting a broad range of topics related to dying and death.*

Gurian, M. 2013. *The Wonder of Aging: A New Approach to Embracing Life After Fifty.* New York: Atria Books. *A look at the emotional, spiritual, and cognitive dimensions of aging—and how to celebrate life after 50.*

Hyams, J. 2011. *Time to Help Your Parents.* London: Piatkus. *A sympathetic overview of the many challenges facing adult children who must care for their aging parents.*

National Institute on Aging. 2010. *Exercise & Physical Activity: Your Everyday Guide from the National Institute on Aging,* book and DVD ed. New York: Hatherleigh Press. *A practical guide to physical activity and exercise, with specific guidelines for safe exercise for older adults.*

Slocum, J., and L. Carlson. 2011. *Final Rights: Reclaiming the American Way of Death.* Hinesburg, VT: Upper Access Publishing. *Discusses how families can assert their rights by taking control of the funeral process. Topics include avoiding being taking advantage of by the funeral industry, green burial, home funerals, and a listing of funeral-related state laws.*

ORGANIZATIONS AND WEBSITES

AARP. Provides information about all aspects of aging, including health promotion, health care, and retirement planning.

http://www.aarp.org

Aging Well. A practical resource for seniors that includes information about diet, exercise, safety, and medical care.

http://www.aging.ny.gov

Aging with Dignity: Five Wishes. Source for an advanced directive that includes designation of a health care proxy (durable power of attorney), the kind of medical treatment you want or don't want, your wishes about pain control, how you want people to treat you, and what you want your loved ones to know when you are dying.

http://www.agingwithdignity.org/five-wishes.php

Alliance for Aging Research. A nonprofit organization supporting medical and psychological research on aging.

http://www.agingresearch.org

Alzheimer's Association. Offers tips for caregivers and patients and information on the causes and treatment of Alzheimer's disease.

http://www.alz.org

American Association of Suicidology. Information and help for people who have lost loved ones to suicide. Contains a variety of resources, including a directory of support groups.

http://www.suicidology.org/suicide-loss-survivors

Arthritis Foundation. Provides information about arthritis, including free brochures, referrals to local services, and research updates.

http://www.arthritis.org

Association for Death Education and Counseling (ADEC). Provides resources for education, bereavement counseling, and care of the dying.

http://www.adec.org

Caring Connections (a program of the National Hospice and Palliative Care Organization). Provides resources for end-of-life decision making with the goal of planning before a crisis occurs. Information about state-specific advance directives. Hotline and multilingual line available.

http://www.caringinfo.org

The Compassionate Friends. Provides grief support after the death of a child, including local chapters and online support groups.

http://www.compassionatefriends.org

The Dougy Center. Offers education about childhood bereavement and support groups for bereaved children, teens, young adults, and parents.

http://www.dougy.org

Dying Well. A website focused on wellness through the end of life.

http://www.dyingwell.org

GRASP: Grief Recovery After a Substance Passing. Website for friends and family of people who have died as a result of substance use. Local and online support groups available.

http://grasphelp.org/

GriefNet. A site where you can communicate with others via e-mail support groups in the areas of death, grief, and major loss.

http://www.griefnet.org

Hospice Foundation of America. Promotes the hospice concept of care through education and leadership.

http://www.hospicefoundation.org

LeadingAge. Provides information about living and care arrangements available for older adults.

http://www.leadingage.org/

Medicare. Provides signup information; "Compare" listings for doctors, providers, hospitals, plans, and suppliers available through the program; and costs and coverage details.

http://www.medicare.gov

National Cancer Institute: Grief, Bereavement and Coping with Loss. Provides extensive information about types of grief reactions, complicated grief, treatment for complicated grief, children and loss, and cultural aspects of grief.

http://www.cancer.gov/cancertopics/pdq/supportivecare/bereavement/Patient

National Council on Aging. Provides helpful information about retirement planning, health promotion, and lifelong learning.

http://www.ncoa.org

National Funeral Directors Association (NFDA). Provides resources related to funerals and funeral costs, body disposition, and bereavement support.

http://www.nfda.org

National Hospice and Palliative Care Organization (NHPCO). Provides information about hospice care and advance directives, including an online national directory of hospices listed by state and city.

http://www.nhpco.org

National Institute on Aging. Provides fact sheets and brochures about aging-related topics.

http://www.nia.nih.gov

http://nihseniorhealth.gov

National Osteoporosis Foundation. Provides information about the causes, prevention, detection, and treatment of osteoporosis.

http://www.nof.org

Nolo Press: Wills and Estate Planning. Provides answers to questions about planning for death, from writing a basic will to organ donation.

http://www.nolo.com

On Our Own Terms: Public Broadcasting System. A companion website to the Bill Moyers PBS series on improving end-of-life care.

http://www.pbs.org/wnet/onourownterms

U.S. Administration on Aging. Provides fact sheets, statistical information, and Internet links to other resources on aging.

http://www.aoa.gov

The following organizations provide information about organ donation and donor cards.

Coalition on Donation

http://www.donatelife.net

Organ Procurement and Transplantation Network

http://www.organdonor.gov/index.html

SELECTED BIBLIOGRAPHY

Alzheimer's Association. 2012. *2013 Alzheimer's Disease Facts and Figures.* Chicago: Alzheimer's Association.

American Cancer Society, 2013. *Hospice Care.* (http://www.cancer.org/acs/groups/cid/documents/webcontent/002868-pdf.pdf)

Americans over 50 at risk for bone fractures. 2005. *FDA Consumer,* January/February.

Centers for Disease Control and Prevention. 2012. Prevalence of doctor-diagnosed arthritis and arthritis-attributable activity limitation—United States, 2010–2012. *Morbidity and Mortality Weekly Report* 55(40): 1089–1092.

Death with Dignity National Center. 2014. *Death with Dignity around the U.S.* (http://www.deathwithdignity.org/advocates/national/).

Doka, K. J., and A. S. Tucci (eds.). 2011. *Beyond Kübler-Ross: New Perspectives on Death, Dying and Grief.* Washington, DC: Hospice Foundation of America.

Green Burial Council. 2014. *FAQs and Fictions* (http://www.greenburialcouncil.org/).

Kirkwood, T. 2010. Why women live longer: Stress alone does not explain the longevity gap. *Scientific American,* 21 October (http://www.scientificamerican.com/article.cfm?id=why-women-live-longer).

Kolata, G. 2006. Live long? Die young? Answer isn't just in genes. *The New York Times,* 31 August.

Konigsberg, R. D. 2011. *The Truth about Grief.* New York: Simon and Schuster.

Mostofsky, E., et al. 2012. Risk of acute myocardial infarction after the death of a significant person in one's life. *Circulation: Journal of the American Heart Association* 125: 491–496.

Moyer, M. 2013. Is the free-radical theory of aging dead? *Scientific American,* 30 January.

Mudge, A. M., et al. 2008. Exercising body and mind: An integrated approach to functional independence in hospitalized older people. *Journal of the American Geriatrics Society* 56(4): 630–635.

National Cancer Institute. 2013. *Grief, Bereavement, and Coping with Loss* (http://www.cancer.gov/cancertopics/pdq/supportivecare/bereavement/HealthProfessional).

National Funeral Directors Association, 2013. *Trends and Statistics* (http://nfda.org/about-funeral-service-/trends-and-statistics.html#cfacts).

National Hospice Foundation. 2013. *The History of Hospice* (http://www.nationalhospicefoundation.org/i4a/pages/index.cfm?pageid=218).

National Hospice and Palliative Care Organization. 2013. *NHPCO's Facts and Figures: Hospice Care in America,* 2013 ed. (http://www.nhpco.org/sites/default/files/public/Statistics_Research/2013_Facts_Figures.pdf).

National Kidney Foundation. 2013. *Organ Donation and Transplantation Statistics* (http://www.kidney.org/news/newsroom/factsheets/Organ-Donation-and-Transplantation-Stats.cfm).

Oregon Health Authority. 2014. *Frequently Asked Questions about the Death with Dignity Act* (http://public.health.oregon.gov/ProviderPartnerResources/EvaluationResearch/DeathwithDignityAct/Pages/faqs.aspx#whatis).

Oregon Public Health Division. 2014. *Death with Dignity Act 2012* (http://public.health.oregon.gov/ProviderPartnerResources/EvaluationResearch/DeathwithDignityAct/Pages/index.aspx).

Shear, M. K., et al. 2011. Complicated grief and related issues for DSM-5. *Depression and Anxiety* 28: 103–117.

Smith, T. J., and B. E. Hillner. 2011. Bending the cost curve in cancer care. *New England Journal of Medicine* 364: 2060–2065.

Stern, C., and Z. Munn. 2010. Cognitive leisure activities and their role in preventing dementia: A systematic review. *International Journal of Evidence-Based Healthcare* 8(1): 2–17.

Syed, F. A., and A. C. Ng. 2010. The pathophysiology of the aging skeleton. *Current Osteoporosis Reports* 8(4): 235–240.

Tufts University. 2006. Pendulum swings on estrogen and women's heart health risk. *Tufts University Health & Nutrition Letter* 24(3): 1–2.

University of Pennsylvania. 2013. Balancing Act: Cell Senescence, Aging Related to Epigenetic Changes. Perelman School of Medicine news release, 30 August.

U.S Department of Health and Human Services, 2014. *The Need is Real: Data* (http://www.organdonor.gov/about/data.html).

Yuhas, D. 2012. Cracks in the plaques: Mysteries of Alzheimer's slowly yielding to new research. *Scientific American,* 6 February.

PHOTO CREDITS

Contents

INDEX